Recent Advances in Nephrology

Recent Advances in Nephrology

Edited by Adriana Jones

hayle
medical

New York

Hayle Medical,
750 Third Avenue, 9th Floor,
New York, NY 10017, USA

Visit us on the World Wide Web at:
www.haylemedical.com

ISBN: 978-1-63241-662-9

Cataloging-in-Publication Data

Recent advances in nephrology / edited by Adriana Jones.
    p. cm.
Includes bibliographical references and index.
ISBN 978-1-63241-662-9
1. Nephrology. 2. Kidneys--Diseases. I. Jones, Adriana.
RC902 .R43 2019
616.61--dc23

Table of Contents

Preface

Every book is a source of knowledge and this one is no exception. The idea that led to the conceptualization of this book was the fact that the world is advancing rapidly; which makes it crucial to document the progress in every field. I am aware that a lot of data is already available, yet, there is a lot more to learn. Hence, I accepted the responsibility of editing this book and contributing my knowledge to the community.

The study of medicine associated with the functioning of kidneys is called nephrology. It includes the study of the prevention, symptoms and treatment of kidney diseases. The physician who is a specialist in the diagnosis, care and treatment of kidney diseases is known as a nephrologist. Examination of the urine is the most common way of diagnosing kidney problems. It is important to check for the presence of blood, protein, pus cells or cancer cells in the urine. Medical ultrasonography, magnetic resonance imaging and computed axial tomography are some of the common tests to assess the structural abnormalities of the kidneys. This book brings forth some of the most innovative concepts and elucidates the unexplored aspects of nephrology. It elucidates new techniques and their applications in a multidisciplinary manner. This book will help the readers in keeping pace with the rapid changes in this field.

While editing this book, I had multiple visions for it. Then I finally narrowed down to make every chapter a sole standing text explaining a particular topic, so that they can be used independently. However, the umbrella subject sinews them into a common theme. This makes the book a unique platform of knowledge.

I would like to give the major credit of this book to the experts from every corner of the world, who took the time to share their expertise with us. Also, I owe the completion of this book to the never-ending support of my family, who supported me throughout the project.

Editor

Annual Decline in Pentraxin 3 Is a Risk of Vascular Access Troubles in Hemodialysis Patients

Kei Nagai,[1,2] **Atsushi Ueda,**[3] **Chie Saito,**[1] **Asako Zempo-Miyaki,**[2] **and Kunihiro Yamagata**[1]

[1]*Department of Nephrology, Faculty of Medicine, University of Tsukuba, 1-1-1 Tennodai, Tsukuba, Ibaraki 305-8575, Japan*
[2]*Comprehensive Human Sciences, Faculty of Medicine, University of Tsukuba, 1-1-1 Tennodai, Tsukuba, Ibaraki 305-8575, Japan*
[3]*Tsukuba University Hospital Hitachi Medical Education and Research Center, Jonan-cho 2-1-1, Hitachi, Ibaraki 317-0077, Japan*

Correspondence should be addressed to Kei Nagai; minkei@hotmail.co.jp

Academic Editor: Jaime Uribarri

Pentraxin 3 (PTX3), a multifunctional modulator of the innate immunoinflammatory response, is higher in patients undergoing hemodialysis than healthy control. Our study focused on annual change in PTX3 levels in patients with chronic hemodialysis, because regularly undergoing hemodialysis for many years modifies vascular inflammatory status. To demonstrate whether annual change in PTX3 is associated with vascular events, we measured blood levels of pentraxins (PTX3 and high-sensitivity C-reactive protein (hsCRP)) at baseline and in the next year in 76 hemodialysis patients and observed 20 patients with vascular access troubles during follow-up years. The annual decline in PTX3, but not hsCRP, is a significant risk of the incidence of vascular access trouble that is a critical and specific complication for hemodialysis patients (hazard ratio; 0.732 per +1 ng/mL/year in PTX3, $^*P = 0.039$). This study is the first to focus on the annual change of pentraxins in a hemodialysis cohort.

1. Introduction

Inflammation in patients with end-stage renal disease (ESRD) receiving hemodialysis (HD) is associated with malnutrition and cardiovascular diseases and resulted in poor clinical outcome [1]. Pentraxin 3 (PTX3) is a multifunctional soluble receptor that modulates the innate immunoinflammatory response and it belongs to the pentraxin-superfamily that includes C-reactive protein (CRP) [2, 3]. Plasma PTX3, similar to CRP, is considered to be an inflammatory marker of endothelial dysfunction and is also linked to increasing cardiovascular mortality risk [4]. However, because different cell types and organs produce PTX3 and CRP [2, 3], PTX3 and CRP may be involved in different pathophysiologic mechanisms [5]. The role of PTX3 has been demonstrated through experiments using PTX3-deficient or PTX3-overexpressing mice, and PTX3 may exert tissue-protective and anti-inflammatory effects [3, 6–9]. However, the functional role of human PTX3 *in vivo* is still under discussion.

Boehme and colleagues first described that the PTX3 levels of HD patients with ESRD are higher than healthy subjects or ESRD patients without receiving HD [9]. It was interesting that spontaneous production of PTX3 in whole-blood samples from HD patients was significantly higher than that in samples from healthy subjects [9]. Otherwise, the mechanism underlying the production and the pathophysiological role of PTX3 in HD patients has not been elucidated fully. To address this issue, we focused on not only baseline PTX3 levels with a single measurement but also annual change in PTX3 levels in patients receiving chronic dialysis, because regularly receiving hemodialysis and continuously uremic condition for many years modify vascular status depending on several factors such as inflammation and oxidative stress [10, 11].

Here we show that the annual decline in PTX3, but not high-sensitive CRP (hsCRP), is a risk of the incidence of vascular access trouble that is a critical and specific complication for HD patients. This study is the first to focus on the annual change of pentraxins in a HD cohort.

TABLE 1: Characteristics of the subjects with stratification by absence or presence of vascular access troubles.

	Total ($N = 76$)		Absence ($N = 56$)		Presence ($N = 20$)	
	Median	IQC	Median	IQC	Median	IQC
Gender (% man)	60	—	64	—	45	—
Diabetes (%)	41	—	38	—	50	—
Age (years)	67	58–77	66	58–77	67	58–77
Dialysis-period (years)	5.4	2.3–9.4	5.8	2.8–9.6	4	2.0–7.4
Body mass index (kg/m^2)	21.9	19.6–24.0	21.2	19.4–24.0	22.5	20.5–24.0
RAS-inhibitor usage (%)	80	—	82	—	72	—
Statin usage (%)	14	—	11	—	22	—
Total protein (g/dL)	6.6	6.3–6.9	6.5	6.3–6.8	6.6	6.2–7.0
Albumin (g/dL)	3.3	3.0–3.4	3.3	3.0–3.5	3.3	3.0–3.4
Calcium (mg/dL)	8.9	8.5–9.8	8.8	8.4–9.8	9	8.6–9.9
Inorganic phosphorus (mg/dL)	5.2	4.6–6.1	5.2	4.6–5.8	5.3	4.6–6.3
Total cholesterol (mg/dL)	165	139–182	167	139–182	158	138–181
LDL-C (mg/dL)	95	77–112	95	73–113	93	77–107
Triglyceride (mg/dL)	93	72–145	93	74–136	97	72–174
Intact parathyroid hormone (pg/mL)	109	70–157	114	75–159	79	48–130
Hemoglobin (g/dL)	11	10.2–11.5	11	10.2–11.5	10.9	10.0–11.9
Ferritin (ng/mL)	65.6	40.8–114.9	66.2	41.1–116.2	62.9	40.6–114.9
Serum iron (mg/dL)	63.5	48.5–84.8	64	48.5–87.8	62	47.3–74.8
β2-microglobulin (mg/L)	29.1	25.5–32.2	28.9	24.7–31.9	29.9	26.8–34.3
PTX3 (ng/mL)	4.2	3.1–5.4	4.1	3.1–5.4	4.2	3.1–5.8
hsCRP (mg/dL)	0.66	0.56–0.73	0.64	0.54–0.72	0.68	0.62–0.75

Data at baseline year was presented as median and interquartile range (IQC). RAS: renin-angiotensin system, LDL-C: low-density lipoprotein cholesterol, PTX3: pentraxin 3, and hsCRP: high-sensitivity C-reactive protein.

2. Materials and Methods

2.1. Subjects and Sampling.

This study was approved by the Ethics Committee of Namegata General Hospital, Namegata, Ibaraki, Japan, and nonhospitalized patients who regularly received HD were enrolled in this observational cohort study. All subjects were approached prospectively and gave informed consent to the study. Exclusion criteria were the presence of clinical signs of acute infection, active vasculitis, active hepatitis, and HIV at the time of evaluation and willingness to participate in the study. Of the 89 subjects initially enrolled in the study during 2011, 4 subjects died, and another 9 subjects did not complete exact one-year follow-up, primarily because they transferred to other hospitals, thus yielding a total of 76 patients who completed the study. Clinical demographic data of the subjects at baseline are given in Table 1. The patients received regular HD treatment 3 times/week and all of them have internal arteriovenous fistula (AVF) or arteriovenous graft (AVG) for hemodialysis. Blood was drawn from the arterial needle before starting a HD session both in baseline year (July 2011) and in the next year (July 2012) with exact one-year interval. Body mass index (BMI) was taken on a dialysis day immediately after a dialysis session. Vascular access troubles were defined as the need for catheter intervention or reoperation to remedy occlusion or stenosis of AVF or AVG or as the replacement of a permanent vascular catheter due to the occlusion of AVF or AVG from baseline year (July 2011) to two years later (the end of 2013).

The patient, who died or transferred to other hospitals after measurement in next year, was censored at the time of death or lost to follow-up. Finally, the mean observed period in all subjects was 2.12 years.

2.2. Laboratory Measurements.

Blood samples were placed in chilled tubes containing ethylenediaminetetraacetic acid (2 mg/mL) or no anticoagulants and centrifuged at 5500 g for 10 min at 4°C; the obtained plasma or serum, respectively, was stored at −80°C until analysis. Plasma concentrations of PTX3 were determined by using a commercial human PTX3 enzyme-linked immunosorbent assay (ELISA) kit system (Perseus Proteomics, Tokyo, Japan). Serum concentrations of hsCRP were determined by using the nephelometric N-latex CRP II kit (Siemens Diagnostics, Erlangen, Germany). Serum level of intact parathyroid hormone was determined by using Elecsys immunoassay systems (Roche Diagnostics, Basel, Switzerland). β2-microglobulin was determined by latex coagulation analysis kit (Eiken Chemical, Tokyo, Japan). Blood count was performed by autoanalyzer (Abbott Japan, Chiba, Japan). Other biochemical parameters were evaluated by using an autochemical analyzer (ci 16200, Toshiba, Japan).

2.3. Statistical Analyses.

Values in tables are expressed as median with interquartile range (IQR). Statistical significance was set at $P < 0.05$. Comparisons between groups were appropriately assessed by the Mann-Whitney U test after normality test. Cox-regression models were performed to

TABLE 2: Comparison of pentraxin levels in baseline year among the subpopulations.

	Mean	SD	Mean	SD	P value
Sex	Male ($N = 45$)		Female ($N = 31$)		
Pentraxin 3	4.627	2.722	4.466	1.27	0.731
hsCRP	0.658	0.126	0.685	0.182	0.474
DM	Non-DM ($N = 45$)		DM ($N = 31$)		
Pentraxin 3	4.946	2.422	4.005	1.83	0.058
hsCRP	0.675	0.18	0.661	0.096	0.656
Age	<65 years ($N = 31$)		≥65 years ($N = 45$)		
Pentraxin 3	4.447	1.898	4.64	2.459	0.701
hsCRP	0.661	0.15	0.674	0.153	0.71
Dialysis-period	<5 years ($N = 34$)		≥5 years ($N = 42$)		
Pentraxin 3	3.961	1.852	5.048	2.416	0.030*
hsCRP	0.66	0.127	0.676	0.168	0.641
Body mass index	≥22 kg/m^2 ($N = 32$)		<22 kg/m^2 ($N = 44$)		
Pentraxin 3	5.175	2.397	3.719	1.689	0.003**
hsCRP	0.649	0.178	0.683	0.127	0.36

Data at baseline year was presented. Values of pentraxin 3 or hsCRP are expressed by ng/mL or mg/dL. DM: diabetes mellitus; hsCRP: high-sensitivity C-reactive protein. *$P < 0.05$, **$P < 0.01$.

assess the risk of incidence of vascular access troubles; these models included age, sex, BMI, dialysis-periods, and presence of diabetes mellitus (DM). All analyses were performed by SPSS version 21.

3. Results

3.1. Comparison of Pentraxin Levels in Baseline Year among Subpopulations in This Study. Characteristic of this study population is shown in Table 1. In the 76 subjects, we observed 45 male patients, 31 patients with DM, 45 patients with age over 65 years, 42 patients with dialysis-period over 5 years, and 44 patients with BMI less than 22 kg/m^2. We next examined differences in baseline levels of pentraxins (i.e., PTX3 and hsCRP) among subpopulations based on sex, presence of DM, age, dialysis-period, or BMI. It was shown that there were higher levels of PTX3 in patients with dialysis-period less than 5 years or BMI over 22 kg/m^2 than the others (Table 2). However, levels of hsCRP are comparable among the subpopulations divided by sex, presence of DM, age, dialysis-period, or BMI (Table 2).

3.2. The Distribution of Annual Changes of PTX3 and hsCRP. Because increased level of PTX3 would be dependent on length of dialysis-period as shown in Table 2, we observed the annual changes in levels of PTX3 and hsCRP from baseline to the next year in this study population (Figure 1). The mean change was +0.010 ng/mL/year or +0.032 mg/dL/year in PTX3 or hsCRP, respectively.

3.3. Annual Changes of PTX3 but Not hsCRP Are a Risk of Vascular Access Troubles. To know the pathophysiological implications of annual change in pentraxin levels in HD patients, we examined whether pentraxins can predict the incidence of vascular events by utilizing cox-regression

model. The number of patients with vascular access trouble during follow-up years (from 2011 to the end of 2013) was twenty. Table 1 shows the characteristics of the patients with stratification by the absence or presence of vascular access events. The level of PTX3 in baseline year in the patients with vascular access troubles is comparable to that without vascular access troubles as well as levels of hsCRP (Figure 2(a)). Interestingly, we observed the inverse trend for annual changes of parameters between hsCRP and PTX3 which is suggesting that annual decline in PTX3 would be related to the incidence of vascular access troubles (Figure 2(b)). Consistent with this result, Table 3 shows that annual decline in PTX3 is a significant risk for the incidence of vascular access troubles (hazard ratio; 0.732 per +1 ng/mL/year in PTX3, *$P = 0.039$) by cox-regression model with adjustment for covariants including dialysis-period and BMI which is crucially involving the level of PTX3, while hsCRP is not significant risk (hazard ratio; 3.605 per +1 mg/mL/year in hsCRP, $P = 0.597$).

4. Discussion

PTX3 is produced by various types of cells and increases rapidly in response to primary local inflammation and innate immunity [8, 9, 12, 13]. In patients with chronic kidney disease and those with ESRD receiving HD, increased, but not increasing, level of PTX3 is strongly predictive of poor clinical outcome and may be independent risk factors of mortality [4]. The subjects in our study had higher level of PTX3 at baseline (mean ± SD; 4.6 ± 2.2 ng/mL) than that of healthy control (0.76 ± 0.2 ng/mL) referred to in the previous observation [9]. Moreover, plasma level of PTX3, but not hsCRP, in patients with longer dialysis-period over five years is higher than that in those with shorter dialysis-period (Table 2). Therefore, we expected that annual change of PTX3

TABLE 3: Cox-regression models for the incidence of vascular access troubles with or without multivariable adjustment.

	Unadjusted			Adjusted by DM, sex, age, dialysis-period, and BMI		
	Hazard ratio	95% C.I.	P value	Hazard ratio	95% C.I.	P value
Baseline PTX3	1.006	0.836–1.211	0.951	1.237	0.936–1.635	0.136
ΔPTX3	0.849	0.680–1.061	0.151	0.732	0.544–0.985	0.039[*]
Baseline hsCRP	3.644	0.469–28.30	0.216	2.713	0.389–18.92	0.314
ΔhsCRP	9.486	0.108–833.2	0.324	3.605	0.033–394.7	0.592

The incidence of vascular access troubles during follow-up years was set as the outcome. Covariants examined in Table 2 were used for adjustment. [*] $P < 0.05$. C.I.: confidential intervals, ΔPTX3: annual change in pentraxin 3 (ng/mL per year), and ΔhsCRP: annual change in high-sensitivity C-reactive protein (mg/dL per year).

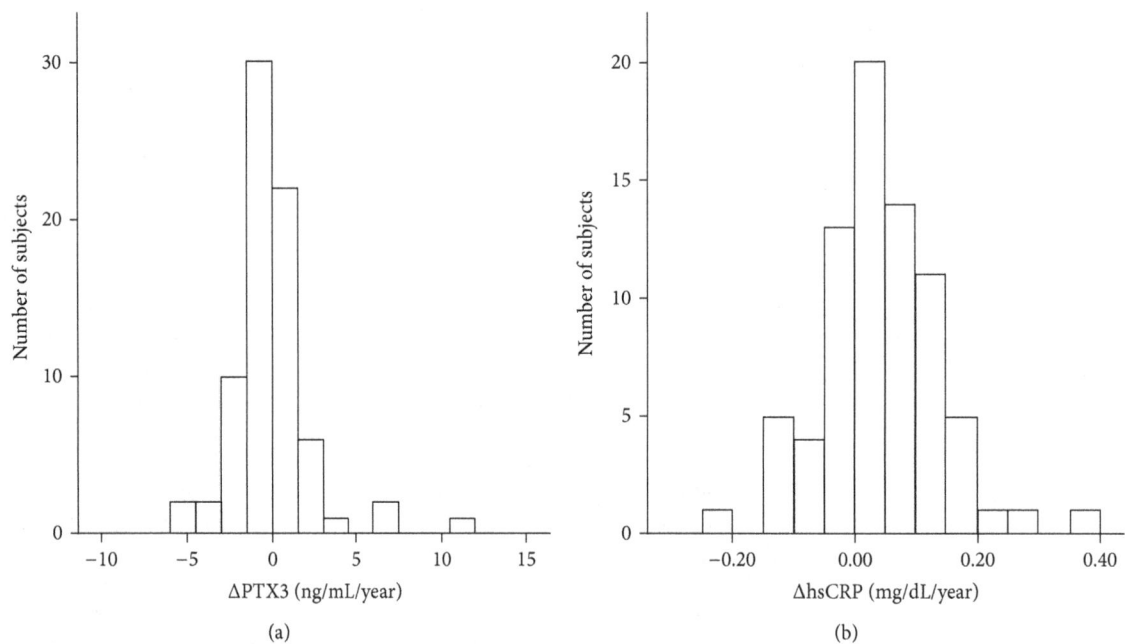

(a)

(b)

FIGURE 1: The annual change in pentraxins in the HD cohort. Distribution of annual change in PTX3 levels (ΔPTX3 (a)) or hsCRP (ΔhsCRP (b)) of the whole subjects is shown.

levels while undergoing chronic dialysis has distinguishing role from that of hsCRP.

Recently, notable results were described in PTX3-deficient murine experiments; the elevation of PTX3 during cardiovascular diseases has recently been postulated to be a compensatory response to protect the body from inflammation [3, 7, 8]. Human PTX3 prevents cells from becoming apoptotic by inhibiting the activation of factor H or by eliminating apoptotic cells quickly before they can secrete proinflammatory factors *in vitro* [14]. In contrast, serum levels of CRP are well recognized as reflection on the generation of proinflammatory cytokines *in vivo*, which cause malnutrition and cardiovascular diseases via several canonical pathways and result in poor prognosis [11]. Taken together, one explanation for high level of PTX3 in patients with long dialysis-period is that HD patients with higher PTX3 live longer because they avoid overproduction of inflammatory factors.

Although cross-sectional studies with a single measurement of pentraxins are available [4, 9], few previous cohort studies focus on the annual changes in PTX3 levels in patients receiving chronic dialysis. To address this complicated accumulation of knowledge about PTX3, a cross-sectional study with a single measurement of PTX3 might not be suitable to assess causality in the observed associations. Therefore, we conducted a longitudinal cohort study in HD patients to know whether annual changes of pentraxin levels could be a risk of the incidence for vascular event in HD patients. Consequently, we here show that annual decline in PTX3 is a risk of the incidence of vascular access trouble with adjustment for physical status represented by BMI that is well-known confounding factor for increased PTX3 [15–17] (Table 2). Though the involvement of PTX3 in the patency of AVF was previously mentioned only briefly [18], our study is the unique observation to support compensatory response of PTX3 to protect the body from vascular thrombotic event.

(a)

(b)

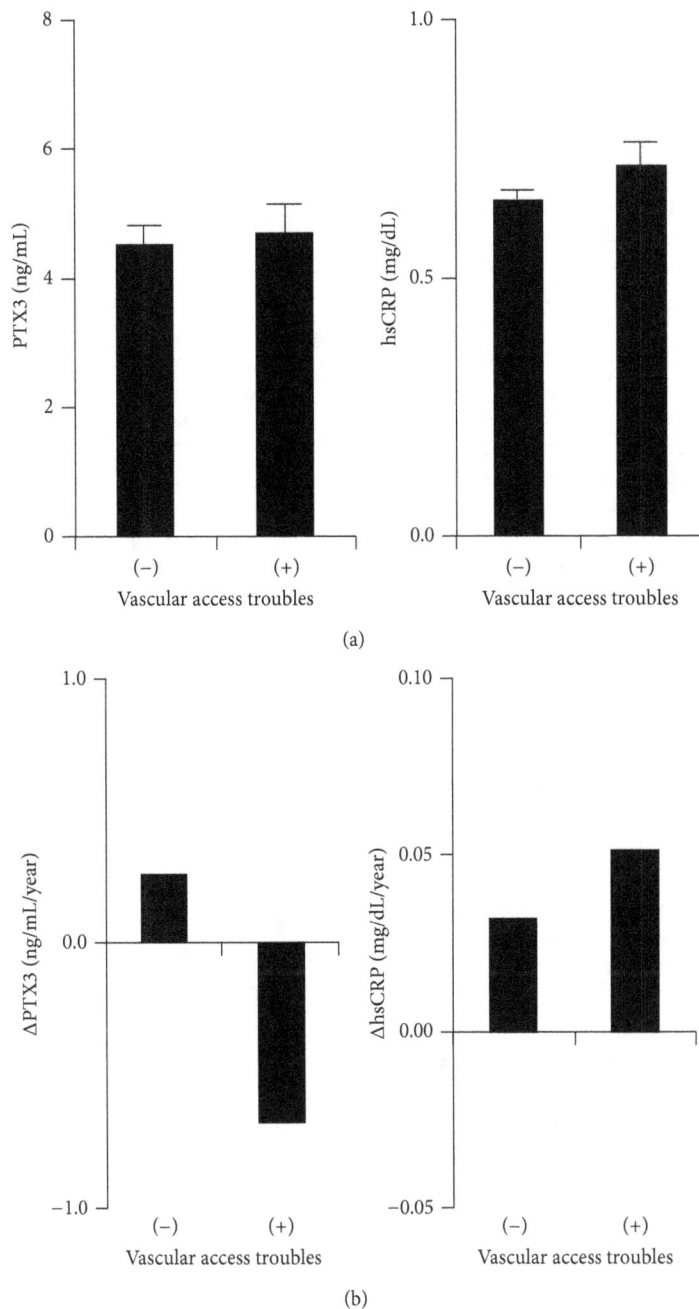

FIGURE 2: Baseline levels and annual change in pentraxins in subjects with vascular access troubles. Mean ± S.E.M. in baseline year (a) or annual change (b) of pentraxins in the subjects without or with vascular access troubles (− or +, N = 56 or 20, resp.) occurred during follow-up years. Significant difference of each parameter between the subjects without or with vascular access troubles was examined by Mann-Whitney U test.

PTX3 is produced by various stimuli including lipopolysaccharide and cytokines such as tumor necrosis factor and interleukin-1β [9, 12]. Moreover, the promoter region of human PTX3 contains binding sites for the redox-sensitive transcription factors including nuclear factor κB, which is critically involved in the regulation pathway of inflammatory mediators in innate immunity [13, 19]. Increased oxidative stress occurs in HD patients [10] and is dependent on many factors including aging, loss of residual renal function,

uremic conditions, and receiving regular HD—all of which were represented in our study cohort. Though we could not determine what the major factor for annual change in PTX3 in this HD cohort was, it was speculated that excessive oxidative-stress would be one of the causes for annually changing PTX3.

Recently, some report suggested a crucial protective role of PTX3 in thrombotic diseases. In acute myocardial infarction, depletion of intracellular PTX3 in neutrophils correlates with increased plasma levels and with platelet-neutrophil aggregates *in vivo* [20]. These phenomena can be explained as follows: PTX3 is released from neutrophils via several stimuli and binds to P-selectin on activated endothelial cells [21] and activated circulating platelets [20] and dampens their proinflammatory and prothrombotic actions [22], thus contributing to its cardioprotective effects in human [20]. In contrast, several prospective studies show that hsCRP levels are positively associated with the incidence of myocardial infraction, stroke, and venous thrombosis [23, 24]. In thrombophilic condition such as essential thrombocythemia and polycythemia, high rate of thrombotic event is observed in the high CRP levels or low PTX3 levels [25]. Altogether, it is considered that PTX3 antagonizes the thrombotic function of CRP likely through a reduction of vascular inflammation.

In this research, by serial measurements of levels of PTX3, here we show that the annual decline in PTX3, but not in hsCRP, is a risk of the incidence vascular access troubles that is a critical complication for HD patients. This is the noteworthy study to focus on the annual change in pentraxins in a HD cohort and to support the evidence for the function of PTX3 to protect bodies from vascular thrombotic events.

References

[1] P. Stenvinkel, "Inflammation in end-stage renal failure: could it be treated?" *Nephrology Dialysis Transplantation*, vol. 17, no. 8, pp. 33–40, 2002.

[2] A. Mantovani, C. Garlanda, A. Doni, and B. Bottazzi, "Pentraxins in innate immunity: from C-reactive protein to the long pentraxin PTX3," *Journal of Clinical Immunology*, vol. 28, no. 1, pp. 1–13, 2008.

[3] G. D. Norata, C. Garlanda, and A. L. Catapano, "The long pentraxin PTX3: a modulator of the immunoinflammatory response in atherosclerosis and cardiovascular diseases," *Trends in Cardiovascular Medicine*, vol. 20, no. 2, pp. 35–40, 2010.

[4] M. Tong, J. J. Carrero, A. R. Qureshi et al., "Plasma pentraxin 3 in patients with chronic kidney disease: associations with renal function, protein-energy wasting, cardiovascular disease, and mortality," *Clinical Journal of the American Society of Nephrology*, vol. 2, no. 5, pp. 889–897, 2007.

[5] B. Bottazzi, A. Doni, C. Garlanda, and A. Mantovani, "An integrated view of humoral innate immunity: pentraxins as a paradigm," *Annual Review of Immunology*, vol. 28, pp. 157–183, 2010.

[6] A. A. M. Dias, A. R. Goodman, J. L. dos Santos et al., "TSG-14 transgenic mice have improved survival to endotoxemia and to CLP-induced sepsis," *Journal of Leukocyte Biology*, vol. 69, no. 6, pp. 928–936, 2001.

[7] M. Salio, S. Chimenti, N. D. Angelis et al., "Cardioprotective function of the long pentraxin PTX3 in acute myocardial infarction," *Circulation*, vol. 117, no. 8, pp. 1055–1064, 2008.

[8] G. D. Norata, P. Marchesi, V. K. Pulakazhi Venu et al., "Deficiency of the long pentraxin PTX3 promotes vascular inflammation and atherosclerosis," *Circulation*, vol. 120, no. 8, pp. 699–708, 2009.

[9] M. Boehme, F. Kaehne, A. Kuehne et al., "Pentraxin 3 is elevated in haemodialysis patients and is associated with cardiovascular disease," *Nephrology Dialysis Transplantation*, vol. 22, no. 8, pp. 2224–2229, 2007.

[10] E. Maggi, R. Bellazzi, F. Falaschi et al., "Enhanced LDL oxidation in uremic patients: an additional mechanism for accelerated atherosclerosis?" *Kidney International*, vol. 45, no. 3, pp. 876–883, 1994.

[11] P. Stenvinkel, O. Heimbürger, B. Lindholm, G. A. Kaysen, and J. Bergström, "Are there two types of malnutrition in chronic renal failure? Evidence for relationships between malnutrition, inflammation and atherosclerosis (MIA syndrome)," *Nephrology Dialysis Transplantation*, vol. 15, no. 7, pp. 953–960, 2000.

[12] V. V. Alles, B. Bottazzi, G. Peri, J. Golay, M. Introna, and A. Mantovani, "Inducible expression of PTX3, a new member of the pentraxin family, in human mononuclear phagocytes," *Blood*, vol. 84, no. 10, pp. 3483–3493, 1994.

[13] A. Altmeyer, L. Klarapfer, A. R. Goodman, and J. Vilcek, "Promoter structure and transcriptional activation of the murine TSG-14 gene encoding a tumor necrosis factor/interleukin-1-inducible pentraxin protein," *The Journal of Biological Chemistry*, vol. 270, no. 43, pp. 25584–25590, 1995.

[14] S. Jaillon, P. Jeannin, Y. Hamon et al., "Endogenous PTX3 translocates at the membrane of late apoptotic human neutrophils and is involved in their engulfment by macrophages," *Cell Death & Differentiation*, vol. 16, no. 3, pp. 465–474, 2009.

[15] T. Miyamoto, A. R. Qureshi, O. Heimbürger et al., "Inverse relationship between the inflammatory marker Pentraxin-3, fat body mass, and abdominal obesity in end-stage renal disease," *Clinical Journal of the American Society of Nephrology*, vol. 6, no. 12, pp. 2785–2791, 2011.

[16] L. Alberti, L. Gilardini, A. Zulian et al., "Expression of long pentraxin PTX3 in human adipose tissue and its relation with cardiovascular risk factors," *Atherosclerosis*, vol. 202, no. 2, pp. 455–460, 2009.

[17] M. E. Suliman, A. R. Qureshi, J. J. Carrero et al., "The long pentraxin PTX-3 in prevalent hemodialysis patients: associations with comorbidities and mortality," *QJM*, vol. 101, no. 5, pp. 397–405, 2008.

[18] C.-Y. Chou, H.-L. Kuo, Y.-F. Yung, Y.-L. Liu, and C.-C. Huang, "C-reactive protein predicts vascular access thrombosis in hemodialysis patients," *Blood Purification*, vol. 24, no. 4, pp. 342–346, 2006.

[19] A. Basile, A. Sica, E. D'Aniello et al., "Characterization of the promoter for the human long pentraxin *PTX3*: role of NF-κB in tumor necrosis factor-α and interleukin-1β regulation," *The Journal of Biological Chemistry*, vol. 272, no. 13, pp. 8172–8178, 1997.

[20] N. Maugeri, P. Rovere-Querini, M. Slavich et al., "Early and transient release of leukocyte pentraxin 3 during acute myocardial infarction," *The Journal of Immunology*, vol. 187, no. 2, pp. 970–979, 2011.

[21] A. Zarbock, K. Singbartl, and K. Ley, "Complete reversal of acid-induced acute lung injury by blocking of platelet-neutrophil aggregation," *Journal of Clinical Investigation*, vol. 116, no. 12, pp. 3211–3219, 2006.

[22] L. Deban, R. C. Russo, M. Sironi et al., "Regulation of leukocyte recruitment by the long pentraxin PTX3," *Nature Immunology*, vol. 11, no. 4, pp. 328–334, 2010.

[23] P. Quist-Paulsen, I. A. Næss, S. C. Cannegieter et al., "Arterial cardiovascular risk factors and venous thrombosis: results from a population-based, prospective study (the HUNT 2)," *Haematologica*, vol. 95, no. 1, pp. 119–125, 2010.

Cost-Effectiveness Analysis for the Treatment of Hyperphosphatemia in Predialysis Patients: Calcium-Based versus Noncalcium-Based Phosphate Binders

B. L. Goh ⓘ,[1] **A. Soraya,**[2] **A. Goh,**[2] **and K. L. Ang ⓘ**[1]

[1]*Clinical Research Centre, Serdang Hospital, Kajang 43000, Malaysia*
[2]*Azmi Burhani Consulting, Petaling Jaya 47820, Malaysia*

Correspondence should be addressed to B. L. Goh; bak.leong@gmail.com

Academic Editor: Jaime Uribarri

Background. Hyperphosphatemia in chronic kidney disease (CKD) patients is often treated with calcium carbonate (CaCO3) despite the fact that CaCO3 is associated with increased calcium load and potentially increased cardiovascular risk. Alternative treatments with noncalcium-based phosphate binders do not increase the calcium load but are more costly. This study analyzes the cost-effectiveness of sevelamer versus CaCO3 for the treatment of hyperphosphatemia in stage III-V predialysis CKD patients in Malaysia. *Methods.* A Markov decision model was adapted to simulate a hypothetical cohort of CKD patients requiring treatment for hyperphosphatemia. Survival was estimated by using efficacy data from the INDEPENDENT-CKD clinical trial. Cost data was obtained from Malaysian studies while health state utilities were derived from literature. Analysis was performed over lifetime duration from the perspective of the Ministry of Health Malaysia with 2013 as reference year. *Results.* In the base case analysis, sevelamer treatment gained 6.37 life years (5.27 QALY) compared to 4.25 life years (3.54 QALY) with CaCO3. At 3% discount, lifetime costs were RM159,901 ($48,750) and RM77,139 ($23,518) on sevelamer and CaCO3, respectively. Incremental cost-effectiveness (ICER) of sevelamer versus CaCO3 was RM47,679 ($14,536) per QALY, which is less than the WHO threshold of three times GDP per capita (RM99,395) per QALY. Sensitivity analyses, both using scenario sensitivity analysis and probabilistic sensitivity analysis, showed the result to be robust. *Conclusions.* Our study finds that sevelamer is potentially cost-effective compared to CaCO3, for the treatment of hyperphosphatemia in predialysis CKD III-V. We propose that sevelamer should be an option in the treatment of Malaysian predialysis patients with hyperphosphatemia, particularly those with high calcium load.

1. Introduction

Treatment of CKD imposes a substantial cost on health care budgets and middle-income countries (MIC) face significant challenges. In Malaysia, a middle-income country, an estimated 9.1% of the adult population suffered from CKD in 2013 [1] and this number is rising largely due to the increasing number of patients diagnosed with type 2 diabetes in recent years caused by changing lifestyles and dietary habits [2, 3]. CKD accounted for 27% of the total US Medicare budget in 2007 [4, 5]. In 2005, Malaysia had spent an estimated RM379 million to provide dialysis services for 13,355 patients [6]. By 2016, the number of CKD Vd patients in Malaysia has tripled to 39,711 [7].

One of the complications that develop in CKD patients is hyperphosphatemia. Studies have shown that elevated serum phosphate increases risk of mortality and cardiovascular disease (CVD) even for patients with early CKD. In fact, high serum phosphate levels are also associated with more rapid decline in renal function [8–10]. Kidney Disease: Improving Global Outcomes (KDIGO) guidelines recommended maintaining serum phosphate in the normal range (0.81 to 1.45 mmol/l) for patients with renal failure, CKD stage III to V (CKD-ND) [11].

Calcium-based binders (CBBs) such as calcium carbonate (CaCO3) are commonly used since they are widely available and cheap. However, clinical studies have shown that the use of oral calcium in the form of supplements or phosphate

TABLE 1: INDEPENDENT-CKD trial patient characteristics.

Patient characteristics	Sevelamer	CaCO3
Subjects (N)	107	105
Mean age (years)	57.4	58.5
Males (%)	61	61
CKD disease stage	Stage 3–4	Stage 3–4
Diabetes (%)	27	29
Hypertension (%)	72.9	76.1
Baseline creatinine clearance (CCr) (ml/min)	31.7	32.7
Baseline phosphorus (mg/dl)	4.82	4.87
Baseline calcium (mg/dl)	9.0	8.8
Baseline parathyroid hormone (PTH) (pg/ml)	200	188

binders may lead to arterial calcification and an increased risk of mortality and CVD events [12–15]. The KDIGO guidelines recommended restricting the dose of CBBs for CKD patients in the presence of arterial calcification [11]. The INDEPENDENT-CKD trial which was performed among 212 patients (107 assigned to sevelamer and 105 assigned to CaCO3) reported that treatment with sevelamer in CKD-ND patients was associated with reductions in mortality and dialysis initiation [16]. Despite concerns regarding the long-term safety of CBBs, CaCO3 is still the first-line treatment for CKD patients in many low and MIC like Malaysia as they cost less than non-CBBs. Data from the Malaysian National Renal Registry indicated that, in 2016, more than 95% of CKD Vd patients were prescribed with CaCO3, and only 17% have a serum phosphate level of less than 1.3 mmol/l, indicating achievement of target based on the KDIGO guidelines was far from satisfactory [7].

There was evidence that non-CBB like sevelamer was cost-effective in two European countries; the value of this information is limited in the local setting due to differences in health systems and cost structures [17–19]. Thus, this study was conducted to determine the cost-effectiveness of sevelamer compared to CaCO3 for treatment of hyperphosphatemia in CKD-ND patients in Malaysia.

2. Methods

We performed an economic evaluation by adapting the previously developed decision-analysis model: the Markov decision model was adapted to simulate a hypothetical cohort of CKD patients requiring treatment for hyperphosphatemia using available Malaysian data [17]. Decision analysis is an approach for decision making taking into account uncertainty and evaluation of the consequences of alternative courses of action in terms of their costs and outcomes. Markov models are a type of decision-analysis model which are used to analyse uncertain processes, such as chronic diseases in which costs and outcomes occur over a long period of time [20]. Markov type decision models have been widely used in cost-effectiveness analysis including the use of sevelamer in dialysis and CKD-ND patients, as well as other chronic kidney disease interventions [17, 21, 22].

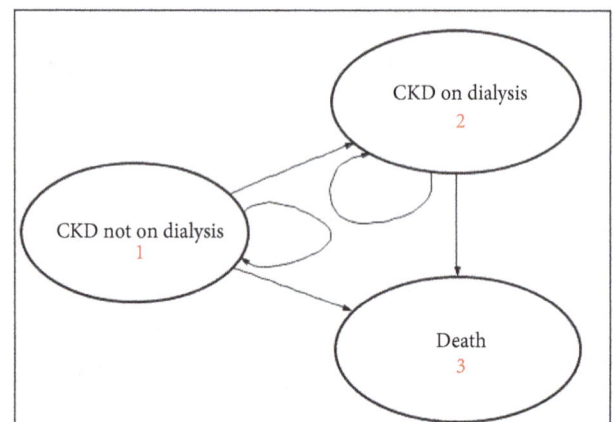

FIGURE 1: State transition diagram of the CLEAR-CKD model.

2.1. Model Overview. The Markov decision model simulates the progression from predialysis CKD to dialysis and death in a hypothetical cohort of CKD-ND patients treated with sevelamer carbonate or CaCO3 for hyperphosphatemia. The model structure is illustrated in Figure 1. The cohort entered the model in the health state "CKD not on Dialysis" and in subsequent one-year cycles, patients could remain alive without dialysis or transition to dialysis or death. Each cycle spent in the health states of "CKD not on Dialysis" or "CKD on dialysis" was associated with an amount of cost and quality of life. In the event of death, the simulated patient no longer incurs any cost nor gains any health outcome. The total duration spent by the cohort in each of the health states was aggregated to obtain the total cost and quality-adjusted life years (QALY) accrued on treatment with sevelamer or CaCO3, respectively. Baseline characteristics of the trial subjects are shown in Table 1. The data inputs are summarized in Table 2.

2.2. Efficacy Data. Transition probabilities between model health states were derived from the survival and dialysis initiation endpoints from the INDEPENDENT-CKD trial which followed patients for a duration of 3 years or until death (Figures 2(a) and 2(b)) [16].

TABLE 2: Base case input values.

Parameter	Sevelamer	CaCO3	Unit	Source
Population characteristics				
Mean age at baseline	57.9	57.9	year	Di Iorio 2012
Baseline serum phosphate level	4.82	4.87	mg/dl	Di Iorio 2012
CKD stage 3	50	50	%	Assumption derived from Di Iorio 2012
CKD stage 4	50	50	%	Assumption derived from Di Iorio 2012
Drug treatment				
Sevelamer dose	2.184	n/a	g/day	Di Iorio 2012
CaCO3 dose	n/a	2.950	g/day	Di Iorio 2012
Drug cost	5.0069	0.0871	RM/g	Sevelamer cost: Sanofi, CaCO3 cost: IMS 2013
Efficacy				
Survival up to 36 months	Figure 2	Figure 2		Modelled from INDEPENDENT-CKD data
Dialysis initiation up to 36 months	Figure 3	Figure 3		Modelled from INDEPENDENT-CKD data
Long-term survival	Figure 2	Figure 2		Modelled from INDEPENDENT-CKD data
Long-term dialysis initiation	Figure 3	Figure 3		Modelled from INDEPENDENT-CKD data
Utility				
Pre-dialysis CKD utility	0.86	0.86		Gorodetskaya 2005; weighted average of utility in stage 4 and 5 CKD
Dialysis utility	0.8	0.8		Bavanandan 2010
Dialysis				
Proportion of patients on HD	88	88	%	21st MDTR 2013
Proportion of patients on CAPD	12	12	%	21st MDTR 2013
HD cost	259.09	259.09	RM/ session	Hooi 2005, IMF 2013
CAPD cost	99.04	99.04	RM/day	Hooi 2005, IMF 2013
Base case modelling parameters				
Cohort size	1000	1000	patient	Assumption
Time horizon	60	60	year	Assumption
Discount rate on costs	3	3	%	Malaysian PE Guidelines 2012
Discount rate on outcomes	3	3	%	Malaysian PE Guidelines 2012

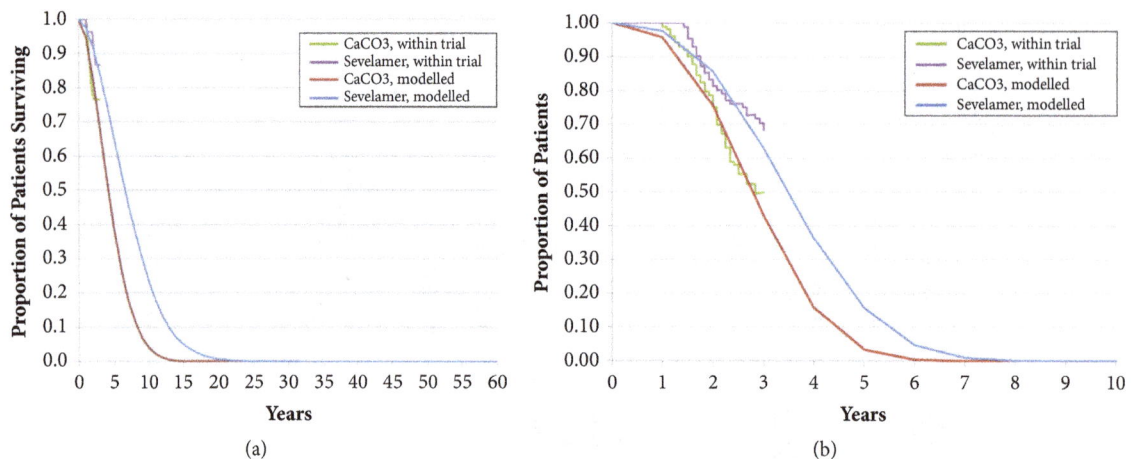

FIGURE 2: (a) Patient survival projected the from INDEPENDENT-CKD trial. Source: Di Iorio 2012, Cornerstone Research Group 2012. (b) Dialysis initiation projected from the INDEPENDENT-CKD trial. Source: Di Iorio 2012, Cornerstone Research Group 2012.

2.3. Health Utility Data. Health utility data inputs in the model required data for the dialysis and predialysis health states. For the quality of life (QOL) of dialysis, we used QOL data of Malaysian dialysis patients [23]. The utility score associated with a predialysis health state was based on a study by Gorodetskaya I et al. [24]. The base case utility input values are listed in Table 2.

2.4. Resource Use and Costs. The perspective of the analysis was that of the provider, i.e., Ministry of Health Malaysia (MOH). Direct medical costs of drugs and dialysis incurred by the MOH were included in the analysis. The costs of other medical resources, i.e., hospitalization, concomitant drugs, treatment of adverse events (AE), and indirect costs (out-of-pocket expenses, productivity losses), were excluded from the analysis.

The medication costs of sevelamer and CaCO3 were calculated by multiplying the average daily drug dose reported in the INDEPENDENT-CKD trial with the latest available unit prices of sevelamer and generic CaCO3 in Malaysia. The cost per gram of sevelamer was derived from the indicative price offered by the drug manufacturer to the MOH whereas the cost of CaCO3 was obtained from the public sector cost of generic CaCO3 in the 3rd quarter of 2013 [25].

The cost of haemodialysis (HD) and continuous ambulatory peritoneal dialysis (CAPD) were obtained from a previous study of the MOH dialysis program conducted in 2001, adjusted to 2013 values by applying general inflation rates obtained from the International Monetary Fund [26, 27]. Dialysis costs were annualized assuming three HD sessions per week (156 HD sessions per year) and daily use of CAPD (365 CAPD days per year) according to the dialysis practice in Malaysia. The base case analysis inputs are listed in Table 2.

Currency conversions from RM to US$ values presented in this study were calculated using the exchange rate on 31 December 2013 of $1 to RM3.28 as the index year of study was 2013 [28].

2.5. Analysis. The model simulated the costs and outcomes over the lifetime of the entire cohort from initiation of CBB therapy to dialysis and/or death. Future costs and QALYs were discounted at 3% per annum to the reference year as recommended by the Malaysian Pharmacoeconomics Guidelines [29]. Analysis was also performed using life years (LY) as health outcome.

We performed scenario sensitivity analysis by varying variables as recommended by guidelines and for key variables that may possibly change the conclusions that are drawn from the base case analysis. The variables that were analysed were discount rate, time horizon, drug dose, utility while on dialysis, and HD cost. As well, a probabilistic sensitivity analysis (PSA) was performed over 10,000 simulations to capture the uncertainty in several parameters in the model, namely, hazard ratios of survival and inception of dialysis, daily doses, and unit costs of sevelamer and CaCO3.

2.6. Assessment Criteria. According to the WHO guidelines, a treatment is cost-effective if the incremental cost-effectiveness ratio (ICER) is below a maximum threshold of 3 times GDP per capita for a country when comparing one treatment against another [30]. The ICER, in this case, compares the cost and QALYs gained from treatment with sevelamer relative to CaCO3 [19, 29, 31, 32]. The ICER was calculated using the following formula:

$$ICER_{sevelamer} = \frac{Cost_{sevelamer} - Cost_{CaCO_3}}{QALY_{sevelamer} - QALY_{CaCO_3}} \quad (1)$$

Based on the IMF's projected GDP per capita for Malaysia of RM33,132 in 2013, treatments with ICER below RM33,132 per QALY would be considered highly cost-effective, ICERs from RM33,132 to RM99,395 could be considered cost-effective while ICERs exceeding RM99,395 are not cost-effective [27, 30].

3. Results

3.1. Base Case Analysis. As shown in Table 3 the lifetime cost of treatment with sevelamer was higher at RM159,901

TABLE 3: Base case results (3% discount on costs and outcomes).

Treatment	Lifetime cost per patient (RM)	Effect (LY)	ICER (Cost per LY gained)	Effect (QALY)	ICER (Cost per QALY gained)
CaCO3	77,139	4.25	-	3.54	-
Sevelamer	159,901	6.37	-	5.27	-
Incremental	82,763	2.12	39,050	1.74	47,679

TABLE 4: Scenario sensitivity analyses results.

No.	Variable	Base case input value	Sensitivity input value	ICER (Cost (RM) per QALY gained)
1a	Undiscounted cost and outcomes	3%	0%	48,033
1b	5% discount rate	3%	5%	47,419
2a	3-year time horizon	60 years	3 years	25,438
2b	10-year time horizon	60 years	10 years	47,586
3a	High sevelamer dose	2.184g	4.8g	65,210
3b	High CaCO3 dose	2.95g	7.5g	47,325
4	Low dialysis utility	0.8	0.72	51,086
5a	Low HD cost	RM259.09	RM197.48	40,627
5b	High HD cost	RM259.09	RM350.00	58,084
6	Exclude dialysis cost	RM259.09	0	14,407

($48,750) compared to RM77,139 ($23,518) per patient on CaCO3. Yet, treatment with sevelamer gained more life years and QALY than CaCO3. In terms of life years, 6.37 years were gained on sevelamer compared to 4.25 years on CaCO3, whereas in terms of QALYs, sevelamer gained 5.27 versus 3.54 QALY gained using CaCO3. Hence, the ICER of treatment with sevelamer relative to CaCO3 was RM39,050 ($11,906) per LY gained and RM47,679 ($14,536) per QALY gained.

At RM47,679 per QALY gained, the ICER of treatment with sevelamer was between one to two times the estimated current Malaysian GDP per capita of RM33,132 and RM66,263, respectively. Based on WHO cost-effectiveness threshold, sevelamer would be considered cost-effective compared to CaCO3 for the treatment of hyperphosphatemia in CKD patients in Malaysia.

3.2. Scenario Sensitivity Analysis. In the scenario sensitivity analysis, the ICER of sevelamer compared to CaCO3 varied from RM14,407 to RM 65,210 per QALY gained, with the ICER being most sensitive to varying the cost of sevelamer (due to higher assumed daily dose of sevelamer), HD cost, and the time horizon. The results of scenario sensitivity analyses are shown in Table 4.

Assuming a high sevelamer dose of 4.8g per day would increase the ICER to RM65, 210 per QALY gained whereas assuming higher HD cost of RM350 per procedure would increase the ICER to RM 58,084 per QALY gained. On the other hand, excluding the cost of dialysis in the extended lifetime of the patient would reduce the ICER to RM 14,407. Overall, none of the one-way sensitivity scenarios exceeded the two times GDP per capita threshold of RM66,263 per QALY gained and sevelamer remained cost-effective. Reducing study duration to a 3-year time horizon lowered the ICER

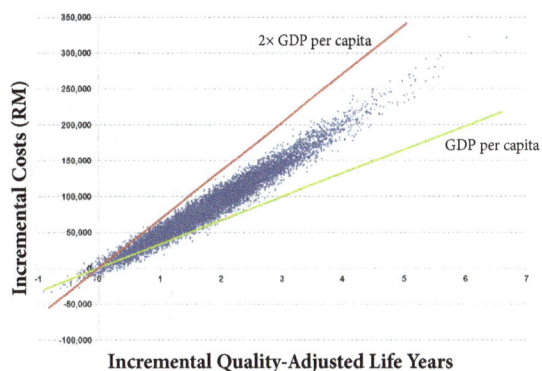

FIGURE 3: Scatter plot of ICER values generated from probabilistic sensitivity analysis.

and sevelamer becomes highly cost-effective at RM25,438 per QALY gained.

3.3. Probabilistic Sensitivity Analyses. Figure 3 illustrates the results of PSA in the form of an ICER scatterplot, which shows that, through 10,000 PSA simulations, the ICER values clustered in a narrow range around the base case ICER value of RM47,679 per QALY gained and between one and two times GDP per capita.

The cost-effectiveness acceptability curve shown in Figure 4 reaffirmed that in most simulations, the ICER would be between one and two times GDP per capita. The results of PSA showed that 98.9% of simulations generated ICERs below two times GDP per capita. Based on the PSA results, sevelamer would very likely be cost-effective for the treatment of hyperphosphatemia in CKD-ND patients in Malaysia as

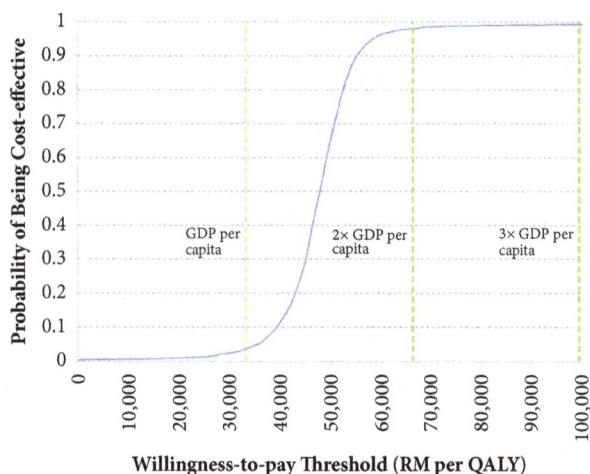

FIGURE 4: Cost-effectiveness acceptability curve.

it was unlikely that the ICER would exceed the WHO cost-effectiveness threshold of three times GDP per capita.

4. Discussion

Our results are consistent with the earlier studies which demonstrated cost-effectiveness of sevelamer in UK and Italy [17, 18]. The ICER is less than twice the GDP per capita for the country.

Our study has a number of strengths. To our knowledge, this study is the first attempt at an evaluation of the relative cost and benefits of sevelamer and CaCO3 in a predialysis population in a developing country setting. Secondly, we utilized Malaysian costs and utility data as inputs where possible. Thirdly, sensitivity analyses were conducted with both scenario and probabilistic sensitivity analyses. The PSA predicted that just 0.4% of simulations would exceed the WHO cost-effectiveness threshold, reinforcing the robustness of the base case findings that sevelamer is cost-effective.

We also note several limitations to the study. Firstly, the analysis was performed using a global cost-effectiveness decision model which comprised only three health states and was based on data from the INDEPENDENT-CKD trial [16]. There was also limited flexibility for customization and long-term efficacy which was based on 36-month follow-up data extrapolated to lifetime by regression modelling. However, as an independent study with a randomized, controlled trial design, it provided a possibly less biased comparative efficacy data from a matched population and remains the best available data in the absence of other head-to-head comparisons of sevelamer and CaCO3 in the local setting.

This study was technically designed to assess cost-effectiveness against the WHO threshold, but it may also be useful to compare our result against previous funding decisions by the Malaysian MOH. Of relevance is a comparison to haemodialysis treatment provided by MOH which has been estimated to cost RM33,642 per annum in 2001 in a previous study [26]. Factoring for inflation and exchange rate changes since 2001, we estimated the current cost of haemodialysis to be RM44,138 per patient per year [26, 28], which is slightly higher than the ICER of sevelamer in the present study at RM39,050 per LY. This means that increasing expenditure on a medication like sevelamer could prevent patients from going on to dialysis, which is a favourable clinical outcome as well as save costs through over the lifetime of patients. Beyond being a good clinical outcome, delay of dialysis treatment would also allow patients with early renal insufficiency to lead better quality and healthier lives which can be defined as priceless to an individual patient. From a societal point of view, renal patients who are not on dialysis have greater potential to contribute fully to the society through their familial, social, and economic contributions.

5. Conclusions

In conclusion, our analysis indicates that sevelamer can be a cost-effective treatment for hyperphosphatemia in Malaysian CKD-ND patients compared to CaCO3 at an ICER of RM47,679 per QALY gained. Results of sensitivity analyses did not substantially differ from the base case results and indicated that the base case results were robust and did not exceed the CE threshold of three times GDP per capita per QALY gained. Further studies incorporating long-term efficacy data, local utilities, cardiovascular disease effects, and adverse events may improve the precision of the results, but we anticipate it would be unlikely to change the overall conclusion. Our results for Malaysia suggest that sevelamer may be cost-effective in middle-income countries. This study finds that sevelamer is potentially cost-effective compared to CaCO3, for the treatment of hyperphosphatemia in predialysis CKD III-V. We propose that sevelamer should be an option in the treatment of Malaysian predialysis patients with hyperphosphatemia, particularly those with high calcium load. However, definitive conclusions about the cost-effectiveness of sevelamer should be confirmed through individual country-level studies incorporating local data.

Ethical Approval

This study was registered and approved by the Ethics Committee of the National Medical Research Register.

Disclosure

However, apart from providing the indicative price of sevelamer in Malaysia, the sponsor did not have any influence over the data collection, analysis, interpretation of data, and manuscript writing.

Acknowledgments

This study received Grant NMRR-11-24-8143 from National Institute of Health Malaysia.

References

[1] L. S. Hooi, L. M. Ong, G. Ahmad et al., "A population-based study measuring the prevalence of chronic kidney disease among adults in West Malaysia," *Kidney International*, vol. 84, no. 5, pp. 1034–1040, 2013.

[2] A. Ramachandran, C. Snehalatha, A. S. Shetty, and A. Nanditha, "Trends in prevalence of diabetes in Asian countries," *World Journal of Diabetes*, vol. 3, no. 6, pp. 110–117, 2012.

[3] C. L. Tam, G. Bonn, S. H. Yeoh, and C. P. Wong, "Investigating diet and physical activity in Malaysia: education and family history of diabetes relate to lower levels of physical activity," *Frontiers in Psychology*, vol. 5, 2014.

[4] Q. Zhang and D. Rothenbacher, "Prevalence of chronic kidney disease in population-based studies: systematic review," *BMC Public Health*, vol. 8, article 117, 2008.

[5] V. Jha, G. Garcia-Garcia, K. Iseki et al., "Chronic kidney disease: global dimension and perspectives," *The Lancet*, vol. 382, no. 9888, pp. 260–272, 2013.

[6] T.-O. Lim, A. Goh, Y.-N. Lim, Z. M. M. Zaher, and A. B. Suleiman, "How public and private reforms dramatically improved access to dialysis therapy in Malaysia," *Health Affairs*, vol. 29, no. 12, pp. 2214–2222, 2010.

[7] B. L. Goh and H. S. Wong, "24th Report of the Malaysian Dialysis and Transplant Registry," 2016.

[8] C.-Y. Hsu and G. M. Chertow, "Elevations of serum phosphorus and potassium in mild to moderate chronic renal insufficiency," *Nephrology Dialysis Transplantation*, vol. 17, no. 8, pp. 1419–1425, 2002.

[9] M. Kanbay, D. Goldsmith, A. Akcay, and A. Covic, "Phosphate - The silent stealthy cardiorenal culprit in all stages of chronic kidney disease: A systematic review," *Blood Purification*, vol. 27, no. 2, pp. 220–230, 2009.

[10] A. Bellasi, M. Mandreoli, L. Baldrati et al., "Chronic kidney disease progression and outcome according to serum phosphorus in mild-to-moderate kidney dysfunction," *Clinical Journal of the American Society of Nephrology*, vol. 6, no. 4, pp. 883–891, 2011.

[11] KDIGO, "KDIGO clinical practice guideline for the diagnosis, evaluation, prevention, and treatment of Chronic Kidney Disease-Mineral and Bone Disorder (CKD-MBD)," *Kidney International Supplements*, vol. S1, no. 130, 2009.

[12] G. M. Chertow, S. K. Burke, and P. Raggi, "Sevelamer attenuates the progression of coronary and aortic calcification in hemodialysis patients," *Kidney International*, vol. 62, no. 1, pp. 245–252, 2002.

[13] S. K. Burke, M. A. Dillon, D. E. Hemken, M. S. Rezabek, and J. M. Balwit, "Meta-analysis of the effect of sevelamer on phosphorus, calcium, PTH, and serum lipids in dialysis patients," *Advances in Chronic Kidney Disease*, vol. 10, no. 2, pp. 133–145, 2003.

[14] D. Russo, I. Miranda, C. Ruocco et al., "The progression of coronary artery calcification in predialysis patients on calcium carbonate or sevelamer," *Kidney International*, vol. 72, no. 10, pp. 1255–1261, 2007.

[15] M. J. Bolland, A. Grey, A. Avenell, G. D. Gamble, and I. R. Reid, "Calcium supplements with or without vitamin D and risk of cardiovascular events: reanalysis of the Women's Health Initiative limited access dataset and meta-analysis," *British Medical Journal*, vol. 342, no. 7804, Article ID d2040, 2011.

[16] B. Di Iorio, A. Bellasi, and D. Russo, "Mortality in kidney disease patients treated with phosphate binders: A randomized study," *Clinical Journal of the American Society of Nephrology*, vol. 7, no. 3, pp. 487–493, 2012.

[17] M. Thompson, S. Bartko-Winters, L. Bernard, A. Fenton, C. Hutchison, and B. Di Iorio, "Economic evaluation of sevelamer for the treatment of hyperphosphatemia in chronic kidney disease patients not on dialysis in the United Kingdom," *Journal of Medical Economics*, vol. 16, no. 6, pp. 744–755, 2013.

[18] M. Ruggeri, F. Cipriani, A. Bellasi, D. Russo, and B. D. Iorio, "Sevelamer is cost-saving vs. calcium carbonate in non-dialysis-dependent CKD patients in Italy: A patient-level cost-effectiveness analysis of the INDEPENDENT study," *Blood Purification*, vol. 37, no. 4, pp. 316–324, 2014.

[19] M. F. Drummond, G. L. Stoddart, and G. W. Torrance, *Methods for the economic evaluation of health care programmes*, Oxford University Press, Oxford, UK, 1997.

[20] A. Gray, *Applied Methods of Cost-Effectiveness Analysis in Health Care*, Oxford University Press, Oxford, UK, 2011.

[21] M. J. Taylor, H. A. Elgazzar, S. Chaplin, D. Goldsmith, and D. A. Molony, "An economic evaluation of sevelamer in patients new to dialysis," *Current Medical Research and Opinion*, vol. 24, no. 2, pp. 601–608, 2008.

[22] J. H. S. You, W.-K. Ming, W.-A. Lin, and Y.-H. Tarn, "Early supplemented low-protein diet restriction for chronic kidney disease patients in Taiwan - A cost-effectiveness analysis," *Clinical Nephrology*, vol. 84, no. 4, pp. 189–197, 2015.

[23] S. Bavanandan, S. Azmi, and A. Goh, "Quality of life of Malaysian dialysis patients on transplant waiting list," in *Proceedings of the ISPOR 4th Asia-Pacific Conference*, Phuket, Thailand, 2010.

[24] I. Gorodetskaya, S. Zenios, C. E. McCulloch et al., "Health-related quality of life and estimates of utility in chronic kidney disease," *Kidney International*, vol. 68, no. 6, pp. 2801–2808, 2005.

[25] IMS Health, *Malaysian Pharmaceutical Audit*, Sanofi Aventis, 2013.

[26] L. S. Hooi, T. O. Lim, A. Goh et al., "Economic evaluation of centre haemodialysis and continuous ambulatory peritoneal dialysis in Ministry of Health hospitals, Malaysia," *Nephrology*, vol. 10, no. 1, pp. 25–32, 2005.

[27] Fund IM, *World Economic Outlook Database*, 2013, https://www.imf.org/external/pubs/ft/weo/2013/02/weodata/index.aspx.

[28] "Bank Negara Malaysia, Exchange Rates," http://www.bnm.gov.my/index.phpAvailable at ?ch=statisticpg=stats_exchangerates.

[29] Pharmaceutical Services Division (Ministry of Health Malaysia), "Pharmacoeconomic Guideline for Malaysia," 2012.

[30] Pharmacoeconomic Guideline for Malaysia, "Cost effectiveness threshold," http://www.who.int/choice/costs/CER_thresholds/en/.

[31] D. Caldwell, "Decision Modelling for Health Economic Evaluation. A Briggs, M Sculpher, K Claxton," *International Journal of Epidemiology*, vol. 36, no. 2, pp. 476-477, 2007.

[32] J. J. Caro, A. H. Briggs, U. Siebert, and K. M. Kuntz, "Modeling good research practices - Overview: A report of the ISPOR-SMDM modeling good research practices task force-1," *Value in Health*, vol. 15, no. 6, pp. 796–803, 2012.

3

High (≥6.5) Spontaneous and Persistent Urinary pH Is Protective of Renal Function at Baseline and during Disease Course in Idiopathic Membranous Nephropathy

Claudio Bazzi,[1] Elena Tagliabue,[2] Sara Raimondi,[2] Virginia Rizza,[3] Daniela Casellato,[4] and Masaomi Nangaku[5]

[1] D'Amico Foundation for Renal Disease Research, 20145 Milan, Italy
[2] Division of Epidemiology and Biostatistics, European Institute of Oncology, 20141 Milan, Italy
[3] Biochemical Laboratory, San Carlo Borromeo Hospital, 20153 Milan, Italy
[4] Nephrology and Dialysis Unit, San Carlo Borromeo Hospital, 20153 Milan, Italy
[5] Division of Nephrology and Endocrinology, University of Tokyo School of Medicine, Tokyo 113-8655, Japan

Correspondence should be addressed to Claudio Bazzi; claudio.bazzi@alice.it

Academic Editor: Danuta Zwolinska

Metabolic acidosis correction in advanced renal failure slows renal function decline attributed to tubulointerstitial damage (TID) reduction. No study evaluated if spontaneous baseline high urinary pH (UpH) is renoprotective in patients with normal renal function and without metabolic acidosis. The study tested this hypothesis in idiopathic membranous nephropathy (IMN). Eighty-five patients (follow-up 81 ± 54 months) measured UpH, serum creatinine, eGFR, protein/creatinine ratio, fractional excretion of albumin, IgG, α1-microglobulin, and urinary N-acetyl-β-D-glucosaminidase (β-NAG)/creatinine ratio. Twenty-eight patients (33%) had UpH ≥ 6.5 and 57 (67%) pH < 6.5; high versus low UpH patients had significantly lower values of the tubulointerstitial damage (TID) markers FE αlm and β-NAG and significantly better baseline renal function. These differences persisted over time in a subset of 38 patients with 5 measurements along 53 ± 26 months. In 29 patients with nephrotic syndrome (NS) treated with supportive therapy (follow-up: 80 ± 52 months) renal function was stable in 10 high and significantly worse in 19 low UpH patients. Steroids + cyclophosphamide treatment in 35 NS patients masks the renoprotection of high UpH. Conclusions. In IMN high and persistent UpH is associated with reduction of the proteinuric markers of tubulointerstitial damage and baseline better renal function in all patients and in NS patients treated only with supportive therapy during disease course. The factors associated with high pH-dependent renoprotection were lower values of TID markers, eGFR ≥ 60 mL/min, BP < 140/90 mmHg, and age < 55 years.

1. Introduction

Metabolic acidosis in CKD is associated with progressive loss of renal function, increased ESRD rate, impaired nutritional parameters, skeletal muscle wasting, bone uremic disease worsening, adverse cardiovascular outcomes, and death [1–5]. Several studies over recent years have evaluated the renoprotective effect of correcting metabolic acidosis (serum bicarbonate < 22 mEq/L) [6] with sodium citrate, sodium bicarbonate, or fruit- and vegetable-rich diet, mainly in patients with advanced renal failure (stage 3-4 CKD) ([7–12]; reviews in [13–18]). These studies showed that the alkalinizing treatment slowed renal function decline, reduced the ESRD rate, ameliorated muscle wasting and nutritional parameters, and reduced the excretion of some urinary markers of kidney injury such as urinary endothelin [8], TGF-β [11], angiotensinogen [12], and the tubulointerstitial damage marker N-acetyl-β-D-glucosaminidase (β-NAG) [8, 9, 11]. The reduced excretion of β-NAG associated with reduction of renal function decline observed after 2 years of Na citrate therapy [8], 5 years of NaHCO$_3$ therapy [9], and one year of fruit- and vegetable-rich diet [10] suggested that the renoprotective effect of metabolic acidosis correction was dependent on reduction of the extent of tubulointerstitial damage (TID) following alkalinizing treatment. The relationship between metabolic acidosis correction, urinary luminal alkalinization, and reduction of TID has been evaluated in several studies. Cell culture and remnant kidney models [19, 20] showed that tubular protein-overload activates complement at the brush border of proximal tubular epithelial cells (PTECs), inducing tubular damage and interstitial inflammatory cells infiltration. These observations were confirmed in experimental models of MN that showed the role of complement activation in PTECs as responsible of tubulointerstitial damage. The mechanisms of complement activation in PTECs have been evaluated in some studies. In a mouse model of protein-overload nephropathy urine luminal alkalinization induced by $NaHCO_3$ feeding attenuates the proteinuria-induced oxidative damage in PTECs. Couser and Nangaku [21] suggested that the protective effect of $NaHCO_3$ is dependent on reduced intratubular complement activation, as shown in some experimental models [22, 23]. Moreover a cell culture study [24] showed that the deposition of C3 and C9 on the surface of HK-2 cells is maximal at acidic pH values and significantly reduced at pH $\geq$ 6.5. A study of patients with glomerular diseases [25] showed that the urinary excretion of complement activation products increased significantly with higher levels of proteinuria in all diseases except minimal change disease and decreased significantly after two weeks of sodium bicarbonate administration. As a whole the results of these studies in experimental models and human diseases suggest that the tubulointerstitial damage is dependent at least on two factors: the tubular load of proteins and the activation of complement in tubular cells whose level is reduced by luminal alkalinization. The studies on metabolic acidosis correction in advanced renal failure showed that the reduction of renal function decline was associated with a reduced excretion of the tubular damage marker β-NAG. The overall conclusion of the studies on metabolic acidosis correction in advanced renal failure is that this treatment is an inexpensive and simple therapeutic strategy with an effective kidney protective value adjunct to blood pressure control with angiotensin-converting enzyme inhibition. The published studies were limited by the inclusion almost exclusively of patients with advanced renal failure (stage 3-4 CKD) and lack of diagnosis in most of them except for hypertensive nephropathy in 2 studies; only one study showed greater improvement in patients with eGFR > 45 mL/min/1.73 m^2. If the renoprotective mechanism does in fact stem from a reduction of tubular damage mediated by reduced complement activation consequent to luminal alkalinization, it would be interesting to evaluate whether high spontaneous and persistent urinary pH is renoprotective not only in patients with advanced renal failure and metabolic acidosis but also in patients with normal renal function without metabolic acidosis. To test this hypothesis we evaluated renal function parameters and some proteinuric markers of tubulointerstitial damage in 85 patients with idiopathic membranous nephropathy (IMN), mainly with normal renal function at biopsy (68% with eGFR $\geq$ 60 mL/min/1.73 m^2) and a rather long follow-up (81±54 months) to assess whether

spontaneous baseline (≥6.5) and persistent high urinary pH is renoprotective in terms of reduced tubulointerstitial damage, better baseline renal function, and slower renal function decline during the disease course. A second aim was to assess whether chronic renal failure (eGFR < 60 mL/min/1.73 m^2), age, and high blood pressure may interfere with the renoprotective effects of spontaneous high pH.

2. Patients

Eighty-five patients with IMN were included in the study; the patients were part of a cohort of 105 IMN patients diagnosed between 1992 and 2005 in the Nephrology and Dialysis Unit of the San Carlo Borromeo Hospital. Inclusion criteria were as follows: typical features of IMN at light and immunofluorescence microscopy; no clinical and/or laboratory signs of secondary MN; clinical presentation with nephrotic syndrome (NS: 82%) or persistent nonnephrotic proteinuria (PP: 18%); at least 6 glomeruli in renal biopsy; follow-up of at least 12 months. Exclusion criteria were as follows: lack of follow-up (N 18); NS with haemodynamic acute reversible renal failure at biopsy (N 2). The baseline clinical and laboratory characteristics of all patients are reported in Table 1. Twenty-nine patients with NS were treated only with supportive therapy: diuretics, antihypertensives (including ACEi/ARBs), statins, antiplatelet agents, and vitamin D3 when indicated. Thirty-five NS patients, besides supportive therapy, were treated soon after diagnosis with steroids and cyclophosphamide for six months according to the Ponticelli protocol [26]. Six NS patients were treated with steroids alone: prednisone 1 mg/kg/day with tapering for 4–12 months. Fifteen patients with PP were treated only with supportive therapy. The patients were screened up until the last planned follow-up clinic visit in 2011; the overall follow-up was 81 ± 54 months (range 12–226). The primary outcome was the level of renal function parameters at baseline and during disease course; a secondary outcome was progression to ESRD.

3. Analytical Methods

Renal biopsies were performed and evaluated by the previously described standard histological and immunofluorescence methods [27]. Total urinary proteins were measured by the Coomassie blue method in second morning urine sample and expressed as protein/creatinine ratio (P/C: mg of proteins/1 g urinary creatinine). Serum (sCr) and urinary creatinine were measured automatically on a Beckman LX20 analyzer using the Jaffè method and expressed in mg/dL. Estimated Glomerular Filtration Rate (eGFR) was calculated according to the 4-variable MDRD formula [28]; the body weight in high and low UpH groups was 62 ± 12 kg (46–83) and 63 ± 9 kg (45–85), respectively. β-NAG was measured in the second morning urine sample by a colorimetric method as described [29] and expressed as the β-NAG/creatinine ratio divided by the eGFR (NAG/C/eGFR) [30], as β-NAG excretion is dependent on the functioning nephron mass; this method of calculation was suggested by Ellam and El Nahas [31] which observed that the urinary excretion of proteins should be adjusted for the functioning nephron mass

TABLE 1: Comparison of baseline and follow-up urinary pH and clinical, functional, and proteinuric parameters in 85 IMN patients with pH ≥ 6.5 (N 28) or pH < 6.5 (N 57).

Parameter	All patients (N = 85) Mean (±SD)	Pts. with pH ≥ 6.5 (N = 28) Mean (±SD)	Pts. with pH < 6.5 (N = 57) Mean (±SD)	p value
Baseline pH	5.96 ± 0.79	6.91 ± 0.36	5.50 ± 0.47	**<0.0001**
Follow-up pH	5.92 ± 0.58 (N 66)	6.44 ± 0.47 (N 23)	5.65 ± 0.47 (N 43)	**<0.0001**
Serum bicarbonate mEq/L	26.8 ± 3.4	27.7 ± 3.8	26.4 ± 3.6	0.13
Age (years)	52 ± 17	52 ± 21	52 ± 15	0.95
sCr (mg/dL)	1.20 ± 0.53	0.99 ± 0.34	1.31 ± 0.57	**0.003**
eGFR (mL/min/1.73 m^2)	73 ± 28	83 ± 28	68 ± 27	**0.03**
eGFR < 60 mL/min/1.73 m^2 (%)	32%	25%	35%	0.35
BP ≥140/90 mmHg (%)	53%	36%	61%	**0.03**
P/C ratio	3731 ± 2573	3649 ± 2288	3772 ± 2721	0.99
FE albumin	0.180 ± 0.170	0.160 ± 0.150	0.190 ± 0.180	0.50
FE IgG	0.05 ± 0.06	0.04 ± 0.06	0.05 ± 0.07	0.27
FE α1m-microglobulin	0.420 ± 0.410	0.290 ± 0.340	0.480 ± 0.440	**0.02**
NAG/C/eGFR	0.30 ± 0.30	0.21 ± 0.23	0.35 ± 0.32	**0.04**

Note: significant p values are in bold.

of whom eGFR may be a reliable index. All patients were measured at biopsy for several urinary proteins of different MW: IgG (MW 150 kDa), albumin (Alb, MW 67 kDa), and α1-microglobulin (α1m : MW 31.8 kDa). The proteins were measured by BNA nephelometer (Behring, Milan, Italy) using rabbit serum antibodies (Behring). The excretion of albumin, IgG, and α1m was expressed as fractional excretion (FE) according to the formula: [(urinary protein/serum protein × sCr/uCr) × 100]. Urinary pH was measured by Multistix (Siemens) soon after urine collection.

4. Statistical Methods

Statistical analysis was performed using SAS 9.2. Patients were divided into two groups based on the second tertile of basal UpH distribution, that is, 6.5. Differences in baseline characteristics between high and low UpH groups were determined using the Mann-Whitney test and the chi-square test for continuous and categorical variables, respectively. Differences in the high and low UpH groups between baseline and last observed creatinine and eGFR values were calculated by the Wilcoxon signed-ranks test for repeated measures. Correlations were assessed using the Spearman rank test. Differences in ESRD rate were evaluated using Kaplan-Meier survival curves; the equality of survival curves was assessed by log-rank test. Multivariate Cox proportional hazard regression analysis was performed on the population as a whole. Statistical significance was defined as $p < 0.05$.

5. Results

5.1. Baseline and Follow-Up pH. At baseline 28 patients (33%) had urinary pH ≥ 6.5 (high pH group: "high UpH") and 57

patients (67%) had pH < 6.5 (low pH group: "low UpH") (Table 1). The baseline pH in high versus low UpH group was 6.91 ± 0.36 and 5.50 ± 0.47, respectively ($p < 0.0001$). Serum bicarbonate was not significantly different between the high and low UpH groups. The percentage of patients with eGFR <60 mL/min/1.73 m^2 was not significantly different between the high and low UpH groups (25% versus 32%, $p = 0.35$). Twenty-three patients in the high UpH group and 43 patients in the low UpH group had several measurements of pH, functional, and proteinuric parameters (on average 5 measurements over time from 6 to 121 months). The baseline values of all functional and proteinuric parameters of patients included or not included in the follow-up study were not significantly different (data not shown). In patients with baseline pH ≥ 6.5 the mean follow-up UpH was significantly higher than in patients with baseline pH < 6.5 (6.45 ± 0.50 versus 5.65 ± 0.40, resp., $p < 0.0001$). Correlation analysis showed that none of the clinical, functional, and proteinuric parameters was correlated with the pH value; it is reasonable to suppose that the different pH levels may be at least partly related to different dietary habits; unfortunately no information is available about the dietary habits of the patients.

5.2. Comparison of Baseline Clinical, Functional, and Proteinuric Parameters in High versus Low UpH Patients. In patients with high versus low UpH (Table 1), at baseline the markers of tubulointerstitial damage FE α1m ($p = 0.02$) and β-NAG/C/eGFR ($p = 0.04$) were significantly lower; the renal function parameters sCr and eGFR were significantly better (sCr: 0.99 ± 0.34 versus 1.31 ± 0.57 mg/dL, $p = 0.003$; eGFR 83 ± 28 versus 68 ± 27, $p = 0.03$). Conversely the proteinuric markers for altered glomerular filtration barrier

TABLE 2: Comparison of functional and proteinuric parameters at baseline and at the last observation in a subset of 38 IMN patients (high UpH group *N* 11, low UpH group *N* 27) with 5 serial measurements along 56 ± 26 months (range 24–121).

Parameter	UpH ≥ 6.5 (*N* = 11)		*p* value	UpH < 6.5 (*N* = 27)		*p* value
	Baseline values Mean (±SD)	Last values Mean (±SD)		Baseline values Mean (±SD)	Last values Mean (±SD)	
Follow-up (months)		57 ± 30			51 ± 25	0.57
Mean follow-up pH		6.32 ± 0.37			5.66 ± 0.43	**0.0001**
sCr (mg/dL)	0.89 ± 0.33	1.23 ± 1.36	0.46	1.27 ± 0.54	2.43 ± 2.13	**0.001**
eGFR mL/min/1.73 m^2	94 ± 32	91 ± 40	0.81	69 ± 27	51 ± 34	**<0.0001**
P/C ratio	2867 ± 2117	2091 ± 3122	0.37	4399 ± 3115	3881 ± 4350	0.43
FE albumin	0.106 ± 0.144	0.165 ± 0.328	0.65	0.179 ± 0.137	0.315 ± 0.454	0.35
FE IgG	0.029 ± 0.064	0.062 ± 0.163	0.97	0.059 ± 0.067	0.150 ± 0.280	0.34
FE αlm	0.195 ± 0.212	0.503 ± 1.183	0.97	0.476 ± 0.495	1.663 ± 2.300	**0.01**
NAG/C/eGFR	0.157 ± 0.228	0.416 ± 0.936	0.70	0.342 ± 0.328	0.791 ± 1.088	0.23
ACE-inhibitors treatment (%)		36%			59%	0.17
Steroid + cyclophosphamide treatment (%)		36%			37%	n.s.

Note: significant *p* values are in bold.

(P/C ratio, FE albumin, and FE IgG) were not significantly different between the two groups. Limiting the analysis to patients with eGFR ≥ 60 mL/min/1.73 m^2 in 21 high UpH versus 37 low UpH sCr was significantly lower (*p* = 0.004), eGFR higher at the limit of significance (*p* = 0.05), and FE αlm significantly lower (*p* = 0.03). Thus spontaneous high UpH was significantly associated at baseline with better renal function and lower values of the proteinuric markers for TID.

5.3. Comparison of Baseline Functional and Proteinuric Parameters between High versus Low UpH Groups in the Subset of 70 Patients with Nephrotic Syndrome. Limiting the analysis to 70 patients with NS in the high UpH (number 25) versus low UpH group (number 45), the sCr was significantly lower (*p* = 0.008) and eGFR higher at the limit of statistical significance (*p* = 0.050); P/C ratio, FE albumin, and FE IgG were not significantly different, while the TID markers FE αlm (*p* = 0.01) and β-NAG/C/GFR (*p* = 0.009) were significantly lower (data not shown).

5.4. Comparison of Functional and Proteinuric Parameters at Baseline and at the Last Measurement in a Subset of 38 Patients (11 High UpH, 27 Low UpH) with 5 Serial Measurements along 56 ± 26 Months (Range 24–121). To assess whether the differences between the high and low UpH group observed at baseline were persistent over time, of the 66 patients with several measurements, a subgroup of 38 patients was selected who had 5 serial measurements of all parameters at least 24 months after baseline (follow-up: 53 ± 26 months; range: 24–121): 11 patients of the high and 27 of the low UpH group. The mean urinary pH during this time was significantly higher in high versus the low UpH group (6.32 ± 0.37 versus 5.66 ± 0.43, *p* = 0.0001). In the high UpH group (follow-up: 57 ± 30 months) the last values of the proteinuric markers of TID and the functional parameters sCr and eGFR were not significantly different from the

baseline values (Table 2). Conversely, in the low UpH group (follow-up: 51 ± 24 months), at the last measurement, sCr was significantly higher (*p* = 0.001), eGFR significantly lower (<0.0001), and FE αlm significantly higher (*p* = 0.01), while β-NAG/C/eGFR was not significantly different. Thus serial measurements of functional and proteinuric parameters during a rather long follow-up confirm that at the last observation spontaneous and persistent high UpH is associated with stable renal function, while low UpH is associated with worse renal function and higher levels of FE αlm.

5.5. Renoprotective Value of Spontaneous Baseline and Persistent High UpH over Time in 29 NS Patients Treated Only with Supportive Therapy. The renoprotective value of spontaneous high UpH was evaluated in 29 NS patients treated only with supportive therapy (10 with high UpH, 19 with low UpH patients). At baseline, the proteinuric TID markers were significantly lower (FE αlm, *p* = 0.01; β-NAG/C/eGFR, *p* = 0.04), sCr was significantly lower (*p* = 0.013), and eGFR was significantly higher (*p* = 0.007) in high versus low UpH patients (Table 3); none of the "glomerular" markers (P/C ratio, FE albumin, and FE IgG) was significantly different between the two groups. At the last observation after a follow-up of 86 ± 55 months, in the high UpH group sCr and eGFR levels were not significantly different from the baseline values (sCr: 0.83 ± 0.12 versus 1.05 ± 0.40, *p* = 0.11; eGFR 97 ± 19 versus 78 ± 29, *p* = 0.12). In the low UpH group, at the last observation after a follow-up of 75 ± 52 months, sCr and eGFR were significantly worse (sCr: 3.30 ± 2.75 versus 1.18 ± 0.39, *p* = 0.027, eGFR: 44 ± 39 versus 69 ± 27, *p* = 0.026), and the TID markers were significantly higher: FE αlm 0.480 ± 0.440 versus 0.290 ± 0.340, *p* = 0.02; β-NAG/C/eGFR 0.35 ± 0.32 versus 0.21 ± 0.23, *p* = 0.04. Progression to ESRD was higher in low versus high UpH patients (37% versus 0%) but the difference did not attain statistical significance (*p* = 0.12). Thus the patients in the

TABLE 3: Baseline and last observation clinical, functional, and proteinuric parameters in 29 IMN with NS patients treated with supportive therapy with UpH ≥ 6.5 (N 10) or UpH < 6.5 (N 19).

Parameter	Patients with pH ≥ 6.5 (N = 10) Mean (±SD)	Patients with pH < 6.5 (N = 19) Mean (±SD)	p value
Baseline pH	7.00 ± 0.33	5.56 ± 0.47	**<0.0001**
Follow-up pH	6.36 ± 0.43	5.75 ± 0.37	**0.005**
BP ≥140/90 mmHg (%)	10%	74%	**0.002**
Baseline sCr (mg/dL)	0.83 ± 0.12$^\wedge$	1.18 ± 0.39§	**0.013**
Last observation sCr (mg/dL)	1.05 ± 0.40$^\wedge$	3.30 ± 2.70§	**0.027**
Baseline eGFR (mL/min/1.73 m^2)	97 ± 19*	69 ± 26°	**0.007**
Last observation eGFR (mL/min/1.73 m^2)	78 ± 30*	44 ± 39°	**0.026**
ESRD (%)	0%	37%	0.12
Follow-up (months)	86 ± 55	75 ± 52	0.49
P/C ratio	3570 ± 1996	4808 ± 3361	0.41
FE Alb	0.103 ± 0.056	0.201 ± 0.150	0.11
FE IgG	0.013 ± 0.011	0.062 ± 0.070	0.07
FE αlm	0.170 ± 0.110	0.499 ± 0.440	**0.01**
NAG/C/eGFR1	0.134 ± 0.06	0.434 ± 0.400	**0.04**

Note: significant p values are in bold.
$^\wedge p = 0.12$; $^\S \mathbf{p = 0.003}$; $^* p = 0.11$; $^\circ \mathbf{p = 0.02}$.

high UpH group treated with supportive therapy have not only significantly better baseline functional parameters and lower TID markers but also stable renal function over time. By contrast, the patients of the low UpH group had worse renal function and increased TID markers both at baseline and during disease course.

5.6. Renal Function over Time in 35 NS Patients Treated with Steroids and Cyclophosphamide. Thirty-five NS patients were treated with steroids and cyclophosphamide according to the Ponticelli protocol [26] (15 with high and 20 with low UpH). At the last observation the sCr and eGFR values of the high UpH group (follow-up: 76 ± 47 months) were improved but not significantly versus baseline values (sCr: 1.16±0.38 versus 2.34 ± 2.50 mg/dL, $p = 0.09$; eGFR: 68 ± 26 versus 61 ± 38 mL/min/1.73 m^2, $p = 0.54$). Also in the low UpH group (follow-up: 112 ± 63 months), at the last observation, sCr and eGFR were not significantly improved versus baseline values (sCr: 1.38 ± 0.63 versus 1.93 ± 1.76 mg/dL, $p = 0.20$; eGFR: 67 ± 24 versus 59 ± 31 mL/min/1.73 m^2, $p = 0.37$). These results suggest that immunosuppressive therapy may mask the renoprotective effect of spontaneous high urinary pH.

5.7. Factors Affecting the Renoprotective Effect of High Urinary pH. Three parameters were considered for their possible influence on renal function and proteinuric markers in high versus low UpH patients: age below or above the median value (< versus ≥55 years), eGFR (≥ versus <60 mL/min/1.73 m^2), and baseline blood pressure (< versus ≥140/90 mmHg). In patients with high versus low UpH and age < 55 years, at baseline sCr was significantly lower ($p = 0.002$) and eGFR was significantly higher ($p = 0.004$); P/C ratio, FE Alb, and FE IgG were not significantly different; FE αlm was significantly lower ($p = 0.02$) and β-NAG/C/eGFR was

lower at the limit of statistical significance ($p = 0.05$). In patients aged ≥55 years none of the parameters was significantly different between high and low UpH. In patients with eGFR ≥ 60 mL/min/1.73 m^2 and high versus low UpH, at baseline sCr was lower ($p = 0.004$) and eGFR was higher at the limit of statistical significance ($p = 0.05$); none of the "glomerular" proteinuric parameters were significantly different; the TID marker FE αlm was significantly lower ($p = 0.03$) while β-NAG/C/eGFR was not significantly different ($p = 0.40$). In patients with eGFR < 60 mL/min/1.73 m^2 none of the parameters was significantly different between the high and low UpH groups. In patients with baseline BP < 140/90 mmHg sCr ($p = 0.006$), FE αlm ($p = 0.01$), and β-NAG/C/eGFR ($p = 0.02$) were significantly lower in high versus low UpH group; eGFR was at the limit of significance ($p = 0.07$). In patients with BP ≥ 140/90 mmHg all parameters were not significantly different between UpH groups. This data suggests that spontaneous high pH is associated with better renal function mainly in patients with age < 55 years, eGFR ≥ 60 mL/min/1.73 m^2, and normal BP; the proteinuric markers for TID were significantly lower in patients with age < 55 years and normal BP, but not in patients with eGFR ≥ 60 mL/min/1.73 m^2.

5.8. Multivariate Cox Regression Analysis. The results of multivariate Cox regression analysis including age, eGFR, fractional excretion of αlm, fractional excretion of IgG, and pH showed that none of the markers was significantly associated with progression.

6. Discussion

The majority of studies showing a reduction in renal function decline following treatment of metabolic acidosis with alkalinizing drugs or foods were performed in patients with advanced renal failure (stages 3-4). Our study evaluated for the first time in a cohort of IMN patients whether high spontaneous baseline and persistent urinary pH may be renoprotective both at baseline and during the disease course in patients without metabolic acidosis. The study was also aimed at assessing which factors might be associated with the renoprotective effect of high UpH. In our cohort, 28 patients had baseline urinary pH ≥ 6.5 significantly higher than in 57 patients with baseline urinary pH < 6.5. In the high UpH group the values of pH remained significantly higher on average in several measurements performed over a mean period of about 5 years compared to patients with low UpH. At baseline, high UpH was associated with significantly lower values of the proteinuric TID markers FE αlm and β-NAG/C/eGFR and better renal function in comparison with patients with low UpH. In patients treated only with supportive therapy, those with high UpH had stable renal function over a period of about 7 years: by contrast patients with low UpH were characterized by significantly worse renal function and significantly higher levels of the TID markers over a period of about 6 years. The ESRD rate was higher in low versus high UpH patients (37% versus 0%) but the difference did not attain a statistical significance ($p = 0.12$). Renal function worsening in low UpH patients cannot be attributed to higher levels of the "glomerular" proteinuric markers for altered filtration barrier (P/C ratio, FE albumin, and FE IgG) known to be associated with progressive renal disease as these markers were not significantly different between low versus high UpH patients. Conversely the significant reduction in high UpH patients of the proteinuric markers of tubulointerstitial damage FE αlm and β-NAG may be possibly dependent on lower complement activation consequent to urinary alkalinization as observed in some experimental models and clinical studies. One functional (eGFR) and two clinical (age, blood pressure) parameters were evaluated as factors that might possibly influence the renoprotective effect of spontaneous high pH: the results showed that, in patients with eGFR ≥ 60 mL/min/1.73 m^2, age < 55 years, and BP < 140/90 mmHg, the baseline functional parameters were significantly better; also the proteinuric TID markers were significantly lower in high versus low UpH, except in patients with eGFR ≥ 60 mL/min/1.73 m^2. By contrast, in patients with eGFR ≤60 mL/min/1.73 m^2, age ≥ 55 years, and BP ≥ 140/90 mmHg both the functional parameters and proteinuric TID markers were not significantly different between high and low UpH. These data suggest that four factors are associated with better renal function in IMN patients with spontaneous and persistently high urinary pH: a less severe tubulointerstitial damage, eGFR ≥ 60 mL/min/1.73 m^2, age < 55 years, and BP < 140/90 mmHg. This observation could suggest that spontaneous high UpH is less powerful in reducing renal function decline and TID markers than the metabolic acidosis correction that reduces renal function decline and TID markers also in patients with advanced renal failure (stages 3-4). The renoprotective effect of spontaneous high urinary pH in IMN patients is a new rather unexpected and interesting observation. If confirmed in prospective controlled trials, the main clinical message could be that, in IMN patients with normal renal function, those with low urinary pH could usefully be given alkalinizing drugs as a cheap and simple treatment strategy, with an effective kidney protective value adjunct to blood pressure control with angiotensin-converting enzyme inhibition. None of our patients with advanced renal failure (stages 3-4) was treated with alkalinizing therapy; obviously our observations do not rule out the possibility that also in IMN patients with advanced renal failure the metabolic acidosis correction with NaHCO$_3$, Na citrate, or alkalinizing foods may be renoprotective.

7. Conclusions

The study shows for the first time that in IMN the patients with high spontaneous and persistent urinary pH (≥6.5) in comparison with patients with lower pH (<6.5) have significantly better renal function at baseline and during disease course in patients treated only with supportive therapy. The main factor associated with high pH-dependent renoprotection is the significant reduction of the tubulointerstitial damage markers FE αlm and β-NAG, possibly dependent on less complement activation in tubular cells due to urinary alkalinization as observed in some experimental and clinical studies.

References

[1] M. Dobre, W. Yang, J. Chen et al., "Association of serum bicarbonate with risk of renal and cardiovascular outcomes in CKD: a report from the Chronic Renal Insufficiency Cohort (CRIC) study," *American Journal of Kidney Diseases*, vol. 62, no. 4, pp. 670–678, 2013.

[2] C. P. Kovesdy, J. E. Anderson, and K. Kalantar-Zadeh, "Association of serum bicarbonate levels with mortality in patients with non-dialysis-dependent CKD," *Nephrology Dialysis Transplantation*, vol. 24, no. 4, pp. 1232–1237, 2009.

[3] V. Menon, H. Tighiouart, N. S. Vaughn et al., "Serum bicarbonate and long-term outcomes in CKD," *The American Journal of Kidney Diseases*, vol. 56, no. 5, pp. 907–914, 2010.

[4] K. L. Raphael, Y. Zhang, G. Wei, T. Greene, A. K. Cheung, and S. Beddhu, "Serum bicarbonate and mortality in adults in NHANES III," *Nephrology Dialysis Transplantation*, vol. 28, no. 5, pp. 1207–1213, 2013.

[5] E. Kanda, M. Ai, M. Yoshida, R. Kuriyama, and T. Shiigai, "High serum bicarbonate level within the normal range prevents the progression of chronic kidney disease in elderly chronic kidney disease patients," *BMC Nephrology*, vol. 14, article 4, 2013.

[6] L. A. Inker, B. C. Astor, C. H. Fox et al., "KDOQI US commentary on the 2012 KDIGO clinical practice guideline for the evaluation and management of CKD," *The American Journal of Kidney Diseases*, vol. 63, no. 5, pp. 713–735, 2014.

[7] I. de Brito-Ashurst, M. Varagunam, M. J. Raftery, and M. M. Yaqoob, "Bicarbonate supplementation slows progression of CKD and improves nutritional status," *Journal of the American Society of Nephrology*, vol. 20, no. 9, pp. 2075–2084, 2009.

[8] S. Phisitkul, A. Khanna, J. Simoni et al., "Amelioration of metabolic acidosis in patients with low GFR reduced kidney endothelin production and kidney injury, and better preserved GFR," *Kidney International*, vol. 77, no. 7, pp. 617–623, 2010.

[9] A. Mahajan, J. Simoni, S. J. Sheather, K. R. Broglio, M. H. Rajab, and D. E. Wesson, "Daily oral sodium bicarbonate preserves glomerular filtration rate by slowing its decline in early hypertensive nephropathy," *Kidney International*, vol. 78, no. 3, pp. 303–309, 2010.

[10] N. Goraya, J. Simoni, C. Jo, and D. E. Wesson, "Dietary acid reduction with fruits and vegetables or bicarbonate attenuates kidney injury in patients with a moderately reduced glomerular filtration rate due to hypertensive nephropathy," *Kidney International*, vol. 81, no. 1, pp. 86–93, 2012.

[11] C. P. Kovesdy, "Metabolic acidosis and kidney disease: does bicarbonate therapy slow the progression of CKD?" *Nephrology Dialysis Transplantation*, vol. 27, no. 8, pp. 3056–3062, 2012.

[12] N. Goraya, J. Simoni, C.-H. Jo, and D. E. Wesson, "A comparison of treating metabolic acidosis in CKD stage 4 hypertensive kidney disease with fruits and vegetables or sodium bicarbonate," *Clinical Journal of the American Society of Nephrology*, vol. 8, no. 3, pp. 371–381, 2013.

[13] N. Goraya, J. Simoni, C.-H. Jo, and D. E. Wesson, "Treatment of metabolic acidosis in patients with stage 3 chronic kidney disease with fruits and vegetables or oral bicarbonate reduces urine angiotensinogen and preserves glomerular filtration rate," *Kidney International*, vol. 86, no. 5, pp. 1031–1038, 2014.

[14] N. Goraya and D. E. Wesson, "Does correction of metabolic acidosis slow chronic kidney disease progression?" *Current Opinion in Nephrology and Hypertension*, vol. 22, no. 2, pp. 193–197, 2013.

[15] M. M. Yaqoob, "Treatment of acidosis in CKD," *Clinical Journal of the American Society of Nephrology*, vol. 8, no. 3, pp. 342–343, 2013.

[16] M. Dobre, M. Rahman, and T. H. Hostetter, "Current status of bicarbonate in CKD," *Journal of the American Society of Nephrology*, vol. 26, no. 3, pp. 515–523, 2014.

[17] W. Chen and M. K. Abramowitz, "Treatment of metabolic acidosis in patients with CKD," *The American Journal of Kidney Diseases*, vol. 63, no. 2, pp. 311–317, 2014.

[18] I. de-Brito Ashurst, E. O'Lone, T. Kaushik, K. McCafferty, and M. M. Yaqoob, "Acidosis: progression of chronic kidney disease and quality of life," *Pediatric Nephrology*, vol. 30, no. 6, pp. 873–879, 2014.

[19] M. Abbate, C. Zoia, D. Rottoli et al., "Antiproteinuric therapy while preventing the abnormal protein traffic in proximal tubule abrogates protein- and complement-dependent interstitial inflammation in experimental renal disease," *Journal of the American Society of Nephrology*, vol. 10, no. 4, pp. 804–813, 1999.

[20] S. Buelli, M. Abbate, M. Morigi et al., "Protein load impairs factor H binding promoting complement-dependent dysfunction of proximal tubular cells," *Kidney International*, vol. 75, no. 10, pp. 1050–1059, 2009.

[21] W. G. Couser and M. Nangaku, "Mechanism of bicarbonate effect in CKD," *Kidney International*, vol. 78, article 817, 2010.

[22] M. Nangaku, J. Pippin, and W. G. Couser, "Complement membrane attack complex (C5b-9) mediates interstitial disease in experimental nephrotic syndrome," *Journal of the American Society of Nephrology*, vol. 10, no. 11, pp. 2323–2331, 1999.

[23] M. Nangaku, J. Pippin, and W. G. Couser, "C6 mediates chronic progression of tubulointerstitial damage in rats with remnant kidneys," *Journal of the American Society of Nephrology*, vol. 13, no. 4, pp. 928–936, 2002.

[24] P. W. Peake, B. A. Pussell, B. Mackinnon, and J. A. Charlesworth, "The effect of pH and nucleophiles on complement activation by human proximal tubular epithelial cells," *Nephrology Dialysis Transplantation*, vol. 17, no. 5, pp. 745–752, 2002.

[25] Y. Morita, H. Ikeguchi, J. Nakamura, N. Hotta, Y. Yuzawa, and S. Matsuo, "Complement activation products in the urine from proteinuric patients," *Journal of the American Society of Nephrology*, vol. 11, no. 4, pp. 700–707, 2000.

[26] C. Ponticelli, P. Altieri, F. Scolari et al., "A randomized study comparing methylprednisolone plus chlorambucil versus methylprednisolone plus cyclophosphamide in idiopathic membranous nephropathy," *Journal of the American Society of Nephrology*, vol. 9, no. 3, pp. 444–450, 1998.

[27] G. D'Amico, F. Ferrario, G. Colasanti, A. Ragni, and M. B. Bosisio, "IgA-mesangial nephropathy (Berger's disease) with rapid decline in renal function," *Clinical Nephrology*, vol. 16, no. 5, pp. 251–257, 1981.

[28] A. S. Levey, L. A. Stevens, C. H. Schmid et al., "A new equation to estimate glomerular filtration rate," *Annals of Internal Medicine*, vol. 150, no. 9, pp. 604–612, 2009.

[29] C. Bazzi, C. Petrini, V. Rizza et al., "Urinary N-acetyl-β-glucosaminidase excretion is a marker of tubular cell dysfunction and a predictor of outcome in primary glomerulonephritis," *Nephrology Dialysis Transplantation*, vol. 17, no. 11, pp. 1890–1896, 2002.

[30] C. Bazzi, V. Rizza, G. Olivieri, D. Casellato, and G. D'Amico, "Tubular reabsorption of high, middle and low molecular weight proteins according to the tubulo-interstitial damage marker N-acetyl-β-d-glucosaminidase in glomerulonephritis," *Journal of Nephrology*, 2014.

[31] T. J. Ellam and M. El Nahas, "Proteinuria thresholds are irrational: a call for proteinuria indexing," *Nephron—Clinical Practice*, vol. 118, no. 3, pp. c217–c224, 2011.

4

Associates of Cardiopulmonary Arrest in the Perihemodialytic Period

Jennifer E. Flythe,[1,2] Nien-Chen Li,[3] Shu-Fang Lin,[3] Steven M. Brunelli,[1,4] Jeffrey Hymes,[3] and Eduardo Lacson Jr.[3]

[1] Department of Medicine, Renal Division, Brigham and Women's Hospital, Boston, MA, USA
[2] Department of Medicine, Division of Nephrology and Hypertension, University of North Carolina Kidney Center, UNC School of Medicine, 7024 Burnett-Womack CB No. 7155, Chapel Hill, NC 27599-7155, USA
[3] Fresenius Medical Care North America, Waltham, MA, USA
[4] DaVita Clinical Research, Minneapolis, MN, USA

Correspondence should be addressed to Jennifer E. Flythe; jflythe@med.unc.edu

Academic Editor: David B. Kershaw

Cardiopulmonary arrest during and proximate to hemodialysis is rare but highly fatal. Studies have examined peridialytic sudden cardiac event risk factors, but no study has considered associates of cardiopulmonary arrests (fatal and nonfatal events including cardiac and respiratory causes). This study was designed to elucidate patient and procedural factors associated with peridialytic cardiopulmonary arrest. Data for this case-control study were taken from the hemodialysis population at Fresenius Medical Care, North America. 924 in-center cardiopulmonary events (cases) and 75,538 controls were identified. Cases and controls were 1:5 matched on age, sex, race, and diabetes. Predictors of cardiopulmonary arrest were considered for logistic model inclusion. Missed treatments due to hospitalization, lower body mass, coronary artery disease, heart failure, lower albumin and hemoglobin, lower dialysate potassium, higher serum calcium, greater erythropoietin stimulating agent dose, and normalized protein catabolic rate (J-shaped) were associated with peridialytic cardiopulmonary arrest. Of these, lower albumin, hemoglobin, and body mass index; higher erythropoietin stimulating agent dose; and greater missed sessions had the strongest associations with outcome. Patient health markers and procedural factors are associated with peridialytic cardiopulmonary arrest. In addition to optimizing nutritional status, it may be prudent to limit exposure to low dialysate potassium (<2 K bath) and to use the lowest effective erythropoietin stimulating agent dose.

1. Introduction

Hemodialysis (HD) patients experience high rates of cardiovascular morbidity and mortality [1]. Cardiac arrest rates among HD patients exceed those of the general population by 30-fold [1–3]. While the vast majority of such arrests occur in unmonitored settings, arrests during and immediately surrounding the HD procedure (i.e., peridialytic) occur in outpatient HD facilities at a rate of ~7 per 100,000 HD sessions [4]. Postperidialytic arrest outcomes are dismal with 1-year survival rates of 9–15% [1, 5]. Prior analyses have identified low dialysate potassium [4, 6] and calcium [7], extremes of serum potassium [7], and traditional risk factors such as diabetes and underlying burden of cardiovascular disease [4] as risk factors for sudden cardiac arrest (SCA) and sudden cardiac death (SCD) among dialysis patients. Risk factors for a broader class of peridialytic events that include respiratory arrest, nonfatal sudden cardiac events, and cardiopulmonary arrest (CPA) are not well-described. While such events, including extreme hypotension, pulmonary embolus, cerebrovascular disorders, seizures, and respiratory arrests (among others), have lower mortality rates than do SCA events, they are nonetheless significant sources of patient morbidity and stress to ambulatory HD facility staff and patients.

We undertook this study to elucidate patient and HD procedural characteristics that associate with CPA. To capture a wide range of peridialytic events, we defined CPA as the absence of a pulse and/or cessation of spontaneous breathing while in the outpatient dialysis facility. Using data from a large, nationally representative 2010 prevalent, in-center patient cohort, we employed a case-control study design in which we matched patients with in-center CPA (cases) to patients without in-center CPA (controls) on the basis of age, gender, race, and diabetes status. To isolate CPA-associated characteristics from perideath-associated characteristics, we performed additional analyses matching CPA cases to non-CPA controls who survived the study year and, separately, to non-CPA controls who died during the study year.

2. Materials and Methods

2.1. Study Design and Study Population. We utilized a case-control study design to elucidate patient and procedural risk factors for peridialytic CPA in the ambulatory setting. CPA was defined as absence of apical or carotid pulse (by corollary, blood pressure) and/or cessation of breathing while on HD or immediately before/after the treatment while in the outpatient dialysis facility, as determined by HD center nursing staff at the time of the event. Routine verification of CPA cases demonstrated >99% concordance between the initial CPA attribution and subsequent adjudication based on medical record review by quality reviewers. In-center HD patients from the 2010 prevalent population of Fresenius Medical Care, North America (FMCNA), were eligible for cohort inclusion. CPA cases were identified from the electronic medical record by screening for HD-associated adverse events. Exclusion criteria were age <18 years, traveling or transient patients, and patients with acute kidney injury. A total of 937 patients with CPA (cases) and 76,202 patients without CPA (eligible controls) were identified from 653 FMCNA facilities where at least one CPA event occurred.

2.2. Data Collection. All study data were obtained from the FMCNA Knowledge Center data warehouse and were collected according to standard clinical protocols [8]. To standardize data reporting across cases and controls, an index date for each control was designated as the date of CPA in the matched case. Demographic data including age, sex, and race were determined as of January 1, 2010. Body mass index and comorbidity status including diabetes, coronary artery disease (CAD), and heart failure were determined as of the CPA event date in cases and at the corresponding index date in matched controls. The following dialytic session data were considered for the 30-day period immediately preceding, but not including, the index date: vascular access type, mean treatment time, mean interdialytic weight gain (IDWG), mean pre-HD heart rate, total number delivered treatments, and total number missed treatments. Biochemical data, erythropoietin stimulating agent (ESA) dose, and estimated dry weight were considered as the last value in the 30 days preceding index date. Dialysate composition was determined from the active physician order on the index date and was categorized based on typical clinical thresholds. Date of death and attributed cause of death were recorded by HD unit staff.

2.3. Statistical Analyses. Baseline subject characteristics were described across cases and controls as counts and proportions for categorical variables and as means and standard deviations for continuous variables. Two-group comparisons were made using Student's t-test of means or contingency table χ^2 test of proportions.

For the primary analysis, each CPA case was randomly matched (without replacement) with up to 5 non-CPA controls on the basis of age (± 3 years), sex, race (white/black/other), and diabetes status. Matching on factors strongly associated with mortality and/or sudden cardiac events was performed to minimize confounding from these previously established, nonmodifiable risk factors. Matching criteria data were available for 924 out of 937 (98.6%) cases and 75,538 out of 76,202 (99.1%) controls. Each of the 924 cases matched to 5 controls with the exception of 2 cases that matched to 4 controls and 1 case that matched to only 1 control; the primary cohort consisted of 4,614 controls (Figure 1).

Candidate CPA predictors were identified based on literature precedent [4, 6, 7, 9–11] and clinical relevance. Univariate logistic regression models (model 1) were used to identify potential CPA risk factors by estimating the CPA odds ratio (OR) for each of the prespecified variables. To identify variables that are independently associated with CPA, 3 additional multivariate logistic models were considered: model 2: multivariate model with inclusion of all covariates; model 3: multivariate model derived through stepwise regression with 0.05 as inclusion and elimination thresholds for significance; and model 4: from model 3 with the addition of quadratic terms for biochemical data to account for nonlinear associations. Model goodness-of-fit was evaluated with Hosmer-Lemeshow testing. The model c-statistic was used to estimate the model predictive capacity of each model. The relative contribution of each model covariate to CPA prediction was ranked according to the magnitude of the respective chi-square value in the final model.

In secondary analyses, two pools of non-CPA matching controls were identified. Control-1s were defined as non-CPA patients who survived 2010, and control-2s were defined as non-CPA patients who died in 2010. Among the 75,538 eligible controls with adequate matching data, 65,484 (86.7%) met criteria for the control-1 pool, and 10,054 (13.3%) met criteria for the control-2 pool. Twenty-five out of 924 cases were unable to be matched to control-2s on the basis of age (± 3 years), sex, race (white/black/other), and diabetes status; 899 cases were included in the secondary analysis. Each of the 899 cases was then similarly matched (random without replacement) to 2 patients from control-1, resulting in 1,798 control-1s for analysis. 879 cases matched with 2 control-2s. The remaining 20 cases matched with only 1 control-2 patient. Thus, a total of 1,778 control-2s were available for analysis (Figure 2). Among the control-1 patients, 169 were in the primary analysis control group while 282 control-2 patients were in the primary analysis control group. CPA cases were then compared to each of control-1s and to control-2s via logistic models constructed similar to the primary analysis.

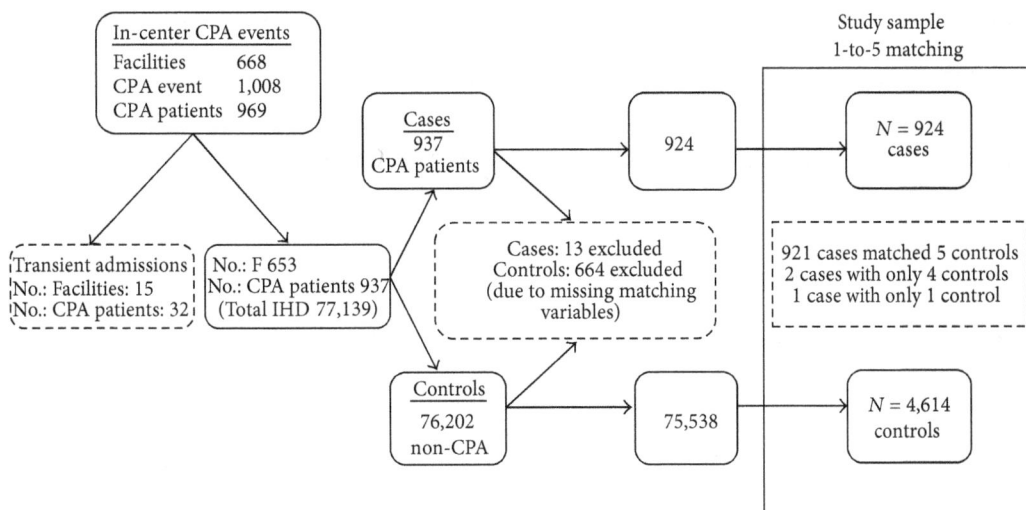

FIGURE 1: Random case-control matching without replacement for primary analysis. CPA, cardiopulmonary arrest; IHD, in-center hemodialysis.

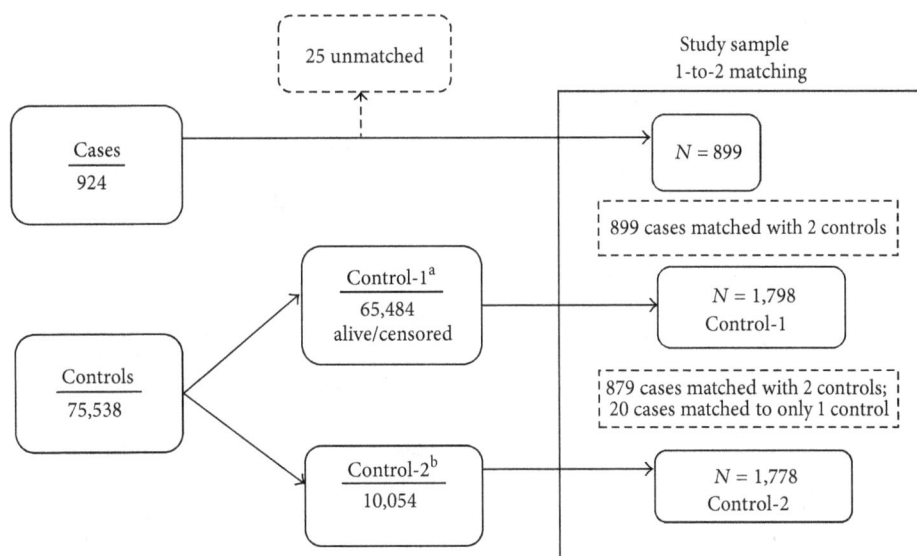

FIGURE 2: Random case-control matching without replacement for secondary analyses. [a] Control-1 included those patients without peridialytic cardiopulmonary arrest who survived 2010. [b] Control-2 included those patients without peridialytic cardiopulmonary arrest who died in 2010.

Effect modification of the associations between CPA and individual prespecified covariates was explored through subgroup analyses. Sensitivity analyses with dialysate bicarbonate alone (versus total buffer) and comparative use of continuous versus categorical variables were performed.

With a large number of CPA events, our study is adequately powered to detect associations between the candidate associate factors and CPA. Assuming a baseline probability of CPA risk of 0.1, we have 90% power ($\alpha = 0.05$) to detect an odds ratio of 1.16 across dichotomized independent variables. All analyses were implemented using SAS v9.3 (http://www.sas.com/).

3. Results

3.1. Baseline Characteristics. Table 1 displays the characteristics of the primary cohort cases and matched controls. For cases, the mean age was 65.7 years; 50.1% were male; 60.2% were white; 34.6% were black; 5.2% were of other racial ancestry; 71.5% were diabetic. Cases and matched controls were well balanced on these matching factors. Overall, the CPA and matched non-CPA controls were similar in terms of estimated dry weight, absolute IDWG, delivered treatment time, dialysate composition (sodium, potassium, calcium, and dialysate buffer concentrations), and the number of

TABLE 1: Characteristics of the primary study cohort across cases and matched controls[a].

Variable	CPA patients (cases) $n = 924$	Non-CPA patients (controls) $n = 4,614$
Matching factors		
Age (years)		
Mean ± SD	65.7 ± 13.2	65.7 ± 13.1
Median [IQR]	66.3 [58.2, 75.5]	66.1 [58.0, 75.3]
(Min, max)	(24.7, 96.2)	(23.3, 95.5)
Male	463 (50.1%)	2309 (50.0%)
Race		
White	556 (60.2%)	2780 (60.3%)
Black	320 (34.6%)	1595 (34.6%)
Other	48 (5.2%)	239 (5.2%)
Diabetes	661 (71.5)	3304 (71.6%)
Other variables		
Weight (kg)	77.5 ± 23.1	79.0 ± 22.0
Body mass index (kg/m^2)		
<18.5	51 (5.8%)	141 (3.1%)
18.6–25	228 (25.9%)	1301 (28.9%)
25.1–29.9	318 (36.1%)	1750 (38.9%)
≥30	284 (32.2%)	1306 (29.0%)
Coronary artery disease	271 (29.3%)	1136 (24.6%)**
Heart failure	326 (35.3%)	1403 (30.4%)**
Vintage[b] (days)	1,088 ± 1,114	1,208 ± 1,205**
<120 days	207 (22.4%)	483 (10.5%)
20 days–<1 year	117 (12.7%)	715 (15.5%)
1 year–<3 years	215 (23.3%)	1440 (31.2%)
3 years–<5 years	165 (17.9%)	862 (18.7%)
5 years or more	193 (20.9%)	1029 (22.3%)
Missing	27 (2.9%)	85 (1.8%)
Access type[c]		
Catheter	416 (46.2%)	1560 (34.8%)****
Fistula	319 (35.4%)	2010 (44.8%)
Graft	166 (18.4%)	919 (20.5%)
IDWG (kg)	3.0 ± 8.7	2.6 ± 4.9
Percent IDWG (%)	4.2 ± 10.5	3.5 ± 5.1**
Patients discharged from hospital within 30 days prior to CPA	54 (5.8%)	182 (3.9%)**
Treatment time[d] (minutes)		
Prescribed time	226 ± 34	223 ± 37*
Delivered time	218 ± 46	219 ± 44
Patients with treatment time shortened > 10 minutes	179 (20.2%)	724 (16.1%)**
Dialysate sodium (mEq/L)	137.8 ± 2.5	137.8 ± 2.5
	$n = 745$	$n = 3,774$
Dialysate calcium (mEq/L)		
<2.3	214 (28.7%)	1057 (28.0%)
2.3–2.5	513 (68.9%)	2566 (68.0%)
>2.5	18 (2.4%)	151 (4.0%)
	$n = 745$	$n = 3,774$

TABLE 1: Continued.

Variable	CPA patients (cases) $n = 924$	Non-CPA patients (controls) $n = 4,614$
Dialysate potassium (mEq/L)		
1	31 (4.2%)	126 (3.3%)
2	564 (75.7%)	2883 (76.4%)
>2	150 (20.1%)	765 (20.3%)
	$n = 745$	$n = 3,774$
Dialysate buffer[e] (mEq/L)		
<41	92 (12.4%)	455 (12.1%)
41–45	602 (80.8%)	2999 (79.5%)
>45	51 (6.9%)	320 (8.5%)
	$n = 745$	$n = 3,774$
Dialysate bicarbonate (mEq/L)	36.5 ± 1.9	36.4 ± 2.3
	$n = 745$	$n = 3,774$
Dialysate acetate (mEq/L)	6.5 ± 2.0	6.6 ± 2.0
	$n = 745$	$n = 3,774$
ESA dose per treatment (units)	11,233 ± 8,656	8,562 ± 7,994****
Number of treatments	10.0 ± 3.6	11.4 ± 2.7****
Number of missed treatments	1.47 ± 2.78	0.87 ± 2.08****
Number of missed treatments due to hospitalization	1.21 ± 2.69	0.63 ± 1.91****
Number of missed treatments due to unexcused absence	0.26 ± 0.87	0.24 ± 0.84
eKt/V	1.45 ± 0.45	1.49 ± 0.40**
Albumin (g/dL)	3.5 ± 0.5	3.7 ± 0.5****
Hemoglobin (g/dL)	10.8 ± 1.5	11.4 ± 1.3****
Phosphorus (mg/dL)	5.0 ± 1.7	5.2 ± 1.7***
Calcium (mg/dL)	8.9 ± 0.8	9.0 ± 0.8***
Potassium (mEq/L)	4.6 ± 0.8	4.7 ± 0.7****
Ferritin (ng/mL)	662 ± 531	676 ± 611
Bicarbonate (mEq/L)	24.1 ± 3.8	23.8 ± 3.5*
Creatinine (mg/dL)	6.5 ± 2.6	7.3 ± 2.8****
nPCR (g/kg/day)	0.86 ± 0.31	0.93 ± 0.29****

[a]*$P < 0.05$; **$P < 0.01$; ***$P < 0.001$; ****$P < 0.0001$; based on two-sample Student's t-testing or chi-square testing as dictated by data type. Values reported as means ± SD or n (%) as dictated by data type.
[b]Vintage defined as number of days from the date of first ever dialysis to the date of event (CPA). For controls, event date was assigned the same index date from the matched CPA case.
[c]Catheter compared to fistula/graft.
[d]Mean treatment time in the 30 days prior to CPA (excludes CPA treatment).
[e]Dialysate buffer = dialysate bicarbonate + dialysate acetate.

missed treatments due to unexcused absences. Compared to controls, CPA cases had shorter dialytic vintage; were more likely to dialyze via catheter; had more CAD and heart failure; had higher % IDWG; and received higher doses of ESA. CPA cases were also more likely to have lower serum albumin, hemoglobin, phosphorus, calcium, potassium, creatinine, normalized protein catabolic rate (nPCR), and eKt/V than controls. Controls were more likely to have lower serum bicarbonate. CPA cases were more likely to have been discharged from the hospital within 30 days prior to the CPA event.

3.2. Primary Analyses. Table 2 displays the CPA model-building results. On univariate analysis (Model 1), CAD, heart failure, catheter access, lower body mass index, larger % IDWG, treatment time shortened by >10 minutes, missed treatments due to hospitalization, greater ESA dose, and higher serum bicarbonate were associated with increased odds of CPA. Longer vintage, higher dialysate calcium, eKt/V, albumin, hemoglobin, phosphorus, serum calcium, serum potassium, and nPCR were associated with decreased odds of CPA. After adjustment for confounders and accounting for nonlinear associations (Model 4), CAD, heart failure, missed HD treatments due to hospitalization, lower dialysate potassium, lower albumin, lower body mass index, lower hemoglobin, higher serum calcium, greater ESA dosing, and both low and high nPCR (J-shaped risk curve; quadratic) were associated with higher CPA odds. Hemoglobin, albumin, body mass index, ESA dosing, and missed treatment sessions due to hospitalization had the greatest predictive influence based on relative chi-square values (Figure 3). Dialysate sodium, calcium, and total buffer were not significantly associated with CPA. Considering dialysate bicarbonate in lieu of total buffer did not result in a significant association with CPA.

The data suggested effect modification of the CPA-serum calcium association on the basis of albumin. At lower albumin levels, higher serum calcium was associated with CPA; however, at higher albumin levels, higher serum calcium was not associated with CPA (data not shown). No effect modification between albumin and other model variables was detected. There was no effect modification of the CPA-serum calcium association by dialysate calcium and no effect modification of the CPA-dialysate potassium association by serum potassium (data not shown).

Timing of death with respect to the CPA event (index) date was compared across cases and controls (Table 3). A total of 299 (32.4%) of CPA cases died on the date of the CPA event compared to 9 (0.2%) of the controls; 548 (59.3%) cases died within one year of CPA compared to 1,333 (28.9%) of controls.

3.3. Secondary Analyses. To mitigate confounding by ambient health status, we matched CPA cases to non-CPA patients who survived 2010 (control-1) and, separately, to non-CPA patients who died in 2010 (control-2). Overall, control-2s were more similar to cases than control-1s (Table 4). Specifically, cases and control-2s were similar in terms of weight, CAD, heart failure, treatment time, shortening of treatment time, ESA dosing, number of missed treatments, eKt/V, albumin, phosphorus, calcium, bicarbonate, and nPCR. Control-1s had greater body weights, less CAD, heart failure, catheter use (compared to graft/fistula), missed treatments, and greater eKt/V, albumin, hemoglobin, phosphorus, calcium, potassium, creatinine, and nPCR compared to CPA cases.

Comparing cases to control-1s in the final model (model 4), lower body mass index, CAD, heart failure, longer vintage, catheter access, more missed treatments due to hospitalization, lower dialysate potassium, higher ESA dosing, and $nPCR^2$ (quadratic) were associated with increased CPA odds; and higher BMI, albumin, hemoglobin, and nPCR were associated with decreased CPA odds (Table 5). Comparing cases to control-2s in the final model (model 4), higher serum calcium was associated with increased CPA odds, and higher hemoglobin, serum potassium, and ferritin were associated with decreased CPA odds (Table 5). Albumin, missed treatments due to hospitalization, ESA dose, hemoglobin, and nPCR had the greatest predictive influence on CPA based on relative chi-square values when comparing cases to control-1s; and serum potassium and hemoglobin had the greatest influence on CPA comparing cases to control-2s (see Supplementary Figures 1(A) and 1(B) in Supplementary Material available online at http://dx.doi.org/10.1155/2014/961978). Consistent with the primary analyses, dialysate total buffer and its bicarbonate component (separately) were not associated with CPA in either control-1 or control-2 secondary analyses.

4. Discussion

Peridialytic CPA is a rare event with a high subsequent fatality rate. In this case-control study inclusive of both cardiac and respiratory events, we demonstrated that comorbidities (CAD and heart failure), health status surrogates (lower body mass index, lower albumin, lower nPCR, lower hemoglobin, and recent hospitalizations), and procedural factors (lower dialysate potassium and higher ESA dosing) were associated with peridialytic CPA. The data suggest that lower hemoglobin, lower albumin, lower body mass index, higher ESA dosing, and greater preevent missed treatment sessions due to hospitalization most strongly associate with ambulatory HD facility CPA.

Multiple studies [4, 6, 10–16] have examined peridialytic SCA and SCD risk factors, but event definition inconsistencies have limited firm conclusions. In the cardiology literature, SCD is defined as the "unexpected natural death from a cardiac cause within a short time period, generally ≤1 hour from the onset of symptoms" [17]. Applying this definition to the general population, SCD occurs at a rate of 1 per 1,000 patient years [18]. The USRDS reports a SCD rate of 59 deaths per 1,000 HD patient years but defines SCD as death from arrhythmia or cardiac arrest of unknown cause [1]. In fact, 51.1 of the 59 deaths per 1,000 years are reported as "cardiac arrest cause unknown," suggesting that the SCD estimate may be inflated in the USRDS data [1, 18]. SCD risk factor investigations have relied on different outcome definitions as exemplified by Genovesi et al.'s definition of sudden death as an unexpected natural death within 1 hour of the onset of symptoms [10] versus Parekh et al.'s definition of SCD as an out-of-hospital death with an underlying cardiac cause [13]. The SCA literature suffers from similar definition discrepancies [4, 6, 10, 16]. Differing outcome specification prevents meta-analysis and renders the study

TABLE 2: Logistic models of peridialytic cardiopulmonary arrest predictors in the matched primary analysis.

	Model 1 (univariate) OR (95% CI)	Model 2 (full multivariate) OR (95% CI)	Model 3 (stepwise) OR (95% CI)	Model 4 (Model 3 + quadratics) OR (95% CI)
Body mass index (kg/m^2)				
<18.5	1.66* (1.05–2.65)	1.95* (1.10–3.44)	2.03*** (1.37–3.00)	1.95*** (1.32–2.89)
18.6–25	1 (ref.)	1 (ref.)	—	—
25.1–29.9	0.81 (0.62–1.04)	0.85 (0.61–1.19)	—	—
≥30	0.84 (0.66–1.06)	0.80 (0.52–1.23)	—	—
Coronary artery disease	1.27** (1.09–1.49)	1.41*** (1.15–1.72)	1.39*** (1.14–1.70)	1.38** (1.13–1.68)
Heart failure	1.25** (1.08–1.45)	1.24* (1.02–1.51)	1.24* (1.03–1.51)	1.27* (1.05–1.54)
Vintage (per 100 days)	0.99* (0.98–1.00)	1.00 (0.99–1.01)	—	—
Catheter vascular access	1.61**** (1.39–1.86)	1.00 (0.82–1.22)	—	—
EDW (kg)	1.00 (0.99–1.00)	1.00 (1.00–1.01)	—	—
Percent IDWG (%)	1.01** (1.004–1.02)	1.00 (0.96–1.04)	—	—
TT shortened > 10 minutes (yes/no)	1.32** (1.10–1.58)	1.14 (0.89–1.45)	—	—
Missed treatment due to hospitalization (yes/no)	1.94**** (1.65–2.28)	1.48*** (1.20–1.84)	1.48*** (1.20–1.82)	1.45*** (1.18–1.80)
Missed treatment due to unexcused absence (yes/no)	1.05 (0.85–1.28)	1.01 (0.77–1.33)	—	—
Dialysate sodium (mEq/L)	0.99 (0.96–1.02)	1.01 (0.97–1.04)	—	—
Dialysate calcium (mEq/L)				
<2.3	1.01 (0.82–1.25)	1.07 (0.83–1.37)	—	—
2.3–2.5	1.00 (ref.)	1.00 (ref.)	—	—
>2.5	0.60 (0.33–1.10)	0.64 (0.32–1.30)	—	—
Dialysate potassium (mEq/L)				
1	1.26 (0.77–2.06)	1.72* (0.99–2.99)	1.73** (1.12–2.68)	1.89** (1.23–2.90)
2	1.00 (ref.)	1.00 (ref.)	—	—
>2	1.00 (0.79–1.28)	0.83 (0.61–1.12)	—	—
Dialysate buffer (mEq/L)			—	—
<41	1.01 (0.75–1.35)	0.95 (0.67–1.34)	—	—
41–45	1.00 (ref.)	1.00 (ref.)	—	—
>45	0.79 (0.55–1.16)	0.77 (0.49–1.19)	—	—
ESA per treatment (per 1000 u)	1.04**** (1.03–1.05)	1.01* (1.00–1.02)	1.01* (1.00–1.03)	1.01* (1.00–1.02)
eKt/V	0.73** (0.59–0.91)	0.93 (0.72–1.22)	—	—
Albumin (g/dL)	0.43**** (0.38–0.50)	0.65*** (0.51–0.81)	0.65**** (0.53–0.81)	0.68*** (0.55–0.85)
Hemoglobin (g/dL)	0.73**** (0.69–0.77)	0.81**** (0.76–0.88)	0.82**** (0.76–0.88)	0.81**** (0.75–0.87)
Phosphorus (mg/dL)	0.93*** (0.89–0.97)	1.01 (0.95–1.07)	—	—
Calcium (mg/dL)	0.84*** (0.77–0.92)	1.17* (1.02–1.33)	1.16* (1.02–1.32)	1.17* (1.04–1.33)
Potassium (mEq/L)	0.78**** (0.71–0.86)	0.85* (0.74–0.98)	—	—
Ferritin (per 100 ng/mL)	1.00 (0.98–1.01)	0.99 (0.97–1.01)	—	—
Bicarbonate (mEq/L)	1.03* (1.01–1.05)	0.99 (0.96–1.01)	—	—
nPCR (g/kg/day)	0.45**** (0.34–0.60)	0.69 (0.47–1.00)	0.62** (0.45–0.88)	0.53*** (0.38–0.75)
nPCR^2 (g/kg/day)	—	—	—	1.99** (1.24–3.20)
c-statistic	—	0.68	0.67	0.68

*$P < 0.05$; **$P < 0.01$; ***$P < 0.001$; ****$P < 0.0001$.
For independent variables with more than 2 categories, P values and confidence intervals were adjusted with multiple comparisons using Bonferroni method. OR, odds ratio; CI, confidence interval; IDWG, interdialytic weight gain; TT, treatment time; nPCR, normalized protein catabolic rate; ESA, erythropoietin stimulating agent; and EDW, estimated dry weight.

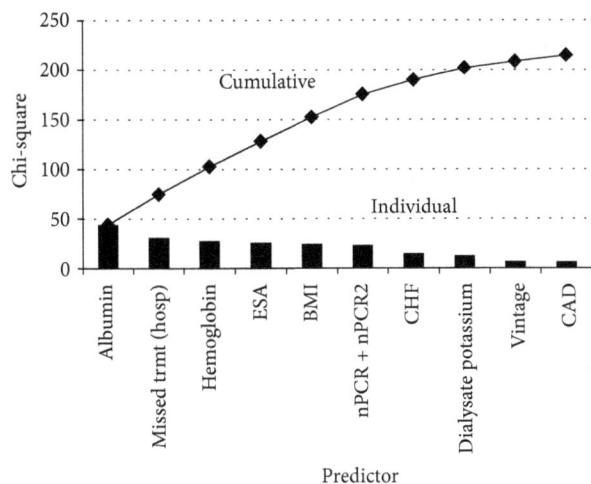

FIGURE 3: Relative contributions of predictors of peridialytic cardiopulmonary arrest in the primary analysis[a]. [a]Based on model 4 chi-square values. nPCR, normalized protein catabolic rate; CAD, coronary artery disease; and ESA, erythropoietin stimulating agent. Note: missed treatment was due to hospitalization.

TABLE 3: Death following peridialytic cardiopulmonary arrest events across cases and controls.

	CPA patients N (%)	Controls[a] N (%)
Death on date of CPA	299 (32.4)	9 (0.2)[****]
Death within 1–30 days following CPA	155 (16.8)	144 (3.1)[****]
Death between 31 and 365 days from CPA	94 (10.2)	1,180 (25.6)[****]
Total deaths at 1 year	548 (59.3)	1,333 (28.9)[****]
Total surviving at 1 year or censored by reasons other than death	376 (40.7)	3,281 (71.1)[****]
Total	924	4,614

[a]For control patients, the reference date is the CPA date for the matched CPA case.
[****]$P < 0.0001$.

of an already rare event even more challenging. In this analysis, we examined associates of CPA, defined as the absence of a pulse or cessation of breathing during HD or immediately preceding or following the HD procedure while the patient is in the dialysis facility. This definition allowed us to investigate a broad class of events associated with not only morbidity and mortality but also significant emotional stress to dialysis facility staff and fellow patients. Better understanding of CPA associates as examined in our study may not only improve patient outcomes but also improve the patient facility experience.

Regardless of the outcome investigated, the peridialytic period is incontrovertibly a high risk period. Interdialytic volume and metabolite accumulation followed by obligate intradialytic electrolyte and fluid shifts may promote a proarrhythmic environment. Numerous studies have demonstrated increased arrhythmias in the peridialytic period [19–22] and

have linked serum and dialysate electrolyte profiles to QT interval abnormalities [23–28]. Conduction abnormalities may be induced by gradient driven electrolyte shifts, transient episodes of hypokalemia and/or hypocalcemia, and/or HD procedure-related myocardial ischemia. Our findings of an association between CPA and lower dialysate potassium support those of other studies [4, 6, 11, 12] and suggest that electrolyte-mediated conduction abnormalities may play important roles in peridialytic CPA.

We hypothesized that other dialysate/serum components such as calcium and bicarbonate might associate with CPA. Consistent with Pun et al., we found an association between higher serum calcium and CPA; however, we found no CPA association with dialysate calcium or the serum-dialysate calcium gradient as did Pun et al. [7]. Such discrepancy may have resulted from our outcome of CPA (versus SCD in Pun et al.'s analysis) [7]. Serum and dialysate bicarbonate levels are also plausible SCD associates as higher dialysate bicarbonate has been linked to increased mortality [29] and SCA [6]. Alkalosis-driven electrolyte shifts could underlie this association; however, we found no association between CPA and serum bicarbonate or dialysate total buffer (bicarbonate + acetate), particularly with adjusted models that included nutritional markers. Furthermore, sensitivity analyses examining dialysate total buffer and dialysate bicarbonate in the models (separately) demonstrated no association between either and CPA risk.

Markers of poor health and chronic inflammation including lower body mass index, lower albumin, lower nPCR, greater ESA dosing, lower hemoglobin, and greater missed treatment due to hospitalizations also associated with CPA in our cohort. These findings should not be surprising given the association of malnutrition and inflammation with poor outcomes among HD patients [30–34] and their association with atherosclerotic cardiovascular disease [35–37]. It is not known if greater inflammation and malnutrition trigger atherosclerosis progression or if they reflect underlying cardiovascular disease burden. Similarly, our finding of an association between CPA risk and lower hemoglobin and higher ESA dosing may stem from ESA resistance related to underlying inflammation, nutrient deficiencies, malignancy, or other systemic illness [38]; all such conditions portend poor outcomes.

To address confounding by ambient health status, we performed secondary analyses in which we matched CPA cases with non-CPA controls who survived 2010 (control-1s) and, separately, with non-CPA controls who died in 2010 (control-2s). Not surprisingly, control-2s were more similar to cases than were control-1s. Comparing CPA cases to patients who died in 2010, we demonstrated that lower hemoglobin, higher serum calcium, lower serum potassium, and lower ferritin are associated with increased odds of peridialytic CPA. These findings suggest that these characteristics play roles beyond that of health status surrogates in their CPA associations.

It must be emphasized that ambulatory HD facility CPA occurrence is dwarfed by community CPA events. Therefore, our study should not detract from the importance of global CPA prevention. However, targeting in-facility CPA represents a unique prevention opportunity given

TABLE 4: Characteristics of the secondary study cohort across cases and matched control-1s and control-2s[a].

Variable	Patients with CPA in 2010 (cases) N = 899	Patients without CPA who survived 2010 (control-1s) N = 1,798	died in 2010 (controls-2s) N = 1,778
Matching factors			
Age (years)			
Mean ± SD	66.1 ± 12.7	66.0 ± 12.5	66.2 ± 12.5
Median [IQR]	66.4 [58.5, 75.5]	66.2 [58.5, 75.4]	66.4 [58.5, 75.5]
(Min, max)	(27.4, 96.2)	(24.5, 94.1)	(24.5, 94.6)
Male	456 (50.7%)	912 (50.7%)	901 (50.7%)
Race			
White	550 (61.2%)	1100 (61.2%)	1095 (61.6%)
Black	306 (34.0%)	612 (34.0%)	602 (33.9%)
Other	43 (4.8%)	86 (4.8%)	81 (4.6%)
Diabetes	649 (72.2%)	1298 (72.2%)	1284 (72.2%)
Other variables			
Weight (kg)	78.8 ± 23.0	81.2 ± 22.4[***]	76.8 ± 23.0
Body mass index (kg/m^2)			
<18.5	47 (5.4%)	32 (1.8%)[****]	95 (5.5%)
18.6–25	240 (27.4%)	554 (31.4%)	461 (26.6%)
25.1–29.9	315 (36%)	763 (43.2%)	607 (35.0%)
≥30	273 (31.2%)	416 (23.6%)	570 (32.9%)
Coronary artery disease	268 (29.8%)	422 (23.5%)[***]	495 (27.8%)
Heart failure	317 (35.3%)	464 (25.8%)[****]	623 (35.0%)
Vintage[b] (days)	1097 ± 1121	1136 ± 1136	1249 ± 1299[**]
Access type[c]			
Catheter	404 (46.1%)	513 (29.5%)[****]	40.7%[*]
Fistula	312 (35.6%)	872 (50.1%)	39.00%
Graft	161 (18.4%)	356 (20.5%)	20.30%
IDWG (kg)	2.5 ± 1.3	2.5 ± 1.1	2.5 ± 1.3
Percent IDWG (%)	3.2 ± 1.6	3.2 ± 1.3	3.3 ± 1.6[*]
Patients discharged from hospital within 30 days prior to CPA	54 (6.0%)	47 (2.6%)[****]	115 (6.5%)
Treatment time[d] (minutes)			
Prescribed time	226 ± 34	222 ± 37[**]	224 ± 38
Delivered time	218 ± 44	219 ± 43	217 ± 44
Time shortened	12 ± 32	7 ± 24[****]	11 ± 30
Patients with treatment time shortened > 10 minutes	174 (20.2%)	242 (13.8%)[****]	338 (19.6%)
Dialysate sodium (mEq/L)	137.8 ± 2.5	137.8 ± 2.2	137.9 ± 2.9
	n = 725	n = 1,477	n = 1,480
Dialysate calcium (mEq/L)			
<2.3	206 (28.4%)	408 (27.6%)	396 (26.8%)
2.3–2.5	501 (69.1%)	1022 (69.2%)	1015 (68.6%)
>2.5	18 (2.5%)	47 (3.2%)	69 (4.7%)
	n = 725	n = 1,477	n = 1,480
Dialysate potassium (mEq/L)			
1	29 (4.0%)	38 (2.6%)	49 (3.3%)
2	550 (75.9%)	1148 (77.7%)	1103 (74.5%)
>2	146 (20.1%)	291 (19.7%)	328 (22.2%)
	n = 725	n = 1,477	n = 1,480
Dialysate buffer[e] (mEq/L)			
<41	88 (12.1%)	174 (11.8%)	198 (13.4%)
41–45	587 (81.0%)	1204 (81.5%)	1174 (79.3%)

TABLE 4: Continued.

Variable	Patients with CPA in 2010 (cases) $N = 899$	Patients without CPA who survived 2010 (control-1s) $N = 1,798$	died in 2010 (controls-2s) $N = 1,778$
>45	50 (6.9%)	99 (6.7%)	108 (7.3%)
	$n = 725$	$n = 1,477$	$n = 1,480$
ESA dose per treatment (units)	$9,313 \pm 7,713$	$6,033 \pm 6,374^{****}$	$9,934 \pm 8,630$
Number of treatments	10.6 ± 3.9	$12.3 \pm 2.2^{****}$	$11.0 \pm 3.5^{**}$
Number of missed treatments	1.5 ± 2.8	$0.56 \pm 1.5^{****}$	1.5 ± 2.9
Number of missed treatments due to hospitalization	1.2 ± 2.7	$0.37 \pm 1.4^{****}$	1.1 ± 2.8
Number of missed treatments due to unexcused absence	0.25 ± 0.86	$0.19 \pm 0.65^{*}$	$0.34 \pm 0.99^{*}$
eKt/V	1.44 ± 0.3	$1.49 \pm 0.3^{**}$	1.46 ± 0.8
Albumin (g/dL)	3.5 ± 0.6	$3.8 \pm 0.4^{****}$	3.5 ± 0.5
Hemoglobin (g/dL)	10.8 ± 1.5	$11.5 \pm 1.2^{****}$	$11.1 \pm 1.5^{****}$
Phosphorus (mg/dL)	5.0 ± 1.7	$5.2 \pm 1.6^{**}$	5.15 ± 1.8
Calcium (mg/dL)	8.9 ± 0.8	$9.0 \pm 0.7^{****}$	8.8 ± 0.8
Potassium (mEq/L)	4.6 ± 0.8	$4.8 \pm 0.7^{****}$	$4.7 \pm 0.8^{***}$
Ferritin (ng/mL)	660 ± 533	662 ± 423	$729 \pm 803^{*}$
Bicarbonate (mEq/L)	24.1 ± 3.8	$23.8 \pm 3.4^{*}$	23.9 ± 3.6
Creatinine (mg/dL)	6.5 ± 2.6	$7.7 \pm 2.8^{****}$	$6.8 \pm 2.6^{**}$
nPCR (g/kg/day)	0.86 ± 0.30	$0.96 \pm 0.28^{****}$	0.89 ± 0.52

[a]$^{*}P < 0.05$; $^{**}P < 0.01$; $^{***}P < 0.001$; $^{****}P < 0.0001$; based on two-sample Student's t-testing or chi-square testing as dictated by data type. Values reported as means $\pm$ SD or n (%) as dictated by data type.
[b]Vintage defined as number of days from the date of first ever dialysis to the date of event (CPA). For controls, event date was assigned the same index date from the matched CPA case.
[c]Catheter compared to fistula/graft.
[d]Mean treatment time in the 30 days prior to CPA (excludes CPA treatment).
[e]Dialysate buffer = dialysate bicarbonate + dialysate acetate.

the feasibility of HD prescription modification and the accessibility of immediate medical intervention. Despite being a relatively rare event, SCA is an important cause of mortality among HD patients. In our cohort, 32.4% of patients who experience CPA died on the CPA event date, and an additional 16.8% died within 30 days. Thus, the identification of high risk subgroups will inform preventive dialytic treatment strategies. HD modifications such as avoidance of low potassium baths (<2 mEq/L) and use of the lowest effective ESA dosing may be important in reducing CPA. Additionally, attention should be paid to nutritional status, underlying illness, and inflammatory processes as these conditions may render HD patients susceptible to peridialytic CPA.

The strengths of our study include its large, nationally representative cohort with a large number of CPA events, the breadth of available covariates, and case-control matched study design. Several limitations of our study deserve mention. As with all observational studies, our study may contain bias due to imperfect control for confounding. We attempted to limit this confounding by matching subjects on age, gender, race, and diabetic status. Such matching accounts for confounding not only from these variables but also from variables that are strongly associated with these variables. Because of data limitations, we were unable to account for additional cardiovascular status markers such as cardiac troponin, cardiac structural abnormalities, residual

renal function, or additional inflammatory markers such as CRP and IL-6. We cannot exclude the possibility of residual confounding related to these variables or other unconsidered variables. In our primary analysis, we allowed CPA cases to match to patients who died later in the study year in efforts to best represent the CPA risk across all patients. It is possible that residual confounding from ambient health status may have influenced results in the primary analysis. Second, we specified CPA as the outcome in all analyses. 67.6% of CPA cases survived beyond the day of CPA, suggesting that the etiology of their CPA may have been respiratory in nature rather than cardiac. Our results should not be extrapolated to other outcomes such as SCA or SCD. On a related note, we lacked data on the breakdown of respiratory versus cardiac CPA events and thus cannot perform event-specific risk factor analyses. Finally, we lacked data regarding the timing of CPA relative to the dialysis treatment and are thus unable to determine whether the identified risk factor-CPA associations differ across the pre-, intra-, and postdialytic time periods.

5. Conclusions

This study demonstrates that, among chronic outpatient HD patients, CAD, heart failure, missed treatments due to hospitalization, lower dialysate potassium, higher ESA dosing, lower albumin, lower body mass index, lower hemoglobin,

TABLE 5: Logistic models of predictors of peridialytic cardiopulmonary arrest in two matched secondary analyses.

Variable	CPA cases versus control-1s		CPA cases versus control-2s	
	Model 1 (univariate) OR (95% CI)	Model 4 (stepwise + quadratics) OR (95% CI)	Model 1 (univariate) OR (95% CI)	Model 4 (stepwise + quadratics) OR (95% CI)
Body mass index (kg/m^2)				
<18.5	2.24** (1.18–4.24)	3.52**** (1.98–6.26)	1.03 (0.62–1.72)	—
18.6–25	1 (ref.)	—	—	—
25.1–29.9	0.66*** (0.49–0.88)	—	1.09 (0.82–1.45)	—
≥30	0.63**** (0.48–0.83)	0.75* (0.60–0.95)	1.08 (0.83–1.42)	—
Coronary artery disease	1.39*** (1.16–1.67)	1.36* (1.07–1.73)	1.11 (0.93–1.33)	—
Heart failure	1.56**** (1.31–1.85)	1.57**** (1.25–1.99)	1.00 (0.85–1.19)	—
Vintage (per 100 days)	1.00 (1.00-1.00)	1.01** (1.00–1.02)	1.00* (1.00-1.00)	—
Catheter vascular access	2.05**** (1.73–2.42)	—	1.24* (1.06–1.47)	—
Percent IDWG	0.99 (0.94–1.06)	—	0.94 (0.89–0.99)*	—
TT shortened > 10 minutes (yes/no)	1.11 (0.82, 1.51)	—	1.03 (0.80–1.33)	—
Missed treatment due to hospitalization (yes/no)	2.02**** (1.54, 2.65)	2.13**** (1.63, 2.79)	1.25 (0.99, 1.56)	—
Missed treatment due to unexcused absence (yes/no)	1.08 (0.78, 1.50)	—	0.82 (0.62, 1.09)	—
Dialysate sodium (mEq/L)	1.00 (0.96–1.04)	—	0.99 (0.95–1.02)	—
Dialysate calcium (mEq/L)		—		
<2.3	1.03 (0.81–1.31)	—	1.05 (0.83–1.35)	—
2.3–2.5	1.00 (ref.)	—	1.00 (ref.)	—
>2.5	0.78 (0.40–1.54)	—	0.53 (0.28–1.01)	—
Dialysate potassium (mEq/L)				
1	1.59 (0.87–2.91)	2.67*** (1.54–4.63)	1.19 (0.67–2.11)	—
2	1.00 (ref.)	—	1.00 (ref.)	—
>2	1.05 (0.80–1.38)	—	0.89 (0.68–1.17)	—
Dialysate buffer (mEq/L)		—		
<41	1.04 (0.74–1.45)	—	0.89 (0.64–1.24)	—
41–45	1.00 (ref.)	—	1.00 (ref.)	—
>45	1.04 (0.67–1.60)	—	0.93 (0.60–1.42)	—
ESA per treatment (per 1000 u)	1.007**** (1.006–1.008)	1.04**** (1.02–1.06)	1.00 (1.00-1.00)	—
eKt/V	0.64** (0.49–0.84)	—	0.95 (0.80–1.12)	—
Albumin (g/dL)	0.21**** (0.17–0.25)	0.40**** (0.30–0.52)	1.01 (0.87–1.17)	—
Hemoglobin (g/dL)	0.67**** (0.63–0.72)	0.78**** (0.72–0.86)	0.87**** (0.83–0.92)	0.87**** (0.82–0.92)
Phosphorus (mg/dL)	0.92** (0.88–0.97)	—	0.96 (0.91–1.00)	—
Calcium (mg/dL)	0.72**** (0.65–0.80)	—	1.04 (0.95–1.15)	1.13* (1.02–1.25)
Potassium (mEq/L)	0.75**** (0.67–0.85)	—	0.82*** (0.74–0.92)	0.84** (0.75–0.93)
Ferritin (per 100 ng/ml)	1.00 (0.98–1.02)	—	0.98* (0.97–1.00)	0.98* (0.97–1.00)
Bicarbonate (mEq/L)	1.00 (1.00–1.05)	—	1.02 (0.99–1.04)	—
nPCR (g/kg/day)	0.25**** (0.18–0.34)	0.43**** (0.28–0.64)	0.79 (0.59–1.04)	—
nPCR^2 (g/kg/day)	—	2.22* (1.18–4.19)	—	—
c-statistic	—	0.77	—	0.58

*$P < 0.05$; **$P < 0.01$; ***$P < 0.001$; ****$P < 0.0001$.

For independent variables with more than 2 categories, P values and confidence intervals were adjusted with multiple comparisons using Bonferroni method. OR, odds ratio; CI, confidence interval; IDWG, interdialytic weight gain; TT, treatment time; nPCR, normalized protein catabolic rate; ESA, erythropoietin stimulating agent; and EDW, estimated dry weight.

lower (and much higher) nPCR, and higher serum calcium are associated with increased odds of ambulatory HD facility CPA. Of these, missed treatments due to hospitalization, albumin, hemoglobin, body mass index, and ESA dosing had the greatest influence on CPA. Further prospective studies are needed to confirm and generalize findings and to explore interventional strategies aimed at mitigating CPA risk among chronic HD patients.

Authors' Contribution

Jennifer E. Flythe and Nien-Chen Li contributed equally to this work.

Acknowledgments

This work was conducted with the support of a KL2 Medical Research Investigator Training award (an appointed KL2 award) from Harvard Catalyst, The Harvard Clinical and Translational Science Center (National Center for Research Resources and the National Center for Advancing Translational Sciences, National Institutes of Health Award 1KL2 TR001100-01 to JEF). The content is solely the responsibility of the authors and does not necessarily represent the official views of Harvard Catalyst, Harvard University and its affiliated academic health care centers, or the National Institutes of Health.

References

[1] USRDS, *Annual Data Report: Atlas of Chronic Kidney Disease and End-Stage Renal Disease in the United States*, 2008.

[2] C. A. Herzog, "Can we prevent sudden cardiac death in dialysis patients?" *Clinical Journal of the American Society of Nephrology* vol. 2, no. 3, pp. 410–412, 2007.

[3] C. A. Herzog, J. M. Mangrum, and R. Passman, "Sudden cardiac death and dialysis patients," *Seminars in Dialysis*, vol. 21, no. 4, pp. 300–307, 2008.

[4] J. A. Karnik, B. S. Young, N. L. Lew et al., "Cardiac arrest and sudden death in dialysis units," *Kidney International*, vol. 60, no. 1, pp. 350–357, 2001.

[5] R. W. Lehrich, P. H. Pun, N. D. Tanenbaum, S. R. Smith, and J. P. Middleton, "Automated external defibrillators and survival from cardiac arrest in the outpatient hemodialysis clinic," *Journal of the American Society of Nephrology*, vol. 18, no. 1, pp. 312–320, 2007.

[6] P. H. Pun, R. W. Lehrich, E. F. Honeycutt, C. A. Herzog, and J. P. Middleton, "Modifiable risk factors associated with sudden cardiac arrest within hemodialysis clinics," *Kidney International*, vol. 79, no. 2, pp. 218–227, 2011.

[7] P. H. Pun, J. R. Horton, and J. P. Middleton, "Dialysate calcium concentration and the risk of sudden cardiac arrest in hemodialysis patients," *Clinical Journal of the American Society of Nephrology*, vol. 8, no. 5, pp. 797–803, 2013.

[8] M. Krishnan, H. M. Wilfehrt, and E. Lacson Jr., "In data we trust: the role and utility of dialysis provider databases in the policy process," *Clinical Journal of the American Society of Nephrology*, vol. 7, no. 11, pp. 1891–1896, 2012.

[9] P. H. Pun, R. W. Lehrich, S. R. Smith, and J. P. Middleton, "Predictors of survival after cardiac arrest in outpatient hemodialysis clinics," *Clinical Journal of the American Society of Nephrology*, vol. 2, no. 3, pp. 491–500, 2007.

[10] S. Genovesi, M. G. Valsecchi, E. Rossi et al., "Sudden death and associated factors in a historical cohort of chronic haemodialysis patients," *Nephrology Dialysis Transplantation*, vol. 24, no. 8, pp. 2529–2536, 2009.

[11] A. J. Bleyer, J. Hartman, P. C. Brannon, A. Reeves-Daniel, S. G. Satko, and G. Russell, "Characteristics of sudden death in hemodialysis patients," *Kidney International*, vol. 69, no. 12, pp. 2268–2273, 2006.

[12] M. Jadoul, J. Thumma, D. S. Fuller et al., "Modifiable practices associated with sudden death among hemodialysis patients in the dialysis outcomes and practice patterns study," *Clinical Journal of the American Society of Nephrology*, vol. 7, no. 5, pp. 765–774, 2012.

[13] R. S. Parekh, L. C. Plantinga, W. H. L. Kao et al., "The association of sudden cardiac death with inflammation and other traditional risk factors," *Kidney International*, vol. 74, no. 10, pp. 1335–1342, 2008.

[14] S. Shastri, N. Tangri, H. Tighiouart et al., "Predictors of sudden cardiac death: a competing risk approach in the hemodialysis study," *Clinical Journal of the American Society of Nephrology*, vol. 7, no. 1, pp. 123–130, 2012.

[15] K. Takeda, A. Harada, S. Okuda et al., "Sudden death in chronic dialysis patients," *Nephrology Dialysis Transplantation*, vol. 12, no. 5, pp. 952–955, 1997.

[16] J.-P. Lafrance, L. Nolin, L. Senécal, and M. Leblanc, "Predictors and outcome of cardiopulmonary resuscitation (CPR) calls in a large haemodialysis unit over a seven-year period," *Nephrology Dialysis Transplantation*, vol. 21, no. 4, pp. 1006–1012, 2006.

[17] D. P. Zipes and H. J. J. Wellens, "Sudden cardiac death," *Circulation*, vol. 98, no. 21, pp. 2334–2351, 1998.

[18] D. Green, P. R. Roberts, D. I. New, and P. A. Kalra, "Sudden cardiac death in hemodialysis patients: an in-depth review," *American Journal of Kidney Diseases*, vol. 57, no. 6, pp. 921–929, 2011.

[19] B. Redaelli, F. Locatelli, D. Limido et al., "Effect of a new model of hemodialysis potassium removal on the control of ventricular arrhythmias," *Kidney International*, vol. 50, no. 2, pp. 609–617, 1996.

[20] S. Sforzini, R. Latini, G. Mingardi, A. Vincenti, and B. Redaelli, "Ventricular arrhythmias and four-year mortality in haemodialysis patients," *The Lancet*, vol. 339, no. 8787, pp. 212–213, 1992.

[21] M. E. Canziani, M. C. Neto, M. A. Saragoça et al., "Hemodialysis versus continuous ambulatory peritoneal dialysis: effects on the heart," *Artificial Organs*, vol. 19, no. 3, pp. 241–244, 1995.

[22] S. Abe, M. Yoshizawa, N. Nakanishi et al., "Electrocardiographic abnormalities in patients receiving hemodialysis," *American Heart Journal*, vol. 131, no. 6, pp. 1137–1144, 1996.

[23] M. Buemi, E. Aloisi, G. Coppolino et al., "The effect of two different protocols of potassium haemodiafiltration on QT dispersion," *Nephrology Dialysis Transplantation*, vol. 20, pp. 1148–1154, 2005.

[24] A. Cupisti, F. Galetta, E. Morelli et al., "Effect of hemodialysis on the dispersion of the QTc interval," *Nephron*, vol. 78, no. 4, pp. 429–432, 1998.

[25] S. Severi, S. Cavalcanti, E. Mancini, and A. Santoro, "Heart rate response to hemodialysis-induced changes in potassium and calcium levels," *Journal of Nephrology*, vol. 14, no. 6, pp. 488–496, 2001.

[26] S. Genovesi, R. Rivera, P. Fabbrini et al., "Dynamic QT interval analysis in uraemic patients receiving chronic haemodialysis," *Journal of Hypertension*, vol. 21, no. 10, pp. 1921–1926, 2003.

[27] S. Genovesi, C. Dossi, M. R. Viganò et al., "Electrolyte concentration during haemodialysis and QT interval prolongation in uraemic patients," *Europace*, vol. 10, no. 6, pp. 771–777, 2008.

[28] S. E. Näppi, V. K. Virtanen, H. H. T. Saha, J. T. Mustonen, and A. I. Pasternack, "QT(c) dispersion increases during hemodialysis with low-calcium dialysate," *Kidney International*, vol. 57, no. 5, pp. 2117–2122, 2000.

[29] F. Tentori, A. Karaboyas, B. M. Robinson et al., "Association of dialysate bicarbonate concentration with mortality in the Dialysis Outcomes and Practice Patterns Study (DOPPS)," *The American Journal of Kidney Diseases*, vol. 62, no. 4, pp. 738–746, 2013.

[30] W. F. Owen Jr., N. L. Lew, Y. Liu, E. G. Lowrie, and J. M. Lazarus, "The urea reduction ratio and serum albumin concentration as predictors of mortality in patients undergoing hemodialysis," *The New England Journal of Medicine*, vol. 329, no. 14, pp. 1001–1006, 1993.

[31] E. G. Lowrie and N. L. Lew, "Death risk in hemodialysis patients: the predictive value of commonly measured variables and an evaluation of death rate differences between facilities," *American Journal of Kidney Diseases*, vol. 15, no. 5, pp. 458–482, 1990.

[32] K. Kalantar-Zadeh, J. D. Kopple, G. Block, and M. H. Humphreys, "A malnutrition-inflammation score is correlated with morbidity and mortality in maintenance hemodialysis patients," *American Journal of Kidney Diseases*, vol. 38, no. 6, pp. 1251–1263, 2001.

[33] P. Goldwasser, N. Mittman, A. Antignani et al., "Predictors of mortality in hemodialysis patients," *Journal of the American Society of Nephrology*, vol. 3, no. 9, pp. 1613–1622, 1993.

[34] J. T. Dwyer, B. Larive, J. Leung et al., "Are nutritional status indicators associated with mortality in the Hemodialysis (HEMO) study?" *Kidney International*, vol. 68, no. 4, pp. 1766–1776, 2005.

[35] P. M. Ridker, M. Cushman, M. J. Stampfer, R. P. Tracy, and C. H. Hennekens, "Plasma concentration of C-reactive protein and risk of developing peripheral vascular disease," *Circulation*, vol. 97, no. 5, pp. 425–428, 1998.

[36] P. M. Ridker and P. Haughie, "Prospective studies of C-reactive protein as a risk factor for cardiovascular disease," *Journal of Investigative Medicine*, vol. 46, no. 8, pp. 391–395, 1998.

[37] P. M. Ridker, J. E. Buring, J. Shih, M. Matias, and C. H. Hennekens, "Prospective study of C-reactive protein and the risk of future cardiovascular events among apparently healthy women," *Circulation*, vol. 98, no. 8, pp. 731–733, 1998.

[38] D. W. Johnson, C. A. Pollock, and I. C. Macdougall, "Erythropoiesis-stimulating agent hyporesponsiveness," *Nephrology*, vol. 12, no. 4, pp. 321–330, 2007.

5

Restless Legs Syndrome in Dialysis Patients: Does the Dialysis Modality Influence its Occurrence and Severity?

Andreia Freire de Menezes ⓘ,[1] Douglas Rafanelle Moura de Santana Motta,[1]
Fernanda Oliveira de Carvalho ⓘ,[1] Eduesley Santana-Santos ⓘ,[2]
Manoel Pacheco de Andrade Júnior,[3] Mirela Farias Figueirôa,[4]
Maria Isabel Teles Farias,[4] and Kleyton de Andrade Bastos[1,3,4]

[1]Postgraduate Program in Health Sciences, Federal University of Sergipe, São Cristóvão, SE, Brazil
[2]Nursing Department, Federal University of Sergipe, São Cristóvão, SE, Brazil
[3]Clinese Clínica de Nefrologia de Sergipe Ltda., Aracaju, SE, Brazil
[4]Department of Medicine, Federal University of Sergipe, São Cristóvão, SE, Brazil

Correspondence should be addressed to Andreia Freire de Menezes; deiamenezes1@hotmail.com

Academic Editor: Anil K. Agarwal

Background. Restless legs syndrome (RLS) is more prevalent in chronic kidney patients than in the general population, but it is often diagnosed late and its predictors are unknown. *Purpose.* To diagnose RLS in a group of chronic kidney patients on dialysis, determine its frequency and severity, compare the prevalence and severity of the condition among dialytic modalities, and identify possible predictive factors in this population. *Methods.* An observational and cross-sectional study with 326 patients who had been on dialysis for more than 3 months, 241 on hemodialysis (HD) and 85 on automatic peritoneal dialysis (APD), using the criteria established by the International Study Group on RLS for the diagnosis and the RLS Rating Scale to determine its severity. *Results.* RLS was diagnosed in 19.3% of the patients, 52.4% with severe or very severe forms. Patients with and without RLS did not differ in clinical and demographic characteristics and dialytic modality; however, patients on APD presented higher RLS severity compared to the HD group. *Conclusions.* RLS is frequent in dialysis patients and occurs predominantly in its most severe forms; the dialytic modality seems to have no influence on its occurrence; however, it is more severe in patients on APD.

1. Introduction

Restless leg syndrome (RLS) is characterized by discomfort, usually in the legs, that causes an overwhelming, irresistible urge to move them, a need that is usually due to unpleasant sensations that worsen during periods of inactivity and that frequently compromises the patient's sleep [1]. It is often diagnosed late, especially when the symptoms are mild or nonspecific [2].

RLS, like other sleep disorders such as insomnia, sleep apnea, and excessive daytime sleepiness, is commonly observed in chronic renal patients, with studies reporting an incidence of 17% to 62% in patients undergoing renal replacement therapy (RRT) [3–8]. The negative impact of these disorders on quality of life (QoL), functional capacity, and survival is well established in the literature [9–15].

The pathophysiology of its occurrence in patients with chronic kidney disease (CKD) is not well established. Authors have proposed several risk factors but the results of the many studies have been inconsistent [6]. The dialytic modality does not seem to interfere in the pathophysiology and incidence of the syndrome [16]; however, recent studies report contrasting results [15, 17].

RLS substantially compromises the quality of life (QoL) of the patient, especially when it occurs in its most severe form and is accompanied by depressive symptoms. Severe forms are usually associated with an increased risk of cardiovascular events and higher mortality [11].

The usual therapeutic measures are generally effective in chronic renal patients, so it is necessary to consider their diagnosis, severity, and identification of possible predictors of their occurrence in this population. And this is what this study aims to accomplish, using a representative sample of patients in a dialysis program.

2. Material and Method

This is an observational, cross-sectional study performed with chronic renal patients enrolled in a dialysis program at a reference unit in the city of Aracaju, Sergipe, Brazil. The patients were aged 18 or over, had been on dialysis for at least three months, were clinically stable, were able to communicate verbally, had no mental deficit, and had not undergone kidney transplantation or surgical amputation of the lower limbs. The local ethics committee approved the study (CAAE 00984012.0.0000.0058), and all patients who met the inclusion criteria signed the free and informed form, agreeing to participate in the study.

Data collection took place between April and July 2012. At that time, there were 430 patients on the dialysis program, of whom 326 agreed to take part in the study: 241 on hemodialysis and 85 on automatic peritoneal dialysis. The HD patient interview was performed at the time of dialysis, which occurs on alternate days with duration of 4 hours for each session; the clinic has 3 sessions per day. The APD patients were interviewed on the day of their monthly consultation with the physician. The data collection was carried out by personal interview by a clinical nurse specialist that was trained to administer the questionnaires. Patients were assessed for the presence of RLS by the four criteria of International Restless Syndrome Study Group (IRLSSG) [2] during the face-to-face interview. The questionnaires took approximately 30–50 min to complete. These criteria include unpleasant sensations in foots or legs which develop or are exacerbated during rest; are aggravate in the evening or at night; and are relieve with movement. Patients who fulfilled all four criteria are considered to have RLS and further evaluated by the self-questionnaire of IRLSSG severity scale.

Those who were diagnosed as having RLS answered another questionnaire with ten questions corresponding to the RLS International Rating Scale [18] translated and validated in Portuguese by Masuko et al. [1]. In this questionnaire, all the answers have a score ranging from 0 (corresponding to "none") to 4 (corresponding to "very large") and the final score represents the sum of the answers of the ten questions, 0 to 10 points, light; 11 to 20 points, moderate; 21 to 30 points, serious; and 31 to 40 points, very serious.

An evaluation form was completed to collect the clinical-demographic information obtained from the electronic medical records of each patient. The following items were included: name, gender, marital status, occupation, schooling, dialysis mode (hemodialysis or peritoneal dialysis), type of vascular access (catheter or arteriovenous fistula), time in dialysis, baseline disease, comorbidities and most recent laboratory exams referring to hemoglobin blood levels, intact parathyroid hormone (iPTH), phosphorus, albumin, and ferritin.

Finally, in order to evaluate the impact of dialysis on the occurrence of RLS and its severity, patients on hemodialysis and peritoneal dialysis were analyzed comparatively.

The information obtained was compared and analyzed using the appropriate statistical methods using the program *Statistical Package for Social Sciences* (SPSS) 16.0 for *Windows* (SPSS Inc., Chicago, Illinois), with $p < 0.05$ being considered for rejection of the null hypothesis.

Descriptive statistics of the studied population were presented in absolute frequency and percentage, in addition to mean and standard deviation and median. In the bivariate statistics, the following tests were applied: Chi-Square and the Odds Ratio (OR) to analyze the relationship between the diagnosis of RLS and categorical independent variables. In the case of ordinal variables, Student's t-tests were conducted, maintaining the same dependent variable (RLS diagnosis).

3. Results

The 326 patients studied had a mean age of 50.4 ± 15.9 years; 191 patients (58.6%) were men; 194 patients (59.5%) lived with a partner; and 203 patients (77.2%) had been on dialysis for over a year. The majority of the patients underwent hemodialysis (73.9%), through an arteriovenous fistula (59.2%). Hypertensive nephrosclerosis was the most common etiology (26.1%) and in 24.2% of patients the cause of CKD was not identified. Systemic arterial hypertension was the main comorbidity identified (271 patients, 83.1%). Sixty-three patients (19.3%) were diagnosed as having RLS.

Tables 1 and 2 show the distribution of patients according to the dialytic modality and clinical-demographic characteristics, segregated according to the diagnosis of RLS. Patients with and without RLS did not differ in the variables studied.

The 63 patients with RLS answered the 10 questions of the International Rating Scale for the disease (1): 7.9% presented mild discomfort, 39.7% moderate discomfort, 32.8% severe discomfort, and 19.6% very severe discomfort. 67.3% of patients reported that their need to move their limbs was moderate to great; however, approximately 45% reported complete relief of discomfort when walking. The majority of patients reported that RLS was associated with impaired sleep quality (67.2%) and fatigue or somnolence (63.8%), of varying degrees of intensity. The symptoms in 39.7% of the cases lasted less than one hour per day; however 43.1% of the individuals reported that they occurred almost daily. For 37.9% of the interviewees, the symptoms of RLS did not affect their ability to perform normal activities, but 72.4% reported mood changes of varying degrees of intensity.

According to the results of the RLS International Rating Scale, most patients (52.4%) had RLS in its severe or very severe forms (Figure 1).

RLS was diagnosed in 17.4% of the individuals who underwent hemodialysis, and in those patients the disease was mild or moderate (54.8%). With regard to patients who underwent peritoneal dialysis, RLS was identified in 24.7% of them and there was greater penetration of severe or very serious disease (66.6), but no statistically significant

TABLE 1: Distribution of hemodialysis patients according to clinical-demographic characteristics, segregated according to the diagnosis of restless legs syndrome (RLS)$^\text{ɛ}$ ($N = 241$).

Characteristics	Population 100% (241)	With RLS 17.4% (42)	Without RLS 82.6 (199)	p^∂ -
Age (average), years	48.9 ± 15.7	48.1 ± 13.7	49.1 ± 16.1	0.71
Male, %	58.5	50.0	60.3	0.22
Arterial hypertension, %	83.1	78.6	84.0	0.40
Diabetes mellitus, %	26.6	19.0	28.1	0.22
Cardiopathy, %	23.2	30.9	21.6	0.19
Peripheral vasculopathy, %	14.9	19.0	14.1	0.41
Having a partner, %	56.4	69.0	53.8	0.07
Years of study, <4, %	51.0	52.4	50.7	0.84
Regular occupation, %	8.3	9.5	8.0	0.75
Time on dialysis, >1 year, %	80.1	80.9	79.9	0.87
Hemoglobin (g/dL)$^\varnothing$	10.8	10.7	10.9	0.70
Parathormone (pg/mL)$^\varnothing$	580.7	621.6	496.1	0.78
Phosphorus (mq/dL)$^\varnothing$	4.8	4.9	4.7	0.13
Albumin (g/dL)$^\varnothing$	3.8	3.8	3.8	0.54
Ferritin (ng/mL)$^\varnothing$	670.3	671.3	625.5	0.94

$^\text{ɛ}$Based on the criteria developed by the International Study Group on Restless Legs Syndrome (18). $^\varnothing$Median of values obtained from blood samples. Significance calculated from mean values. $^\partial$Significance level $p < 0.05$.

TABLE 2: Distribution of peritoneal dialysis patients according to clinical-demographic characteristics, segregated according to the diagnosis of restless legs syndrome (RLS)$^\text{ɛ}$ ($N = 85$).

Characteristics	Population 100% (85)	With RLS 24.7% (21)	Without RLS 75.3% (64)	p^∂ -
Age (average), years	56.5 ± 15.3	59.3 ± 13.8	53.0 ± 17.5	0.14
Male, %	57.1	71.4	54.7	0.18
Arterial hypertension, %	83.9	90.5	81.2	0.50
Diabetes mellitus, %	32.1	38.0	32.8	0.66
Cardiopathy, %	28.6	23.8	34.4	0.37
Peripheral vasculopathy, %	16.1	19.0	18.7	1.00
Having a partner, %	73.2	61.9	70.3	0.47
Years of study, <4, %	58.9	47.6	65.6	0.14
Regular occupation, %	16.1	19.0	15.6	0.74
Time on dialysis, >1 year, %	67.9	61.9	68.7	0.56
Hemoglobin (g/dL)$^\varnothing$	11.0	11.9	11.1	0.60
Parathormone (pg/mL)$^\varnothing$	457.7	355.5	396.0	0.41
Phosphorus (mq/dL)$^\varnothing$	4.9	3.9	4.84	0.33
Albumin (g/dL)$^\varnothing$	3.5	3.4	3.4	0.40
Ferritin (ng/mL)$^\varnothing$	704.3	723.5	746.8	0.59

$^\text{ɛ}$Based on the criteria developed by the International Study Group on Restless Legs Syndrome (18). $^\varnothing$Median values. $^\partial$Significance level, $p < 0.05$.

differences were observed between the two groups in terms of prevalence ($p = 0.11$).

4. Discussion

In this study we diagnosed RLS in 19.3% of the chronic renal patients who were in a dialysis program, and in 52.4% of them the disease was characterized as severe or very serious. No independent predictor of this syndrome was identified in the study population. Additionally, it was verified that patients with RLS on peritoneal dialysis presented different profiles in terms of the prevalence and severity of the disease compared to those on hemodialysis but with no statistical significance.

It is estimated that RLS has a prevalence in the general population varying from 2 to 15%, depending on the characteristics of the individuals and the diagnostic criteria used, and that it is a common disorder in chronic renal patients in renal replacement therapy RRT [19]. Studies report rates of diagnosis of the disease in this population ranging from

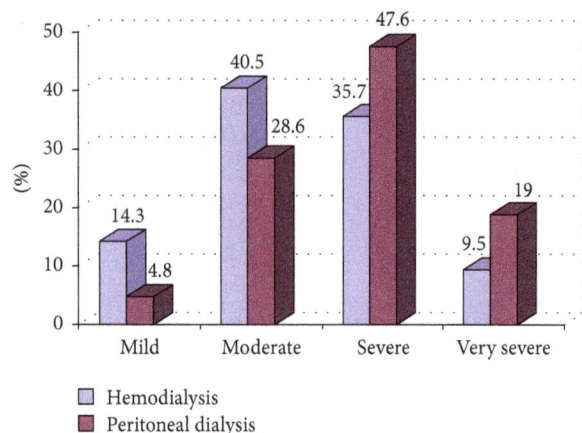

FIGURE 1: Percentage distribution of patients with restless legs syndrome in terms of their severity, according to the dialysis modality ($N = 63$).

17 to 62% [3–7]. The pathophysiology of RLS is still obscure, and its genesis may be uremia, as well as iron deficiency. It is thought to be a peripheral disorder, but studies of dopamine metabolism in the brain raise the possibility of central nervous system (CNS) origin, more specifically by the organic deficiency of hypothalamic dopaminergic cells that are the source of dopamine for the spinal cord [20]. Iron acts as a cofactor for the enzyme tyrosine hydroxylase, an important step in the synthesis of dopamine in the CNS. Thus, low levels of serum iron would cause a decrease in dopamine production, which, in itself, could lead to RLS [21].

As reported for the general population, a strong association between RLS and serum levels of iron and ferritin has been reported in chronic renal failure, which is generally below 40 ng/mL [3, 13, 22–24]; however, more recent studies have not confirmed these findings [21, 25]. Additionally, in dialysis patients it has been suggested that anemia, regardless of iron stores, may be the major cause of RLS development [14]. Patients with altered renal function produce less erythropoietin, with a consequent reduction of erythropoiesis, which, in a not yet fully understood way, reduces the cotransport of iron to the CNS and medulla [21].

Regarding hemoglobin and hematocrit levels, the results diverge, in a study with hemodialysis patients only; there was a relationship between RLS in dialysis patients and a decrease in hemoglobin ($p < 0.005$) [26]; however, other recent studies have not found any type of association [13, 17]. In a recent meta-analysis by Mao et al. [27], in which 23 studies were included, dialysis patients with RLS had markedly lower levels of hemoglobin (Hb)/iron compared to non-RLS in global populations.

The median values of the laboratory test results for hemoglobin, iPTH, albumin, and phosphorus were in agreement with that recommended for this population. The median ferritin was above the recommended level. However, in 59.2% of the patients, the values were within the normal range, with only 14 patients (4.3%) having ferritin levels < 100 ng/mL, two of whom were diagnosed as having RLS (3.2% of RLS cases) [28]. However, it should be borne in mind that

this marker reflects iron stores more accurately when they are reduced, since inflammation is highly prevalent in this population, and liver disease contributes to its elevation [29]. In addition, dialysis patients generally have strict hematimetric and iron store control, with the almost continuous use of erythropoiesis and iron supplementation agents.

CKD combined with hemodialysis, the most common dialysis modality, are among the chronic pathologies and therapies that most affect patients' QoL, with depression being a relatively common psychiatric disorder in this population. More broadly, a complex interaction between depression, QoL, clinical complications, and survival is observed in dialysis patients [30]. It has been shown that RLS can add to this effect and further substantially compromise the QoL of those it affects, with the most important factors being its severity and the presence of depressive symptoms [31]. Tuncel et al. [13] reported that the presence of RLS in hemodialysis patients negatively affects QoL and contributes to the occurrence of depression. In a cross-sectional study, Szentkiralyi et al. [12] found that those with chronic kidney disease and RLS had a higher prevalence of depressive symptoms than those without RLS (56% versus 22%, $p < 0.001$).

In this series, we did not study the associations between RLS, QoL, and depression; however, in our previous study, in the same place, Salman [32] reported a significant lowering of the QoL level among 114 chronic hemodialysis patients, mainly in regard to physical aspects. Depression, with a prevalence of 28.9%, was the highest predictor of QoL, being associated with lower scores in all dimensions of the evaluation instrument used. A similar result was found in a recent study. Of the 400 patients interviewed, 19.3% had depressive symptoms and the main independent factors were poor sleep quality, unemployment, diabetes, hypoalbuminemia, low education, and pruritus [26].

In the present analysis, we observed that the majority of patients had severe or very severe RLS, and it was notable that 67.2% of them reported impaired sleep quality, 63.8% reported drowsiness, 62.1% reported that the symptoms affected the performance of routine activities, and 72.4% reported having mood changes. These results corroborate current data showing that RLS is associated with poor sleep quality, excessive daytime sleepiness, depressive symptoms, and increased risk of obstructive sleep apnea [26].

Increased severity of RLS has been associated with an increased risk of cardiovascular events and increased mortality and is thought to play a role in the pathogenesis of hypertension during sleep [11, 14]. Considering what has been reported in the literature, it is plausible that, due to the intensity of the symptoms observed in our patients, there is a substantial impairment in their QoL [13, 31] and a higher cardiovascular risk [11, 14].

Considering that in the bivariate analysis there was no evidence of an association between the characteristics, a multivariate analysis to identify possible independent predictors for RLS was not performed, since no statistical significance was found in the bivariate analysis between the characteristics considered and restless leg syndrome. When segregating patients according to the dialysis modality, although there is no statistical significance in terms of numbers, the severity profile of the disease appears to be different. There was a higher prevalence of RLS (24.7 versus 17.4%) and a higher percentage of patients perceived to be more severe (66.7 versus 45.2%) in patients on peritoneal dialysis than in those on hemodialysis. The quantitative study of individuals on peritoneal dialysis (85 patients) submitted to RLS evaluation in this study contrasts with the majority of publications in which only hemodialysis patients are considered in the analysis, perhaps because this is the predominant modality in most countries [32, 33]. Recent studies report contrasting results: Al-Jahdali [17] reported a significantly higher prevalence of RLS in APD patients than in hemodialysis patients (69 versus 46%). However, Merlino et al. [15], investigating 86 patients (67.4% on hemodialysis), identified a higher prevalence of RLS in hemodialysis patients (19%) than in patients on APD (10.7%).

5. Conclusions

RLS is a common disease in dialysis patients and occurs predominantly in its most severe forms and should be investigated early and routinely in these patients, in order to apply the known effective therapeutic measures and prevent its well described negative outcomes. The dialytic modality does not seem to influence the occurrence of RLS and we did not identify other factors independently associated with it in this population. Further studies are needed to confirm whether other clinical-demographic factors predict its onset.

It is worth noting that this study presents a high number of patients compared to the articles already published; however, it presents the limitation of not being multicentric, and the lack of association between the characteristics considered and RLS did not allow us to identify independent predictors through a multivariate analysis.

Care of a dialysis patient should include special attention to the diagnosis and treatment of RLS, as it has a high prevalence in relation to the general population and presents in a severe form in this population, particularly in those on APD. Additional studies are needed in an attempt to identify possible predictors, since the characteristics analyzed in this study were not associated with the diagnosis.

Conflicts of Interest

The authors have no relevant affiliations or financial involvement with any organization or entity with a financial interest in or financial conflict with the subject matter or materials discussed in the manuscript.

References

[1] A. H. Masuko, L. B. C. Carvalho, M. A. C. Machado, J. F. Morais, L. B. F. Prado, and G. F. Prado, "Translation and validation into the Brazilian Portuguese of the restless legs syndrome rating scale of the International Restless Legs Syndrome Study Group," *Arquivos de Neuro-Psiquiatria*, vol. 66, no. 4, pp. 832–836, 2008.

[2] R. P. Allen, D. Picchietti, W. A. Hening, C. Trenkwalder, A. S. Walters, and J. Montplaisi, "Restless legs syndrome: diagnostic criteria, special considerations, and epidemiology. A report from the restless legs syndrome diagnosis and epidemiology workshop at the National Institutes of Health," *Sleep Medicine*, vol. 4, no. 2, pp. 101–119, 2003.

[3] D. S. C. Hui, T. Y. H. Wong, F. W. S. Ko et al., "Prevalence of sleep disturbances in Chinese patients with end-stage renal failure on continuous ambulatory peritoneal dialysis," *American Journal of Kidney Diseases*, vol. 36, no. 4, pp. 783–788, 2000.

[4] M. L. Thorp, "Restless legs syndrome," *International Journal of Artificial Organs*, vol. ;4, pp. 755-756, 2001.

[5] I. Mucsi, M. Z. Molnar, C. Ambrus et al., "Restless legs syndrome, insomnia and quality of life in patients on maintenance dialysis," *Nephrology Dialysis Transplantation*, vol. 20, no. 3, pp. 571–577, 2005.

[6] D. Kavanagh, S. Siddiqui, and C. C. Geddes, "Restless Legs Syndrome in Patients on Dialysis," *American Journal of Kidney Diseases*, vol. 43, no. 5, pp. 763–771, 2004.

[7] A. Kawauchi, Y. Inoue, T. Hashimoto et al., "Restless legs syndrome in hemodialysis patients: Health-related quality of life and laboratory data analysis," *Clinical Nephrology*, vol. 66, no. 6, pp. 440–446, 2006.

[8] M. G. Bastos, "Kirsztajn GM: Chronic kidney disease: importance of early diagnosis, immediate referral and structured interdisciplinary approach to improve outcomes in patients not yet on dialysis," *Jornal Brasileiro de Nefrologia*, vol. 33, pp. 93–108, 2011.

[9] R. L. Benz, M. R. Pressman, E. T. Hovick, and D. D. Peterson, "Potential novel predictors of mortality in end-stage renal disease patients with sleep disorders," *American Journal of Kidney Diseases*, vol. 35, no. 6, pp. 1052–1060, 2000.

[10] S. Happe, G. Klösch, B. Saletu, and J. Zeitlhofer, "Treatment of idiopathic restless legs syndrome (RLS) with gabapentin," *Neurology*, vol. 57, no. 9, pp. 1717–1719, 2001.

[11] F. Portaluppi, P. Cortelli, G. C. Buonaura, M. H. Smolensky, and F. Fabbian, "Do restless legs syndrome (RLS) and periodic limb movements of sleep (PLMS) play a role in nocturnal hypertension and increased cardiovascular risk of renally impaired patients?" *Chronobiology International*, vol. 26, no. 6, pp. 1206–1221, 2009.

[12] A. Szentkiralyi, M. Z. Molnar, M. E. Czira et al., "Association between restless legs syndrome and depression in patients with chronic kidney disease," *Journal of Psychosomatic Research*, vol. 67, no. 2, pp. 173–180, 2009.

[13] D. Tuncel, F. Ö. Orhan, H. Sayarlioglu, I. O. IsIk, U. Utku, and A. Dinc, "Restless legs syndrome in hemodialysis patients: Association with depression and quality of life," *Sleep and Breathing*, vol. 15, no. 3, pp. 311–315, 2011.

[14] G. La Manna, F. Pizza, E. Persici et al., "Restless legs syndrome enhances cardiovascular risk and mortality in patients with end-stage kidney disease undergoing long-term haemodialysis treatment," *Nephrology Dialysis Transplantation*, vol. 26, no. 6, pp. 1976–1983, 2011.

[15] G. Merlino, S. Lorenzut, G. Romano et al., "Restless legs syndrome in dialysis patients: A comparison between hemodialysis and continuous ambulatory peritoneal dialysis," *Neurological Sciences*, vol. 33, no. 6, pp. 1311–1318, 2012.

[16] L. Janzen, J. A. Rich, and L. M. Vercaigne, "An overview of levodopa in the management of restless legs syndrome in a dialysis population: Pharmacokinetics, clinical trials, and complications of therapy," *Annals of Pharmacotherapy*, vol. 33, no. 1, pp. 86–92, 1999.

[17] H. Al-Jahdali, "A comparison of sleep disturbances and sleep apnea in patients on hemodialysis and chronic peritoneal dialysis," *Saudi Journal of Kidney Diseases and Transplantation*, vol. 22, no. 5, pp. 922–930, 2011.

[18] A. S. Adabag, A. Ishani, H. E. Bloomfield, A. K. Ngo, and T. J. Wilt, "Efficacy of N-acetylcysteine in preventing renal injury after heart surgery: a systematic review of randomized trials," *European Heart Journal*, vol. 30, no. 15, pp. 1910–1917, 2009.

[19] R. P. Allen, M. Bharmal, and M. Calloway, "Prevalence and disease burden of primary restless legs syndrome: Results of a general population survey in the United States," *Movement Disorders*, vol. 26, no. 1, pp. 114–120, 2011.

[20] S. Clemens, D. Rye, and S. Hochman, "Restless legs syndrome: revisiting the dopamine hypothesis from the spinal cord perspective," *Neurology*, vol. 67, no. 1, pp. 125–130, 2006.

[21] G. S. Goffredo Filho, C. C. Gorini, A. S. Purysko, H. C. Silva, and I. E. F. Elias, "Restless legs syndrome in patients on chronic hemodialysis in a Brazilian city: Frequency, biochemical findings and comorbidities," *Arquivos de Neuro-Psiquiatria*, vol. 61, no. 3 B, pp. 723–727, 2003.

[22] C. J. Earley, J. R. Connor, J. L. Beard, E. A. Malecki, D. K. Epstein, and R. P. Allen, "Abnormalities in CSF concentrations of ferritin and transferrin in restless legs syndrome," *Neurology*, vol. 54, no. 8, pp. 1698–1700, 2000.

[23] R. P. Allen, P. B. Barker, F. Wehrl, H. K. Song, and C. J. Earley, "MRI measurement of brain iron in patients with restless legs syndrome," *Neurology*, vol. 56, no. 2, pp. 263–265, 2001.

[24] M. H. Silber and J. W. Richardson, "Multiple blood donations associated with iron deficiency in patients with restless legs syndrome," *Mayo Clinic Proceedings*, vol. 78, no. 1, pp. 52–54, 2003.

[25] J.-M. Kim, H.-M. Kwon, C. S. Lim, Y. S. Kim, S.-J. Lee, and H. Nam, "Restless legs syndrome in patients on hemodialysis: Symptom severity and risk factors," *Journal of Clinical Neurology*, vol. 4, no. 4, pp. 153–157, 2008.

[26] S. M. H. A. Araujo, V. M. S. D. Bruin, L. A. Nepomuceno et al., "Restless legs syndrome in end-stage renal disease: Clinical characteristics and associated comorbidities," *Sleep Medicine*, vol. 11, no. 8, pp. 785–790, 2010.

[27] S. Mao, H. Shen, S. Huang, and A. Zhang, "Restless legs syndrome in dialysis patients: A meta-analysis," *Sleep Medicine*, vol. 15, no. 12, pp. 1532–1538, 2014.

[28] "KDOQI, Foundation NK: KDOQI Clinical Practice Guidelines and Clinical Practice Recommendations for Anemia in Chronic Kidney Disease," in *American Journal of Kidney Diseases*, pp. S11–145, 47, 2006.

[29] K. V. Kowdley, P. Belt, L. A. Wilson et al., "Serum ferritin is an independent predictor of histologic severity and advanced fibrosis in patients with nonalcoholic fatty liver disease," *Hepatology*, vol. 55, no. 1, pp. 77–85, 2012.

[30] P. L. Kimmel, "Psychosocial factors in dialysis patients," *Kidney International*, vol. 59, no. 4, pp. 1599–1613, 2001.

[31] S. Happe, J. P. Reese, K. Stiasny-Kolster et al., "Assessing health-related quality of life in patients with restless legs syndrome," *Sleep Medicine*, vol. 10, no. 3, pp. 295–305, 2009.

[32] S. M. Salman, "Restless legs syndrome in patients on hemodialysis," *American Journal of Kidney Diseases*, vol. 22, pp. 368–372, 2011.

[33] M. Malaki, F. S. Mortazavi, S. Moazemi, and M. Shoaran, "Insomnia and limb pain in hemodialysis patients: what is the share of restless leg syndrome?" *Saudi Journal of Kidney Diseases and Transplantation*, vol. 23, no. 1, pp. 15–20, 2012.

6

Prognostic Importance of Fibroblast Growth Factor-23 in Dialysis Patients

Nilgül Akalin,[1] **Yıldız Okuturlar,**[2] **Özlem Harmankaya,**[1] **Asuman Gedıkbaşi,**[3] **Selçuk Sezıklı,**[2] **and Sibel Koçak Yücel**[1]

[1] *Department of Nephrology, Bakırköy Dr. Sadi Konuk Training and Research Hospital, Istanbul 34147, Turkey*
[2] *Department of Internal Medicine, Bakırköy Dr. Sadi Konuk Training and Research Hospital, Istanbul 34147, Turkey*
[3] *Department of Biochemistry, Bakırköy Dr. Sadi Konuk Training and Research Hospital, Istanbul 34147, Turkey*

Correspondence should be addressed to Nilgül Akalin; nilnef@hotmail.com

Academic Editor: Laszlo Rosivall

Introduction. In this study, we aimed to demonstrate the correlation of FGF-23 levels with bone-mineral metabolism, anemia, and the treatment in dialysis patients. *Methods.* Eighty-nine patients with similar age, gender, dialysis duration, and dialysis adequacy who were receiving hemodialysis replacement therapy for at least 6 months were included in the study. Serum iron, iron binding capacity, ferritin, hemoglobin (Hb), hematocrit (Htc), calcium (Ca), phosphorus (P), intact parathormone (iPTH), and FGF-23 levels were studied. In addition, active vitamin D and phosphate binders calcimimetic therapies that patients have received in the last 6 months were recorded. *Results.* It was determined that there was a positive correlation between serum FGF-23 values and PTH values ($P < 0,01$) and Ca∗P values ($P < 0,01$). A positive correlation was found between serum FGF-23 values and Ca values at a rate of 24,6% ($P < 0,05$) and between P values at a rate of 59,1% ($P < 0,01$). A positive correlation was determined between serum FGF-23 values and hemoglobin (Hb) values ($P < 0,05$) and hematocrit (Htc) values ($P < 0,05$). In multivariate analysis, no significant correlation was found between serum FGF-23 levels and Hb and Htc. *Conclusion.* The effects of high serum FGF-23 levels on different parameters may be correlated with the development of refractory secondary hyperparathyroidism.

1. Introduction

Fibroblast growth factor-23 (FGF-23) is a hormone that has been shown to play a role on the mineralization, vitamin D metabolism, parathyroid gland functions, and phosphate excretion from the kidney. Studies trying to show a correlation between FGF-23 and development of cardiovascular disease and mortality have reported contradictory results [1, 2]. Considering increasing FGF-23 levels with the progression of chronic kidney disease, its effects on the mineral metabolism, and possible relationship with the development of cardiovascular disease, it is thought that FGF-23 might be a prognostic factor [3]. FGF-23, which increases in parallel with the increase of phosphate levels from the early stages of chronic kidney disease, is known to contribute to the development of secondary hyperparathyroidism by leading

to suppression of 1,25(OH)2 D levels and increased phosphate excretion [4].

In addition to predicting the prognosis in chronic kidney disease, determination of the correlation between decreased glomerular filtration rate and increased levels of FGF-23 may be an important target, especially in treatment of secondary hyperparathyroidism. In the studies conducted with hemodialysis studies, FGF-23 levels >7500 ng/L have been found to be important in prediction of refractory secondary hyperparathyroidism; however, effects of the secondary hyperparathyroidism treatment on FGF-23 levels is yet to be cleared [5]. In the secondary analysis of the Achieve trial [6], 91 hemodialysis patients were administered low-dose of calcitriol analogues calcimimetic agent cinacalcet and FGF-23 levels were observed to decrease by 9,7% in cinacalcet group.

In Accelerated Mortality on Renal Replacement study [7], phosphate binder therapy was found to be correlated with decreased FGF-23 levels. However, place of vitamin D and calcimimetic in the treatment is unclear.

In this study, we aimed to demonstrate the correlation between FGF-23 and the parameters that have effects on morbidity and mortality in dialysis patients as well as the effect of vitamin D and phosphorus binding calcimimetic on FGF-23.

2. Materials and Methods

A total of 89 patients followed up and treated in the Nephrology Polyclinic who were receiving hemodialysis replacement therapy for at least 6 months were included in the study. Patients were divided into two groups according to serum PTH level being below or above 300 pg/mL. Patients were included provided they were similar in terms of age, gender, disease etiology, and dialysis duration and having dialysis adequacy. Patients with chronic and active inflammatory disease (e.g., malignancy, collagen tissue disease, and diabetic foot) and incompliant patients in the treatment were excluded from the study.

Following an overnight fasting, venous blood samples were simultaneously collected from all the patients. Serum LDL-cholesterol, albumin, uric acid, high sensitive C- reactive protein, iron (Fe), iron binding capacity, ferritin, hemoglobin (Hb), hematocrit (Htc), calcium (Ca), phosphorus (P), intact PTH (iPTH), and FGF-23 levels were studied. In addition, Ca∗P ratio was calculated in each patient and averages of active vitamin D and phosphate binders calcimimetic therapies that patients have received in last 6 months were defined. These therapies were recorded. Patients' Kt/V and urea reduction ratio (URR) values were recorded in order to evaluate hemodialysis adequacy.

Total cholesterol, triglycerides, high-density lipoprotein (HDL), and low-density lipoprotein (LDL) cholesterol were analyzed with Architect c16200 Integrated System (Abbott Diagnostics Europe, Wiesbaden, Germany). Plasma levels of high sensitive CRP were measured with Siemens Immulite 2000 device using two-way chemiluminometric immunoassay method.

Serum iPTH levels were determined by Siemens Immulite 2000 immunoassay system (Siemens Healthcare Diagnostics, USA) (normal range < 149 pg/mL). Patients' Kt/V and URR values were recorded in order to evaluate hemodialysis adequacy. $Kt/V = -\ln[(R-0{,}008 \times t) + (4-3{,}5 \times R)]\Delta BW/BW$ (R: ratio of postdialysis urea to predialysis urea; t: dialysis duration; BW: body weight) formula model was used for calculation of Kt/V. [URR = (postdialysis urea/predialysis urea)] formula was used for calculation of URR values. Kt/V >1,4 and URR >70% were considered as dialysis adequacy.

Serum FGF-23 levels were determined and venous blood samples were collected in tubes from the antecubital vein followed by an overnight fasting. The tubes were centrifuged at 2000 g (10 min) to remove the serum. Aliquots of serum samples were stored at −80°C until FGF-23 assaying.

Serum FGF-23 levels were determined using Human FGF-23 ELISA Kit (cat. number EZHFGF-23-32K) purchased from Millipore (USA) following the manufacturer's instructions. Millipore Human FGF-23 ELISA Kit employs the quantitative sandwich enzyme immunoassay technique. Intra-assay and interassay coefficients of variation were 7,2% and 5,3%, respectively. FGF-23 levels were expressed as pg/mL.

This study was approved by the Ethics Committee of Bakırköy Medical Hospital and conducted in accordance with the principles of the Declaration of Helsinki. All participants gave their written informed consent prior to participation in the study.

2.1. Statistical Analysis. In this study, statistical analyses were performed using NCSS (Number Cruncher Statistical System) 2007 Statistical Software (Utah, USA) package program.

In evaluation of the data, one-way variance analysis was used in the descriptive statistical methods (mean, standard deviation, median, and interquartile range). Conformity of variables to a normal distribution was provided by applying the logarithmic transformation for FGF-23 and a square root transformation for PTH. Independent t-test was used for comparison of two groups and Mann-Whitney U test for comparison of the variables with nonnormal distribution. Comparison of the qualitative data was performed using Chi-square test. Lineer regression analysis was carried out in order to define the parameters that affect FGF-23 levels. $P < 0{,}05$ values were considered as statistically significant.

3. Results

Patients followed up in the Nephrology Polyclinics who were receiving dialysis replacement therapy for at least 6 months were included in the study. Hemodialysis patients were divided into 2 groups as having serum iPTH above or below 300 pg/mL.

Mean age and gender distribution of the patients with serum iPTH levels above and below <300 pg/mL were found with no significant difference between both groups (Table 1).

No significant difference was found between the patient groups that developed etiology of end stage kidney disease (Table 1).

Mean dialysis duration of patients with serum iPTH levels above and below <300 pg/mL were found with no significant difference between both groups (Table 1).

When the patients were divided into 2 groups as having serum iPTH above or below 300 pg/mL, serum levels of FGF-23 were found to be significantly higher in the group with iPTH >300 pg/mL ($P = 0{,}029$; Table 1). In the logistic analysis carried out with Ca∗P and PTH a statistical correlation was found ($P = 0{,}0001$; Table 1).

Existence of Vitamin D therapy was found to be statistically higher in >300 iPTH group ($n = 7$; 83,90%) than in <300 iPTH group ($n = 7$; 21,2%) ($P = 0{,}0001$) (Table 2). Existence of Ca-containing phosphorus binding therapy was found to be statistically higher in >300 iPTH group ($n = 53$; 94,6%) than in <300 iPTH group ($n = 21$; 63,6%) ($P = 0{,}0001$) (Table 2).

TABLE 1: The relationships of demographic features and comparison of serum parathormone levels with fibroblast growth factor-23, calcium, and phosphorus in the dialysis patients.

	PTH < 300 pg/mL	PTH > 300 pg/mL	P
Age; mean ± SD	47,94 ± 14,21	46,88 ± 16,57	**0,394**
Gender; n (%)			
Male	17 (51,50)	24 (42,90)	**0,506**
Female	16 (48,50)	32 (57,10)	
Dialysis duration (years); mean ± SD	3,03 ± 1,91	4,71 ± 3,03	**0,587**
Etiology; n (%)			
Hypertension	14 (42,40)	25 (44,70)	**0,923**
Postrenal KBH	7 (21,30)	7 (12,50)	
Glomerulonephritis	12 (36,40)	23 (41,10)	
Unknown	—	1 (1,80)	
FGF-23$_{Log 10}$ (ng/mL); mean ± SD	159,40 ± 3,66	741,31 ± 4,77	**0,001****
Calcium (mg/dL); mean ± SD	8,61 ± 0,99	8,58 ± 0,93	**0,871**
Phosphorus (mg/dL); mean ± SD	4,38 ± 1,07	5,62 ± 1,54	**0,0001**
Ca∗P (mg^2/dL^2) mean ± SD	37,77 ± 10,61	48,46 ± 14,75	**0,001**

Data are presented as n(%). PTH: parathormone; KBH: chronic renal diseases; FGF-23 $_{Log 10}$: fibroblast growth factor; Ca: calcium; P: phosphorus.
** Statistical significance positive correlation ($P < 0,01$).

TABLE 2: The treatment received according to serum levels of parathormone.

Therapy	PTH < 300 pg/mL	PTH > 300 pg/mL	P
Vitamin D			
No	26 (78,80)	9 (16,10)	**0,0001**
Yes	7 (21,20)	47 (83,90)	
Calcium-containing phosphorus binding			
No	12 (36,40)	3 (5,40)	**0,0001**
Yes	21 (63,60)	53 (94,60)	

Data are presented as n(%). PTH: parathormone.

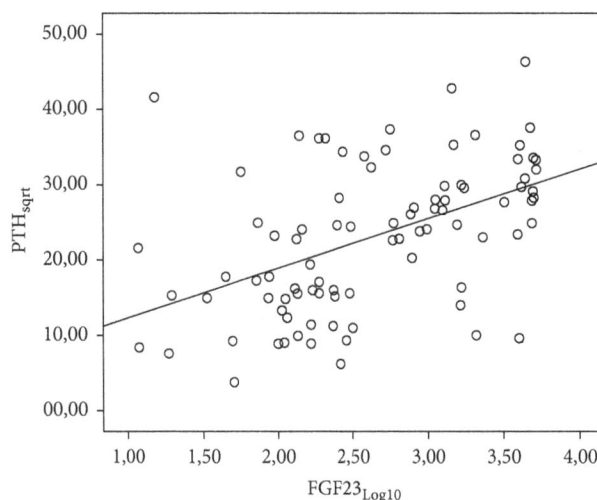

FIGURE 1: Relationship between FGF-23 and iPTH values.

According to the results of univariate analysis, a statistically significant positive correlation was determined between FGF-23 values and iPTH values at a level of 48,0% (r: 0,480; P: 0,001; $P < 0,01$) and a statistically significant positive correlation between FGF-23 values and Ca∗P values at a level of 62,3% (r: 0,623; P: 0,001; $P < 0,01$) (Table 3; Figures 1 and 2).

A statistically significant positive correlation was determined between FGF-23 values and Ca values at a level of 24,6% (r: 0,246; P: 0,021; $P < 0,05$) and a statistically significant positive correlation between FGF-23 values and P values at a level of 59,1% (r: 0,591; P: 0,001; $P < 0,01$) (Table 3, Figure 3).

A statistically significant positive correlation was determined between FGF-23 values and Hb values at a level of 24,7% (r: 0,247; P: 0,020; $P < 0,05$) and a statistically significant positive correlation between FGF-23 values and Htc values at a level of 24,6% (r: 0,246; P: 0,020; $P < 0,05$) (Table 3).

In multivariate analysis, it was observed that the correlation between Hb and Htc values and FGF-23 values becomes insignificant in the model with the effect of the other variables. It was determined that the effects of iPTH and Ca∗P values were significant at the level of $P < 0,01$ (Table 3).

4. Discussion

Fibroblast growth factor-23 has an important effect on mineral metabolism. Serum FGF-23 levels begin to rise as glomerular filtration rate falls under 90 mL/min/per 1,73 square meters. It was shown that serum FGF-23 levels increased before PTH began to rise in chronic kidney disease [8].

Increased serum FGF-23 levels lead to a decrease in calcitriol production, resulting in secretion of PTH. In our study, we demonstrated a positive correlation between serum

Table 3: Evaluation of factors affecting $FGF23_{Log10}$ value.

	Univariate test results		Linear regression analysis results			
	r	P	P	B	95% CI	
					Lower	Upper
Constant	—	—	$0{,}001^{**}$	1,070	0,673	1,467
PTH_{Sqrt}	0,480	$0{,}001^{**}$	$0{,}007^{**}$	0,018	0,005	0,032
Ca∗P	0,623	$0{,}001^{**}$	$0{,}001^{**}$	0,025	0,016	0,035
Ca	0,246	$0{,}021^{*}$	—	—	—	—
P	0,591	$0{,}001^{**}$	—	—	—	—
Hemoglobin	0,247	$0{,}020^{*}$	0,965	−0,009	−0,433	0,414
Hematocrit	0,246	$0{,}020^{*}$	0,742	0,004	−0,020	0,028

PTH: parathormone; Ca: calcium.
* Statistical significance positive correlation ($P < 0{,}05$).
** Statistical significance positive correlation ($P < 0{,}01$).

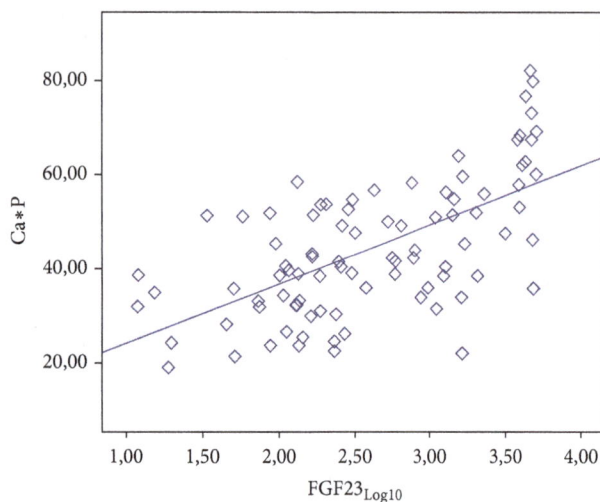

Figure 2: Relationship between FGF-23 and Ca∗P values.

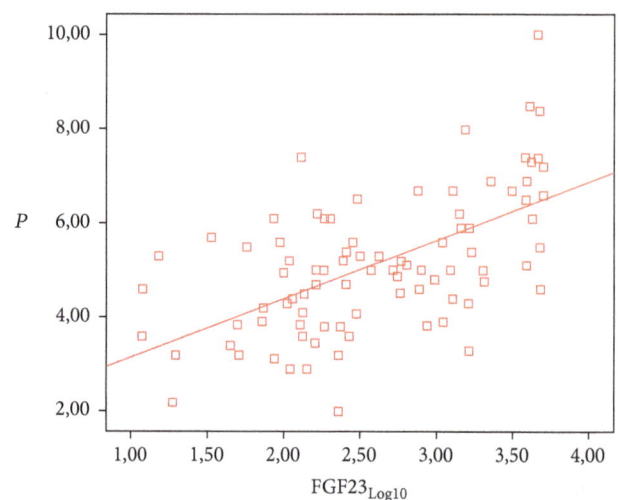

Figure 3: Relationship between FGF-23 and P values.

FGF-23 and PTH levels. Although the duration of dialysis replacement therapy was the same in all the patients, there were differences between the serum FGF-23 levels of the patients. Today, despite similar duration of disease, etiology, and demographic features, studies conducted in the patients with chronic kidney disease and dialysis patients are trying to explain the differences between the serum FGF-23 levels. Some studies reported that high serum FGF-23 levels had an effect in prediction of resistance to vitamin D therapy and refractory secondary hyperparathyroidism [9]. However, its mechanism of action is yet to be explained. Besides phosphate retention, FGF-23 contributes to progression of parathyroid hyperplasia. Therefore, a correlation has been considered between refractory secondary hyperparathyroidism and FGF-23 levels and importance of FGF-23 in the treatment was begun to be emphasized.

Knowledge about the effects of active vitamin D and calcium-containing phosphorus binding therapies on the serum FGF-23 levels is controversial. In this study, we found serum PTH levels to be elevated in the patients with high serum FGF-23 levels, despite administration of high doses of active vitamin D and calcium-containing phosphorus binding therapies. As it was stated by Gogusev et al. [10], it might be caused by the paradoxical correlation between the serum FGF-23 levels and secondary hyperparathyroidism. According to this opinion, this might be caused by insufficient suppression of parathyroid secretion by the parathyroid gland that remains unresponsive to the calcitriol therapy as well as elevated FGF-23 levels that remain unresponsive in refractory secondary hyperparathyroidism [10, 11]. Although the doses and duration of the therapies were similar in all of the patients in our study, high serum levels in the patients with elevated serum PTH and FGF-23 levels could be insufficient in suppression of PTH secretion and resulted in the development of secondary hyperparathyroidism.

There were some studies indicating that serum FGF-23 levels increased following administration of regular active vitamin D and phosphorus binding treatment compared to pretreatment in hemodialysis patients with severe secondary hyperparathyroidism [12, 13]. However, when we compared the patients with high serum FGF-23 levels, patients with severe secondary hyperparathyroidism, and patients with low and/or normally controlled secondary hyperparathyroidism in this study, we found that the doses of active vitamin D and phosphorus binding treatments were similar. Results obtained from the studies on this issue are controversial. Today, explanation of the FGF23-Klotho axis is becoming increasingly important in order to reveal unknown aspect of the treatment of refractory secondary hyperparathyroidism.

Recent studies have shown that coreceptors Klotho and FGFR1c, which activate FGF-23, decreased in uremic parathyroid hyperplasia, and high serum FGF-23 levels could be explained by Klotho-FGFR1c complexes of secondary hyperparathyroidism [14, 15]. Klotho is produced by the kidneys; therefore, it was seen to decrease in parallel with the loss of the renal functions in chronic kidney disease. Besides mineral metabolism, Klotho FGFR1c-FGF23 axis is considered to be a predictor of progression of kidney disease and to be related to morbidity and mortality. However, this was not fully proven with the current studies.

Secondary hyperparathyroidism contributes to anemia by inhibition of red blood cell production, increasing the fragility and leading to bone marrow fibrosis. Anemia is an important determinant of morbidity and mortality in every stage of kidney disease [16]. Considering the positive correlation between the serum FGF-23 levels and PTH, FGF-23 is believed to contribute to the development of anemia in dialysis patients [16]. However, in our study, we did not determine any correlation between high serum parathormone levels and FGF-23 levels and anemia. This result can be attributed to the regular treatment received by the patient. When the effects of different parameters are excluded, determination of correlation between FGF-23 levels and anemia in the group determined to have high serum FGF-23 levels can support our thought. Correlation between the serum ferritin and FGF-23 levels and effects of the parenteral iron therapy on FGF-23 metabolism are yet to be clarified [17]. In this study, all the patients were receiving parenteral iron therapy at different doses. We found no significant difference between the patients with severe secondary hyperparathyroidism high serum FGF-23 levels and the patients with controlled secondary hyperparathyroidism and low and/or normal serum FGF-23 levels in terms of serum iron and ferritin levels and iron binding capacity.

Gutiérrez et al. [18] found that elevated serum FGF-23 levels were not correlated with mortality in the patient group with low serum phosphorus levels, but they were positively correlated with mortality in the patient group with higher serum phosphorus levels. In another study supporting the aforementioned study, the positive effects of high FGF-23 and phosphorus levels on mortality were attributed to more protein intake of the dialysis patients by the authors [19]. In our study, although albumin values were similar in the patients with low and/or normal or high serum FGF-23 levels, C-reactive protein, P, and Ca*P values were found to be higher in the patients with high serum FGF 23 levels. Given the different studies, this might indicate increased risk for calcification and inflammation and it might cause negative effects on morbidity. In the studies investigating the effects of FGF-23 on morbidity and mortality, it was reported that FGF-23 might cause peripheral vascular and tissue proliferation by increasing Ca*P ratio, cellular proliferation, and inflammation and by decreasing calcitriol production and by the toxic effects that we could not explain yet [20, 21].

In this study, we demonstrated that serum FGF-23 levels affected especially the phosphorus metabolism. Besides FGF-23 being a biomarker of phosphate metabolism, we believe that it might also be a biomarker for chronic kidney disease. With a better understanding of the FGF23-Klotho axis, we believe that new approaches might be developed in the treatment of refractory secondary hyperparathyroidism.

5. Conclusions

Elevated serum FGF-23 levels prior to determination of iPTH levels in chronic kidney disease and higher FGF-23 levels in patients with refractory secondary hyperparathyroidism assert the importance of FGF23-Klotho axis. We believe that elucidation of FGF23-Klotho will provide a different approach in the treatment of refractory secondary hyperparathyroidism.

References

[1] B. D. Parker, L. J. Schurgers, V. M. Brandenburg et al., "The associations of fibroblast growth factor 23 and uncarboxylated matrix Gla protein with mortality in coronary artery disease: the heart and soul study," *Annals of Internal Medicine*, vol. 152, no. 10, pp. 640–648, 2010.

[2] M. A. I. Mirza, A. Larsson, H. Melhus, L. Lind, and T. E. Larsson, "Serum intact FGF23 associate with left ventricular mass, hypertrophy and geometry in an elderly population," *Atherosclerosis*, vol. 207, no. 2, pp. 546–551, 2009.

[3] D. Fliser, B. Kollerits, U. Neyer et al., "Fibroblast growth factor 23 (FGF23) predicts progression of chronic kidney disease: the Mild to Moderate Kidney Disease (MMKD) Study," *Journal of the American Society of Nephrology*, vol. 18, no. 9, pp. 2600–2608, 2007.

[4] K. Nakai, H. Komaba, and M. Fukagawa, "New insights into the role of fibroblast growth factor 23 in chronic kidney disease," *Journal of Nephrology*, vol. 23, no. 6, pp. 619–625, 2010.

[5] O. Gutierrez, T. Isakova, E. Rhee et al., "Fibroblast growth factor-23 mitigates hyperphosphatemia but accentuates calcitriol deficiency in chronic kidney disease," *Journal of the American Society of Nephrology*, vol. 16, no. 7, pp. 2205–2215, 2005.

[6] J. B. Wetmore, S. Liu, R. Krebill, R. Menard, and L. D. Quarles, "Effects of cinacalcet and concurrent low-dose vitamin D on FGF23 levels in ESRD," *Clinical Journal of the American Society of Nephrology*, vol. 5, no. 1, pp. 110–116, 2010.

[7] T. Isakova, O. M. Gutiérrez, Y. Chang et al., "Phosphorus binders and survival on hemodialysis," *Journal of the American Society of Nephrology*, vol. 20, no. 2, pp. 388–389, 2009.

[8] J. H. Ix, M. G. Shlipak, C. L. Wassel, and M. A. Whooley, "Fibroblast growth factor-23 and early decrements in kidney function: the heart and soul study," *Nephrology Dialysis Transplantation*, vol. 25, no. 3, pp. 993–997, 2010.

[9] S. Nakanishi, J. J. Kazama, T. Nii-Kono et al., "Serum fibroblast growth factor-23 levels predict the future refractory hyperparathyroidism in dialysis patients," *Kidney International*, vol. 67, no. 3, pp. 1171–1178, 2005.

[10] J. Gogusev, P. Duchambon, B. Hory et al., "Depressed expression of calcium receptor in parathyroid gland tissue of patients with hyperparathyroidism," *Kidney International*, vol. 51, no. 1, pp. 328–336, 1997.

[11] H. Komaba, S. Goto, H. Fujii et al., "Depressed expression of Klotho and FGF receptor 1 in hyperplastic parathyroid glands from uremic patients," *Kidney International*, vol. 77, no. 3, pp. 232–238, 2010.

[12] H. Nishi, T. Nii-Kono, S. Nakanishi et al., "Intravenous calcitriol therapy increases serum concentrations of fibroblast growth factor-23 in dialysis patients with secondary hyperparathyroidism," *Nephron Clinical Practice*, vol. 101, no. 2, pp. c94–c99, 2005.

[13] A. L. E. Cancela, R. B. Oliveira, F. G. Graciolli et al., "Fibroblast growth factor 23 in hemodialysis patients: effects of phosphate binder, calcitriol and calcium concentration in the dialysate," *Nephron—Clinical Practice*, vol. 117, no. 1, pp. c74–c82, 2011.

[14] M.-H. Lafage-Proust, "Does the downregulation of the FGF23 signaling pathway in hyperplastic parathyroid glands contribute to refractory secondary hyperparathyroidism in CKD patients," *Kidney International*, vol. 77, no. 5, pp. 390–392, 2010.

[15] C. Kumata, M. Mizobuchi, H. Ogata et al., "Involvement of alpha-klotho and fibroblast growth factor receptor in the development of secondary hyperparathyroidism," *American Journal of Nephrology*, vol. 31, no. 3, pp. 230–238, 2010.

[16] D. S. Rao, M.-S. Shih, and R. Mohini, "Effect of serum parathyroid hormone and bone marrow fibrosis on the response to erythropoietin in uremia," *The New England Journal of Medicine*, vol. 328, no. 3, pp. 171–175, 1993.

[17] H. Sliem, G. Tawfik, F. Moustafa, and H. Zaki, "Relationship of associated secondary hyperparathyroidism to serum fibroblast growth factor-23 in end stage renal disease: a case-control study," *Indian Journal of Endocrinology and Metabolism*, vol. 15, no. 2, pp. 105–109, 2011.

[18] O. M. Gutiérrez, M. Mannstadt, T. Isakova et al., "Fibroblast growth factor 23 and mortality among patients undergoing hemodialysis," *The New England Journal of Medicine*, vol. 359, no. 6, pp. 584–592, 2008.

[19] E. Ashikaga, H. Honda, H. Suzuki et al., "Impact of fibroblast growth factor 23 on lipids and atherosclerosis in hemodialysis patients," *Therapeutic Apheresis and Dialysis*, vol. 14, no. 3, pp. 315–322, 2010.

[20] G. Jean, E. Bresson, J.-C. Terrat et al., "Peripheral vascular calcification in long-haemodialysis patients: associated factors and survival consequences," *Nephrology Dialysis Transplantation*, vol. 24, no. 3, pp. 948–955, 2009.

[21] P. Kocełak, M. Olszanecka-Glinianowicz, and J. Chudek, "Fibroblast growth factor 23—structure, function and role in kidney diseases," *Advances in Clinical and Experimental Medicine*, vol. 21, no. 3, pp. 391–401, 2012.

7

Automated Fluid Management for Treatment of Rhabdomyolysis

Christian M. Beilstein, John R. Prowle, and Christopher J. Kirwan

Adult Critical Care Unit, The Royal London Hospital, Barts Health NHS Trust, Whitechapel Road, London E1 1BB, UK

Correspondence should be addressed to Christopher J. Kirwan; christopher.kirwan@bartshealth.nhs.uk

Academic Editor: Frank Park

Purpose. Fluid therapy aimed at increasing urine output is a commonly employed strategy to prevent acute kidney injury (AKI) in critically ill patients with rhabdomyolysis. Automated fluid management has the potential to optimise urine output while avoiding fluid accumulation in rhabdomyolysis patients. *Methods.* In a single centre clinical service evaluation we compared a convenience sample of critically ill adults with rhabdomyolysis treated with automated fluid management using the RenalGuard® device to patients managed with manual fluid adjustment following our standard rhabdomyolysis protocol. Primary outcome was number of hours with urine output >2 mL/kg during first 48 h of therapy. *Results.* Eight patients treated with RenalGuard were compared to 28 patients treated with manual fluid management. Number of hours of target urine output was greater in the RenalGuard versus the Standard group (176/312 (56.4%) versus 534/1305 (40.9%); $p < 0.01$). Urine output was significantly higher in the first 24 h in the RenalGuard group (median (IQR) 4033 mL (3682–7363) versus 2913 mL (2263–4188 mL); $p < 0.01$). Fluid balance, electrolyte, diuretics, and bicarbonate use were comparable between groups. *Conclusions.* Automated fluid management resulted in a higher urine output more quickly in the treatment of rhabdomyolysis. Further research is needed to analyse the effect of diuresis-matched hydration for the prevention of AKI in rhabdomyolysis.

1. Introduction

Rhabdomyolysis is the dissolution of striped muscle and has numerous causes. The leakage of muscle-cell contents including electrolytes, myoglobin, and Creatine Phosphokinase (CK) into the blood stream has toxic effects on the kidneys in a number of ways and may lead to acute kidney injury (AKI). Renal injury is understood to be caused by intrarenal vasoconstriction, direct tubular toxicity, and tubular obstruction by Tamm-Horsfall protein containing casts all of which are precipitated by the presence of myoglobin. AKI is reported to complicate between 13 and 50% of cases of rhabdomyolysis [1]. Whilst peak myoglobin predicts AKI better, serum CK remains elevated for longer following rhabdomyolysis and is therefore more widely used to guide therapy [2, 3]. A CK level of greater 5000 U/l is widely accepted as threshold indicating serious muscle injury [4, 5].

The prevention of AKI in patients with significant rhabdomyolysis includes treating the underlying cause (e.g., fasciotomy to relieve compartment syndrome), fluid resuscitation (hypovolaemia is common at diagnosis), and maintaining high urine output with alkalinisation of the urine to prevent precipitation of casts in the renal tubules [6–8]. High volume haemofiltration or super high flux haemodialysis has been used for extracorporeal elimination of myoglobin in severe cases [9, 10].

Rhabdomyolysis is common in our critical care unit (about 7% of all admissions [11]) and treatment is a protocolled high fluid output/input strategy for any patient with a CK greater than 5000 U/l. The protocol targets a urine output of greater than 2 mL per kg estimated body weight (EBW) per hour, a urine pH of greater than 6, and allows the use of loop diuretics and intravenous sodium bicarbonate 1.26% to achieve this. The aim is to replace 100% urine output of the previous hour in the following hour. Our concern is that the delay in manual fluid replacement results in episodic hypovolaemia as it is always "behind" the previous hours output.

The RenalGuard System (PLC Medical Systems, Milford, Massachusetts, USA) works by replacing the patient's urine output millilitre-for-millilitre, minute-by-minute. This accurate, automated real-time replacement reduces the risk of over- or underhydration (i.e., episodic hypovolaemia) relative to standard infusion in the presence of desired high volume diuresis. RenalGuard has previously been tested and evaluated in patients at risk for developing acute kidney injury following coronary or peripheral angiography. It is believed that maintaining a high urine flow rate leads to lower concentration and a faster transit of potentially toxic molecules trough the kidneys, respectively, [12]. There are promising results which suggest a 50–80% relative risk reduction for the development of contrast-induced nephropathy [13, 14].

The aim of this clinical service evaluation is to demonstrate that the RenalGuard device can be safely and practically incorporated into a rhabdomyolysis treatment protocol for critically ill patients that will perform better than the established standard protocol. Our primary outcome measure was number of hours of urine output greater than 2 mL/kg/h. Secondary outcomes were primarily focused on safety (in terms of fluid balance and electrolyte disturbance) and usability, achieving daily set fluid balance, use of electrolyte substitution, loop diuretics and sodium bicarbonate, and premature protocol cessation.

2. Methods

2.1. Governance. This was a prospective clinical service evaluation audit of a commercial medical device and was registered as an audit with the Clinical Effectiveness Unit, Barts Health NHS Trust. All patients were managed using our existing clinical protocol for fluid therapy in rhabdomyolysis.

2.2. Setting. This single-center study was conducted in a 44-bedded general adult critical care unit in East London, United Kingdom. The case mix is split between medical (40%), surgical (30%), and major trauma (30%) patients.

2.3. Outcome Measures. Primary outcome measure: number of hours with urine output greater 2 mL/kg estimated body weight within the first 48 hours using a "standard" rhabdomyolysis protocol versus one incorporating the RenalGuard. Secondary outcome measures were the maintenance of a set fluid balance, the need for electrolyte replacement, the administration of loop diuretics and bicarbonate, and premature protocol cessation.

2.4. Patient Groups. Patients already on or with acute indications for renal replacement therapy or patients with a diagnosis of diabetes insipidus were excluded from use of out rhabdomyolysis management protocol. A convenience sample of patients from 01.01.2015 to 31.04.2015 with a CK greater than 5000 U/l were commenced on rhabdomyolysis treatment using the RenalGuard device if the RebalGuard was not in use already and also if there was a member of the investigating team present to support setting it up.

The final decision regarding management of rhabdomyolysis protocol was with the treating clinician. Data from patients with a transient CK rise of <48 hours were prospectively excluded from our analysis as they would not receive 48 h of protocolled therapy. We compared automated fluid management with the RenalGuard to manual fluid management using the same therapeutic protocol. For our comparison group we audited charts from ICU patients with more than one CK measurement of >5000 U/l in our electronic clinical records system between 01.01.2014 and 31.12.2014. Patients were excluded if they required RRT, had a CK > 5000 U/I for less than 48 hours, and the treatment protocol stopped before 48 hours of treatment had occurred at the instruction of the treating clinician.

2.5. Protocol Application. Rhabdomyolysis protocol using manual fluid management was initiated and implemented by the clinical team without any external intervention and discontinued when the CK fell below 5000 U/l.

The RenalGuard protocol required the investigators to help set up and use the RenalGuard device for the bedside nurse who then followed the protocol independently. The use of the RenalGuard was discontinued by one of the following scenarios: CK fell below 5000 U/l, at the treating clinician's discretion or after 72 h of therapy. If required, the rhabdomyolysis protocol using manual fluid management was continued thereafter.

2.6. Observation Period. We collected observations on all patients for the first 48 hours after the first CK measurement of >5000 U/l.

2.7. Data Collection. All data was collected from the bedside charts, medical notes, and electronic records, retrospectively for the standard group and prospectively for the RenalGuard group. Baseline data included demographic information, diagnosis, and serum Creatinine value on admission to the critical care unit. At 12 h intervals following the diagnosis of rhabdomyolysis, total fluid input, output, and balance were recorded along with hourly urine output, electrolyte, and metabolic indicators from blood gas analysis. In both groups, hours off the ward (e.g., in radiology) were not counted to allow correct calculation of the primary outcome measure as the protocol was paused during these times. We also collected the dose of intravenous electrolyte substitution, loop diuretic, and sodium bicarbonate 1.26%. In addition we recorded >1 L deviations from the set fluid balance, new onset pulmonary oedema, and premature protocol cessation.

2.8. Data Analysis. The number of hours where the target urine output was >2 mL/kg was calculated for every 12-hour period. Average urine output (absolute and per kg) was calculated for every 24-hour period, fluid balance as well as deviation from a set target balance for the whole observation period (48 hours). Data is presented as median (interquartile range) for continuous variables and absolute or relative frequencies as percentages for categorical variables. Serial measures were analysed comparing the area under the

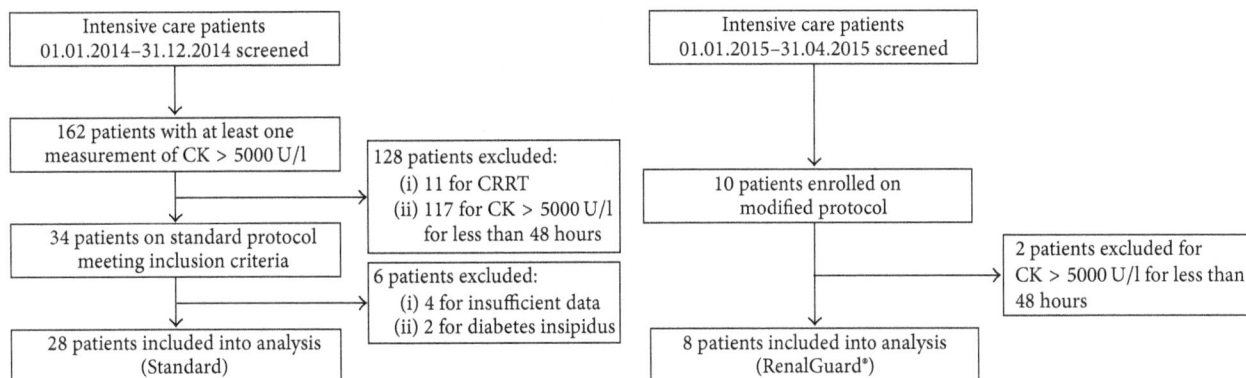

FIGURE 1: Recruitment flow chart.

TABLE 1: Baseline Characteristics (median, interquartile range) and number (percentage); ICU, Intensive Care Unit, IQR, interquartile range; CK, Creatine Phosphokinase; U/l, international units per Litre.

	Manual	RenalGuard
Number (n)	28	8
Age (median, IQR) (years)	31 (21.5–43)	44 (24.5–63)
Gender (n, %)		
Female	6 (21.4)	1 (12.5)
Male	22 (78.6)	7 (87.5)
BMI (median, IQR) (kg/m^2)	24.9 (22.2–26.9)	25 (23.5–29.5)
Creatinine at ICU admission (median, IQR) (mmol/L)	102 (75–133)	99 (92–112)
Peak CK (median, IQR) (U/l)	14 431 (9372–21578)	13 965 (10606–33225)
Primary cause of rhabdomyolysis (n, %)		
Seizure	1 (3.6)	1 (12.5)
Trauma	21 (75.0)	5 (62.5)
Muscle/limb ischaemia	4 (14.3)	2 (25.0)
Postoperative	2 (7.1)	0 (0.0)

curve using the trapezoid method as described by Matthews et al. [15]. Differences in between groups were compared using Mann–Whitney U test and Pearson's chi-square (χ^2) test with continuous and categorical date, respectively. All statistical analysis was carried out using IBM SPSS Statistics 22 (IBM Corp, USA) and Microsoft Excel 2011 (Microsoft Corp, USA).

3. Results

3.1. Baseline Characteristics. We compared 8 patients using automated fluid management with RenalGuard to 28 patients who received manual rhabdomyolysis treatment (Figure 1). Baseline characteristics were comparable (Table 1).

3.2. Hours within Urine Output Target. The urine output target of 2 mL/kg EBW/hour was reached in the first 48 hours in 56.4% hours (176 of 312) in the RenalGuard group and 40.9% (534 of 1305) in the Standard group ($p < 0.01$). The RenalGuard group produced on average more hours of higher urine output more quickly that the standard group ($p = 0.0003$) (Figure 2).

3.3. Urine Output. Urine output in the first 24 hours was significantly higher in the RenalGuard group in comparison to the standard group (Table 2). There was no significant difference in the second 24 hours of the observation period.

3.4. Fluid Balance, Electrolyte Replacement, Loop Diuretic, and Sodium Bicarbonate Administration. Fluid balance at 48 hours was comparable in both groups as was deviation from clinician set daily fluid balance. Electrolyte replacement, dose of loop diuretics, and number of sodium bicarbonate administrations during the protocol period were also comparable (Table 3). Creatinine and blood urea nitrogen (BUN) trends can be found in Table 4. There were no significant differences in acid-base status, electrolytes, or Creatinine Phosphokinase levels at 48 hours between groups (data not shown).

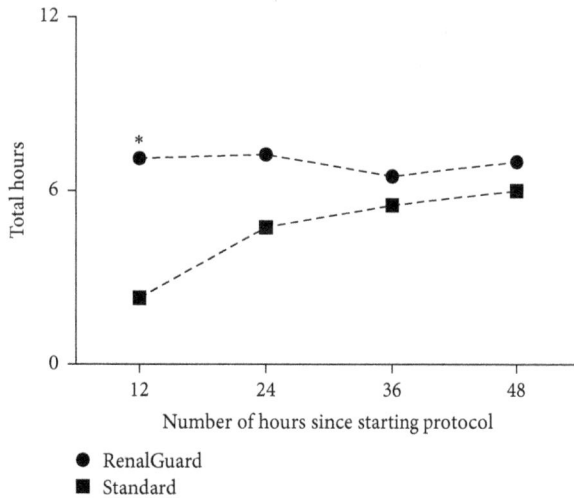

FIGURE 2: The number of hours of urine output >2 mL/kg in each 12 hours of treatment ($^*p < 0.01$).

TABLE 2: Comparison of urine output between groups (median, interquartile range).

	Manual	RenalGuard	p value
Absolute urine output (mL)			
First 24 hours	3006 (2263–4188)	4054 (3682–7363)	0.01
Second 24 hours	4228 (3246–7655)	4311 (3173–11263)	0.58
Observation period (48 hours)	7228 (6044–9454)	7834 (7103–20259)	0.22
Urine output (mL/kg/h)			
First 24 hours	1.6 (1.2–2.2)	2.6 (1.7–4.4)	0.03
Second 24 hours	2.4 (1.9–2.8)	2.3 (1.6–6.7)	0.88
Observation period (48 hours)	1.9 (1.7–2.6)	2.3 (1.7–6.0)	0.41

3.5. Protocol Cessation. The RenalGuard protocol was stopped prematurely in two cases, one for haemodynamic instability and one for the initiation of renal replacement therapy, and both are included in the analysis. A third patient, who is also included in the analysis, had the RenalGuard protocol discontinued at 48 hours of treatment by the treating clinician due to concerns over excessive urine output (30 865 mL over 48 hours) even though the fluid balance had not deviated from the set target. In the remaining 5 patients the RenalGuard was discontinued in line with our rhabdomyolysis protocol for CK lower 5000 U/l after at least 48 hours of treatment in 4. A further case switched to the standard protocol after 72 hours. One patient had a brief interruption of the protocol to change a blocked urinary catheter but was still included in the final analysis. There were no episodes of hypotension requiring the institution of new vasopressors nor were there any episodes of pulmonary oedema requiring invasive or noninvasive ventilation.

4. Discussion

In critically ill patients with rhabdomyolysis, incorporating automatic fluid management using the RenalGuard device increased the number of hours with urine output >2 mL/kg/h in the first 48 hours of treatment. This was primarily due to a reduction in time taken to achieve target urine output compared to a standard protocol in the first 24 hours (Figure 2). These findings are supported by the observation that absolute urine output and urine output per kg per hour were only significantly higher in the RenalGuard group in the first 24 hours of therapy but not thereafter. However, overall, an average target urine output of 2 mL/kg per hour was reached in the RenalGuard group for the whole 48 hours but not in the control group. We hypothesise that automatic urine output replacement might be superior by eliminating the need for error-prone manual calculations and delayed infusion pump adjustments, by avoiding transient intravascular hypovolaemia.

Fluid balances at 48 hours as well as Creatinine trends were similar in both groups. Electrolyte replacement and the administration of loop diuretics and sodium bicarbonate did not significantly differ between the groups demonstrating safety and the efficacy of an automated fluid management approach.

4.1. Strengths and Limitations. This single centre service evaluation is with only a small number of patients aimed at demonstrating that we could use the RenalGuard to implement our current Rhabdomyolysis treatment protocol safely and effectively; these goals were achieved and we were able to easily employ this device to provide comparable management to our current standard of care. To our knowledge, this is the first application of the RenalGuard in critically ill patients with significant rhabdomyolysis. As this was not a trial, small sample size, lack of prospective randomisation, and the use of retrospectively collected control data mean that any findings are susceptible to bias and random effects; therefore, the results can only be taken as hypothesis generating only. In particular the mandatory presence and surveillance by an investigator of patients using RenalGuard during the initial stages of treatment may have enforced better compliance with treatment protocols. Finally, the study was too small to analyse any effect of the different protocols on kidney function and development of AKI, which is the overall intent of fluid administration in Rhabdomyolysis.

5. Conclusions and Future Research

We have demonstrated that the use of a protocol incorporating RenalGuard is effective at rapidly increasing urine output without the need for additional electrolyte replacement and diuretic administration and can achieve results at least comparable to manual fluid management in these patients. A randomised trial would be required to assess the effect of diuresis-matched hydration on prevention of acute kidney injury in severe rhabdomyolysis to demonstrate a therapeutic benefit of automated fluid management to these patients our preliminary data would support further study of the

TABLE 3: Fluid balance, electrolyte replacement, and furosemide and sodium bicarbonate administration (median, interquartile range). Deviation from fluid balance is a delta from set target so positive and negative changes do not cancel each other out.

	Manual	RenalGuard	p value
Actual fluid balance at 48 hours (mL)	2024 (178–4096)	2215 (1278–5170)	0.39
Deviation (above or below) from set target balance (mL)	1720 (−201–2595)	1253 (528–3545)	0.87
Magnesium (g)	0 (0–10)	5 (0–12.5)	0.79
Potassium (mmol)	40 (0–160)	0 (0–40)	0.26
Phosphate (mmol)	0 (0–40)	20 (0–50)	0.69
Sodium bicarbonate 1.26% (n, %)	13 (46.4)	4 (50.0)	0.93
Furosemide (mg)	98 (0–110)	60 (30–102)	0.67

TABLE 4: Creatinine and blood urea nitrogen (BUN) trends in mmol/L, respectively, median (interquartile range).

Patient number	BUN (mmol/L)			Creatinine (mmol/L)		
	First	Maximal	Last	First	Maximal	Last
1	13	24	6	92	232	55
2	6.3	5.3	4.9	121	163	25
3	3.5	9.8	5	149	149	95
4	2.2	5.6	5.6	102	102	49
5	5.7	4.8	4.8	107	107	69
6	4.8	11.2	7.2	77	116	88
7	8.4	16.1	15.8	88	388	188
8	5.4	5.4	3.7	96	96	82
RenalGuard	6 (5–8)	8 (5–12)	5 (5-6)	99 (92–112)	115 (103–160)	66 (56–87)
Manual				102 (75–133)	113 (86–156)	57 (48–67)

RenalGuard device in this context as well as in other groups of critically ill patients who might benefit from precise fluid management.

Competing Interests

The authors have no competing interests in regard to this paper.

Acknowledgments

John R. Prowle has received consulting and speaker fees for Baxter Ltd (Europe) and Nikisso Ltd (Japan). Christopher J. Kirwan has received Speaker fees for Baxter Ltd (Europe).

References

[1] X. Bosch, E. Poch, and J. M. Grau, "Rhabdomyolysis and acute kidney injury," *The New England Journal of Medicine*, vol. 361, no. 1, pp. 62–72, 2009.

[2] A. R. de Meijer, B. G. Fikkers, M. H. de Keijzer, B. G. M. Van Engelen, and J. P. H. Drenth, "Serum creatine kinase as predictor of clinical course in rhabdomyolysis: a 5-year intensive care survey," *Intensive Care Medicine*, vol. 29, no. 7, pp. 1121–1125, 2003.

[3] S. Kasaoka, M. Todani, T. Kaneko et al., "Peak value of blood myoglobin predicts acute renal failure induced by rhabdomyolysis," *Journal of Critical Care*, vol. 25, no. 4, pp. 601–604, 2010.

[4] P. Brancaccio, G. Lippi, and N. Maffulli, "Biochemical markers of muscular damage," *Clinical Chemistry and Laboratory Medicine*, vol. 48, no. 6, pp. 757–767, 2010.

[5] C. V. R. Brown, P. Rhee, L. Chan, K. Evans, D. Demetriades, and G. C. Velmahos, "Preventing renal failure in patients with rhabdomyolysis: do bicarbonate and mannitol make a difference?" *The Journal of Trauma—Injury, Infection and Critical Care*, vol. 56, no. 6, pp. 1191–1196, 2004.

[6] L. Brochard, F. Abroug, M. Brenner et al., "An official ATS/ERS/ESICM/SCCM/SRLF statement: prevention and management of acute renal failure in the ICU patient: an international consensus conference in intensive care medicine," *American Journal of Respiratory and Critical Care Medicine*, vol. 181, no. 10, pp. 1128–1155, 2010.

[7] A. I. Gunal, H. Celiker, A. Dogukan et al., "Early and vigorous fluid resuscitation prevents acute renal failure in the crush victims of catastrophic earthquakes," *Journal of the American Society of Nephrology*, vol. 15, no. 7, pp. 1862–1867, 2004.

[8] N. Iraj, S. Saeed, H. Mostafa et al., "Prophylactic fluid therapy in crushed victims of Bam earthquake," *The American Journal of Emergency Medicine*, vol. 29, no. 7, pp. 738–742, 2011.

[9] L. Zhang, Y. Kang, P. Fu et al., "Myoglobin clearance by continuous venous-venous haemofiltration in rhabdomyolysis with acute kidney injury: a case series," *Injury*, vol. 43, no. 5, pp. 619–623, 2012.

[10] T. Naka, D. Jones, I. Baldwin et al., "Myoglobin clearance by super high-flux hemofiltration in a case of severe rhabdomyolysis: a case report," *Critical Care*, vol. 9, no. 2, pp. R90–R95, 2005.

[11] N. Chakkalakal, R. Taylor, G. Marshall et al., "Rhabdomyolysis and acute kidney injury: incidence, treatments, and outcomes in the ICU," *Intensive Care Medicine*, vol. 39, 2014.

[12] C. Briguori, "Renalguard system: a dedicated device to prevent contrast-induced acute kidney injury," *International Journal of Cardiology*, vol. 168, no. 2, pp. 643–644, 2013.

[13] C. Briguori, G. Visconti, A. Focaccio et al., "Renal insufficiency after contrast media administration trial II (REMEDIAL II): RenalGuard system in high-risk patients for contrast-induced acute kidney injury," *Circulation*, vol. 124, pp. 1260–1269, 2011.

[14] J.-F. Dorval, S. R. Dixon, R. B. Zelman, C. J. Davidson, R. Rudko, and F. S. Resnic, "Feasibility study of the RenalGuard™ balanced hydration system: a novel strategy for the prevention of contrast-induced nephropathy in high risk patients," *International Journal of Cardiology*, vol. 166, no. 2, pp. 482–486, 2013.

[15] J. N. S. Matthews, D. G. Altman, M. J. Campbell, and P. Royston, "Analysis of serial measurements in medical research," *British Medical Journal*, vol. 300, no. 6719, pp. 230–235, 1990.

8

Clinical Use of Diuretics in Heart Failure, Cirrhosis, and Nephrotic Syndrome

Ahmed Hassaan Qavi,[1] **Rida Kamal,**[1] **and Robert W. Schrier**[2]

[1]*Shifa College of Medicine, Shifa Tameer-e-Millat University, Pitras Bukhari Road, Sector H-8/4, Islamabad 44000, Pakistan*
[2]*Division of Renal Diseases and Hypertension, University of Colorado School of Medicine, 12700 East 19th Avenue C281, Research Building 2, Room 7001, Aurora, CO 80045, USA*

Correspondence should be addressed to Ahmed Hassaan Qavi; ahmed.h.qavi@gmail.com

Academic Editor: Kazunari Kaneko

Diuretics play significant role in pharmacology and treatment options in medicine. This paper aims to review and evaluate the clinical use of diuretics in conditions that lead to fluid overload in the body such as cardiac failure, cirrhosis, and nephrotic syndrome. To know the principles of treatment it is essential to understand the underlying pathophysiological mechanisms that cause the need of diuresis in the human body. Various classes of diuretics exist, each having a unique mode of action. A systemic approach for management is recommended based on the current guidelines, starting from thiazides and proceeding to loop diuretics. The first condition for discussion in the paper is cardiac failure. Treatment of ascites in liver cirrhosis with spironolactone as the primary agent is highlighted with further therapeutic options. Lastly, management choices for nephrotic syndrome are discussed and recommended beginning from basic sodium restriction to combined diuretic therapies. Major side effects are discussed.

1. Background

Choosing the suitable use of diuretics in patients with heart failure, nephrotic syndrome and cirrhosis requires an understanding of the pathophysiology of these edematous conditions. These diseases lead to sodium and water retention in patients, causing detrimental effects in their morbidity and mortality. Heart failure decreases cardiac output and cirrhosis causes progressive systemic arterial vasodilation, which eventually leads to ascites [1]. Nephrotic syndrome causes retention through defective glomerular barriers, induction of the distal nephron and altered capillary permeability [2]. It also leads to hypoalbuminemia, which decreases plasma oncotic pressure, thereby indirectly causing edema [3].

The body fluid volume regulation hypothesis suggests a common circulation pathway for the three disorders [4]. According to this, the underfilling due to low cardiac output or peripheral vasodilation leads to activation of sympathetic nervous system and nonosmotic arginine vasopressin release. Consequently, diminished water and sodium delivery at collecting duct sites in addition to renal adrenergic activity induces renin angiotensin aldosterone system, which enhances tubular reabsorption [1, 4–6].

The cortical collecting tubules are the primary site to contribute to the edema formation in nephrotic syndrome. These are primarily made up of principal and intercalated cells which function to reabsorb sodium and water and excrete potassium. Sodium retention is caused primarily by transcriptional induction of Na/K/ATPase pump. This activation is independent of aldosterone and vasopressin [7]. The electrochemical gradient setup by the Na/K/ATPase pump drives sodium through the apical membranes containing epithelial sodium channels (ENaC). Defective glomerular filtration barrier leaks plasma proteases such as plasmin, prostasin, and kallikrein that cause proteolytic activation of ENaC [8, 9]. Enhanced sodium retention through the aforementioned mechanisms along with proteinuria and hypoalbuminemia via impaired glomerular filtration barrier leads to asymmetrical extracellular volume expansion [2, 9].

As described previously, two pathophysiological processes cause edema formation. Firstly, shifts in capillary pressures promote movement of fluid from the vascular compartment into the interstitium. Secondly, the kidneys cause retention of sodium and water [10]. Consequently, there is marked expansion of the total extracellular volume with plasma volume kept close to normal levels. Clinically these events have great significance. Tissue perfusion is returned to normal through appropriate compensation at the price of expanding the degree of edema in most edematous disorders that cause water and sodium retention [10]. Diuretic therapy drains the edema fluid causing recovery from symptoms due to edema but infrequently results in a decrease in tissue perfusion. On the other hand, primary renal dysfunction leads to inappropriate renal fluid retention where both plasma and interstitial volumes are swelled. Hence, diuretic therapy may not cause any significantly adverse effects as superfluous fluid is excreted [10].

The pharmacology of the various classes of diuretics is important to know for clinical application. All classes of diuretics have different mechanisms of action; however various forms of diuretics from one class have similar pharmacological characteristics [11]. For instance, since all loop diuretics operate similarly, addition of another loop diuretic after one with appropriate dosage failing to show response is not warranted. Instead, a combination therapy with administration of different classes of diuretic is recommended [11, 12].

Thiazide diuretics work by blocking the sodium-chloride transporter [12] and loop diuretics act by inhibiting the sodium-potassium-chloride pump in the thick ascending limb of the loop of Henle [13]. Amiloride and triamterene block apical sodium channels in the distal nephron [14, 15]. All diuretics but spironolactone reach these luminal transport sites through the tubular fluid. Spironolactone competitively binds receptors at the aldosterone-dependent sodium-potassium exchange site in the distal convoluted renal tubule. Except osmotic diuretics, all diuretics are actively secreted into the urine by proximal tubule cells. Loops, thiazides, and acetazolamide are secreted through the organic-acid pathway while amiloride and triamterene are secreted through the organic-base pathway [12, 14, 15]. These drugs escape ultrafiltration at the glomerulus due to their high protein binding, more than 95% [11, 12]. Figure 1 outlines the basic management strategies employed in the three main edematous conditions.

2. Use of Diuretics in Heart Failure

Heart failure is the foremost cause of morbidity among the elderly Americans. It accounts for more than 1 million hospital admissions annually in the US [16]. After hospitalization, 50% of heart failure patients are readmitted to hospitals within 6 months and 25–30% expire at 1 year [17]. Numerous clinical trials have all failed to deduce a universal drug therapy strategy to treat acute heart failure by decreasing mortality or rehospitalization rates [18]. The Acute Heart Failure Registry (ADHERE), comprising of over 105, 000 hospitalized patients, showed 90% of them being treated with intravenous loop diuretics and 30% showed

resistance to diuretic therapy [19]. These patients were suffering from signs and symptoms that included breathlessness (89%), pulmonary rales (67%), and peripheral edema (66%) [19].

Diuretics are well established as the first-line therapy for heart failure patients with congestion [20]. A meta-analysis assessing the benefits of diuretics in chronic heart failure showed a decrease in mortality (3 trials, 202 patients) and worsening heart failure (2 trials, 169 patients) in patients compared to placebo. A few clinical trials (4 trials, 169 patients) also demonstrated that diuretics improved exercise tolerance in patients with chronic heart failure compared to active controls [20]. Diuretics have also established their superiority over device-based strategies. In a randomized controlled trial (RCT) involving 188 hospitalized patients with acute decompensated heart failure, poor renal function, and persistent congestion, treatment with intravenous diuretics was compared to ultrafiltration. Diuretics proved to be more efficacious in the preservation of renal function and had lesser adverse effects than ultrafiltration. The serious adverse effects compared were renal and heart failure, anemia, thrombocytopenia, and gastrointestinal hemorrhage [21].

Mild congestive heart failure is initially managed with a thiazide diuretic [11]. However, loop diuretics (e.g., furosemide, torsemide, or bumetanide) are the principal drugs used in the treatment of heart failure [22]. Severe heart failure causes decrease in the rate of absorption of loop diuretics. Hence, peak response arises 4 hours or more after the dose has been administered [23]. Furosemide has a variable oral absorption from 10% to 100% while bumetanide and torsemide have closer to 100% absorptive capacity [12, 22]. Studies show that patients suffering from heart failure (New York Heart Association (NYHA) class II or III) have 1/3rd to 1/4th the natriuretic response to maximally effective dose of loop diuretics. Administering moderate doses at decreased intervals can elevate the response. However giving large doses causes no change in response [12].

Loop diuretics are administered by a threshold type dose-response curve. Furosemide is started with 20 mg and can be incremented up to 40 mg according to the diuretic response. Maximum single oral doses of furosemide for patients with normal glomerular filtration range from 40 to 80 mg and the maximum daily dose is 600 mg. If maximum dose has already been given, it is recommended to increase the frequency of the dose to 2 or 3 times a day. Bumetanide is given at a dose ranging from 2 to 3 mg per day (initial oral dose: 0.5 to 1.0 mg, maximum dose: 10 mg per day) while torsemide is given at 20 to 50 mg per day (initial oral dose: 5 to 10 mg, maximum: 200 mg per day) [24, 25].

Several studies [26–29] have provided evidence that torsemide and bumetanide are more effective than furosemide in the treatment of heart failure. These agents showed superiority in reducing symptoms such as dyspnea and fatigue and resulted in an increased weight loss. Significant decrease in the rates of hospital readmissions and all-cause mortality was also seen [26–29]. These results can be attributed to the higher bioavailability of torsemide and bumetanide over furosemide as described above. Torsemide,

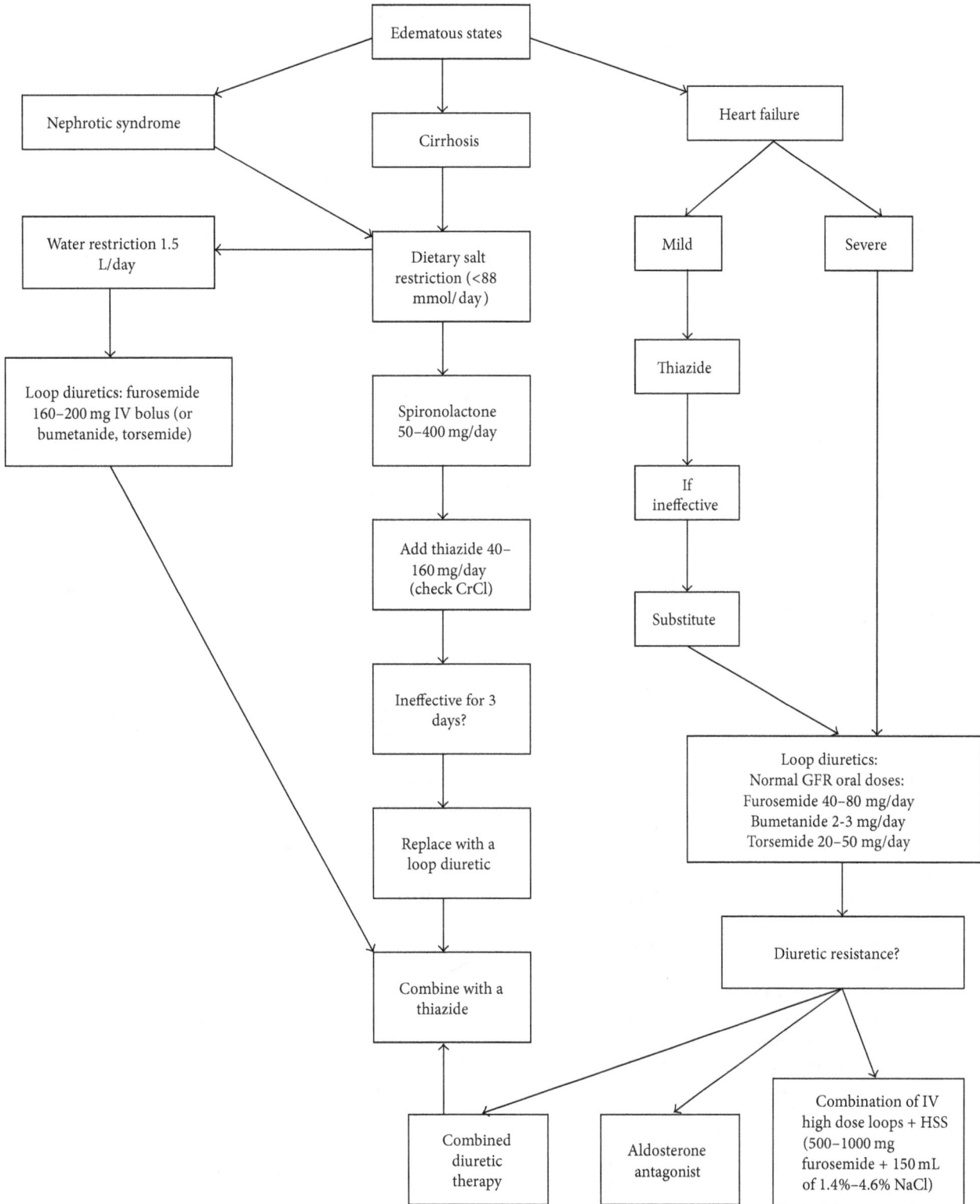

FIGURE 1: Management of edematous states with diuretics. Abbreviations: HSS: hypertonic saline solution [11, 12, 24, 25, 30–33].

in addition, has a longer half-life than both furosemide and bumetanide [26].

Intravenous diuretics are considered to be more potent than oral doses and are used in advanced heart failure.

Furosemide is initially administered at a dose ranging from 20 to 40 mg or up to 2.5 times the previously unsuccessful oral dose. In case of a lack of response, the dose can be doubled and repeated at 2-hour intervals till maximum allowed dose levels are reached. The maximum intravenous doses in patients with normal glomerular filtration are 160 to 200 mg of furosemide, 20 to 40 mg of torsemide, or 1 to 2 mg of bumetanide. If a patient has renal dysfunction, higher maximum bolus doses are recommended: 160 to 200 mg of furosemide, 100 to 200 mg of torsemide, or 4 to 8 mg of bumetanide [25].

A Cochrane meta-analysis of 8 trials (254 patients) demonstrated poor evidence to confer supremacy of continuous infusion of loop diuretics over bolus injection in congestive heart failure patients. The results showed an insignificant increase in diuretic effect and better safety profile of the continuous infusion form [39]. A recent single-center, pilot RCT showed that continuous furosemide infusion could lead to better diuresis and greater reduction in b-type natriuretic peptide (BNP) levels for inpatients as compared with bolus injections of furosemide. Nonetheless, the continuous infusion was associated with worsening renal function, longer hospitalizations, and higher rates of adverse episodes during follow-up [40]. A recent large review and meta-analysis (10 trials, 518 patients) showed meaningful differences in neither the efficacy nor the safety of continuous infusion of loop diuretic compared with bolus injections in patients with acute decompensated heart failure [41]. Another meta-analysis to resolve the disparity in previous studies was done, which included 18 RCTs (936 patients). Results failed to exhibit a significant increase in diuresis with the continuous infusion form. However, this review described that, by administering a loading dose and following it up with continuous loop diuretic infusion, a substantial diuresis is achieved in hospitalized patients [42]. All trials and reviews agreed that further, larger studies are warranted to examine if the explored benefits can convert into improved clinical outcomes [39–42].

Combination diuretic therapy (CDT), comprising of loop plus a thiazide diuretic, is recommended for overcoming diuretic resistance in patients with severe volume overload, refractory to adequate dosage (IV furosemide, 160 to 320 mg per day) of intravenous loop diuretic [30]. This approach produces diuretic synergy via "sequential nephron blockade." Thiazide diuretics block distal tubule sodium reabsorption and can thereby antagonize the renal adaptation to chronic loop diuretic therapy. This improves diuretic resistance secondary to rebound sodium retention. The use of CDT has been shown to result in weight loss, symptomatic improvement, decrease in systemic congestion, hospital discharge, and prevention of readmission. However, careful inspection and frequent monitoring of electrolytes and renal function tests is essential with initiation of CDT as this therapy can lead to severe hypokalemia. Metolazone at a starting dose of 2.5 mg daily is advised for 2 to 3 times weekly dosing in outpatient setting. A 10 mg initial daily dose of metolazone is suggested for inpatients with a 3-day limit to the drug course [30].

Clinical trials such as the Randomized Aldactone Evaluation Study (RALES trial) and the Eplerenone Post-Acute Myocardial Infarction Heart Failure Efficacy and Survival Study (EPHESUS trial) have demonstrated benefits of using aldosterone antagonists (spironolactone or eplerenone) in addition to loop diuretics [43, 44]. The RALES trial demonstrated a 30% reduction in all-cause mortality, with a mean spironolactone dose of 26 mg per day and a 35% reduction in hospitalization for heart failure [43, 45]. In a patient suffering from decompensated heart failure with fluid overload who shows resistance to loop diuretics, natriuretic doses of aldosterone antagonists (spironolactone 50 to 100 mg per day) can be considered as an option [46]. The EPHESUS trial also showed the benefit of eplerenone in decreasing morbidity in dose ranging from 25 to 50 mg per day in patients with heart failure after an acute myocardial infarction and left ventricular systolic dysfunction [44]. One meta-analysis (8 trials, 3929 patients) ascertained that the additional use of an aldosterone antagonist (spironolactone, eplerenone, or canrenone) in treating chronic heart failure patients (NYHA class I to II) reduces mortality and rehospitalization rates and improves heart function with the reversal of left ventricle remodeling [47].

Another positive approach towards diuretic resistant heart failure is the combination of intravenous high-dose loop diuretics with hypertonic saline solutions. Studies have shown this treatment to be efficacious as well as well-tolerated (serum creatinine <2.5 mg/dL) providing symptomatic relief as well as decreasing rehospitalization and long-term mortality [31, 48, 49]. One RCT enrolled 170 patients with refractory congestive heart failure (NYHA class IV) who were unresponsive to high-dose oral furosemide. Treating these patients with intravenous infusion of furosemide (500 to 1000 mg) plus hypertonic saline solution (150 mL of 1.4%–4.6% NaCl) twice a day in 30 minutes showed better daily diuresis and natriuresis in addition to improvement in the quality of life through the relief of signs and symptoms of congestion. Long-term benefit in reduction of mortality rate was also observed when compared with the group receiving intravenous bolus of furosemide (500 to 1000 mg) twice a day, without hypertonic saline solution (55% v 13% survival rate) [31].

Effectiveness of V2 receptor antagonists to treat water retention and hyponatremia in severe heart failure is encouraging. Conivaptan can be used parenterally for inpatients for 4 days while tolvaptan is administered orally for the first day to treat hyponatremia and serum sodium levels are monitored every 6 to 8 hours [1]. The use of tolvaptan may be an effective alternative in the short-term but its use may be limited by its price [48]. Evidence also suggests that tolvaptan can effectively correct chronic hyponatremia for as long as 2 years with minimal side effects (increased urination, thirst) [1, 50].

3. Use of Diuretics in Cirrhosis with Ascites

The usually advised first-line therapy includes sodium restriction to 88 mmol/d (2000 mg sodium per day) [51]. Oral diuretics and total abstinence from alcohol are both considered the second line of treatment [11]. Spironolactone is the first-line diuretic recommended for a patient with cirrhosis and edema, initiating with a dose of 50 mg. With its long half-life, doses are altered after 3 to 4 days. Maximum titration sometimes requires higher doses, up to 400 mg per day. However, this may cause gynecomastia [11, 12]. Spironolactone when used alone was as effective as its combined therapy with furosemide [32]. Amiloride can be used as an alternative, initiating with 5 mg per day and titrating up to 20 mg per day. However it is not as effective as spironolactone [51].

In case of an inadequate response to spironolactone, thiazide diuretics are added to the regimen. Depending upon the patient's renal status, doses of 40 mg per day to a maximum of 160 mg per day can be used. Thiazides are terminated if the patient does not respond after 3 days and replaced with a loop diuretic. In patients with renal impairment, frequent doses of moderate amounts are preferred instead of a single large dose. If results are not desirable, spironolactone and thiazides may be added to the regimen. Dietary salt restriction should be ordered in all patients [11, 12].

In comparing the efficacy of furosemide and spironolactone in a randomized comparative study, the activity of the renin angiotensin system proved to alter the action of these diuretics. Patients with high renin and aldosterone levels failed to respond to furosemide but were successfully treated with 300 mg per day of spironolactone [52]. When compared to furosemide, the long acting torsemide produced greater urinary output [53]. Similar results were obtained in an RCT conducted over 70 days with torsemide when compared to furosemide [54]. Administration of octreotide in combination with diuretics not only suppressed both plasma glucagon levels and renin angiotensin system, thereby improving portal and systemic hemodynamics [55].

In a prospective cohort study, human serum albumin was administered to patients who had serum albumin concentration less than 3.5 g/dL and were being treated with furosemide and spironolactone. The body weight loss recorded was dependent upon the amount of human serum albumin administered instead of the dose of diuretics [56]. A reduction in plasma renin concentration was observed in patients treated with human serum albumin combined with diuretic therapy [57].

Combined therapy of 200 mg per day of potassium canrenoate and 50 mg per day of furosemide was more effective when compared with sequential therapy in patients with moderate ascites. Complications such as hyperkalemia were more profound in patients being treated with sequential therapy [58]. Potassium canrenoate and spironolactone are both in the aldosterone antagonist family, having a common metabolite called canrenone spironolactone is more potent and has in addition sulfur-containing metabolites, which have a high renal clearance, thereby allowing access to their site of activity via the renal tubular fluid [59]. For treatment of tense ascites in hospitalized patients, therapeutic paracentesis along with plasma expanders has replaced diuretic therapy and results in fewer complications. However, maintenance diuretics must be given afterwards to prevent recurrence [60].

4. Use of Diuretics in Nephrotic Syndrome

Nephrotic syndrome is defined by the presence of proteinuria, edema, hyperlipidemia, and hypoalbuminemia. The incidence of nephrotic syndrome is about 3 new cases per 100,000 each year in adults [33]. Besides the management of underlying disease, treatment of nephrotic syndrome includes limiting proteinuria and inducing diuresis to reduce fluid overload. The key to effective treatment is to create a negative sodium balance. Patients are asked to restrict their dietary sodium intake (<100 mmol per day; 3 g per day), restrict their fluid intake (1.5 liters per day), and take diuretics. Edema should be toned down gradually by avoiding vigorous diuresis that may lead to electrolyte disturbances, acute renal injury, and thromboembolism secondary to hemoconcentration [33].

Due to low serum albumin levels, the diffusion of diuretics in the extracellular compartment is increased. Therefore, a combination of albumin and diuretic may be needed to achieve adequate levels of loop diuretic at the active site. An infusion of 30 mg of furosemide with 25 g of albumin may improve the diuresis. The tubular secretion of furosemide is not affected by this combined therapy. However, this may not apply to patients with serum albumin concentrations of less than 2 g/dL. Therefore, in such patients combined therapies may be theoretically beneficial [61–63]. Moreover, with lesser creatinine clearance, larger doses of diuretic are required to achieve adequate free, unbound drug at the site of action [11, 12].

Coadministration of furosemide with albumin was approved in an RCT with results showing greater urine output and sodium excretion [64]. A meta-analysis revealed that the combination of furosemide and albumin in hypoalbuminic patients demonstrated significant results only within the first 8 hours with respect to greater urine volume and sodium excretion. Results in the next 24 hours were not significant [65]. Another study had conflicting results and concluded that furosemide and albumin combinations should be reserved for diuretic resistant patient with severe hypoalbuminemia [66].

The challenge is to administer the right amount of dose that will reach the active site. The largest dose, also known as the ceiling dose, is an IV bolus of furosemide, 160 to 200 mg or the equivalent of bumetanide and torsemide. Administering such doses yields maximum results however it must be noted that maximum effect is only 20% of filtered sodium [11].

There is evidence indicating that the addition of thiazides with loop diuretics increases overall effectiveness [11]. Metolazone-furosemide combination of diuretics was compared with the thiazide-furosemide combination and it was concluded that similar results occurred with both combinations [67]. Choice of combination diuretics depends highly upon the pharmacokinetics of the drug. Metolazone's action does not differ much from thiazides except for the fact that its elimination half-life is much longer at up to 2 days [11]. In a study assessing the long-term effect of metolazone in patients with nephrotic syndrome, loss of edema and improved control of blood pressure was observed. Moreover, addition of furosemide enhanced diuresis [68].

In a prospective study assessing treatment of children with severe edema and nephrotic syndrome, diuretics were used alone in patients with volume expansion contrary to the regimen of diuretics with albumin in patients with volume contraction. The rationale was the fluid overload associated

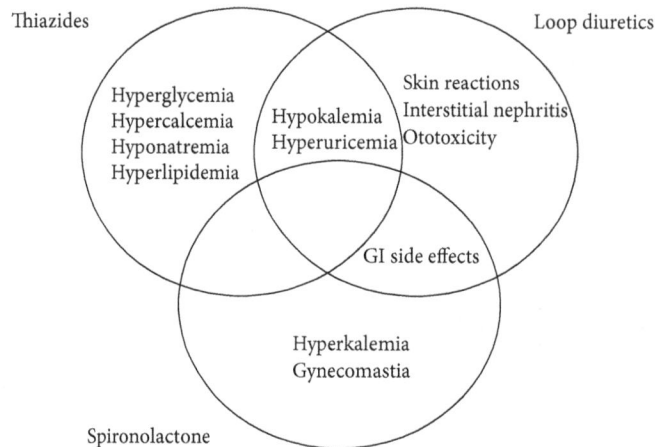

FIGURE 2: Adverse effects of major diuretics [11, 12, 34–38].

with albumin administration. Patients with volume expansion were given IV furosemide at 1 mg/kg per dose up to 40 mg twice daily and oral spironolactone at 2.5 mg/kg per dose divided twice daily up to 100 mg. The study concluded that treatment with diuretics alone in pediatric age group was safe and effective [69]. Three children were given a combination of mannitol and furosemide, which led to promising results of 10–30% weight reduction and edema in a week [70].

5. Adverse Effects of Diuretics

Thiazide diuretics are known to cause hypokalemia that may result in arrhythmias [34, 35]. The hypokalemic state causes increased blood glucose levels. Correction of potassium levels resolves this glucose intolerance. Thiazides compete with uric acid in renal tubular secretion, which ultimately precipitates hyperuricemia. This state can be managed by taking uric acid lowering drugs such as allopurinol along with thiazides [36]. Loop diuretics are known to cause interstitial nephritis and skin reactions. Loops have to be carefully monitored, especially in high doses as they can precipitate transient ototoxicity. Administering loop diuretics is also associated with hypokalemia, which could cause cardiac arrhythmias and lead to mortality [37]. Loop and thiazide diuretics deplete the body of not only potassium but also magnesium. Their synergistic use results in even further losses of these cations. Oral supplementation and/or potassium-sparing diuretics are used to recover from these losses [11, 12]. The mineralocorticoid receptor antagonist spironolactone, but not eplerenone, can result in gynecomastia [11, 12]. Increased incidence of hyperkalemia was observed with spironolactone. Gastrointestinal side effects and gynecomastia were more pronounced when a combination of spironolactone and furosemide was used compared to a combination of amiloride and furosemide [38].

Figure 2 illustrates the common side effects of the main diuretics.

6. Conclusions

Effective and adequate diuresis can be achieved in patients with cardiac failure, cirrhosis, and nephrotic syndrome with ideal therapeutic approach of diuretics therapy. Therapy should be directed first to the primary disease mechanism and later to the patient [11, 12]. Each underlying disorder influences the action of the diuretic being administered; therefore, correct choice of drug is essential for successful management [12].

References

[1] R. W. Schrier, "Use of diuretics in heart failure and cirrhosis," *Seminars in Nephrology*, vol. 31, no. 6, pp. 503–512, 2011.

[2] A. Doucet, G. Favre, and G. Deschênes, "Molecular mechanism of edema formation in nephrotic syndrome: therapeutic implications," *Pediatric Nephrology*, vol. 22, no. 12, pp. 1983–1990, 2007.

[3] N. Perico and G. Remuzzi, "Edema of the nephrotic syndrome: the role of the atrial peptide system," *American Journal of Kidney Diseases*, vol. 22, no. 3, pp. 355–366, 1993.

[4] R. W. Schrier, A. K. Gurevich, and M. A. Cadnapaphornchai, "Pathogenesis and management of sodium and water retention in cardiac failure and cirrhosis," *Seminars in Nephrology*, vol. 21, no. 2, pp. 157–172, 2001.

[5] R. W. Schrier and R. G. Fassett, "Pathogenesis of sodium and water retention in cardiac failure," *Renal Failure*, vol. 20, no. 6, pp. 773–781, 1998.

[6] R. W. Schrier, "Water and sodium retention in edematous disorders: role of vasopressin and aldosterone," *The American Journal of Medicine*, vol. 119, no. 7, supplement 1, pp. S47–S53, 2006.

[7] G. Deschênes, V. Guigonis, and A. Doucet, "Molecular mechanism of edema formation in nephrotic syndrome," *Archives de Pediatrie*, vol. 11, no. 9, pp. 1084–1094, 2004.

[8] P. Svenningsen, H. Andersen, L. H. Nielsen, and B. L. Jensen, "Urinary serine proteases and activation of ENaC in kidney—implications for physiological renal salt handling and hypertensive disorders with albuminuria," *Pflugers Archiv*, vol. 467, no. 3, pp. 531–542, 2014.

[9] E. C. Siddall and J. Radhakrishnan, "The pathophysiology of edema formation in the nephrotic syndrome," *Kidney International*, vol. 82, no. 6, pp. 635–642, 2012.

[10] A. C. Guyton, "The microcirculation and the lymphatic system," in *Textbook of Medical Physiology*, chapter 16, Saunders, Philadelphia, Pa, USA, 8th edition, 1991.

[11] D. C. Brater, "Update in diuretic therapy: clinical pharmacology," *Seminars in Nephrology*, vol. 31, no. 6, pp. 483–494, 2011.

[12] D. C. Brater, "Diuretic therapy," *The New England Journal of Medicine*, vol. 339, no. 6, pp. 387–395, 1998.

[13] D. H. Ellison, "Diuretic drugs and the treatment of edema: from clinic to bench and back again," *American Journal of Kidney Diseases*, vol. 23, no. 5, pp. 623–643, 1994.

[14] K. Besseghir and B. Rennick, "Renal tubule transport and electrolyte effects of amiloride in the chicken," *Journal of Pharmacology and Experimental Therapeutics*, vol. 219, no. 2, pp. 435–441, 1981.

[15] S. T. Kau, "Handling of triamterene by the isolated perfused rat kidney," *Journal of Pharmacology and Experimental Therapeutics*, vol. 206, no. 3, pp. 701–709, 1978.

[16] D. Lloyd-Jones, R. Adams, M. Carnethon et al., "Heart disease and stroke statistics—2009 update: a report from the American Heart Association Statistics Committee and Stroke Statistics Subcommittee," *Circulation*, vol. 119, no. 3, pp. 480–486, 2009.

[17] S. A. Hunt, W. T. Abraham, M. H. Chin et al., "2009 focused update incorporated into the ACC/AHA 2005 guidelines for the diagnosis and management of heart failure in adults: a report of the American College of Cardiology Foundation/American Heart Association Task Force on Practice Guidelines Developed in Collaboration With the International Society for Heart and Lung Transplantation," *Journal of the American College of Cardiology*, vol. 53, no. 15, pp. e1–e90, 2009.

[18] G. M. Felker, P. S. Pang, K. F. Adams et al., "Clinical trials of pharmacological therapies in acute heart failure syndromes: lessons learned and directions forward," *Circulation: Heart Failure*, vol. 3, no. 2, pp. 314–325, 2010.

[19] M. Gheorghiade and G. Filippatos, "Reassessing treatment of acute heart failure syndromes: the ADHERE Registry," *European Heart Journal*, vol. 7, supplement, pp. B13–B19, 2005.

[20] R. F. Faris, M. Flather, H. Purcell, P. A. Poole-Wilson, and A. J. Coats, "Diuretics for heart failure," *Cochrane Database of Systematic Reviews*, no. 2, Article ID CD003838, 2012.

[21] B. A. Bart, S. R. Goldsmith, K. L. Lee et al., "Ultrafiltration in decompensated heart failure with cardiorenal syndrome," *The New England Journal of Medicine*, vol. 367, no. 24, pp. 2296–2304, 2012.

[22] D. Shchekochikhin, F. Al Ammary, J. Lindenfeld, and R. Schrier, "Role of diuretics and ultrafiltration in congestive heart failure," *Pharmaceuticals*, vol. 6, no. 7, pp. 851–866, 2013.

[23] M. R. Vasko, D. B. Cartwright, J. P. Knochel, J. V. Nixon, and D. C. Brater, "Furosemide absorption altered in decompensated congestive heart failure," *Annals of Internal Medicine*, vol. 102, no. 3, pp. 314–318, 1985.

[24] D. C. Brater, B. Day, A. Burdette, and S. Anderson, "Bumetanide and furosemide in heart failure," *Kidney International*, vol. 26, no. 2, pp. 183–189, 1984.

[25] S. A. Hunt, W. T. Abraham, M. H. Chin et al., "2009 focused update incorporated into the ACC/AHA 2005 Guidelines for the Diagnosis and Management of Heart Failure in Adults: a report of the American College of Cardiology Foundation/American Heart Association Task Force on Practice Guidelines: developed in collaboration with the International Society for Heart and Lung Transplantation," *Journal of the American College of Cardiology*, vol. 53, no. 15, pp. e1–e90, 2009.

[26] K. A. Wargo and W. M. Banta, "A comprehensive review of the loop diuretics: should furosemide be first line?" *Annals of Pharmacotherapy*, vol. 43, no. 11, pp. 1836–1847, 2009.

[27] J. J. Dinicolantonio, "Should torsemide be the loop diuretic of choice in systolic heart failure?" *Future Cardiology*, vol. 8, no. 5, pp. 707–728, 2012.

[28] M. D. Murray, M. M. Deer, J. A. Ferguson et al., "Open-label randomized trial of torsemide compared with furosemide therapy for patients with heart failure," *The American Journal of Medicine*, vol. 111, no. 7, pp. 513–520, 2001.

[29] J. Cosín and J. Díez, "Torasemide in chronic heart failure: results of the TORIC study," *European Journal of Heart Failure*, vol. 4, no. 4, pp. 507–513, 2002.

[30] J. C. Jentzer, T. A. Dewald, and A. F. Hernandez, "Combination of loop diuretics with thiazide-type diuretics in heart failure," *Journal of the American College of Cardiology*, vol. 56, no. 19, pp. 1527–1534, 2010.

[31] G. Licata, P. Di Pasquale, G. Parrinello et al., "Effects of high-dose furosemide and small-volume hypertonic saline solution infusion in comparison with a high dose of furosemide as bolus in refractory congestive heart failure: long-term effects," *American Heart Journal*, vol. 145, no. 3, pp. 459–466, 2003.

[32] J. Santos, R. Planas, A. Pardo et al., "Spironolactone alone or in combination with furosemide in the treatment of moderate ascites in nonazotemic cirrhosis. A randomized comparative study of efficacy and safety," *Journal of Hepatology*, vol. 39, no. 2, pp. 187–192, 2003.

[33] R. P. Hull and D. J. A. Goldsmith, "Nephrotic syndrome in adults," *British Medical Journal*, vol. 336, no. 7654, pp. 1185–1189, 2008.

[34] H. Velázquez and F. S. Wright, "Control by drugs of renal potassium handling," *Annual Review of Pharmacology and Toxicology*, vol. 26, pp. 293–309, 1986.

[35] D. Siegel, S. B. Hulley, D. M. Black et al., "Diuretics, serum and intracellular electrolyte levels, and ventricular arrhythmias in hypertensive men," *Journal of the American Medical Association*, vol. 267, no. 8, pp. 1083–1089, 1992.

[36] D. A. Sica, B. Carter, W. Cushman, and L. Hamm, "Thiazide and loop diuretics," *The Journal of Clinical Hypertension*, vol. 13, no. 9, pp. 639–643, 2011.

[37] H. A. Cooper, D. L. Dries, C. E. Davis, Y. L. Shen, and M. J. Domanski, "Diuretics and risk of arrhythmic death in patients with left ventricular dysfunction," *Circulation*, vol. 100, no. 12, pp. 1311–1315, 1999.

[38] M. Hafizullah, K. Bangash, and F. Abbas, "Comparative efficacy and tolerability of lasoride and spiromide in congestive cardiac failure," *Journal of Postgraduate Medical Institute (Peshawar, Pakistan)*, vol. 14, no. 1, pp. 36–42, 2011.

[39] D. R. Salvador, N. R. Rey, G. C. Ramos, and F. E. Punzalan, "Continuous infusion versus bolus injection of loop diuretics

in congestive heart failure," *Cochrane Database of Systematic Reviews*, no. 3, Article ID CD003178, 2005.

[40] A. Palazzuoli, M. Pellegrini, B. Franci et al., "Short and long-term effects of continuous versus intermittent loop diuretics treatment in acute heart failure with renal dysfunction," *Internal and Emergency Medicine*, vol. 10, no. 1, pp. 41–49, 2015.

[41] M.-Y. Wu, N.-C. Chang, C.-L. Su et al., "Loop diuretic strategies in patients with acute decompensated heart failure: a meta-analysis of randomized controlled trials," *Journal of Critical Care*, vol. 29, no. 1, pp. 2–9, 2014.

[42] F. Alqahtani, I. Koulouridis, P. Susantitaphong, K. Dahal, and B. L. Jaber, "A meta-analysis of continuous vs intermittent infusion of loop diuretics in hospitalized patients," *Journal of Critical Care*, vol. 29, no. 1, pp. 10–17, 2014.

[43] "Effectiveness of Spironolactone added to an angiotensin-converting enzyme inhibitor and a loop diuretic for severe chronic congestive heart failure (the Randomized Aldactone Evaluation Study [RALES])," *The American Journal of Cardiology*, vol. 78, no. 8, pp. 902–907, 1996.

[44] B. Pitt, G. Bakris, L. M. Ruilope, L. DiCarlo, and R. Mukherjee, "Serum potassium and clinical outcomes in the eplerenone post-acute myocardial infarction heart failure efficacy and survival study (EPHESUS)," *Circulation*, vol. 118, no. 16, pp. 1643–1650, 2008.

[45] B. Pitt, F. Zannad, W. J. Remme et al., "The effect of spironolactone on morbidity and mortality in patients with severe heart failure," *The New England Journal of Medicine*, vol. 341, no. 10, pp. 709–717, 1999.

[46] M. Eng and S. Bansal, "Use of natriuretic-doses of spironolactone for treatment of loop diuretic resistant acute decompensated heart failure," *International Journal of Cardiology*, vol. 170, no. 3, pp. e68–e69, 2014.

[47] L.-J. Hu, Y.-Q. Chen, S.-B. Deng, J.-L. Du, and Q. She, "Additional use of an aldosterone antagonist in patients with mild to moderate chronic heart failure: a systematic review and meta-analysis," *British Journal of Clinical Pharmacology*, vol. 75, no. 5, pp. 1202–1212, 2013.

[48] J. L. Morales-Rull, J. C. Trullàs, and F. Formiga, "Alternatives to conventional diuretic therapy in heart failure," *Medicina Clinica*, vol. 142, supplement 1, pp. 42–48, 2014.

[49] A. Tuttolomondo, A. Pinto, G. Parrinello, and G. Licata, "Intravenous high-dose furosemide and hypertonic saline solutions for refractory heart failure and ascites," *Seminars in Nephrology*, vol. 31, no. 6, pp. 513–522, 2011.

[50] T. Berl, F. Quittnat-Pelletier, J. G. Verbalis et al., "Oral tolvaptan is safe and effective in chronic hyponatremia," *Journal of the American Society of Nephrology*, vol. 21, no. 4, pp. 705–712, 2010.

[51] G. A. Perri, "Ascites in patients with cirrhosis," *Canadian Family Physician*, vol. 59, no. 12, pp. 1297–1299; e538–e540, 2013.

[52] R. M. Pérez-Ayuso, V. Arroyo, R. Planas et al., "Randomized comparative study of efficacy of furosemide versus spironolactone in nonazotemic cirrhosis with ascites. Relationship between the diuretic response and the activity of the renin-aldosterone system," *Gastroenterology*, vol. 84, no. 5, part 1, pp. 961–968, 1983.

[53] F. Fiaccadori, G. C. Pasetti, G. Pedretti, P. Pizzaferri, and G. F. Elia, "Comparative analysis of torasemide and furosemide in liver cirrhosis," *Cardiology*, vol. 84, no. 2, pp. 80–86, 1994.

[54] F. Fiaccadori, G. Pedretti, G. Pasetti, P. Pizzaferri, and G. Elia, "Torasemide versus furosemide in cirrhosis: a long-term, double-blind, randomized clinical study," *The Clinical Investigator*, vol. 71, no. 7, pp. 579–584, 1993.

[55] G. Kalambokis, M. Economou, P. Kosta, K. Papadimitriou, and E. V. Tsianos, "The effects of treatment with octreotide, diuretics, or both on portal hemodynamics in nonazotemic cirrhotic patients with ascites," *Journal of Clinical Gastroenterology*, vol. 40, no. 4, pp. 342–346, 2006.

[56] T. Nakamura, M. Sata, K. Hiroishi et al., "Contribution of diuretic therapy with human serum albumin to the management of ascites in patients with advanced liver cirrhosis: a prospective cohort study," *Molecular and Clinical Oncology*, vol. 2, no. 3, pp. 349–355, 2014.

[57] T. Nakamura, M. Sata, K. Suzuki et al., "Open-labeled randomized controlled trial to compare diuretic therapy with recombinant human serum albumin and diuretic therapy for therapeutic treatment of ascites in patients with advanced liver cirrhosis: an exploratory trial," *Hepatology Research*, vol. 44, no. 5, pp. 502–514, 2014.

[58] P. Angeli, S. Fasolato, E. Mazza et al., "Combined versus sequential diuretic treatment of ascites in non-azotaemic patients with cirrhosis: results of an open randomised clinical trial," *Gut*, vol. 59, no. 1, pp. 98–104, 2010.

[59] A. Dasgupta, M. J. Johnson, and T. K. Sengupta, "Clinically insignificant negative interferences of spironolactone, potassium canrenoate, and their common metabolite canrenone in new dimension vista LOCI digoxin immunoassay," *Journal of Clinical Laboratory Analysis*, vol. 26, no. 3, pp. 143–147, 2012.

[60] P. Gines, V. Arrovo, and J. Rodes, "Pharmacotherapy of ascites associated with cirrhosis," *Drugs*, vol. 43, no. 3, pp. 316–332, 1992.

[61] M. Inoue, K. Okajima, K. Itoh et al., "Mechanism of furosemide resistance in analbuminemic rats and hypoalbuminemic patients," *Kidney International*, vol. 32, no. 2, pp. 198–203, 1987.

[62] A. Rane, J. P. Villeneuve, W. J. Stone, A. S. Nies, G. R. Wilkinson, and R. A. Branch, "Plasma binding and disposition of furosemide in the nephrotic syndrome and in uremia," *Clinical Pharmacology and Therapeutics*, vol. 24, no. 2, pp. 199–207, 1978.

[63] E. Keller, G. Hoppe-Seyler, and P. Schollmeyer, "Disposition and diuretic effect of furosemide in the nephrotic syndrome," *Clinical Pharmacology & Therapeutics*, vol. 32, no. 4, pp. 442–449, 1982.

[64] A. Ghafari, A. Mehdizadeh, I. Alavi-Darazam, E. Rahimi, C. Kargar, and N. Sepehrvand, "Co-administration of albumin-furosemide in patients with the nephrotic syndrome," *Saudi Journal of Kidney Diseases and Transplantation*, vol. 22, no. 3, pp. 471–475, 2011.

[65] G. D. Kitsios, P. Mascari, R. Ettunsi, and A. W. Gray, "Co-administration of furosemide with albumin for overcoming diuretic resistance in patients with hypoalbuminemia: a meta-analysis," *Journal of Critical Care*, vol. 29, no. 2, pp. 253–259, 2014.

[66] R. J. Elwell, A. P. Spencer, and G. Eisele, "Combined furosemide and human albumin treatment for diuretic-resistant edema," *Annals of Pharmacotherapy*, vol. 37, no. 5, pp. 695–700, 2003.

[67] E. H. Garin, "A comparison of combinations of diuretics in nephrotic edema," *American Journal of Diseases of Children*, vol. 141, no. 7, pp. 769–771, 1987.

[68] R. R. Paton and R. E. Kane, "Long-term diuretic therapy with metolazone of renal failure and the nephrotic syndrome," *The Journal of Clinical Pharmacology*, vol. 17, no. 4, pp. 243–251, 1977.

9

The Role of Renal Replacement Therapy in the Management of Pharmacologic Poisonings

Aibek E. Mirrakhimov,[1] Aram Barbaryan,[2] Adam Gray,[1] and Taha Ayach[3]

[1]Department of Medicine, University of Kentucky College of Medicine, Lexington, KY, USA
[2]Department of Internal Medicine, University of Kansas Medical Center, Kansas City, KS, USA
[3]Division of Nephrology, Bone and Mineral Metabolism, University of Kentucky College of Medicine, Lexington, KY, USA

Correspondence should be addressed to Aibek E. Mirrakhimov; amirrakhimov1@gmail.com

Academic Editor: Alessandro Amore

Pharmacologic toxicities are common and range from mild to life-threatening. The aim of this study is to review and update the data on the role of renal replacement therapy (RRT) in the management of various pharmacologic poisonings. We aim to provide a focused review on the role of RRT in the management of pharmacological toxicities. Relevant publications were searched in MEDLINE with the following search terms alone or in combination: pharmacologic toxicity, hemodialysis, hemofiltration, renal replacement therapy, toxicology, poisonings, critical illness, and intensive care. The studies showed that a pharmacologic substance should meet several prerequisites to be deemed dialyzable. These variables include having a low molecular weight (<500 Da) and low degree of protein binding (<80%), being water-soluble, and having a low volume of distribution (<1 L/kg). RRT should be strongly considered in critically ill patients presenting with toxic alcohol ingestion, salicylate overdose, severe valproic acid toxicity, metformin overdose, and lithium poisoning. The role of RRT in other pharmacologic toxicities is less certain and should be considered on a case-by-case basis.

1. Introduction

Pharmacological substances carry an intrinsic risk of toxicity as the result of either idiosyncrasy or overdose. For example, there were 2,188,013 cases of human exposures to various toxic substances resulting in 20,749 cases of serious adverse reactions and 1,552 deaths in 2013 [1]. In such cases, hemodialysis was used in more than 2,290 cases [2]. In the year 2014, pharmaceutical toxicities were responsible for 61.4% of cases and nonpharmacological exposures accounted for 14.1% of registered cases in 2014 [2].

The goal of this article is to review the data and evidence on the use of RRT in the management of certain pharmacologic overdoses. First, we review and discuss the different factors that would affect dialyzability of drugs and toxins. Second, we discuss different extracorporeal treatment modalities with focus on hemodialysis and hemofiltration treatments.

Third, we review the role of RRT in the management of specific drugs and poisons including toxic alcohols, salicylate, lithium, metformin, valproic acid, and dabigatran. Lastly, we discuss the role of RRT in the management of less common miscellaneous cases of intoxication.

It is important to mention that the management of the toxicities mentioned above is complex and usually requires measures in addition to dialysis.

2. Removal of Drugs and Toxins by Extracorporeal Therapies

The use of extracorporeal techniques to remove toxins is justified if there is an indication of severe toxicity. The extent to which a drug is affected by extracorporeal therapies is determined primarily by several physicochemical

TABLE 1: Optimal physicochemical properties for extracorporeal removal of drugs.

	Hemodialysis	Hemofiltration	Hemoperfusion
Molecular weight	<500 Da	<40 KDa	<40 KDa
Protein binding	Low (<80%)	Low	Low or high
Volume of distribution	<1 L/Kg	<1 L/Kg	<1 L/Kg
Solubility	Water	Water	Water or lipid
Endogenous clearance	<4 mL/Kg/min	<4 mL/Kg/min	<4 mL/Kg/min

characteristics of the drug which are summarized in Table 1. These include molecular size, protein binding, volume of distribution, water solubility, and endogenous clearance. In addition to these properties of the drug, technical aspects of the procedure may also determine the extent to which a drug is removed [3, 4].

2.1. Molecular Weight. Dialysis is dependent upon the use of a synthetic dialytic membrane with fixed pore size. The movement of drugs or other solutes is largely determined by the size of these molecules in relation to the pore size of the membrane. As a general rule, smaller molecular weight substances will pass through the membrane more easily than larger molecular weight substances.

2.2. Protein Binding. Another important factor determining drug removal during dialysis is the concentration gradient of unbound (free) drug across the dialysis membrane. Because the primary binding proteins for most drugs (mainly albumin) are of large molecular size, the drug protein complex is often unable to cross the dialysis membrane. Drugs with a high degree of protein binding will have a low plasma concentration of unbound drug available for dialysis and therefore lower clearance.

2.3. Volume of Distribution. The efficacy of toxin removal is also influenced by its theoretical volume of distribution (VD). A drug with a large VD is distributed widely throughout tissues and is present in relatively small amounts in the blood. Factors that contribute to a large VD include a high degree of lipid solubility and low plasma protein binding. Drugs with a large volume of distribution (>1 L/kg) are likely to be minimally dialyzed.

2.4. Water Solubility. The dialyzate used for hemodialysis is an aqueous solution. In general, drugs with high water solubility will be dialyzed to a greater extent than those with high lipid solubility. Highly lipid-soluble drugs tend to be distributed throughout tissues, and therefore only a small fraction of the drug is present in plasma and is accessible for dialysis.

2.5. Endogenous Clearance. This includes renal and nonrenal (mainly hepatic) clearance of the drug. Dialysis will have a limited impact if the rate of drug removal is significantly faster by endogenous routes (>4 mL/Kg/min). It is generally accepted that use of extracorporeal treatment is justified, if at least 30% can be added to total body clearance by such treatment.

3. Extracorporeal Treatment Modalities

The extracorporeal techniques most frequently employed for the removal of toxins are intermittent hemodialysis, continuous renal replacement therapy, and hemoperfusion. There are a few reports on the use of molecular adsorbent recirculating system (MARS) in poisoning, specifically for those toxins that are strongly protein bound; however, the use of MARS is limited by its availability, technical applicability, and high costs.

3.1. Intermittent Hemodialysis. During hemodialysis (HD), toxins and other solutes are cleared from the blood by diffusion against a steep concentration gradient through a semipermeable membrane into dialyzate. In addition to its specific properties (Table 1), the clearance of a toxic substance during HD depends also on membrane surface area and type, as well as on blood and dialyzate flow rates. HD comes in standard as well as high-efficiency or high-flux modalities. The major difference is the pore size of the membrane, the type of membrane, and the amount of dialyzate flow that occurs. Increasing blood and dialyzate flow rates can increase the concentration gradient between blood and dialyzate, thus optimizing the rates of diffusion and elimination. Clearances can also be enhanced by increasing dialyzer efficiency or membrane surface area. Larger-solute removal can be enhanced by increasing dialyzer flux when intermittent HD is used (for toxins >500 d and up to 10,000 d) or by switching to hemofiltration, which is usually applied continuously as discussed later.

The major drawback of HD is the risk of rebound toxicity after cessation of the treatment, due to redistribution of the toxin between body compartments. Extending the HD session beyond 4 hours can to some extent ameliorate rebound; however, this may not be easily feasible. An alternative or adjunctive solution is to increase dialysis session frequency or switch to continuous therapy after initial HD treatment specifically for substances with higher volume of distribution.

Intermittent HD is usually the first-choice extracorporeal modality because of its common availability, the rapidity of toxin removal, and the low molecular weight of the common agents of poisoning [5].

3.2. Continuous Renal Replacement Therapy (CRRT). The use of CRRT has become common practice in Intensive Care Unit (ICU) settings during the last 2 decades for treatment of acute kidney injury. The term CRRT is commonly used to describe all continuous modalities of hemofiltration. Continuous venovenous hemofiltration (CVVH) is the most commonly used of the CRRT modalities, where dialysis occurs by convective transport. In continuous venovenous hemodiafiltration (CVVHDF), diffusive transport of molecules is combined with convective removal in order to mainly improve the clearance of small solutes [6].

The main advantage of CRRT is its applicability in hemodynamically unstable patients. It can be easily set up and run by regular ICU staff, thereby avoiding the need for specially trained dialysis nurses and technicians. The membranes used in CRRT are typically more permeable compared to standard intermittent HD membranes. Most high-flux HD membranes allow for the clearance of molecules up to 10,000 Da. CRRT membranes allow for the clearance of molecules as large as 20,000–40,000 Da and therefore would be the preferred modality for larger toxins removal. Another advantage of CRRT is the ability to avoid rebound of toxins removed from intravascular space, due to continuous nature of the procedure and slower rate of clearance, leading to less dramatic decreases in plasma drug levels and slower reequilibration of toxins between intracellular and intravascular spaces [5, 7].

Although CRRT gives better longer-term solute clearances (over the course of several days), it is less efficient in the short term and does not provide the rapidity of elimination afforded by intermittent HD when minimizing toxin exposure is a high priority. Other disadvantages of CRRT include the requirement for intensive anticoagulation which can place a patient at risk for bleeding and it is more associated with electrolyte disturbances. Finally, CRRT is not available at many smaller hospitals, possibly due to high equipment, training, and staffing costs [4, 8].

There are abundant case reports as well as a few small case series in the medical literature documenting the use of CRRT in the treatment of poisonings, but specific techniques and the clinical outcomes vary considerably. Therefore, one cannot draw definitive conclusions regarding benefit. Some patients, particularly those who are hemodynamically unstable and are not candidates for conventional HD, may warrant a trial of CRRT. If it is logistically possible, an ideal combination may be initial use of intermittent HD for rapid reduction of toxin levels followed by continuous therapy to ameliorate any postdialysis rebound when this is predicted. Controlled trials to better clarify the role of CRRT in treatment of poisonings would be beneficial, though such studies would be extremely difficult to conduct in this field [8].

3.3. Hemoperfusion. Hemoperfusion consists of the passage of anticoagulated blood through a cartridge containing an adsorbent material such as activated charcoal or a resin. In order to be removed by hemoperfusion, the toxic substance must have binding affinity to the sorbent in the cartridge and a low volume of distribution (Table 1). Water-soluble and lipid-soluble substances with molecular weights ranging from 100 to 40,000 daltons are well adsorbed with hemoperfusion.

In general, hemoperfusion is preferred to hemodialysis for the removal of chemicals that are lipid-soluble or are highly protein bound. However, the advantage of hemoperfusion over HD has lessened with the advent of high-flux dialysis membranes. Additionally, there is generally greater expertise and availability with respect to hemodialysis than hemoperfusion [42].

4. Renal Replacement Therapy in the Management of Specific Pharmacologic Poisonings

4.1. Toxic Alcohol Ingestion. Methanol, ethylene glycol, diethylene glycol, and isopropyl alcohol (also known as isopropanol) are alcohols commonly used in household solutions such as various cleaners, disinfectants, solvents, and antifreeze solutions as well as machine fluids [43–45]. There were 52,430 exposures to alcohols resulting in 174 fatalities in 2013 [46]. The vast majority of methanol, ethylene glycol, and isopropyl alcohol toxicities arise either as a result of suicidal attempts or after drinking the toxic alcohol as a substitute for ethanol [43]. However, the vast majority of diethylene glycol toxicities are the result of the introduction of diethylene glycol into various pharmacologic substances as a substitution for more expensive and less toxic substances [45].

To understand the basic pathogenesis of methanol, ethylene glycol, diethylene glycol, and isopropyl alcohol toxicities, it is important to briefly review the metabolism in vivo. When ingested, both methanol and ethylene glycol undergo an initial biochemical reaction catalyzed by alcohol dehydrogenase (the same enzyme metabolizing ethanol), which converts the parent alcohol into formaldehyde and glycolaldehyde, respectively. The final products of methanol and ethylene glycol metabolism are formic acid and oxalic acid, respectively [43]. The metabolism of methanol and ethylene glycol disrupts cellular energy metabolism leading to cellular damage [47, 48]. These end products result in classic features of toxicity such as retinal toxicity caused by methanol and renal injury mediated by oxalic acid.

The first step of diethylene glycol metabolism also involves the alcohol dehydrogenase enzyme which converts diethylene glycol into 2-hydroxyethoxyacetaldehyde [45]. Aldehyde dehydrogenase enzyme, in turn, converts 2-hydroxyethoxyacetaldehyde into 2-hydroxyethoxyacetic acid. The pathogenesis of diethylene glycol toxicity was first believed to involve the in vivo formation of ethylene glycol as the result of metabolism. However, further animal studies showed that the major toxic metabolite is 2-hydroxyethoxyacetic acid and that the metabolic conversion of diethylene glycol into ethylene glycol does not occur in vivo [45].

The first step of isopropyl alcohol in vivo metabolism also involves the enzyme alcohol dehydrogenase, which converts it into acetone. Acetone, in turn, undergoes several intermediate metabolic steps with the end product being glucose [44]. It is important to note that, in the vast majority of cases, isopropyl alcohol appears to be less toxic than methanol and ethylene glycol which are associated with greater toxicities and mortality rates [44, 47, 48].

The clinical presentations of methanol, ethylene glycol, and isopropyl alcohol overlap and include CNS depression, altered mental status, and seizures. Retinal toxicity and blindness are more specific for methanol intoxication, and acute kidney injury and hypocalcemia are more typical for ethylene glycol intoxication. Laboratory testing and diagnosis of methanol and ethylene glycol are based on the presence of

Methanol → Formaldehyde → Formic acid (toxic) → CO₂+H₂O

Ethylene glycol → Glycolaldehyde → Glycolic acid → Glyoxylic acid

Alcohol dehydrogenase

Aldehyde dehydrogenase

Glycolate oxidase

Folic acid

Lactate dehydrogenase → Oxalic acid (toxic) → Calcium oxalate

Pyridoxine → Glycine

Thiamine → Alpha-hydroxy-beta-ketoadipate

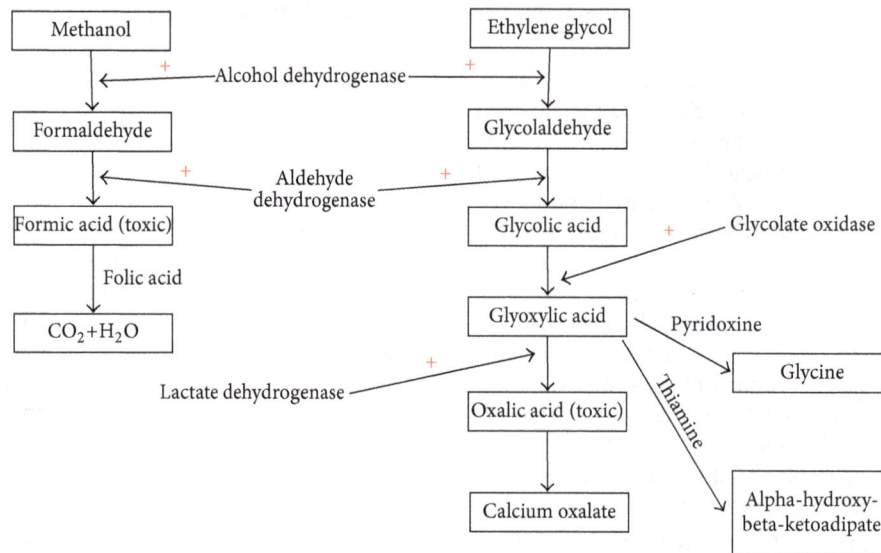

FIGURE 1: An overview of in vivo methanol and ethylene glycol metabolism.

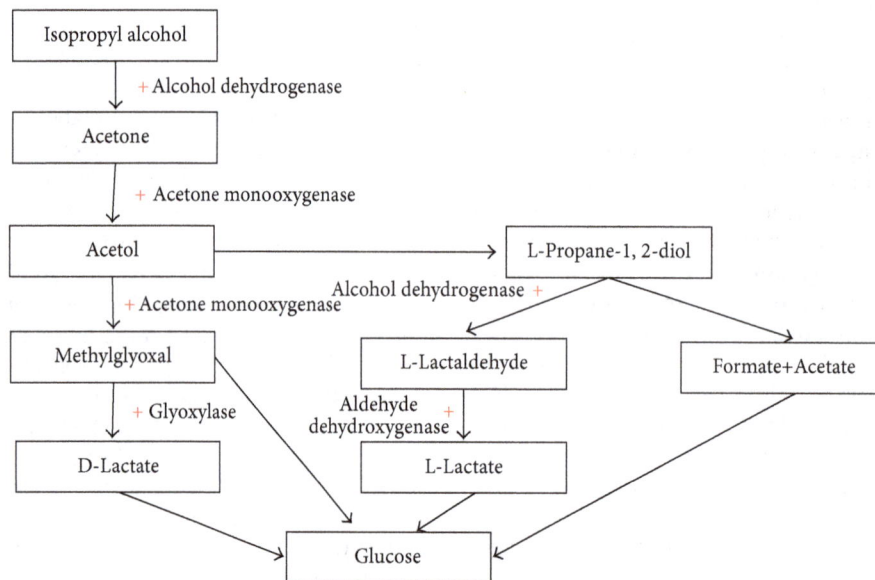

Isopropyl alcohol → Acetone → Acetol → Methylglyoxal → D-Lactate → Glucose

+ Alcohol dehydrogenase

+ Acetone monooxygenase

+ Acetone monooxygenase

L-Propane-1, 2-diol

Alcohol dehydrogenase +

L-Lactaldehyde

Formate+Acetate

Aldehyde dehydroxygenase

+ Glyoxylase

L-Lactate

FIGURE 2: An overview of in vivo isopropyl alcohol metabolism.

a high anion gap metabolic acidosis, presence of a serum osmolal gap (a difference between measured osmolality and calculated osmolality ≥ 10), and measuring the levels of the toxic alcohols which is used for confirmation (typically these tests are not time sensitive, and treatment should not be withheld in any patient suspected of having toxic alcohol ingestion). Isopropyl alcohol laboratory findings include the presence of a high serum osmolal gap, presence of ketone bodies in the blood and/or urine (because of acetone), and typically the absence of a high anion gap metabolic acidosis. A brief overview of the in vivo metabolism of methanol and ethylene glycol is presented in Figure 1 and an overview of isopropyl alcohol metabolism is presented in Figure 2.

The management of methanol and ethylene glycol poisoning includes supportive care, respiratory support if needed (mechanical ventilation), the use of cofactors to stimulate formation of less toxic metabolites (see Figures 1 and 2), and the use of either an alcohol dehydrogenase inhibitor (fomepizole) or ethanol, which work by displacing the toxic alcohol and preventing it from being metabolized by alcohol dehydrogenase. Ethanol is less desirable and should only be used in cases of fomepizole unavailability. It is important to remember that fomepizole and ethanol have no effect on the metabolism and clearance of toxic metabolites such as formic acid and glycolic acid. Therefore, inhibition of alcohol dehydrogenase will not translate into an improved outcome once the parent alcohol has been metabolized.

RRT should be considered in cases of ongoing hemodynamic instability despite appropriate management and especially in the presence of severe metabolic acidosis, acute kidney injury, and target organ damage (retinal toxicity in methanol and acute kidney injury in ethylene glycol toxicity) [45, 47]. The small size, low VD, and low protein binding for these alcohols make them readily dialyzable, making standard hemodialysis the first-line therapy for extracorporeal elimination except in cases where hemodialysis is not available or in the setting of significant hemodynamic compromise where CRRT would be indicated [8]. Consensus guidelines recommend hemodialysis when the levels of parent alcohols exceed 50 mg/dL, although some patients without evidence of target organ damage, acute kidney injury, and metabolic acidosis may be managed without hemodialysis. Hemodialysis should also be considered in patients with ethylene glycol poisoning that have a persistent hyperosmolar state (despite appropriate management) [49] and levels of glycolic acid above 8 mmol/L [50]. It is important to mention that, in cases of methanol poisoning, hemodialysis enhances the clearance of methanol (the endogenous clearance of methanol is slow after alcohol dehydrogenase inhibition) [48], but it only marginally increases the clearance of formic acid [9]. Also, hemodialysis may be less costly than therapy with fomepizole; however, it is essential to remember that hemodialysis is associated with more complications and should be limited to patients with clear indications [51]. End goals of hemodialysis in these patients should be normalization of acid base status, resolution of hyperosmolar states, and a decreased blood level of parent toxic alcohols (less than 25 mg/dL). Redistribution of methanol and ethylene glycol can occur after hemodialysis and the serum electrolytes, osmolality, and acid base status should be monitored for additional 12–36 hours after the last hemodialysis treatment [47, 48].

Literature on the role of hemodialysis in the management of diethylene glycol is scant [45], and it is unclear whether the active toxic metabolite is removed by hemodialysis. Nevertheless, hemodialysis should be considered in patients with progressive clinical deterioration despite appropriate care and persistent high anion gap metabolic acidosis.

In cases of isopropyl alcohol toxicity, the role of hemodialysis is less clear [44]. Isopropyl alcohol intoxication generally has a more favorable outcome compared to methanol and ethylene glycol poisonings and the vast majority of patients will improve with supportive therapy and alcohol dehydrogenase inhibition. In the rare patient with hemodynamic instability and an isopropyl alcohol level above 4,000 mg/dL (which is usually due to a massive ingestion), hemodialysis may be considered.

When considering renal replacement therapy in these patients, it is important to note that both fomepizole and ethanol are cleared by hemodialysis and the doses of fomepizole and ethanol should be adjusted accordingly.

An overview of the clinical presentations, major laboratory findings, general principles of management, and indications for hemodialysis among patients with toxic alcohol

ingestion is presented in Table 2. A summary of toxic alcohol pharmacokinetics and the utility of hemodialysis is presented in Table 3.

4.2. Salicylate Toxicity. Salicylates are a group of pharmacologic agents which includes aspirin, bismuth salicylate, and local skin preparations such as salicylic acid and methyl salicylate (topical preparations occasionally cause toxicity if used excessively or in patients with skin damage leading to increased absorption) [10, 52, 53].

Analgesics including aspirin are the most common etiology of all drug poisonings in the USA, and salicylate poisoning caused 34 out of 2,113 deaths due to poisonings reported in 2013 [51]. The major mechanism of action of aspirin is via inhibition of cyclooxygenase enzyme resulting in decreased production of thromboxane A2 and various prostaglandins [11]. However, with higher dosages, other biochemical alterations may occur such as uncoupling of oxidative phosphorylation in the electron transport chain resulting in heat release and stimulation of the respiratory center in the medulla. A decrease in blood pH will favor formation of lipid-soluble salicylic acid which easily penetrates the blood brain barrier and undergoes renal reabsorption [54]. When used therapeutically, aspirin has a high degree of protein binding which significantly decreases in cases of overdose and poisoning.

Patients with salicylate toxicity typically present with tinnitus, gastrointestinal complications (nausea, vomiting, bleeding, and liver toxicity), hyperthermia (via uncoupling of oxidative phosphorylation), pulmonary edema, and a mixed acid-base disorder (high anion gap metabolic acidosis and respiratory alkalosis via stimulation of respiratory center in the brainstem) [54, 55].

Recent consensus panel guidelines on the management of severe salicylate toxicity recommend intermittent hemodialysis over other modalities of extracorporeal removal [12]. Hemodialysis should be strongly considered in patients with an altered mental status (which may be reflective of high salicylate content in the CNS), pulmonary edema, hypoxemia, fluid overload states or presence of a medical condition limiting the administration of sodium bicarbonate (such as congestive heart failure), presence of either acute or chronic kidney failure (since it will limit the amount of sodium bicarbonate administration and endogenous salicylate clearance), salicylate levels > 90 mg/dL in acute toxicity and normal renal function and levels > 80 mg/dL in acute toxicity, and impaired renal function and in cases of failure of appropriate management [12]. A summary of aspirin pharmacokinetics and the utility of hemodialysis is presented in Table 3.

4.3. Lithium Toxicity. Lithium has been used in the management of bipolar disorder since the nineteenth century [56]. The exact mechanism of action of lithium is not clear, but it may involve modulation of intracellular signaling pathways [57]. The major route of lithium elimination is renal excretion, but it is important to note that about 80% of filtered lithium is reabsorbed [13].

TABLE 2: The features of toxic alcohol poisonings.

Type of toxic alcohol	Core clinical features	Core laboratory features	General principles of treatment	Indications for RRT
Methanol	CNS depression AMS Seizures Visual changes/retinal toxicity Hemodynamic instability	HAGMA High osmolal gap Elevated lactic acid (formic acid mediated inhibition of mitochondrial electron transport chain)	Supportive care Fomepizole Ethanol (if fomepizole is unavailable) Folic acid or folinic acid	pH < 7.3 Methanol level > 50 mg/dL Visual changes AKI Severe electrolyte derangements Hemodynamic instability and progression despite appropriate care
Ethylene glycol	CNS depression AMS Seizures AKI Calcium oxaluria	HAGMA High osmolal gap Hypocalcemia Electrolyte abnormalities AKI Calcium oxalate crystals in the urine Falsely elevated lactic acid (glycolic acid can be mistaken for lactic acid)	Supportive care Fomepizole Ethanol (if fomepizole is unavailable) Thiamine Pyridoxine	pH < 7.3 Ethylene glycol level > 50 mg/dL Glycolic acid level > 8 mmol/L Refractory hyperosmolarity AKI Severe electrolyte derangements Hemodynamic instability and progression despite appropriate care
Diethylene glycol	CNS depression AMS Seizures AKI Gastrointestinal symptoms Peripheral neuropathy	HAGMA High osmolal gap Elevated liver enzymes	Supportive care Fomepizole Ethanol (if fomepizole is unavailable) Thiamine Pyridoxine	Hemodynamic instability and progression despite appropriate care Persistent HAGMA
Isopropyl alcohol	CNS depression AMS Hemodynamic instability in advanced cases	High osmolal gap Increased ketones in the blood and urine Absence of HAGMA Falsely elevated creatinine (due to acetone cross reactivity)	Supportive care Fomepizole Ethanol (if fomepizole is unavailable)	Hemodynamic instability and progression despite appropriate care Isopropyl alcohol level > 4000 mg/dL

CNS: central nervous system.
AMS: altered mental status.
HAGMA: high anion gap metabolic acidosis.
AKI: acute kidney injury.

Lithium has a narrow therapeutic window and is associated with numerous side effects [57]. Several clinical scenarios of lithium toxicity can occur such as acute overdose in a suicidal patient, acute on chronic toxicity in patients taking lithium whose renal function has declined (e.g., patients with gastroenteritis, decreased oral intake, and patients concomitantly taking other medications such as nonsteroidal anti-inflammatory drugs and angiotensin converting enzyme inhibitors), and chronic toxicity in patients who slowly accumulate the medication and develop toxicity [14, 57]. Lithium was responsible for 6,610 cases of toxicities including 5 fatalities in the year 2013 [1].

Patients with chronic lithium poisoning typically develop nephrogenic diabetes insipidus and urinary concentrating defects, neurologic symptoms (ataxia, tremors, and altered mental status), hyperparathyroidism, hypothyroidism, and weight gain [14]. Patients with more acute presentations tend to have more pronounced gastrointestinal symptoms such as nausea, vomiting, diarrhea, cardiac arrhythmias, and neurologic symptoms.

Laboratory findings of acute lithium intoxication may include a negative anion gap and an osmolal gap [15]. Also it is important to assess kidney function since acute kidney insults often precipitate lithium toxicity.

The management of lithium intoxication includes stopping the offending medication, supportive care, and, in selected cases, renal replacement therapy such as hemodialysis [15]. Hemodialysis should be considered in patients with lithium levels > 4 mEq/L regardless of symptomatology and in patients with lithium levels > 2.5 mEq/L who either

TABLE 3: Summary of pharmacological and clearance properties of some pharmacological substances*.

Substance	Molecular weight (daltons)	Protein binding (%)	Volume of distribution (L/kg)	Metabolism and excretion (%)	Clearance without hemodialysis (mL/min)	Clearance with hemodialysis (mL/min)
Methanol	~32	Minimal	~0.6–0.77	~95 hepatic ~2.5 respiratory ~1 renal	~11.3	~125–215
Ethylene glycol	~62	Minimal	0.5–0.8	~80 hepatic ~20 renal	Up to 27	145–230
Diethylene glycol	~62	Minimal	~1	30–50 hepatic 50–70 renal	Unknown	Unknown
Isopropyl alcohol	~60	Minimal	~0.45–0.55	80 hepatic 20 renal	Unknown	~137 (isopropyl alcohol) ~165 (acetone)
Aspirin	~180	~49 (~90 with therapeutic use and ~30 in overdose)	~0.15	~80 hepatic ~20 renal	0.6–25	3–100
Lithium	~74	0	~0.3–1	>95 renal	20–40	70–170
Valproic acid	~144	~80–90 (continuously decreases with higher valproic acid concentrations)	~0.1–0.5	Predominantly hepatic	5–10	~50–90
Metformin	~129	Minimal	~1.1	>90 renal	~7	Up to 170
Dabigatran	471	~35	~0.85	>80 renal	Dependent on renal function	Decreases dabigatran concentration by at least 40%

*Adapted from [5–20].

are symptomatic or have some clinical factors (advanced kidney disease and decompensated congestive heart failure) limiting the use of intravenous hydration. The end points of hemodialysis in patients with lithium toxicity are resolution of clinical symptoms of toxicity and lithium levels < 1 mEq/L [15]. However, it is important to monitor lithium levels after the cessation of hemodialysis, since lithium tissue stores can be redistributed into the bloodstream [15, 16]. Most cases of lithium intoxication treated with hemodialysis require at least a second session of hemodialysis following rebound. This rebound can be avoided by use of CRRT as described above preferably after the initial hemodialysis session for rapid reduction of lithium level [8, 15].

A summary of lithium pharmacokinetics and the utility of hemodialysis is presented in Table 3.

4.4. Valproic Acid Poisoning. Valproic acid is used for the management of epilepsy, bipolar disorder, migraine headaches, and peripheral neuropathy. The mechanism of action includes modulation of gamma aminobutyric acid activity and sodium channel blockade [17]. Valproic acid is a fatty acid and its toxicity is believed to involve the inhibition of mitochondrial beta oxidation [18]. Valproic acid has a favorable molecular weight and volume of distribution to be cleared by hemodialysis, though the degree of protein binding is high at therapeutic concentrations. However, the degree of protein binding decreases with extra therapeutic concentrations due to protein saturation, thus making it amenable for hemodialysis [19]. Valproic acid was responsible for 7,776 toxicities including 2 fatalities in the year 2013 [1].

Clinical manifestations may include altered mental status, tremors, myoclonus, hypotension, tachycardia, and respiratory depression [58]. Classic laboratory abnormalities include hyperammonemia, presence of an osmolal gap, hypernatremia, high anion gap metabolic acidosis, and elevated liver enzymes.

Management of acute valproic acid intoxication includes supportive care, administration of naloxone to help against respiratory depression, and antidote therapy with carnitine supplementation to offset the inhibitory effects on mitochondrial fatty acid oxidation. RRT should be strongly considered in patients with severe toxicity including those with cerebral edema (patients with papilledema, focal neurologic deficits, altered mental status, imaging findings, etc.) and hemodynamic instability and in those with valproic acid levels > 1300 mg/L. RRT should also be considered in patients with valproic acid levels > 900 mg/L, respiratory depression, hyperammonemia, and severe metabolic acidosis (pH < 7.1). Intermittent HD is the preferred modality of RRT in valproic acid poisoning. If hemodialysis is not available, then intermittent hemoperfusion or continuous renal replacement therapy is an acceptable alternative. The end point of hemodialysis includes clinical stabilization and valproic acid levels < 100 mg/L [19]. As in many other cases of intoxication, it is important to monitor valproic acid levels after the cessation of hemodialysis, since redistribution of the medication can cause reemergence of toxicity. A summary of valproic acid pharmacokinetics and the utility of hemodialysis is presented in Table 3.

4.5. Metformin Poisoning. Metformin is the most commonly used oral antihyperglycemic agent worldwide [58]. Besides treatment of type 2 diabetes mellitus and prediabetes, it is often used in the management of polycystic ovarian syndrome [59]. Metformin's mechanism of action includes decreased hepatic and intestinal gluconeogenesis, enhanced glucose utilization, and modulation of mitochondrial oxidation of fatty acids [20, 59]. The majority of overdose cases occur in patients with renal disease (either acute or chronic), advanced liver disease, and acute concurrent illness [20]. Metformin was responsible for 8,829 toxicities including 12 fatalities in the year 2013 [1].

The pharmacokinetics of metformin are generally favorable for hemodialysis and extracorporeal elimination such as a low molecular weight and minimal protein binding except with high volume of distribution [20, 21]. Clinical manifestations of metformin poisoning are nonspecific and may include gastrointestinal symptoms such as nausea, vomiting, diarrhea, abdominal pain, altered mental status, and hemodynamic instability. Laboratory features of metformin poisoning include a high anion gap metabolic acidosis due to accumulation of lactic acid. The initial mechanism of lactic acidosis involves modulation of gluconeogenesis [20]. However, later, hemodynamic deterioration may underlie the perpetuation of lactic acidosis.

Treatment of metformin poisoning includes supportive care and RRT. The low molecular weight, negligible plasma protein binding, and rapid transport of drug from cells to serum allow for drug removal by hemodialysis despite a relatively large VD. It is unclear whether hemodialysis improves mortality in patients with metformin poisoning. Furthermore, its efficacy may be suboptimal in patients who present after tissue redistribution occurs as that leads to a large volume of distribution. Nevertheless, hemodialysis should be strongly considered in patients with advanced renal failure, decompensated congestive heart failure, severe metabolic acidosis (pH < 7.1), and hemodynamic and clinical decline despite supportive care [20]. Whenever possible, prolonged sessions of hemodialysis should be undertaken; alternatively CRRT can be considered [22]. A summary of metformin pharmacokinetics and the utility of hemodialysis is presented in Table 3.

4.6. Dabigatran Poisoning. Dabigatran is a non-vitamin K oral anticoagulant used in the management of nonvalvular atrial fibrillation, venous thromboembolism, and postprocedural deep venous thrombosis prophylaxis [23]. Dabigatran

represents an alternative to vitamin K antagonists in the vast majority of patients with the above-mentioned conditions. Dabigatran is predominantly excreted by the kidneys and is contraindicated in patients with advanced renal disease typically defined as creatinine clearance < 30 mL/min.

The major adverse effect related to the use of dabigatran is bleeding which may be minor or life-threating, such as in case of intracranial hemorrhage. Until recently, the management of bleeding in patients taking dabigatran was supportive [24]. However, recently, a monoclonal antibody, idarucizumab, has been shown to be effective in the management of patients with dabigatran related bleeding [25].

Before the availability of idarucizumab, RRT was used in the bleeding patient taking dabigatran. Several case reports highlighted the efficacy of RRT in the management of patients with dabigatran related bleeding [26]. In a small study, intermittent hemodialysis enhanced elimination of dabigatran more efficiently than CRRT, though dabigatran levels may rebound after cessation of hemodialysis via the effect of redistribution [27]. Dabigatran levels should be repeated and repeat hemodialysis should be considered in patients with a rebound increase in dabigatran concentration. Alternatively, longer duration hemodialysis sessions or CRRT may be considered specifically that most patients with dabigatran toxicity are critically ill with life-threatening bleeding or are in need for an emergent surgery, where CRRT would be more tolerated. However, it is important that the vast majority of patients with dabigatran poisoning do not have advanced renal disease and do not receive renal replacement therapy. Therefore, a dialysis vascular catheter must be inserted which may be difficult in an overanticoagulated patient and result in more bleeding and other complications. Thus, RRT should be considered in patients with severe bleeding and patients on dabigatran requiring emergent surgery when idarucizumab is not available. It is important to note that RRT does not have a role in the management of other non-vitamin K anticoagulants.

A summary of dabigatran pharmacokinetics and the utility of hemodialysis is presented in Table 3.

4.7. Miscellaneous Pharmacologic Poisonings. RRT has been effective in the management of various medication related toxicities [28–41, 60–66]. It is important to note that scientific data is limited to case reports and case series. RRT should be considered in patients with severe toxicity after failure of supportive care. A summary of some of these medications and the role of hemodialysis in the management of these toxicities is presented in Table 4.

5. Conclusion

The use of RRT should be considered in patients with toxic alcohol poisoning, salicylate toxicity, lithium overdose, and metformin poisoning as well as valproic acid toxicity. The role of RRT in the management of dabigatran toxicity is likely limited to cases with severe bleeding when idarucizumab is not available. RRT use should also be considered in the management of other drug toxicities on a case-by-case basis.

TABLE 4: Role of hemodialysis in the management of miscellaneous pharmacological poisonings.

Medication	Therapeutic use	Classic toxicity	Treatment	Efficacy of hemodialysis (HD)
Carbamazepine	Epilepsy Trigeminal neuralgia Bipolar disorder	Altered mental status Seizures Hemodynamic instability Arrhythmias	Supportive	May reduce carbamazepine level by about 50% [21–23]
Phenobarbital	Epilepsy	Altered mental status	Supportive	May reduce phenobarbital level by up to 59% after 4 h HD [24–26]
Phenytoin	Epilepsy Cardiac arrhythmias	Horizontal nystagmus Ataxia Altered mental status Arrhythmias Hypersensitivity reactions	Supportive	Should be considered in patients with severe poisoning not responding to supportive care [27]
Baclofen	Spasticity	Muscle hypotonia Altered mental status Hemodynamic instability	Supportive	Conventional HD can decrease the concentration by up to 79% [28–30]
Eptifibatide	Antiplatelet agent Acute coronary syndrome	Bleeding	Supportive Platelet transfusion	Limited to patients with renal failure experiencing ongoing severe bleeding not responding to supportive care [31]
Diltiazem Atenolol	Hypertension Cardiac arrhythmias	Bradycardia Hemodynamic instability	Supportive	HD may be considered in unstable patient with renal failure not responding to supportive care [32, 33]
Lisinopril	Hypertension Heart failure Renal disease	Acute kidney injury Hyperkalemia Hemodynamic instability Angioedema	Supportive	HD may be considered in unstable patient with renal failure not responding to supportive care [34]
Theophylline	Obstructive pulmonary disease	Arrhythmias Altered mental status Seizures	Supportive	HD may be considered in unstable patient with renal failure not responding to supportive care [35, 36]
Cefepime	Antibiotic	Neurotoxicity Altered mental status	Supportive	HD may be considered in unstable patient with renal failure not responding to supportive care [37]
Metronidazole	Antibiotic	Altered mental status Seizures Neuropathy Gastrointestinal symptoms	Supportive	HD should be considered in patient with metronidazole overdose and renal failure [38]
Dapsone	Antibiotic	Hypersensitivity reactions Methemoglobinemia	Supportive Methylene blue	HD should be considered in patients not responding to conventional therapy [39]
Isoniazid	Antibiotic	Neurotoxicity Seizures Liver toxicity	Supportive Pyridoxine	HD should be considered in patients not responding to conventional therapy [40]
Acetaminophen	Analgesic	Liver failure	Supportive N-Acetylcysteine Liver transplant	HD may be considered in unstable patients with metabolic acidosis [41]

Additional Points

Why is this topic important? It critically reviews the scientific literature on the management of pharmacological toxidromes. What does this review attempt to show? It attempts to show the role of hemodialysis in the management of pharmacological poisonings. What are the key findings? Hemodialysis should be strongly considered in patients with toxic alcohol ingestion, salicylate overdose, severe valproic acid toxicity, metformin overdose, and lithium poisoning. Hemodialysis should be considered on case-by-case basis in the management of toxidromes secondary to other pharmacological agents. How is patient care impacted? Hemodialysis in the management of various pharmacological toxidromes which can be fatal should be considered. Early consultation with nephrologist regarding hemodialysis initiation is advised.

References

[1] J. B. Mowry, D. A. Spyker, L. R. Cantilena Jr., N. McMillan, and M. Ford, "2013 annual report of the American Association of Poison Control Centers' National Poison Data System (NPDS): 31st annual report," *Clinical Toxicology*, vol. 52, no. 10, pp. 1032–1283, 2014.

[2] S. H. Rhyee, L. Farrugia, S. L. Campleman, P. M. Wax, and J. Brent, "The toxicology investigators consortium case registry—the 2014 experience," *Journal of Medical Toxicology*, vol. 11, no. 4, pp. 388–409, 2015.

[3] J. M. Orlowski, S. Hou, and J. B. Leikin, "Extracorporeal removal of drugs and toxins," *Clinical Toxicology*, 1st Edition, pp. 43–50, 2001.

[4] D. Goldfarb, "Principles and techniques applied to enhance elimination," in *Goldfrank's Toxicologic Emergencies*, L. Nelson, N. A. Lewin, M. A. Howland, R. S. Hoffman, L. R. Goldfrank, and N. E. Flomenbaum, Eds., pp. 135–148, McGraw-Hill, 9th edition, 2010.

[5] N. S. Kanagasundaram and A. Lewington, "Dialytic therapies for drug overdose and poisoning," in *Comprehensive Clinical Nephrology*, chapter 98, pp. 1116–1121, 5th edition, 2014.

[6] G. Villa, Z. Ricci, and C. Ronco, "Renal Replacement Therapy," *Critical Care Clinics*, vol. 31, no. 4, pp. 839–848, 2015.

[7] L. G. Forni and P. J. Hilton, "Continuous hemofiltration in the treatment of acute renal failure," *New England Journal of Medicine*, vol. 336, no. 18, pp. 1303–1309, 1997.

[8] Z. Kim and D. S. Goldfarb, "Continuous renal replacement therapy does not have a clear role in the treatment of poisoning," *Nephron—Clinical Practice*, vol. 115, pp. c1–c6, 2010.

[9] W. Kerns II, C. Tomaszewski, K. McMartin et al., "Formate kinetics in methanol poisoning," *Journal of Toxicology—Clinical Toxicology*, vol. 40, no. 2, pp. 137–143, 2002.

[10] J. E. Davis, "Are one or two dangerous? Methyl salicylate exposure in toddlers," *Journal of Emergency Medicine*, vol. 32, no. 1, pp. 63–69, 2007.

[11] J. Y. Wick, "Aspirin: a history, a love story," *Consultant Pharmacist*, vol. 27, no. 5, pp. 322–329, 2012.

[12] D. N. Juurlink, S. Gosselin, J. T. Kielstein et al., "Extracorporeal treatment for salicylate poisoning: systematic review and recommendations from the EXTRIP workgroup," *Annals of Emergency Medicine*, vol. 66, no. 2, pp. 165–181, 2015.

[13] M. E. Ward, M. N. Musa, and L. Bailey, "Clinical pharmacokinetics of lithium," *Journal of Clinical Pharmacology*, vol. 34, no. 4, pp. 280–285, 1994.

[14] R. F. McKnight, M. Adida, K. Budge, S. Stockton, G. M. Goodwin, and J. R. Geddes, "Lithium toxicity profile: a systematic review and meta-analysis," *The Lancet*, vol. 379, no. 9817, pp. 721–728, 2012.

[15] M. M. Sood and R. Richardson, "Negative anion gap and elevated osmolar gap due to lithium overdose," *Canadian Medical Association Journal*, vol. 176, no. 7, pp. 921–923, 2007.

[16] F. Eyer, R. Pfab, N. Felgenhauer et al., "Lithium poisoning: pharmacokinetics and clearance during different therapeutic measures," *Journal of Clinical Psychopharmacology*, vol. 26, no. 3, pp. 325–330, 2006.

[17] R. M. Nanau and M. G. Neuman, "Adverse drug reactions induced by valproic acid," *Clinical Biochemistry*, vol. 46, no. 15, pp. 1323–1338, 2013.

[18] M. F. B. Silva, C. C. P. Aires, P. B. M. Luis et al., "Valproic acid metabolism and its effects on mitochondrial fatty acid oxidation: a review," *Journal of Inherited Metabolic Disease*, vol. 31, no. 2, pp. 205–216, 2008.

[19] M. Ghannoum, M. Laliberté, T. D. Nolin et al., "Extracorporeal treatment for valproic acid poisoning: systematic review and recommendations from the EXTRIP workgroup," *Clinical Toxicology*, vol. 53, no. 5, pp. 454–465, 2015.

[20] K. T. Kopec and M. J. Kowalski, "Metformin-Associated Lactic Acidosis (MALA): case files of the Einstein Medical Center medical toxicology fellowship," *Journal of Medical Toxicology*, vol. 9, no. 1, pp. 61–66, 2013.

[21] A. J. Scheen, "Clinical pharmacokinetics of metformin," *Clinical Pharmacokinetics*, vol. 30, no. 5, pp. 359–371, 1996.

[22] S. I. Rifkin, C. McFarren, R. Juvvadi, and S. S. Weinstein, "Prolonged hemodialysis for severe metformin intoxication," *Renal Failure*, vol. 33, no. 4, pp. 459–461, 2011.

[23] G. J. Hankey and J. W. Eikelboom, "Dabigatran etexilate: a new oral thrombin inhibitor," *Circulation*, vol. 123, no. 13, pp. 1436–1450, 2011.

[24] R. Alikhan, R. Rayment, D. Keeling et al., "The acute management of haemorrhage, surgery and overdose in patients receiving dabigatran," *Emergency Medicine Journal*, vol. 31, no. 2, pp. 163–168, 2014.

[25] C. V. Pollack Jr., P. A. Reilly, J. Eikelboom et al., "Idarucizumab for dabigatran reversal," *New England Journal of Medicine*, vol. 373, no. 6, pp. 511–520, 2015.

[26] C. Chai-Adisaksopha, C. Hillis, W. Lim, K. Boonyawat, K. Moffat, and M. Crowther, "Hemodialysis for the treatment of dabigatran-associated bleeding: a case report and systematic review," *Journal of Thrombosis and Haemostasis*, vol. 13, no. 10, pp. 1790–1798, 2015.

[27] J. Bouchard, M. Ghannoum, A. Bernier-Jean et al., "Comparison of intermittent and continuous extracorporeal treatments for the enhanced elimination of dabigatran," *Clinical Toxicology*, vol. 53, no. 3, pp. 156–163, 2015.

[28] J. L. Harder, M. Heung, A. M. Vilay, B. A. Mueller, and J. H. Segal, "Carbamazepine and the active epoxide metabolite are effectively cleared by hemodialysis followed by continuous venovenous hemodialysis in an acute overdose," *Hemodialysis International*, vol. 15, no. 3, pp. 412–415, 2011.

[29] A. Ozhasenekler, S. Gökhan, C. Güloğlu, M. Orak, and M. Ustündağ, "Benefit of hemodialysis in carbamazepine intoxications with neurological complications," *European Review for Medical and Pharmacological Sciences*, vol. 16, supplement 1, pp. 43.-47, 2012.

[30] A. Azak, G. Koçak, B. Huddam, and M. Duranay, "Is conventional hemodialysis enough to manage carbamazepine intoxication?" *Blood Purification*, vol. 33, no. 4, pp. 225–226, 2012.

[31] B. F. Palmer, "Effectiveness of hemodialysis the extracorporeal therapy of phenobarbital overdose," *American Journal of Kidney Diseases*, vol. 36, no. 3, pp. 640–643, 2000.

[32] F. Jacobs and F. G. Brivet, "Conventional haemodialysis significantly lowers toxic levels of phenobarbital," *Nephrology Dialysis Transplantation*, vol. 19, no. 6, pp. 1663–1664, 2004.

[33] K. Hoyland, M. Hoy, R. Austin, and M. Wildman, "Successful use of haemodialysis to treat phenobarbital overdose," *BMJ Case Reports*, vol. 2013, 2013.

[34] M. Ghannoum, S. Troyanov, P. Ayoub, V. Lavergne, and T. Hewlett, "Successful hemodialysis in a phenytoin overdose: case report and review of the literature," *Clinical Nephrology*, vol. 74, no. 1, pp. 59–64, 2010.

[35] V.-C. Wu, S.-L. Lin, S.-M. Lin, and C.-C. Fang, "Treatment of baclofen overdose by haemodialysis: A Pharmacokinetic Study," *Nephrology Dialysis Transplantation*, vol. 20, no. 2, pp. 441–443, 2005.

[36] M. Brvar, M. Vrtovec, D. Kovač, G. Kozelj, T. Pezdir, and M. Bunc, "Haemodialysis clearance of baclofen," *European Journal of Clinical Pharmacology*, vol. 63, no. 12, pp. 1143–1146, 2007.

[37] M.-J. Hsieh, S.-C. Chen, T.-I. Weng, C.-C. Fang, and T.-J. Tsai, "Treating baclofen overdose by hemodialysis," *American Journal of Emergency Medicine*, vol. 30, no. 8, pp. 1654.e5–1654.e7, 2012.

[38] R. T. Sperling, D. S. Pinto, K. K. L. Ho, and J. P. Carrozza Jr., "Platelet glycoprotein IIb/IIIa inhibition with eptifibatide: prolongation of inhibition of aggregation in acute renal failure and reversal with hemodialysis," *Catheterization and Cardiovascular Interventions*, vol. 59, no. 4, pp. 459–462, 2003.

[39] C. P. Snook, K. Sigvaldason, and J. Kristinsson, "Severe atenolol and diltiazem overdose," *Journal of Toxicology—Clinical Toxicology*, vol. 38, no. 6, pp. 661–665, 2000.

[40] S.-H. S. Huang, R. G. Tirona, C. Ross, and R. S. Suri, "Case report: atenolol overdose successfully treated with hemodialysis," *Hemodialysis International*, vol. 17, no. 4, pp. 652–655, 2013.

[41] T. W. Belay and A. R. Nusair, "Apparent lisinopril overdose requiring hemodialysis," *American Journal of Health-System Pharmacy*, vol. 70, no. 14, pp. 1226–1229, 2013.

[42] A. S. Shalkham, B. M. Kirrane, R. S. Hoffman, D. S. Goldfarb, and L. S. Nelson, "The availability and use of charcoal hemoperfusion in the treatment of poisoned patients," *American Journal of Kidney Diseases*, vol. 48, no. 2, pp. 239–241, 2006.

[43] J. A. Kraut, "Diagnosis of toxic alcohols: limitations of present methods," *Clinical Toxicology*, vol. 53, no. 7, pp. 589–595, 2015.

[44] R. J. Slaughter, R. W. Mason, D. M. G. Beasley, J. A. Vale, and L. J. Schep, "Isopropanol poisoning," *Clinical Toxicology*, vol. 52, no. 5, pp. 470–478, 2014.

[45] L. J. Schep, R. J. Slaughter, W. A. Temple, and D. M. G. Beasley, "Diethylene glycol poisoning," *Clinical Toxicology*, vol. 47, no. 6, pp. 525–535, 2009.

[46] H. K. Tan, "Molecular adsorbent recirculating system (MARS)," *Annals of the Academy of Medicine Singapore*, vol. 33, no. 3, pp. 329–335, 2004.

[47] D. G. Barceloux, E. P. Krenzelok, K. Olson, W. Watson, and H. Miller, "American academy of clinical toxicology practice guidelines on the treatment of ethylene glycol poisoning," *Journal of Toxicology—Clinical Toxicology*, vol. 37, no. 5, p. 537, 1999.

[48] D. G. Barceloux, G. R. Bond, E. P. Krenzelok, H. Cooper, and J. A. Vale, "American Academy of Clinical Toxicology practice guidelines on the treatment of methanol poisoning," *Journal of Toxicology—Clinical Toxicology*, vol. 40, no. 4, pp. 415–446, 2002.

[49] A. Pizon and D. Brooks, "Hyperosmolality: another indication for hemodialysis following acute ethylene glycol poisoning," *Clinical Toxicology*, vol. 44, no. 2, pp. 181–183, 2006.

[50] W. H. Porter, P. W. Rutter, B. A. Bush, A. A. Pappas, and J. E. Dunnington, "Ethylene glycol toxicity: the role of serum glycolic acid in hemodialysis," *Journal of Toxicology—Clinical Toxicology*, vol. 39, no. 6, pp. 607–615, 2001.

[51] M. A. Darracq, L. L. Rentmeester, R. F. Clark, C. A. Tomaszewski, A. B. Schneir, and F. L. Cantrell, "Cost of hemodialysis versus fomepizole-only for treatment of ethylene glycol intoxication," *Clinical Toxicology*, vol. 51, no. 3, p. 188, 2013.

[52] J. Herres, D. Ryan, and M. Salzman, "Delayed salicylate toxicity with undetectable initial levels after large-dose aspirin ingestion," *American Journal of Emergency Medicine*, vol. 27, no. 9, pp. 1173–e1, 2009.

[53] A. Wong, K. Mac, A. Aneman, J. Wong, and B. S. Chan, "Modern Intermittent Haemodialysis (IHD) is an effective method of removing salicylate in chronic topical salicylate toxicity," *Journal of Medical Toxicology*, vol. 12, no. 1, pp. 130–133, 2015.

[54] J. B. Hill, "Salicylate intoxication," *New England Journal of Medicine*, vol. 288, no. 21, pp. 1110–1113, 1973.

[55] J. K. Glisson, T. S. Vesa, and M. R. Bowling, "Current management of salicylate-induced pulmonary edema," *Southern Medical Journal*, vol. 104, no. 3, pp. 225–232, 2011.

[56] A. D. Strobusch and J. W. Jefferson, "The checkered history of lithium in medicine," *Pharmacy in History*, vol. 22, no. 2, pp. 72–76, 1980.

[57] R. Oruch, M. A. Elderbi, H. A. Khattab, I. F. Pryme, and A. Lund, "Lithium: a review of pharmacology, clinical uses, and toxicity," *European Journal of Pharmacology*, vol. 740, pp. 464–473, 2014.

[58] M. D. Sztajnkrycer, "Valproic acid toxicity: overview and management," *Journal of Toxicology—Clinical Toxicology*, vol. 40, no. 6, pp. 789–801, 2002.

[59] J. Hajjar, M. A. Habra, and A. Naing, "Metformin: an old drug with new potential," *Expert Opinion on Investigational Drugs*, vol. 22, no. 12, pp. 1511–1517, 2013.

[60] S. Okada, S. Teramoto, and R. Matsuoka, "Recovery from theophylline toxicity by continuous hemodialysis with filtration," *Annals of Internal Medicine*, vol. 133, no. 11, p. 922, 2000.

[61] J. Kneser, P. Wehmeier, R. Lichtinghagen, M. M. Hoeper, and J. T. Kielstein, "Successful treatment of life threatening theophylline intoxication in a pregnant patient by hemodialysis," *Clinical Nephrology*, vol. 80, no. 1, pp. 72–74, 2013.

[62] L.-Y. Mani, S. Kissling, D. Viceic et al., "Intermittent hemodialysis treatment in cefepime-induced neurotoxicity: case report, pharmacokinetic modeling, and review of the literature," *Hemodialysis International*, vol. 19, no. 2, pp. 333–343, 2015.

[63] A. M. Burda, C. B. Fischbein, T. Howe, T. R. Sigg, and M. A. Wahl, "Hemodialysis clearance of metronidazole following overdose," *Annals of Pharmacotherapy*, vol. 39, no. 7-8, p. 1366, 2005.

[64] G. Thunga, K. G. Sam, D. Patel et al., "Effectiveness of hemodialysis in acute dapsone overdose—a case report," *American Journal of Emergency Medicine*, vol. 26, no. 9, pp. 1070.e1–1070.e4, 2008.

[65] K. Skinner, A. Saiao, A. Mostafa et al., "Isoniazid poisoning: pharmacokinetics and effect of hemodialysis in a massive ingestion," *Hemodialysis International*, vol. 19, no. 4, pp. E37–E40, 2015.

[66] M. L. A. Sivilotti, D. N. Juurlink, J. S. Garland et al., "Antidote removal during haemodialysis for massive acetaminophen overdose," *Clinical Toxicology*, vol. 51, no. 9, pp. 855–863, 2013.

10

Clinicopathological Correlation in Asian Patients with Biopsy-Proven Lupus Nephritis

Bancha Satirapoj, Pamila Tasanavipas, and Ouppatham Supasyndh

Division of Nephrology, Department of Medicine, Phramongkutklao Hospital and College of Medicine, Bangkok 10400, Thailand

Correspondence should be addressed to Bancha Satirapoj; satirapoj@yahoo.com

Academic Editor: Richard Fatica

A total of 244 patients with lupus nephritis (219 women (89.8%) with a female to male ratio of 9 : 1) were included in the study. Clinical and laboratory findings at renal biopsy are clinically valuable in identifying different renal classifications of lupus pathology, activity, and chronicity index. Patients with class IVG had significantly higher proportions of microscopic hematuria, proteinuria, hypertension, impaired renal function, anemia, hypoalbuminuria, and positive anti-DNA antibody. All of these findings correlated well with high activity index and chronicity index of lupus pathology. Considering these correlations may help to determine the clinicopathologic status of lupus patients.

1. Introduction

Renal involvement is one of the most severe complications of systemic lupus erythematosus (SLE) and the clinical presentation of lupus nephritis (LN) is highly variable, ranging from mild asymptomatic proteinuria to rapidly progressive glomerulonephritis [1, 2]. The renal morphological expression can vary considerably among patients or within an individual over time [3, 4]. Performing renal biopsies to accurately determine the prognosis and to guide treatment in LN patients is greatly needed. Recently, the International Society of Nephrology/Renal Pathology Society (ISN/RPS) 2003 classification of LN was proposed [5].

It has been generally agreed upon that renal morphological lesions and some clinical and laboratory features are correlated. Several studies are available on the clinicopathological correlation in LN subjects mainly from developed countries [6, 7]. However, very few publications are currently available concerning the demographic, clinical, and pathological features of LN and their correlations in Thailand [8]. Therefore, this study aimed to assess the clinical and basic laboratory features of Thai patients with biopsy-proven LN class according to ISN/RPS 2003 classification, renal pathological activity, and chronicity index in patients with LN. Clinical records were reviewed and information regarding renal function, serological activity, and urinary protein is collected and compared across histological classes.

2. Methods

2.1. Subjects. Patients with LN who underwent renal biopsy between 2010 and 2013 in Phramongkutklao and Siriraj Hospitals, Bangkok, Thailand, were included in this study. All patients met the American College of Rheumatology (ACR) revised criteria for the classification of SLE [9]. For inclusion, patients had to have adequate renal biopsy samples for histological diagnosis, including >10 glomeruli. For the patients who had repeated biopsies, samples and clinical records at the time of the first biopsy were used. Consequently, data of 244 patients were available in the study. For included patients, clinical records and laboratory parameters at the time of biopsy were collected. The research followed the tenets of the Declaration of Helsinki; informed consent was obtained, and the research was approved by the institutional review board.

2.2. Renal Pathological Diagnosis. Renal biopsy-confirmed LN cases were classified according to the 2003 ISN/RPS classification [5]. Data regarding immunofluorescence findings were available for 100% of the patients. Activity indices (AIs) and chronicity indices (CIs) were calculated (maximum

TABLE 1: The demographic and clinical findings at renal biopsy by LN class.

	Total ($N = 244$)	Class II ($N = 7$)	Class III ($N = 38$)	Class IVG ($N = 117$)	Class IVS ($N = 39$)	Class V ($N = 43$)
Female (n, %)	219 (89.8%)	5 (71.4%)	35 (92.1%)	106 (90.6%)	34 (87.2%)	39 (90.7%)
Age (years)	34 ± 12	42 ± 9.8	34.7 ± 13.2	32 ± 11.4[†]	33 ± 11.1	38.6 ± 12.5
Current immunosuppressive agents (n, %)						
Prednisolone	226 (92.6%)	6 (85.7%)	37 (97.4%)	104 (88.9%)	38 (97.4%)	41 (95.3%)
Azathioprine	72 (29.5%)	2 (28.6%)	9 (23.7%)	31 (26.5%)	14 (35.9%)	16 (37.2%)
Cyclophosphamide	85 (34.8%)	2 (28.6%)	14 (36.8%)	40 (34.2%)	13 (33.3%)	16 (37.2%)
Mycophenolate mofetil	39 (16%)	1 (14.3%)	8 (21.1%)	19 (16.2%)	7 (17.9%)	4 (9.3%)
Current antihypertensive agents (n, %)						
ACEI/ARB	102 (41.8%)	4 (57.1%)	12 (31.6%)	45 (38.5%)	19 (48.7%)	22 (51.2%)
CCB	59 (24.2%)	3 (42.9%)	3 (7.9%)[*]	36 (30.8%)	9 (23.1%)	8 (18.6%)
BB	15 (6.1%)	—	—	8 (6.8%)	5 (12.8%)	2 (4.7%)
Extrarenal manifestation (n, %)						
Arthritis	134 (54.9%)	2 (28.6%)	28 (73.7%)	59 (50.4%)	20 (51.3%)	25 (58.1%)
Malar rash	112 (45.9%)	2 (28.6%)	16 (42.1%)	57 (48.7%)	20 (51.3%)	17 (39.5%)
Discoid rash	60 (24.6%)	1 (14.3%)	6 (15.8%)	28 (23.9%)	10 (25.6%)	15 (34.9%)
Photosensitivity rash	45 (18.4%)	1 (14.3%)	7 (18.4%)	20 (17.1%)	8 (20.5%)	9 (20.9%)
Oral ulcer	66 (27%)	—	11 (28.9%)	39 (33.3%)	6 (15.4%)	10 (23.3%)
AIHA	79 (32.4%)	—	13 (34.2%)	45 (38.5%)	10 (25.6%)	11 (25.6%)
Leukopenia	86 (35.2%)	1 (14.3%)	18 (47.4%)	44 (37.6%)	11 (28.2%)	12 (27.9%)
Thrombocytopenia	64 (26.2%)	1 (14.3%)	8 (21.1%)	30 (25.6%)	14 (35.9%)	11 (25.6%)
Serositis	50 (20.5%)	—	6 (15.8%)	32 (27.6%)	8 (20.5%)	4 (9.3%)
CNS	11 (4.5%)	—	—	7 (6%)	—	4 (9.3%)

Data are mean ± SD, median with interquartile range and percentages; [†]$P < 0.05$ versus class V and [*]$P < 0.05$ versus class II. ACEI: angiotensin converting enzyme inhibitor, AIHA: autoimmune hemolytic anemia, ARB: angiotensin type 1 receptor blocker, BB: beta-blockers, CCB: calcium channel blocker, CNS: central nervous system.

scores, 24 for AI and 12 for CI) and interstitial fibrosis was evaluated for each biopsy specimen and was graded semiquantitatively using a scoring system from 0 to 3 (0 = no changes, 1 = mild, 2 = moderate, and 3 = severe) [10].

2.3. Data Collection. Demographic data (sex, age, and duration of disease), extrarenal SLE manifestations, systolic blood pressure (SBP), diastolic blood pressure (DBP), anti-dsDNA antibody, anti-nuclear antibodies, and biochemical parameters white blood cells, hemoglobin, blood urea nitrogen, serum creatinine and estimated glomerular filtration rate (GFR), serum albumin, serum complement, urine protein creatinine ratio (UPCR), and previous immunosuppressive treatments at the time of kidney biopsy were obtained from the patient records. Nephrotic syndrome was defined as clinical edema, an increase in the UPCR of ≥3.5 g/gCr and serum cholesterol of >200 mg/dL, and a decrease in serum albumin to ≤3.0 g/dL. Nephrotic range proteinuria was defined as UPCR of ≥3.5 g/gCr.

2.4. Statistical Analysis. Data with normal distribution and nonnormal distribution were summarized as mean ± SD and median and range, respectively. Categorical variables were presented as percentage. For multiple comparisons,

univariate analysis of variance (ANOVA) with post hoc analysis by Dunnett t was used followed by the least significance difference test. Pearson's correlation and Chi square tests were used to compare frequency variables and correlation among different variables. Multivariate model using a stepwise regression analysis was performed to correct for confounders. A backward stepwise elimination process was used to remove any other covariates. All statistical evaluations were performed using the SPSS Program, version 12.0 (SPSS, Chicago, IL, USA). A P value of <0.05 was considered statistically significant.

3. Results

A total of 244 patients were included in this study. The mean patient age at renal biopsy was 34.0 ± 12.0 years. Significant differences of mean age were observed between LN classes and in particular mean age was significantly low in patients with class IVG compared with patients with class V. Of the 244 patients, 219 (89.8%) were female with a female to male ratio of 9 : 1. Various treatment regimens were used, all of which included prednisolone (92.6%), cyclophosphamide (34.8%), azathioprine (29.5%), and mycophenolate mofetil (MMF) (16.0%) (Table 1).

TABLE 2: Renal findings at renal biopsy by LN class.

	Total (N = 244)	Class II (N = 7)	Class III (N = 38)	Class IVG (N = 117)	Class IVS (N = 39)	Class V (N = 43)
Levels of clinical and laboratory findings						
SBP (mmHg)	138.9 ± 22.7	118.4 ± 14.7	131.1 ± 17.9	144.2 ± 22.8[*]	139.3 ± 22.3[*]	134.6 ± 23.9
DBP (mmHg)	85.8 ± 14.4	76.1 ± 10.7	81 ± 12.1	89.5 ± 14.2[†*]	86.1 ± 14.8	81.1 ± 13.9
Hemoglobin (g/dL)	10.7 ± 2.2	12.5 ± 1.3	11.2 ± 2.2	10 ± 2.2[†*]	10.7 ± 1.5[†]	12 ± 1.9
BUN (mg/dL)	27.9 ± 21.4	14.7 ± 4.7	18.4 ± 12.3	33.5 ± 24.3[†*]	28.8 ± 17.4	22.2 ± 19.6
Serum creatinine (mg/dL)	1.3 ± 1	1.2 ± 0.8	0.9 ± 0.5	1.5 ± 1.1[†]	1.3 ± 1	1.1 ± 1.1
Estimated GFR (mL/min/1.73 m^2)	80.2 ± 38.3	76 ± 32.4	98.2 ± 31.7	68.4 ± 37.2[†]	82 ± 36.9	95.3 ± 38.2
Serum cholesterol (mg/dL)	287.2 ± 107.6	225.7 ± 45.7	249.5 ± 74.5	296.2 ± 105.6	302 ± 138.3	297.3 ± 113.9
Serum albumin (g/dL)	2.9 ± 0.7	3.9 ± 0.5	3 ± 0.8[*]	2.8 ± 0.6[*]	2.9 ± 0.6[*]	2.9 ± 0.6[*]
UPCR (g/g creatinine)	4.4 ± 3.2	1.3 ± 0.5[†]	3.4 ± 2.4[*]	4.7 ± 3.3[*]	4.2 ± 2.4[*]	5.1 ± 3.8[*]
Percentages of clinical and laboratory findings						
Hypertension (n, %)	163 (66.8%)	3 (42.9%)	18 (47.4%)	92 (78.6%)[†]	26 (66.7%)	24 (55.8%)
Microscopic hematuria (n, %)	157 (64.3%)	4 (57.1%)	24 (63.2%)[†]	86 (73.5%)[†]	29 (74.4%)[†]	14 (32.6%)
GFR < 50 mL/min/1.73 m^2	68 (27.9%)	2 (28.6%)	5 (13.2%)	44 (37.6%)[†]	10 (25.6%)	7 (16.3%)
Nephrotic range proteinuria (n, %)	125 (51.2%)	—	14 (36.8%)	67 (57.3%)[*]	19 (48.7%)[*]	25 (58.1%)[*]
Nephrotic syndrome (n, %)	74 (30.3%)	—	7 (18.4%)	39 (33.3%)[*]	10 (25.6%)	18 (41.9%)[*]
Anti-dsDNA (n, %)	190 (77.9%)	3 (42.9%)	33 (86.8%)[*]	92 (80.7%)[*]	32 (86.5%)[*]	30 (69.8%)

Data are mean ± SD, median with interquartile range and percentages; [†] $P < 0.05$ versus class V and [*] $P < 0.05$ versus class II. BUN: blood urea nitrogen, DBP: diastolic blood pressure, and GFR: glomerular filtration rate. UPCR: urine protein creatinine ratio and SBP: systolic blood pressure.

3.1. Clinical and Laboratory Parameters Associated with Each LN Class (Tables 1 and 2). In patients with LN class II, blood pressure was well controlled and renal function was well preserved: mean serum creatinine was 1.2 ± 0.8 mg/dL and mean estimated GFR was 76 ± 32.4 mL/min/1.73 m^2. Urinary findings were microscopic hematuria (57.1%) and mild degree of proteinuria with mean urinary protein of 1.3 ± 0.5 g/gCr. Importantly, no patients with nephrotic syndrome or nephrotic range protein were detected. Patients with serologically active anti-dsDNA antibody comprised 42.9%.

Data were compared between class III and other classes. In class III, blood pressure was well controlled. Renal function was well preserved and no significant difference was observed with classes II and IV: mean serum creatinine was 0.9 ± 0.5 mg/dL and mean estimated GFR was 98.2 ± 31.7 mL/min/1.73 m^2. Microscopic hematuria was significantly higher in patients with class III (63.2%) than in patients with class V (32.1%). Urinary protein excretion was moderate: mean urinary protein was 3.4 ± 2.4 g/gCr, and frequency of nephrotic syndrome was 18.4%. Significant differences were found in levels of proteinuria in class III and class II. Serologically active anti-dsDNA antibody (86.8%) in patients with class III was significantly higher than in patients with class II (42.9%).

Patients with class IVG had the most severe nephritis as follows: SBP, 144.2 ± 22.8 mmHg; DBP, 89.5 ± 14.2 mmHg; serum creatinine, 1.5 ± 1.1 mg/dL; estimated GFR, 68.4 ± 37.2 mL/min/1.73 m^2; urinary protein, 4.7 ± 3.3 g/gCr; serum albumin, 2.8 ± 0.6 g/dL; and hemoglobin, 10 ± 2.2 g/dL. At the time of renal biopsy, 92 (78.6%) patients were hypertensive

(blood pressure ≥ 140/90 mmHg) and 44 (37.6%) patients exhibited impaired GFR (GFR < 50 mL/min/1.73 m^2). In comparison with other classes, patients with class IVG had a significant increase in serum creatinine, blood pressure, proteinuria, and frequency of microscopic hematuria and a significant decrease in estimated GFR, serum albumin, and hemoglobin (Tables 1 and 2). A significantly high frequency of nephrotic syndrome (33.3%) and active anti-dsDNA antibody (80.7%) were observed. Data were similar between classes IVG and IVS, but patients with class IVS tended be less severe nephritis profiles including blood pressure, renal function, serum albumin, hemoglobin, and frequency of nephrotic syndrome.

In class V, blood pressure was well controlled. Renal function was significantly higher in class V patients than patients with class IVG (estimated GFR 95.3 ± 38.2 versus 68.4 ± 37.2 mL/min/1.73 m^2, $P < 0.05$). Microscopic hematuria was significantly lower in patients with class V (32.6%) than in patients with class IVG (73.5%) and class IVS (74.4%). Urinary protein excretion was high: mean urinary protein was 5.1 ± 3.8 g/gCr, and a significantly high frequency of nephrotic syndrome (41.9%) was observed compared with class II. However, no significant differences were found in levels of proteinuria in class V with class IV. Serologically active anti-dsDNA antibody in patients with class V was 69.8%.

3.2. Renal Pathological Findings. The relative frequency of each class was as follows: class II (mesangial proliferative LN) 2.9%, class III (focal proliferative LN) 15.6%, class

TABLE 3: The renal pathological findings at renal biopsy by LN class.

	Total (N = 244)	Class II (N = 7)	Class III (N = 38)	Class IVG (N = 117)	Class IVS (N = 39)	Class V (N = 43)
Activity index						
Endocapillary proliferation	184 (75.4%)	1 (14.3%)	34 (89.5%)[†*]	108 (92.3%)[†*]	39 (100%)[†*]	2 (4.7%)
Glomerular leukocyte infiltration	148 (60.7%)	1 (14.3%)	20 (52.6%)[†*]	92 (78.6%)[†*]	30 (76.9%)[†*]	5 (11.6%)
Hyaline thrombi	154 (63.1%)	0 (0%)	17 (44.7%)[†*]	100 (85.5%)[†*]	33 (84.6%)[†*]	4 (9.3%)
Fibrinoid necrosis	41 (16.8%)	1 (14.3%)	6 (15.8%)	23 (19.7%)[†]	11 (28.2%)[†]	0 (0%)
Cellular crescent	94 (38.5%)	0 (0%)	15 (39.5%)[†]	58 (49.6%)[†*]	20 (51.3%)[†*]	1 (2.3%)
Interstitial inflammation	150 (61.5%)	3 (42.9%)	22 (57.9%)	78 (66.7%)[†]	28 (71.8%)	19 (44.2%)
Total activity index (Max 24)	6.8 ± 4.3	1.1 ± 2.2	$4.4 \pm 2.3^{†*}$	$9.4 \pm 3.1^{†*}$	$8.6 \pm 2.9^{†*}$	1.2 ± 1.8
Median (IQR)	7 (3, 10)	0 (0, 1)	4 (3, 6)	9 (7, 11.5)	8 (6, 11)	1 (0, 1)
Chronicity index						
Sclerotic glomeruli	121 (49.6%)	4 (57.1%)	16 (42.1%)	55 (47%)	26 (66.7%)	20 (46.5%)
Fibrous crescent	53 (21.7%)	0 (0%)	5 (13.2%)	33 (28.2%)[†]	15 (38.5%)[†*]	0 (0%)
Tubular atrophy	121 (49.6%)	1 (14.3%)	12 (31.6%)	64 (54.7%)	23 (59%)[*]	21 (48.8%)
Interstitial fibrosis	139 (57%)	1 (14.3%)	14 (36.8%)	73 (62.4%)[*]	27 (69.2%)[*]	24 (55.8%)
Total chronicity index (Max 12)	2.5 ± 2.3	1.1 ± 1.5	1.6 ± 1.9	2.9 ± 2.4	$3 \pm 2.1^{*}$	2.2 ± 2.3
Median (IQR)	2 (0, 4)	1 (0, 2)	1 (0, 3)	3 (1, 4)	3 (2, 4)	2 (0, 3)

Data are mean ± SD, median with interquartile range and percentages; [†]$P < 0.05$ versus class V and [*]$P < 0.05$ versus class II.

IVG (diffuse global proliferative LN) 50%, class IVS (diffuse segmental proliferative LN) 16%, and class V (membranous LN) 17.6%. Patients of class III + V were considered to be class III and patients of class IV + V were considered to be class IV. No class VI was diagnosed at the initial renal biopsy. Patients with classes III and IV had a higher activity index, percentage of endocapillary proliferation, glomerular leukocyte infiltration, hyaline thrombi, fibrinoid necrosis, cellular crescents, and interstitial inflammation (Table 3). Patients with class IV had a higher chronicity index, percentage of fibrous crescents, tubular atrophy, and interstitial fibrosis (Table 3).

3.3. Clinical Parameters Associated with Renal Pathological Activity and Chronicity Index. Univariate analysis was performed to assess the relationship between clinical parameters with renal pathological activity and chronicity index. SBP, DBP, BUN, serum creatinine, UPCR, and presence of serositis, microscopic hematuria, and anti-dsDNA were positively correlated with renal pathological activity index, whereas age, estimated GFR, hemoglobin, and serum albumin were negatively correlated with renal pathological activity index. After multiple regression analyses, significant correlations were found among age, DBP, serum creatinine, estimated GFR, hemoglobin, serum albumin, UPCR, and presence of microscopic hematuria and anti-dsDNA antibody with renal pathological activity index (Table 4).

Renal pathological chronicity index was positively correlated significantly with SBP, DBP, BUN, serum creatinine, UPCR, and presence of serositis but negatively correlated with estimated GFR, hemoglobin, and serum albumin. After multiple regression analyses, significant correlations were found among serum creatinine, estimated GFR, hemoglobin, UPCR, and presence of microscopic hematuria and anti-dsDNA antibody with renal pathological chronicity index (Table 5).

4. Discussion

The study demonstrated the correlation of various demographic and laboratory findings in cases of biopsy-proven LN with the pathological features on renal biopsies. One of the most common findings was class IVG (48%). At renal biopsy, a higher microscopic hematuria, impaired GFR, proteinuria, anemia, hypoalbuminemia and hypertension, and the presence of positive anti-DNA antibody were all associated with the worst class, that is, class IV. These parameters were also correlated with high renal pathological activity and chronicity index in patients with LN.

Renal survival is mainly determined by the severity of renal involvement and renal classification [11]. The discrepancy may be related to differences in ethnicity or to different severity of renal disease in LN at biopsy. Several clinical characteristics related to lupus classification in our study confirmed those previously reported [12–14]. Initially, significant differences were observed in the degree of nephritic and nephrotic features including microscopic hematuria, high blood pressure, impaired renal function, high proteinuria, and presence of anti-dsDNA antibody between LN classes II and IVG/IVS. Importantly, no patients with nephrotic syndrome or nephrotic range proteinuria were detected in class II. Unfortunately, the data in our series offered no way of distinguishing among the different clinical findings among patients with LN classes III and IV. Additionally, there was no difference in all extrarenal manifestations among each class.

Our patients with class IV or V had massive proteinuria with lower serum albumin levels than those of patients with class II. Regarding the difference between class IV and class V, no statistical difference was found in proteinuria, serum albumin, and cholesterol levels in this study, suggesting that all clinical features of nephrotic syndrome

TABLE 4: Univariate and multivariate regression analyses demonstrating clinical factors showing correlation with renal pathological activity index (AI).

	Univariate regression			Multivariate regression $R^2 = 0.386$		
	Beta	SE.	P value	Beta	SE.	P value
Age (yrs)	−0.09	0.02	<0.001	−0.10	0.02	<0.001
SBP (mmHg)	0.05	0.01	<0.001			
DBP (mmHg)	0.08	0.02	<0.001	0.05	0.02	0.001
Serositis	1.97	0.68	0.004			
Anti-dsDNA	2.23	0.69	0.001	1.18	0.57	0.039
Blood urea nitrogen (mg/dL)	0.08	0.01	<0.001			
Serum creatinine (mg/dL)	1.43	0.27	<0.001	−0.98	0.43	0.024
Estimated GFR (mL/min/1.73 m^2)	−0.04	0.01	<0.001	−0.05	0.01	<0.001
Hemoglobin (g/dL)	−0.81	0.12	<0.001	−0.40	0.12	0.001
Serum albumin (g/dL)	−1.21	0.40	0.003			
UPCR (g/g creatinine)	0.21	0.09	0.016	0.18	0.07	0.014
Microscopic hematuria	2.50	0.56	<0.001	1.44	0.48	0.003

Independent variables in the multivariate model were chosen using a stepwise regression analysis where all significant variables listed in the univariate analysis were included.
DBP: diastolic blood pressure, GFR: glomerular filtration rate, SBP: systolic blood pressure, and UPCR: urine protein creatinine ratio.

TABLE 5: Univariate and multivariate regression analyses demonstrating clinical factors showing correlation with renal pathological chronicity index (CI).

	Univariate regression			Multivariate regression $R^2 = 0.409$		
	Beta	SE.	P value	Beta	SE.	P value
Age (yrs)	0.01	0.01	0.762			
SBP (mmHg)	0.02	0.01	0.001			
DBP (mmHg)	0.03	0.01	0.006			
Serositis	0.86	0.37	0.020			
Anti-dsDNA	0.64	0.38	0.092	0.67	0.30	0.026
Blood urea nitrogen (mg/dL)	0.04	0.01	<0.001			
Serum creatinine (mg/dL)	1.17	0.13	<0.001	0.62	0.21	0.004
Estimated GFR (mL/min/1.73 m^2)	−0.03	0.00	<0.001	−0.02	0.01	0.008
Hemoglobin (g/dL)	−0.37	0.07	<0.001	−0.20	0.06	0.002
Serum albumin (g/dL)	−0.39	0.22	0.077			
UPCR (g/g creatinine)	0.13	0.05	0.005	0.12	0.04	0.003
Microscopic hematuria	−0.58	0.31	0.063	−1.06	0.26	<0.001

Independent variables in the multivariate model were chosen using a stepwise regression analysis where all significant variables listed in the univariate analysis were included.
DBP: diastolic blood pressure, GFR: glomerular filtration rate, SBP: systolic blood pressure, and UPCR: urine protein creatinine ratio.

may be unimportant to define LN class IV and class V, whereas significant differences were observed in nephritic parameters including microscopic hematuria, anemia, high blood pressure, and impaired renal function between LN classes V and IV in initial biopsy finding. The results from our study on biopsy-proven cases of LN largely concur with the previously reported study [15]. Finally, our findings indicated that, at the same level of proteinuria without microscopic hematuria, anemia, high blood pressure, and impaired renal function might prefer diagnosis of LN class V compared with LN class IV.

Histological activity and chronicity index were strongly predictive for renal function outcome [16] and these measurements were used to grade the individual morphologic components in a given biopsy as a guide to treat and predict the renal survival in patients with LN [17, 18]. Previous studies have shown that serum creatinine and proteinuria had a significant positive correlation with high activity and chronicity index on pathological features of LN [13, 14]. Our results support this finding; advanced age and nephritic parameters including blood pressure, serum creatinine, estimated GFR, hemoglobin, serum albumin, UPCR, and presence of microscopic hematuria and anti-dsDNA antibody had a significant positive correlation with high renal pathological activity and chronicity index. We speculated that all nephritic features might reflect renal activity and chronicity scores, especially immunologic disease activities in patients with SLE.

Our study had several limitations, including its retrospective design and assessment of a small number of patients in LN class II. Furthermore, a possibility of differences in immunosuppressive agents may have occurred before inclusion and during the follow-up period. Evaluation of other clinical factors potentially affecting clinical features, such as other medications and socioeconomic status, would be interesting but was undetermined in this study. Larger prospective trials are still required to ascertain consistent baseline clinical markers.

In conclusion, this study indicates that clinical and laboratory findings at renal biopsy are clinically valuable in identifying different renal classifications of lupus pathology, activity, and chronicity index. Our results suggest that patients with class IVG had significantly higher proportions of microscopic hematuria, proteinuria, hypertension, impaired renal function, anemia, hypoalbuminuria, and positive anti-DNA antibody. All of these findings correlated well with high activity index and chronicity index of lupus pathology.

Acknowledgments

The authors would like to thank Dr. Ratana Chawanasuntorapoj, Division of Nephrology, Department of Medicine, Faculty of Medicine, Siriraj Hospital, Mahidol University, Bangkok, Thailand, for providing data. This work was supported by grant from Department of Medicine, Phramongkutklao Hospital and College of Medicine, Bangkok, Thailand.

References

[1] R. Cervera, M. A. Khamashta, J. Font et al., "Morbidity and mortality in systemic lupus erythematosus during a 10-year period: a comparison of early and late manifestations in a cohort of 1,000 patients," *Medicine*, vol. 82, no. 5, pp. 299–308, 2003.

[2] B. Satirapoj, J. Wongchinsri, N. Youngprang et al., "Predictors of renal involvement in patients with systemic lupus erythematosus," *Asian Pacific Journal of Allergy and Immunology*, vol. 25, no. 1, pp. 17–25, 2007.

[3] F. Yu, Y. Tan, L.-H. Wu, S.-N. Zhu, G. Liu, and M.-H. Zhao, "Class IV-G and IV-S lupus nephritis in Chinese patients: a large cohort study from a single center," *Lupus*, vol. 18, no. 12, pp. 1073–1081, 2009.

[4] K. I. Dibbs, Y. Sadovsky, X.-J. Li, S. S. Koide, S. Adler, and A.-R. Fuchs, "Estrogenic activity of RU 486 (mifepristone) in rat uterus and cultured uterine myocytes," *American Journal of Obstetrics and Gynecology*, vol. 173, no. 1, pp. 134–140, 1995.

[5] J. J. Weening, V. D. D'Agati, M. M. Schwartz et al., "The classification of glomerulonephritis in systemic lupus erythematosus revisited," *Journal of the American Society of Nephrology*, vol. 15, no. 2, pp. 241–250, 2004.

[6] Z. Shariati-Sarabi, A. Ranjbar, S. M. Monzavi, H. Esmaily, M. Farzadnia, and A. A. Zeraati, "Analysis of clinicopathologic correlations in Iranian patients with lupus nephritis," *International Journal of Rheumatic Diseases*, vol. 16, no. 6, pp. 731–738, 2013.

[7] S. Chen, Z. Tang, Y. Zhang, Z. Liu, H. Zhang, and W. Hu, "Significance of histological crescent formation in patients with diffuse proliferative lupus nephritis," *American Journal of Nephrology*, vol. 38, no. 6, pp. 445–452, 2014.

[8] P. Parichatikanond, N. D. Francis, P. Malasit et al., "Lupus nephritis: clinicopathological study of 162 cases in Thailand," *Journal of Clinical Pathology*, vol. 39, no. 2, pp. 160–166, 1986.

[9] M. C. Hochberg, "Updating the American College of Rheumatology revised criteria for the classification of systemic lupus erythematosus," *Arthritis and Rheumatism*, vol. 40, no. 9, p. 1725, 1997.

[10] H. A. Austin III, L. R. Muenz, K. M. Joyce et al., "Prognostic factors in lupus nephritis. Contribution of renal histologic data," *The American Journal of Medicine*, vol. 75, no. 3, pp. 382–391, 1983.

[11] M. Faurschou, H. Starklint, P. Halberg, and S. Jacobsen, "Prognostic factors in lupus nephritis: diagnostic and therapeutic delay increases the risk of terminal renal failure," *Journal of Rheumatology*, vol. 33, no. 8, pp. 1563–1569, 2006.

[12] I. G. Okpechi, C. R. Swanepoel, N. Tiffin, M. Duffield, and B. L. Rayner, "Clinicopathological insights into lupus nephritis in South Africans: a study of 251 patients," *Lupus*, vol. 21, no. 9, pp. 1017–1024, 2012.

[13] H. Nasri, A. Ahmadi, A. Baradaran et al., "Clinicopathological correlations in lupus nephritis; a single center experience," *Journal of Nephropathology*, vol. 3, no. 3, pp. 115–120, 2014.

[14] F. Mitjavila, V. Pac, I. Moga et al., "Clinicopathological correlations and prognostic factors in lupus nephritis," *Clinical and Experimental Rheumatology*, vol. 15, no. 6, pp. 625–631, 1997.

[15] Q. Chen, Z. Liu, W. Hu, H. Chen, C. Zeng, and L. Li, "Class V lupus nephritis: a clinicopathologic study in 152 patients," *Journal of Nephrology*, vol. 16, no. 1, pp. 126–132, 2003.

[16] S. Emre, I. Bilge, A. Sirin et al., "Lupus nephritis in children: prognostic significance of clinicopathological findings," *Nephron*, vol. 87, no. 2, pp. 118–126, 2001.

[17] A. J. Howie, N. Turhan, and D. Adu, "Powerful morphometric indicator of prognosis in lupus nephritis," *QJM*, vol. 96, no. 6, pp. 411–420, 2003.

[18] B. H. Rovin and S. V. Parikh, "Lupus nephritis: the evolving role of novel therapeutics," *The American Journal of Kidney Diseases*, vol. 63, no. 4, pp. 677–690, 2014.

11

Hyperuricemia: An Early Marker for Severity of Illness in Sepsis

Sana R. Akbar,[1] **Dustin M. Long,**[2] **Kashif Hussain,**[3] **Ahmad Alhajhusain,**[3] **Umair S. Ahmed,**[1] **Hafiz I. Iqbal,**[1] **Ailia W. Ali,**[3] **Rachel Leonard,**[4] **and Cheryl Dalton**[1]

[1]*Division of Nephrology, Department of Medicine, West Virginia University School of Medicine, Morgantown, WV, USA*
[2]*Division of Biostatistics, West Virginia University School of Medicine, Morgantown, WV, USA*
[3]*Division of Pulmonary and Critical Care Medicine, Department of Medicine, West Virginia University School of Medicine, Morgantown, WV, USA*
[4]*Department of Medicine, West Virginia University School of Medicine, Morgantown, WV, USA*

Correspondence should be addressed to Sana R. Akbar; sakbar@hsc.wvu.edu

Academic Editor: Danuta Zwolinska

Background. Uric acid can acutely activate various inflammatory transcription factors. Since high levels of oxyradicals and lower antioxidant levels in septic patients are believed to result in multiorgan failure, uric acid levels could be used as a marker of oxidative stress and poor prognosis in patients with sepsis. *Design.* We conducted a prospective cohort study on Medical Intensive Care Unit (MICU) patients and hypothesized that elevated uric acid in patients with sepsis is predictive of greater morbidity. The primary end point was the correlation between hyperuricemia and the morbidity rate. Secondary end points were Acute Kidney Injury (AKI), mortality, Acute Respiratory Distress Syndrome (ARDS), and duration of stay. *Results.* We enrolled 144 patients. 54 (37.5%) had the primary end point of hyperuricemia. The overall morbidity rate was 85.2%. The probability of having hyperuricemia along with AKI was 68.5% and without AKI was 31.5%. Meanwhile the probability of having a uric acid value <7 mg/dL along with AKI was 18.9% and without AKI was 81.1% (p value < 0.0001). *Conclusion.* We report that elevated uric acid levels on arrival to the MICU in patients with sepsis are associated with poor prognosis. These patients are at an increased risk for AKI and ARDS.

1. Introduction

In humans uric acid is the final oxidative product of purine metabolism through the action of xanthine oxidase or xanthine dehydrogenase. Approximately two-thirds of uric acid is excreted by the kidney, and the rest is excreted by the gastrointestinal tract. In addition some uric acid is degraded in the body after reaction with oxidants or peroxynitrite [1]. Uric acid occurs predominantly as a urate anion under physiologic pH. In the kidney, urate is filtered readily by the glomerulus and subsequently reabsorbed by the proximal tubular cells of the kidney; normal fractional excretion of uric acid is approximately 10% [2]. Normal levels of blood uric acid are typically 3.4–7.2 mg/dL for men and 2.4–6.1 mg/dL for women. Since the last century elevated uric acid levels have been noted to be associated with atherosclerosis [3–7], hypertension, hyperinsulinemia [8, 9], and chronic kidney disease [10]. Uric acid has been shown to be elevated in hypoxic states such as chronic heart failure [11, 12] and

obstructive pulmonary disease [13, 14]. Hyperuricemia is defined as the accumulation of serum uric acid beyond its solubility point in water and develops due to uric acid overproduction, undersecretion, or both [15].

Uric acid can induce acute inflammation of the renal epithelial cells via uric acid crystals. Uric acid can also have an impact in the human body by its noncrystal effects. It may cause endothelial dysfunction and cause an afferent renal arteriolopathy and tubulointerstitial fibrosis in the kidney by activating the renin-angiotensin-aldosterone system [16], activate various inflammatory transcription factors [17], and induce systemic cytokine production such as tumor necrosis factor alpha [18] and local expression of chemokines such as monocyte chemotactic protein 1 in the kidney and cyclooxygenase 2 (COX-2) in blood vessels [19]. Experimentally induced hyperuricemia in rats leads to reduced urinary nitrite levels and systemic and glomerular hypertension [20, 21]. Other in vitro experimental studies have shown that uric acid decreases nitric oxide production [22] and also may lead to nitric oxide depletion [23]. The noncrystal effects of uric acid remain contentious because, under physiologic concentrations, urate is a powerful antioxidant that can scavenge superoxide, hydroxyl radicals, and singlet oxygen [24].

Sepsis is a serious medical condition characterized by a whole-body inflammatory state (systemic inflammatory response syndrome) and the presence of a known or suspected infection that has severe consequences [25]. Hence majority of intensive care unit patients undergo ischemic-reperfusion injury and inflammation to varying degrees during their hospitalization. Uric acid may be a factor playing a role in these processes since it has both oxidant and antioxidant properties. Since high levels of oxyradicals and lower antioxidant levels in patients with sepsis are believed to result in multiorgan failure, the measurement of uric acid levels could be possibly used as a marker of oxidative stress in patients with sepsis. Hence we decided to conduct a prospective cohort study in Medical Intensive Care Unit (MICU) patients admitted with sepsis to see if there is any significance of serum uric acid with respect to the morbidity rate. We hypothesized that elevated uric acid levels at the early hours of sepsis can predict an increased risk of morbidities as a single test.

2. Materials and Methods

2.1. Study Design. We conducted a prospective cohort study among patients admitted to the Medical Intensive Care Unit (MICU) at Ruby Memorial Hospital, West Virginia University (Morgantown, West Virginia), between January 2014 and July 2014. Patients or their Medical Power of Attorneys provided written informed consent and all the protocol was approved by the West Virginia University Office of Research Integrity and Compliance (West Virginia University Institutional Review Board). Funding for this study was provided through the West Virginia Clinical and Translational Science Institute Pilot Grants Program.

2.2. Enrollment Criteria. Inclusion criteria were age >18 years and admission to the MICU with a working diagnosis of sepsis based on the Society of Critical Care Medicine, Surviving Sepsis Campaign 2012 definition [26]. Exclusion criteria were as follows: (1) pregnant females and (2) patients from an outside facility that have already been in the MICU for more than 24 hours.

2.3. Data Collection and Definitions. Patients being admitted to the MICU were screened for sepsis. Sepsis was defined based on the Society of Critical Care Medicine, Surviving Sepsis Campaign 2012 definition [26]. Once the patient met the inclusion criteria then blood samples were obtained for uric acid, basic metabolic profile, complete blood count, lactic acid, phosphorus, albumin, and arterial blood gas. Repeat samples for arterial blood gas and basic metabolic profile were obtained at 24 and 48 hours. Subsequently, the electronic health records were reviewed to gather the remaining data such as the patients' age, sex, weight, race, body mass index, vital signs, comorbidities, ventilation status, need for renal replacement therapy, and hospital course over a 72-hour

period. During the course of the study all patients continued to receive standard of care for their illnesses by the MICU team. For the purpose of our study we defined hyperuricemia as a uric acid level ≥7 mg/dL in both males and females. We defined Acute Kidney Injury (AKI) as an absolute ≥0.3 mg/dL increase in serum creatinine over a 48-hour time period from the baseline creatinine based on the Acute Kidney Injury Network (AKIN) definition [27]. We used as the baseline creatinine value the patients' creatinine value at the time of initial presentation to the MICU. We calculated the Acute Physiology and Chronic Health Evaluation (APACHE) II score based on Knaus et al. [28] definition to help assess the severity of disease in the MICU patient population. Acute Respiratory Distress Syndrome (ARDS) was defined per the Berlin definition [29].

2.4. Clinical Outcomes. The primary end point was the correlation between hyperuricemia in patients presenting with sepsis and the morbidity rate. We hypothesized that elevated uric acid in patients presenting to the MICU with sepsis is predictive of a greater morbidity rate. Hyperuricemia in general is defined as a serum urate level of >7 mg/dL (420 uM) in men and >6 mg/dL (300 uM) in women. For the purpose of our study we defined hyperuricemia as a uric acid level ≥7 mg/dL in both males and females. Secondary end points were Acute Kidney Injury (AKI), mortality, Acute Respiratory Distress Syndrome (ARDS), and duration of stay in MICU. AKI was defined as an absolute ≥0.3 mg/dL increase in serum creatinine over a 48-hour time period from the baseline creatinine based on the Acute Kidney Injury Network (AKIN) definition. We used as the baseline creatinine value the patients' creatinine value at the time of initial presentation to the MICU. Additional end points included need for renal replacement therapy and the patients' stability to be transferred to a lower level of care.

2.5. Statistical Analyses. Percentages of measures by uric acid level were compared using Chi squared tests for association. For APACHE II scores, linear regression was performed to assess the linear association with uric acid. All analyses were performed in SAS 9.4.

3. Results

3.1. Baseline Characteristics. We enrolled and collected samples from 144 patients. The median age was 60.5 years. The most prevalent comorbidities were Diabetes, coronary artery disease, and cerebrovascular accident. Overall there were 57.6% males and 42.4% females and 39.6% of the enrolled patient population were ≥65 years of age. Our patient population was predominantly Caucasian (97.2%) (see Table 1). Also to note was that 47.8% of the overall patient population had a body mass index (BMI) ≥30 (see Table 1 and Figure 1). The BMI distribution in the overall population is given in Figure 1.

3.2. Acute Kidney Injury and Acute Respiratory Distress Syndrome. Amongst 144 patients, 54 (37.5%) had the primary end point of hyperuricemia. Within this subset of patients

TABLE 1: Baseline characteristics.

| Characteristics | Overall N (%) | Uric acid | | p value* |
		High N (%)	Low N (%)	
Age				0.8519
<30 years old	10 (6.9%)	3 (5.6%)	7 (7.8%)	
30–65 years old	77 (53.5%)	30 (55.6%)	47 (52.2%)	
≥65 years old	57 (39.6%)	21 (38.9%)	36 (40.0%)	
Sex				0.9653
Females	61 (42.4%)	23 (42.6%)	38 (42.2%)	
Males	83 (57.6%)	31 (57.4%)	52 (57.8%)	
Ethnicity				0.2436
Caucasian	140 (97.2%)	51 (94.4%)	89 (98.9%)	
Black	3 (2.1%)	2 (3.7%)	1 (1.1%)	
BMI				0.0195
18.5–24.9	37 (27.2%)	12 (22.6%)	25 (30.1%)	
25–29.9	34 (25.0%)	8 (15.1%)	26 (31.3%)	
≥30	65 (47.8%)	33 (62.3%)	32 (38.6%)	
Comorbidities				
DM	53 (36.8%)	22 (40.7%)	31 (34.4%)	0.4482
CAD	37 (25.7%)	15 (27.8%)	22 (24.4%)	0.6576
Severe pulmonary disease	23 (16.0%)	7 (13.0%)	16 (17.8%)	0.4452
CHF	14 (9.7%)	8 (14.8%)	6 (6.7%)	0.1101
CVA	24 (16.7%)	7 (13.0%)	17 (19.9%)	0.3556
h/o malignancy	23 (16.0%)	10 (18.5%)	13 (14.4%)	0.5182

*Chi square test.

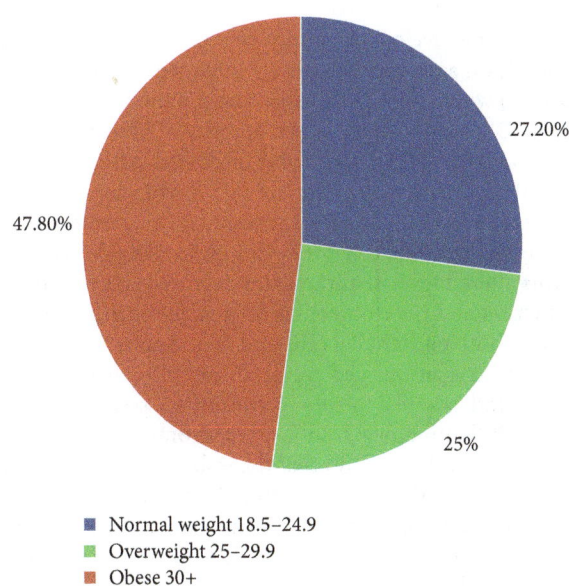

FIGURE 1: BMI distribution of the total patient population.

The probability of having hyperuricemia along with AKI is about 68.5% and without AKI is about 31.5%. Meanwhile the probability of having a uric acid value <7 mg/dL along with AKI is 18.9% and without AKI about 81.1%. These probabilities are statistically significant with a p value of <0.0001. Of the 37 patients who had hyperuricemia and AKI, only 3 (8.1%) needed renal replacement therapy; meanwhile for the overall sample 2.08% ended up having renal replacement therapy in the first 48 hrs of their MICU hospitalization.

The most prevalent comorbidities among patients with hyperuricemia were Diabetes Mellitus (40.7%), coronary artery disease (27.8%), and history of a malignancy (18.5%). Meanwhile the most prevalent comorbidities in patients with hyperuricemia who incurred AKI were Diabetes (43.3%), coronary artery disease (32.4%), and Congestive Heart Failure (21.6%) (see Figure 2).

3.3. *Severity of Illness.* Elevated lactic acid levels can be used as a marker for indicating impaired tissue oxygenation, leading to increased anaerobic metabolism and suggesting the presence of hemodynamic instability resulting in lack of appropriate organ perfusion. In our lab elevated lactic acid level was considered as any level >2.2 mmol/L. Of the patients with hyperuricemia 35.2% had an elevated lactic acid level. Our data is suggestive of an association between high uric acid levels and elevated lactic acid levels; however the results are not statistically significant most likely due to the small sample size.

the overall morbidity rate was 85.2% of which AKI accounted for 68.5% and 83.8% had ARDS. Of those with ARDS 70.6% required mechanical ventilation. In terms of ARDS, although a high percentage of patients incurred this in our sample population, the incidence was not statistically significant most likely due to the small sample size of the study population.

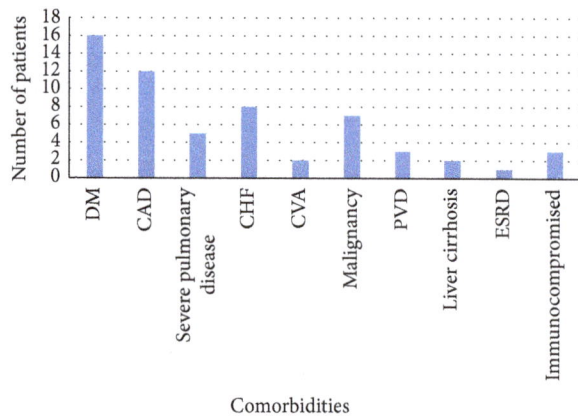

FIGURE 2: Comorbidities in patients with hyperuricemia and AKI.

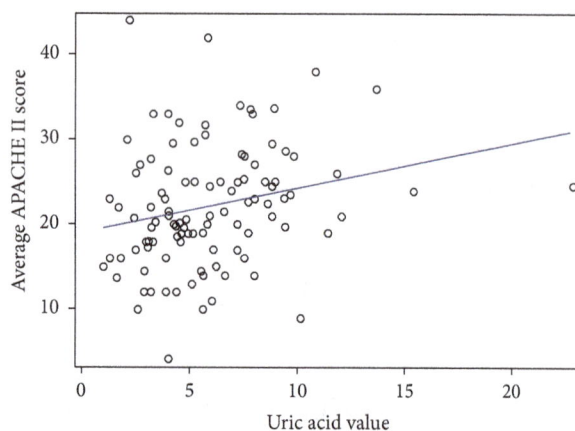

FIGURE 3: Uric acid levels and APACHE II score.

The Acute Physiology and Chronic Health Evaluation (APACHE) II score helps predict the severity of disease and the prognosis of the patients in the intensive care unit. For the purpose of our study we defined an elevated APACHE II score as any value ≥20 as scores of ≥20 have been associated with a greater than 35% predictive mortality rate. Of the 144 study patients 40 patients were excluded while calculating the APACHE II score as they did not have an arterial blood gas result. In our study of the patients with hyperuricemia 83.3% had an APACHE II score ≥20 while only 16.7% had an APACHE II score <20. The probability of having a uric acid level <7 mg/dL with an APACHE II score of ≥20 was 54.4% and with an APACHE II score of <20 was 45.6%. These probabilities are statistically significant with a p value of 0.0034. In addition a linear correlation between the APACHE II score and uric acid value was noted, p value of 0.014 (see Figure 3).

Hypoalbuminemia is a common problem associated with patients with acute and chronic medical conditions. The normal albumin values are 3.5–4.5 g/dL. We defined hypoalbuminemia as levels ≤3.5 gm/dL. Based on this of the patients with hyperuricemia 88.5% had hypoalbuminemia while 91.7% of those with a uric acid level <7 mg/dL had a low albumin level. The results were not statistically significant as the p value was 0.5367.

Hypophosphatemia has been hypothesized to be associated with early sepsis and the presence of elevated inflammatory cytokines. As per our results the overall incidence of hypophosphatemia in our sample population was only 16.7% and in the subgroup with hyperuricemia 7.4% had a serum phosphorus level of ≤2.5 mg/dL. Although of the nonhyperuricemic patients 22.2% had a low phosphorus level and these values are significantly different with p value of 0.0209, no correlation between hypophosphatemia and elevated uric acid levels was noted in our study.

Duration of stay in the MICU helps indirectly identify the degree of severity of illness of the ICU patients. We found that overall 75% and 54.2% of our enrolled patients were still in the MICU and not transferred to a lower level of care at 48 and 72 hours, respectively. The probability of having hyperuricemia and still being in the MICU at 48 and 72 hours was 81.5% and 64.8%, respectively, while the probability of having a uric acid level <7 mg/dL and being in the MICU at 48 and 72 hours was 71.1% and 47.8%, respectively. These probabilities are different with a p value of 0.1209 and 0.0464, respectively. For those with AKI, there was no difference in still being in the MICU by uric acid level, 82.4% versus 86.5% at 48 hours and 70.6% versus 70.6% at 72 hours. While not significant, there was a higher probability of still being in the MICU for those with ARDS and high uric acid levels compared to those with ARDS and low uric acid levels, 93.6% versus 81.5% (p value = 0.20) at 48 hours and 77.4% versus 68.5% (p value = 0.38).

4. Discussion

In this prospective cohort study, we report that elevated uric acid levels on arrival to the MICU in patients with sepsis are associated with a poor prognosis; that is, an increased risk for AKI, ARDS, marks an increased severity of illness measured as per the APACHE II score and increased duration of stay in the MICU. One may postulate that during sepsis there is an increased level of antioxidant response to counterbalance the excessive proinflammatory cytokines and oxidative stress, and this altered level of antioxidant defense leads to immune dysfunction and poor outcomes. In a systemic inflammatory response, both endothelial cells and neutrophils are activated to release oxygen-derived free radicals [30]. It seems that these oxyradicals play a role in causing or propagating the systemic inflammatory response syndrome (SIRS) in life-threatening conditions and that the imbalance in redox state reflects both oxidative stress and tissue damage [31, 32]. Serum uric acid, like other antioxidants such as albumin, bilirubin, or vitamins A, C, and E, is a powerful free radical scavenger and increases in response to acute oxidative stress [33, 34]. Uric acid formation may even provide a significant antioxidant defense mechanism against nitration by peroxynitrite in rat heart during hypoxia [35]. Hence uric acid is believed to be an important marker of oxidative stress.

The mechanisms for increased uric acid in sepsis are unknown and could be due to increased production as well as decreased excretion. Severe sepsis and septic shock may induce ischemia or hypoxia in multiple organs, which further increases the change in xanthine/hypoxanthine to uric acid through activation of xanthine oxidase in microvascular endothelium [36, 37]. When uric acid accumulates in blood vessels and deposits on the endothelium of vessels, the release of vasorelaxation factors is hampered [3], and vascular contraction interfered, leading to a series of pathophysiological processes and dysfunction of internal organs especially the kidney. Development of AKI during sepsis increases patient morbidity, predicts higher mortality, has a significant effect on multiple organ functions, is associated with an increased length of stay in the intensive care unit, and hence consumes considerable healthcare resources [25].

The first important finding of our study is that hyperuricemia is associated with AKI in patients with early sepsis. The development of AKI has significant effect on prognosis. For example, whereas the acute operative and postoperative mortality rate after cardiovascular surgery varies between 1 and 2%, this increases to 10 to 38% if renal insufficiency occurs and to >50% if dialysis is required [38, 39]. In general the septic patient population is a very complex subset of patients and majority of the time they have multiple organ involvement and are very sick patients. They are at risk for developing AKI due to changes in hemodynamics, exposure to various medications, changes in the functional capacity of other organs such as the heart and liver, and numerous other factors. Uric acid may be one of the factors contributing to it too.

Uric acid can cause AKI due to several mechanisms ranging from direct tubular toxicity from crystal induced injury to indirect injury secondary to the release of vasoactive mediators and oxidative stress. Uric acid can cause AKI secondary to renal vasoconstriction which occurs in response to the activation of the renin-angiotensin system, catecholamine release, oxidative stress, release of proinflammatory markers, and decreased nitric oxide levels. Renal vasoconstriction occurs in rats with experimentally induced hyperuricemia and is characterized by a marked increase in resistance of the afferent (and, to a lesser extent, efferent) arterioles and a reduction in single nephron GFR [40]. Uric acid strongly inhibits nitric oxide release from endothelial cells [41]. Khosla et al. [41] have demonstrated a reduction in plasma nitrites (metabolites of NO) in hyperuricemic rats that can be rescued by allopurinol. Uric acid levels have been shown by Zoccali et al. [42] to correlate with endothelial dysfunction [42]. Uric acid stimulates an inflammatory response via increasing various proinflammatory markers such as MCP and CRP. Hyperuricemic rats have a significant increase in macrophage infiltration in their kidneys independent of crystal deposition [20]. Despite having both oxidative and antioxidative properties, it appears that in periods of significant degrees of stress such as sepsis uric acids' protective antioxidative properties get overwhelmed and that despite increased levels of oxidative stress leading to increased uric acid levels the uric acid is more injurious than beneficial to the human body. Hence uric acid may be an early marker of impending AKI in patients with sepsis and could be used to predict the risk for AKI in septic patients. This further raises the question of whether the treatment of hyperuricemia in early sepsis could potentially decrease the risk for AKI.

Increased uric acid levels play a role not only in the occurrence of AKI but also in the progression of CKD. Uric

acid levels are increased in subjects with renal disease as the result of reduction in GFR and renal urate excretion. Chonchol et al. have reported that uric acid levels are associated strongly with prevalent CKD [43]. Because of progressive loss of GFR, patients with CKD have decreased renal clearance of uric acid and thus greater serum uric acid levels than the general population [44].

The second important finding of our study is that hyperuricemia correlated with an elevated APACHE II score. This coincides with Jabs et al. [45] findings as they too found that plasma uric acid levels increased in relation to higher APACHE II scores. Chuang et al. [46] also found that an increase in serum uric acid had a positive correlation with total antioxidant capacity and APACHE II scores in patients with severe sepsis and septic shock. This suggests that uric acid may be an important contributor to total antioxidant capacity and that hyperuricemia may be an early predictive marker of poorer clinical outcomes in patients with sepsis. This raises the question then in the management of patients with early sepsis if the hyperuricemia should be treated to decrease the degree of injury that it may cause and decrease the morbidity and mortality rate in this patient population. Although it is known that uric acid has both oxidant and antioxidant properties the overall impact on the human body appears to be more injurious than protective. Hence perhaps the MICU can use uric acid level as a single marker to predict the severity of illness in critically ill patients presenting to the MICU rather than the slew of tests and variables needed to calculate the APACHE II score.

The third important finding of our study was that hyperuricemia noted in the septic population correlated with an increased probability of having the patient still in the MICU at 72 hours. This again suggests that uric acid may indeed be considered as a marker of severity of illness like the APACHE II score and can help predict that those with an elevated uric acid level at initial presentation are more likely to be still in the MICU at 72 hours versus those with a uric acid level less than 7 mg/dL. Thus raising thoughts that will treatment of hyperuricemia improve patient outcomes and decrease length of stay in the MICU?

In our study we found that although there was a high incidence of ARDS noted in this septic patient population, there was no statistically significant association of hyperuricemia with ARDS. Thus although uric acid levels may be used to predict severity of illness, length of stay in the MICU, and risk for AKI, it cannot at least at this time help us predict the incidence of ARDS. This could potentially be due to the small patient population that we had for our study, especially since increasing uric acid levels have been reported by Nagaya et al. [47] to correlate with clinical severity of primary pulmonary hypertension and has an independent association with long-term mortality of patient with primary pulmonary hypertension. Also from our study we found that although a high percentage of our patient populations were obese and a high percentage of those with hyperuricemia were obese, the results were not statistically significant. This was most likely due to the small sample size.

We acknowledge several limitations of this study, including modest sample size, enrollment of patients from the MICU and not the surgical intensive care unit, predominant Caucasian patient population, and short follow-up period. By virtue of the single-center study design, the results may not be generalizable to other MICU settings. If we had a larger sample size, perhaps the linear correlation between hyperuricemia with ARDS, obesity, and lactic acid levels may have become more apparent. Given the fact that the study center was located in West Virginia which is ranked as number two in terms of the state with the highest obesity rate in the USA, there could be potentially some degree of effect on our study results as hyperuricemia has been believed to often precede the development of obesity. So the possibility that our patient population already had an elevated uric acid level prior to being septic may be a factor increasing their risk of overall morbidity and degree of illness severity. Hence possibly we should test and potentially treat the general population for hyperuricemia to improve patient outcomes, which is a thought. Also to note is that our patient population was predominantly Caucasian, so the generalizability of the results is limited. The other limitations include that we did not have the baseline creatinine on the patients from prior to admission and hence did not know for certain what percentage of the patients had CKD prior to presentation. This is an important factor as patients with CKD are often noted to have an elevated uric acid level and it is debatable that elevated uric acid levels are injurious to the renal parenchyma as well as that CKD has been associated with decreased uric acid excretion and subsequently results in elevated uric acid levels. Thus, in order to minimize the degree of potential errors we used the patients' admission creatinine as the baseline value to mark the occurrence of AKI. Other potential limitations include the fact that we only followed the patients for 72 hours and that we did not trend the uric acid level during the course of the hospital stay to see if there was a potential change which was reflective of the patients hospital course. Throughout the analysis of the data we considered all the above-mentioned limitations especially the sample size and selection bias as it may have influenced our study results to a certain degree. Subsequently our study sets the stage for further randomized control trials that are multicenter and encompass a greater sample size and population diversity to help better elucidate and confirm our findings.

5. Conclusion

Our study findings simply demonstrate that hyperuricemia may be associated with poorer clinical outcomes in patients admitted to the MICU with sepsis. Serum uric acid levels may be potentially used as a sole marker of severity of illness as well as a predictor of morbidity in patients presenting to the MICU with sepsis. Further studies are needed to confirm our observations and elucidate the underlying mechanisms for hyperuricemia in sepsis.

Disclaimer

The content is solely the responsibility of the authors and does not necessarily represent the official views of the NIH.

Acknowledgment

The project described was supported by the West Virginia Clinical and Translational Science Institute Pilot Grants Program under the National Institute of General Medical Services, U54GM104942.

References

[1] W. Doehner, N. Schoene, M. Rauchhaus et al., "Effects of xanthine oxidase inhibition with allopurinol on endothelial function and peripheral blood flow in hyperuricemic patients with chronic heart failure: results from 2 placebo-controlled studies," *Circulation*, vol. 105, no. 22, pp. 2619–2624, 2002.

[2] N. L. Edwards, "The role of hyperuricemia and gout in kidney and cardiovascular disease," *Cleveland Clinic Journal of Medicine*, vol. 75, supplement 5, pp. S13–S16, 2008.

[3] A. G. Ioachimescu, D. M. Brennan, B. M. Hoar, S. L. Hazen, and B. J. Hoogwerf, "Serum uric acid is an independent predictor of all-cause mortality in patients at high risk of cardiovascular disease: a Preventive Cardiology Information System (PreCIS) database cohort study," *Arthritis and Rheumatism*, vol. 58, no. 2, pp. 623–630, 2008.

[4] D. B. Corry and M. L. Tuck, "Uric acid and the vasculature," *Current Hypertension Reports*, vol. 8, no. 2, pp. 116–119, 2006.

[5] P. Patetsios, W. Rodino, W. Wisselink, D. Bryan, J. D. Kirwin, and T. F. Panetta, "Identification of uric acid in aortic aneurysms and atherosclerotic artery," *Annals of the New York Academy of Sciences*, vol. 800, pp. 243–245, 1996.

[6] J. Fang and M. H. Alderman, "Serum uric acid and cardiovascular mortality, the NHANES I epidemiologic follow up study, 1971–1992," *Journal of the American Medical Association*, vol. 283, no. 18, pp. 2404–2410, 2000.

[7] P. Verdecchia, G. Schillaci, G. Reboldi, F. Santeusanio, C. Porcellati, and P. Brunetti, "Relation between serum uric acid and risk of cardiovascular disease in essential hypertension: the PIUMA study," *Hypertension*, vol. 36, no. 6, pp. 1072–1078, 2000.

[8] T. Nakagawa, P. Cirillo, W. Sato et al., "The conundrum of hyperuricemia, metabolic syndrome, and renal disease," *Internal and Emergency Medicine*, vol. 3, no. 4, pp. 313–318, 2008.

[9] L. G. Hunsicker, S. Adler, A. Caggiula et al., "Predictors of the progression of renal disease in the Modification of Diet in Renal Disease Study," *Kidney International*, vol. 51, no. 6, pp. 1908–1919, 1997.

[10] K. Iseki, S. Oshiro, M. Tozawa, C. Iseki, Y. Ikemiya, and S. Takishita, "Significance of hyperuricemia on the early detection of renal failure in a cohort of screened subjects," *Hypertension Research*, vol. 24, no. 6, pp. 691–697, 2001.

[11] F. Leyva, S. Anker, J. W. Swan et al., "Serum uric acid as an index of impaired oxidative metabolism in chronic heart failure," *European Heart Journal*, vol. 18, no. 5, pp. 858–865, 1997.

[12] S. D. Anker, F. Leyva, P. A. Poole-Wilson, W. J. Kox, J. C. Stevenson, and A. J. S. Coats, "Relation between serum uric acid and lower limb blood flow in patients with chronic heart failure," *Heart*, vol. 78, no. 1, pp. 39–43, 1997.

[13] A. Braghiroli, C. Sacco, M. Erbetta, V. Ruga, and C. F. Donner, "Overnight urinary uric acid: creatinine ratio for detection of sleep hypoxemia: Validation study in chronic obstructive pulmonary disease and obstructive sleep apnea before and

after treatment with nasal continuous positive airway pressure," *American Review of Respiratory Disease*, vol. 148, no. 1, pp. 173–178, 1993.

[14] N. M. Elsayed, J. M. Nakashima, and E. M. Postlethwait, "Measurement of uric acid as a marker of oxygen tension in the lung," *Archives of Biochemistry and Biophysics*, vol. 302, no. 1, pp. 228–232, 1993.

[15] N. L. Edwards, "The role of hyperuricemia and gout in kidney and cardiovascular disease," *Cleveland Clinic Journal of Medicine*, vol. 75, no. 5, pp. 13–16, 2008.

[16] M. Mazzali, J. Kanellis, L. Han et al., "Hyperuricemia induces a primary renal arteriolopathy in rats by a blood pressure-independent mechanism," *The American Journal of Physiology—Renal Physiology*, vol. 282, no. 6, pp. F991–F997, 2002.

[17] H. J. Han, M. J. Lim, Y. J. Lee, J. H. Lee, I. S. Yang, and M. Taub, "Uric acid inhibits renal proximal tubule cell proliferation via at least two signaling pathways involving PKC, MAPK, $cPLA_2$, and NF-κB," *American Journal of Physiology—Renal Physiology*, vol. 292, no. 1, pp. F373–F381, 2007.

[18] M. G. Netea, B. J. Kullberg, W. L. Blok, R. T. Netea, and J. W. M. Van der Meer, "The role of hyperuricemia in the increased cytokine production after lipopolysaccharide challenge in neutropenic mice," *Blood*, vol. 89, no. 2, pp. 577–582, 1997.

[19] D. H. Kang, T. Nakagawa, L. Feng et al., "A role for uric acid in the progression of renal disease," *Journal of the American Society of Nephrology*, vol. 13, no. 12, pp. 69–78, 2002.

[20] M. Mazzali, J. Hughes, Y.-G. Kim et al., "Elevated uric acid increases blood pressure in the rat by a novel crystal-independent mechanism," *Hypertension*, vol. 38, no. 5, pp. 1101–1106, 2001.

[21] L. G. Sánchez-Lozada, E. Tapia, R. López-Molina et al., "Effects of acute and chronic L-arginine treatment in experimental hyperuricemia," *The American Journal of Physiology—Renal Physiology*, vol. 292, no. 4, pp. F1238–F1244, 2007.

[22] S. Zharikov, K. Krotova, H. Hu et al., "Uric acid decreases NO production and increases arginase activity in cultured pulmonary artery endothelial cells," *The American Journal of Physiology—Cell Physiology*, vol. 295, no. 5, pp. C1183–C1190, 2008.

[23] C. Gersch, S. P. Palii, K. M. Kim, A. Angerhofer, R. J. Johnson, and G. N. Henderson, "Inactivation of nitric oxide by uric acid," *Nucleosides, Nucleotides and Nucleic Acids*, vol. 27, no. 8, pp. 967–978, 2008.

[24] B. N. Ames, R. Cathcart, E. Schwiers, and P. Hochstein, "Uric acid provides an antioxidant defense in humans against oxidant- and radical-caused aging and cancer: a hypothesis," *Proceedings of the National Academy of Sciences of the United States of America*, vol. 78, no. 11, pp. 6858–6862, 1981.

[25] A. Zarjou and A. Agarwal, "Sepsis and acute kidney injury," *Journal of the American Society of Nephrology*, vol. 22, no. 6, pp. 999–1006, 2011.

[26] R. Dellinger, M. Levy, A. Rhodes et al., "Surviving sepsis campaign: international guidelines for management of severe sepsis and septic shock," *Critical Care Medicine*, vol. 41, no. 2, pp. 580–637, 2013.

[27] A. Khwaja, "KDIGO clinical practice guidelines for acute kidney injury," *Nephron Clinical Practice*, vol. 120, no. 4, pp. c179–c184, 2012.

[28] W. A. Knaus, E. A. Draper, D. P. Wagner, and J. E. Zimmerman, "APACHE II: a severity of disease classification system," *Critical Care Medicine*, vol. 13, no. 10, pp. 818–829, 1985.

[29] V. M. Ranieri, G. D. Rubenfeld, B. T. Thompson et al., "Acute respiratory distress syndrome. The Berlin definition," *Journal of the American Medical Association*, vol. 307, no. 23, pp. 2526–2533, 2012.

[30] H. C. Cowley, P. J. Bacon, H. F. Goode, N. R. Webster, J. G. Jones, and D. K. Menon, "Plasma antioxidant potential in severe sepsis: a comparison of survivors and non-survivors," *Critical Care Medicine*, vol. 24, no. 7, pp. 1179–1183, 1996.

[31] J. M. Alonso de Vega, J. Díaz, E. Serrano, and L. F. Carbonell, "Oxidative stress in critically ill patients with systemic inflammatory response syndrome," *Critical Care Medicine*, vol. 30, no. 8, pp. 1782–1786, 2002.

[32] J. M. Alonso de Vega, J. Díaz, E. Serrano, and L. F. Carbonell, "Plasma redox status relates to severity in critically ill patients," *Critical Care Medicine*, vol. 28, no. 6, pp. 1812–1814, 2000.

[33] C. Pascual, W. Karzai, A. Meier-Hellmann et al., "Total plasma antioxidant capacity is not always decreased in sepsis," *Critical Care Medicine*, vol. 26, no. 4, pp. 705–709, 1998.

[34] K. L. MacKinnon, Z. Molnar, D. Lowe, I. D. Watson, and E. Shearer, "Measures of total free radical activity in critically ill patients," *Clinical Biochemistry*, vol. 32, no. 4, pp. 263–268, 1999.

[35] R.-J. Teng, Y.-Z. Ye, D. A. Parks, and J. S. Beckman, "Urate produced during hypoxia protects heart proteins from peroxynitrite-mediated protein nitration," *Free Radical Biology and Medicine*, vol. 33, no. 9, pp. 1243–1249, 2002.

[36] A. Meneshian and G. B. Bulkley, "The physiology of endothelial xanthine oxidase: from urate catabolism to reperfusion injury to inflammatory signal transduction," *Microcirculation*, vol. 9, no. 3, pp. 161–175, 2002.

[37] L. S. Terada, D. M. Guidot, J. A. Leff et al., "Hypoxia injures endothelial cells by increasing endogenous xanthine oxidase activity," *Proceedings of the National Academy of Sciences of the United States of America*, vol. 89, no. 8, pp. 3362–3366, 1992.

[38] G. M. Chertow, J. M. Lazarus, C. L. Christiansen et al., "Preoperative renal risk stratification," *Circulation*, vol. 95, no. 4, pp. 878–884, 1997.

[39] M. Hilberman, B. D. Myers, B. J. Carrie, G. Derby, R. L. Jamison, and E. B. Stinson, "Acute renal failure following cardiac surgery," *Journal of Thoracic and Cardiovascular Surgery*, vol. 77, no. 6, pp. 880–888, 1979.

[40] L. G. Sánchez-Lozada, E. Tapia, J. Santamaría et al., "Mild hyperuricemia induces glomerular hypertension in normal rats," *The American Journal of Physiology—Renal Physiology*, vol. 283, no. 5, pp. F1105–F1110, 2002.

[41] U. M. Khosla, S. Zharikov, J. L. Finch et al., "Hyperuricemia induces endothelial dysfunction," *Kidney International*, vol. 67, no. 5, pp. 1739–1742, 2005.

[42] C. Zoccali, R. Maio, F. Mallamaci, G. Sesti, and F. Perticone, "Uric acid and endothelial dysfunction in essential hypertension," *Journal of the American Society of Nephrology*, vol. 17, no. 5, pp. 1466–1471, 2006.

[43] M. Chonchol, M. G. Shlipak, R. Katz et al., "Relationship of uric acid with progression of kidney disease," *The American Journal of Kidney Diseases*, vol. 50, no. 2, pp. 239–247, 2007.

[44] M. E. Suliman, R. J. Johnson, E. García-López et al., "J-shaped mortality relationship for uric acid in CKD," *American Journal of Kidney Diseases*, vol. 48, no. 5, pp. 761–771, 2006.

12

Estimating Renal Function in the Elderly Malaysian Patients Attending Medical Outpatient Clinic: A Comparison between Creatinine Based and Cystatin-C Based Equations

Maisarah Jalalonmuhali◉,[1] Salma Mohamed Abouzriba Elagel,[2] Maw Pin Tan,[1] Soo Kun Lim,[1] and Kok Peng Ng[1]

[1]Department of Medicine, University of Malaya Medical Centre, 59100 Kuala Lumpur, Malaysia
[2]Management and Science University, 40100 Shah Alam, Selangor, Malaysia

Correspondence should be addressed to Maisarah Jalalonmuhali; mai_jalal@yahoo.com

Academic Editor: Jaime Uribarri

Background. To assess the performance of different GFR estimating equations, test the diagnostic value of serum cystatin-C, and compare the applicability of cystatin-C based equation with serum creatinine based equation for estimating GFR (eGFR) in comparison with measured GFR in the elderly Malaysian patients. *Methods.* A cross-sectional study recruiting volunteered patients 65 years and older attending medical outpatient clinic. 51 chromium EDTA (^{51}Cr-EDTA) was used as measured GFR. The predictive capabilities of Cockcroft-Gault equation corrected for body surface area (CGBSA), four-variable Modification of Diet in Renal Disease (4-MDRD), and Chronic Kidney Disease Epidemiology Collaboration (CKD-EPI) equations using serum creatinine (CKD-EPIcr) as well as serum cystatin-C (CKD-EPIcys) were calculated. *Results.* A total of 40 patients, 77.5% male, with mean measured GFR 41.2 ± 18.9 ml/min/1.73 m^2 were enrolled. Mean bias was the smallest for 4-MDRD; meanwhile, CKD-EPIcr had the highest precision and accuracy with lower limit of agreement among other equations. CKD-EPIcys equation did not show any improvement in GFR estimation in comparison to CKD-EPIcr and MDRD. *Conclusion.* The CKD-EPIcr formula appears to be more accurate and correlates better with measured GFR in this cohort of elderly patients.

1. Background

Prevalence of chronic kidney disease (CKD) in the elderly is increasing globally as life expectancy continues to improve [1]. According to the latest report from the Department of Statistics Malaysia, life expectancy at birth in Malaysia is 72.7 years for male and 77.4 years for female [2]. From previous literatures, we know that serum creatinine alone is imprecise to assess kidney function in the elderly [3]. Apart from age, the level can also be affected by gender, muscle mass, diet, and tubular creatinine secretion particularly at reduced glomerular filtration rate (GFR); this is especially important in older people. Serum creatinine based equation such as Cockcroft-Gault corrected for body surface area (CGBSA), four-variable Modification of Diet in Renal Disease (4-MDRD), and

Chronic Kidney Disease Epidemiology Collaboration (CKD-EPI) equation is widely used to overcome the shortcomings of serum creatinine alone in estimating GFR [4–6].

In this part of the world, creatinine based formula remained an important tool for assessment of kidney function. The main bulk of patients are being treated at the peripheral hospitals and clinics by the primary healthcare practitioner. A small proportion will present to major hospitals during illnesses and later transferred over back to the community for further management. This is partly due to the difficulty transporting elderly patients to major hospitals which are usually situated in the cities. Therefore, the use of GFR estimating equations in the out-patient settings will help the healthcare practitioner in deciding the need and timing of referrals for subspecialty management.

TABLE 1: Different eGFR formula according to gender.

eGFR methods	Gender	Equations
Cockcroft-Gault BSA (CGBSA)	Male	$((140 - \text{Age}) \times \text{mass}\,(\text{kg}) \times 1.23)/\text{Serum Creatinine}\,(\mu\text{mol/L})$ $\Big\}$ $\times 1.73/\text{BSA}$
	Female	$((140 - \text{Age}) \times \text{mass}\,(\text{kg}) \times 1.04)/\text{Serum Creatinine}\,(\mu\text{mol/L})$
4-MDRD	Male	$175 \times (\text{Serum Creatinine}/88.4)^{-1.154} \times \text{Age}^{-0.203} \times \{1.212 \text{ if Black}\}$
	Female	$175 \times (\text{Serum Creatinine}/88.4)^{-1.154} \times \text{Age}^{-0.203} \times \{1.212 \text{ if Black}\} \times 0.742$
		(Serum Creatinine in μmol/L)
CKD-EPIcr (creatinine)	Male	$141 \times \min (\text{SCr}/0.9, 1)^{-0.411} \times \max (\text{SCr}/0.9, 1)^{-1.209} \times 0.993^{\text{Age}} \times \{1.159 \text{ if Black}\}$
	Female	$141 \times \min (\text{SCr}/0.7, 1)^{-0.329} \times \max (\text{SCr}/0.7, 1)^{-1.209} \times 0.993^{\text{Age}} \times \{1.159 \text{ if Black}\} \times 1.018$
CKD-EPIcys (cystatin-c)	Male	$133 \times \min (\text{Scys}/0.8, 1)^{-0.499} \times \max (\text{Scys}/0.8, 1)^{-1.328} \times 0.996^{\text{Age}}$
	Female	$133 \times \min (\text{Scys}/0.8, 1)^{-0.499} \times \max (\text{Scys}/0.8, 1)^{-1.328} \times 0.996^{\text{Age}} \times 0.932$

Serum cystatin-C is a small molecular weight protein produced by all nucleated cells, freely filtered by glomerulus then reabsorbed and completely degraded (but not secreted) by proximal tubules [7, 8]. It is present in serum, saliva, semen, urine, and cerebrospinal fluid and the level is not affected by muscle mass, and hence it is ideal to be used in elderly patients especially those with malnutrition. In a meta-analysis by Dharnidharka et al., serum cystatin-C was found to be superior to serum creatinine as a marker of GFR [9]. The use of cystatin-C in estimating GFR in this country is still very limited mainly due to its availability. It is interesting to look at the performance of different creatinine based equations against cystatin-C based equation in estimating GFR in our multiethnic elderly cohort.

2. Methods

This is a cross-sectional study recruiting elderly patients aged 65 years and older seen in University of Malaya Medical Centre (UMMC) medical outpatient clinic. Participation in this study is on voluntary basis and a written informed consent was taken from each participant. Patients were excluded if they have any of the following: (a) acute kidney injury, (b) inability to consent, (c) history of limb amputation, (d) physical disability rendering weight and height measurement difficult, (e) oedema, fluid overload, and nephrotic syndrome, and (f) physical condition that renders phlebotomy for blood samples and/or peripheral line insertion difficult. The study was approved by UMMC Medical Ethics Committee (UMEC) in accordance with the Helsinki Declaration under MECID number 20145-324.

2.1. GFR Measurement. GFR was determined using plasma clearance of 51 chromium ethylenediamine tetraacetic acid (^{51}Cr-EDTA), which was injected as a single bolus intravenously into patients. Four blood samples were taken at 2 hours, 2.5 hours, 3 hours, and 4 hours after ^{51}Cr-EDTA injection from the opposite upper limb. Patient's height and weight were measured for body surface area (BSA) calculation. GFR was calculated using the slope-intercept method and normalized to BSA, which was calculated using du Bois formula. The result was then corrected using Brochner-Mortensen equation.

Volume distribution (Vd) is calculated by

Vd

$$= \frac{\text{Standard activity}\,(\text{cpm}) \times \text{weight of dose} \times 100\,\text{ml}}{\text{Po}\,(\text{cpm}) \times \text{weight of standard}} \quad (1)$$

(i) Standard activity is calculated using computer generated chromium result.

(ii) Weight of dose is calculated from weight of syringe and dose before injection – after injection.

(iii) Po (zero time plasma activity) is corrected by extrapolating the curve to zero time.

Slope clearance (C-slope) is calculated by

$$\frac{\text{C-slope}}{\text{slope intercept}} = \frac{0.693}{\text{T}^{1/2}} \times \text{Vd} \quad (2)$$

Normalized GFR is calculated by

$$\text{Normalized GFR} = \frac{\text{C-slope}}{\text{Patient's BSA}} \times 1.73 \quad (3)$$

2.2. GFR Estimation. Table 1 showed the different equations used for comparison in this study. All patients had their serum creatinine and serum cystatin-C blood test withdrawn during the peripheral venous access insertion. Measurement of serum creatinine was performed using enzymatic creatinine assay based on the enzymatic reaction [10] with normal adult reference range of 53–97 μmol/L for male and 44–71 μmol/L for female. The creatinine values were adjusted to isotope dilution mass spectrometry (IDMS) traceable assay. Measurement of serum cystatin-C was performed at an independent pathology laboratory outside the hospital using an automated particle-enhanced immune-nephelometry method with normal reference range of 0.85 mg/l or less using N Latex Cystatin-C from Siemens Healthcare Diagnostics Products GmbH (Germany). N Latex Cystatin-C values were then converted to eGFR based on the Hoek equation. The adjusted Hoek equation to calculate the eGFR is GFR (ml/min/1.73 m^2) = −4.32 + 80.35/cys-C [11].

2.3. Statistical Analysis. SPSS version 20.0 was used to calculate baseline characteristics frequency, mean, median, range, and standard deviation. Mean GFR were given with a 95% confidence interval (CI) unless indicated otherwise. P values < 0.05 were considered significant. Pearson's correlation coefficients (r) were calculated between ^{51}Cr-EDTA clearance and estimated GFR by a linear correlation analysis. Pairwise comparison of the mean was performed using paired t-test.

Bias, precision, and accuracy within 30% of the measured GFR were determined. Bias is defined as mean difference between estimated GFR and the measured GFR (^{51}Cr-EDTA). The precision of the estimates was determined as SD of the mean difference between measured GFR and eGFR. Accuracy was determined by integrating precision and bias and was calculated as the percentage of GFR estimates within 30% of the measured GFR. Moreover, a graphical analysis was carried out using Bland and Altman plots. This was used to assess the limits of agreement between the eGFR and the measured GFR.

Accuracy is the most important determinants for a good estimated GFR and best supported by lower bias, greater precision, and lower limits of agreement. However, as we understand that bias, precision and limits of agreement may be affected by the overall means and outliers; therefore, the individual parameter may not reflect the best estimated GFR.

3. Results

A total of 40 elderly patients with mean age of 73.1 ± 5.9 years and predominantly male 31 (77.5%) were recruited. Mean serum creatinine was 165.7 ± 60 μmol/L, cystatin-C was 1.6 ± 0.5 mg/l, and mean measured GFR was 41.2 ± 18.9 ml/min/ 1.73 m^2. 34 out of 40 patients (85%) had measured GFR $<$ 60 ml/min/1.73 m^2 with mean of 34.97 ± 10.2 ml/min/1.73 m^2 with 13 (32.5%) of them with measured GFR of $<$30 ml/min/ 1.73 m^2. Baseline demographics of study population are shown in Table 2.

All the eGFR equations, namely, CGBSA, 4-MDRD, CKD-EPIcr, and CKD-EPIcys, correlated well with measured GFR (^{51}Cr-EDTA). The 4-MDRD equation had the lowest bias followed by CKD-EPIcr, CKD-EPIcys, and CGBSA with bias of -2.76, -3.09, 4.51, and -7.97 ml/min/1.73 m^2, respectively. In this study we found that CKD-EPIcr seems to be more precise (8.18 ml/min/1.73 m^2) followed by CKD-EPIcys (8.26 ml/min/1.73 m^2), 4-MDRD (8.70 ml/min/1.73 m^2), and CGBSA (10.68 ml/min/1.73 m^2). CKD-EPIcr was found to have the higher accuracy as compared to the others. The performances of the estimated GFR equations are tabulated in Table 3 for reference.

The differences between estimated and measured GFR were illustrated using a graphical technique according to Bland and Altman plot (Figures 1(a)–1(d)). These figures display the span between +2SD and −2SD of the mean difference (limits of agreement between 2 methods), which represent 95% CI. Smaller limits of agreement were found for the CKD-EPIcr (32.67 ml/min/1.73 m^2), followed by CKD-EPIcys (33.06 ml/min/1.73 m^2), 4-MDRD (34.76 ml/min/ 1.73 m^2), and CGBSA (42.69 ml/min/1.73 m^2) equation.

TABLE 2: Patient's baseline characteristics.

Characteristic ($n = 40$)	Mean $\pm$ SD (median) or n (%)
Male	31 (77.5%)
Age (year)	73.1 ± 5.9
Age category	
<75	28 (70.0%)
≥75	12 (30.0%)
Weight (kg)	69.16 ± 13.32
BMI (kg/m^2)	26.5 ± 4.6
BSA (m^2)	1.70 ± 0.2
Serum creatinine (umol/l)	165.7 ± 60.0
Serum cystatin-C (mg/l)	1.6 ± 0.5
Measured GFR (ml/min/1.73 m^2)	41.2 ± 18.9
CKD staging (ml/min/1.73 m^2)	
<60	34 (85.0%)
≥60	6 (15.0%)
Medical history	
Diabetes mellitus	17 (42.5%)
Hypertension	28 (70.0%)

Limits of agreement can also be affected by the extreme outliers. Therefore, a sum of all the parameters has to be considered to determine the more accurate eGFR equation in comparison with ^{51}Cr-EDTA in our study cohort.

Overall, we can conclude that CGBSA, 4-MDRD, CKD-EPIcr, and CKD-EPIcys have an excellent correlation with measured GFR and it can be used in our daily clinical practice. Further analysis revealed that CKD-EPIcr seems to perform better as compared to other equations in the elderly populations with reasonably low bias, greater precision, and accuracy. It is further supported by lower limits of agreement and less scattering of the Bland-Altman plot. CKD-EPIcys equation unexpectedly did not perform very well in our study probably because of the different standardization of the cystatin-C value used in the original CKD-EPIcys equation.

4. Discussion

It has been shown that GFR decreases with aging, age-related changes in the renal function, and progressive loss of muscle mass with aging (sarcopenia) [12, 13]. Accurate measurement of renal function is mandatory for appropriate drug dosing and contrast related procedure. Apart from that, it is a well-known fact that CKD in the elderly populations is associated with frailty and poor physical performance [14]. Frailty and its progression have a significant impact on the mortality among the elderly [15]. Hence, an accurate GFR measurement is an important clinical assessment in daily clinical practice particularly in this cohort.

Direct GFR measurement is the gold standard of kidney function assessment. However, it is costly and time consuming and the need for multiple bloods sampling makes it impractical. Since GFR estimation in elderly is a topic of ongoing debate, we conducted this study to evaluate

TABLE 3: Correlation coefficient (r), mean, bias, precision, and accuracy for CGBSA, 4-MDRD, CKD-EPIcr, and CKD-EPIcys equations.

	Correlation coefficient (r)	Mean GFR (ml/min/1.73 m^2)	Range (IQR) Lower	Upper	Mean difference (bias)	SD of mean bias (precision)	Accuracy within 30%
Measured GFR		41.2	17.7	98.3			
CGBSA	0.861*	33.2	15.4	65.6	−7.97	10.68	85
4-MDRD	0.889*	38.4	14.0	86.0	−2.76	8.70	90
CKD-EPIcr	0.902*	38.1	14.0	85.0	−3.09	8.18	95
CKD-EPIcys	0.928*	46.1	16.0	108.0	4.90	8.26	81

*Significantly correlates with $P < 0.001$ (bias: mean difference of estimated GFR and measured GFR; accuracy: n percentage of GFR estimates within n% of measured GFR; IQR: interquartile range).

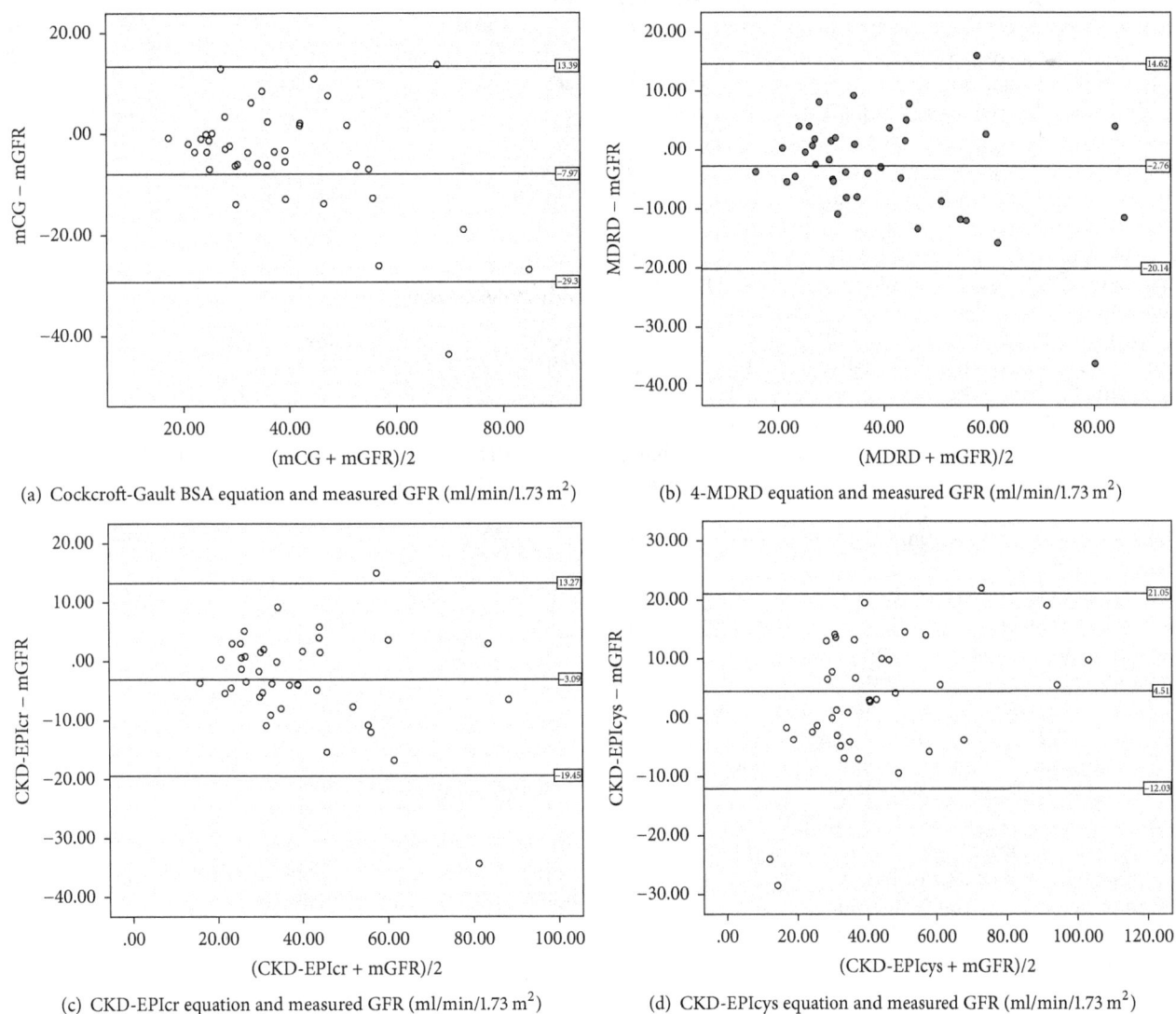

(a) Cockcroft-Gault BSA equation and measured GFR (ml/min/1.73 m^2)

(b) 4-MDRD equation and measured GFR (ml/min/1.73 m^2)

(c) CKD-EPIcr equation and measured GFR (ml/min/1.73 m^2)

(d) CKD-EPIcys equation and measured GFR (ml/min/1.73 m^2)

FIGURE 1: (a–d) Bland and Altman analysis of GFR estimates. In this analysis, the differences between estimated and measured GFR are plotted against the average of the estimated and measured GFR for each individual patient.

the performance of different GFR estimating equations in comparison with gold standard radio-labelled measurement of ^{51}Cr-EDTA clearance in our multiethnic cohort of elderly patients. We have also included Cockcroft-Gault equation into this study because it is still commonly used by many even until now. One must remember that Cockcroft-Gault equation intends to measure the creatinine clearance. In contrast, other eGFR equations are measuring the GFR instead. Tubular secretion, extrarenal clearance of creatinine, and drugs affecting the renal handling of creatinine will result in inaccurate creatinine clearance. That is why creatinine clearance always gives higher values than GFR, while Cockcroft-Gault equation provides lower values than GFR equations. Age and weight are the main reasons of discrepancy. Therefore, Cockcroft-Gault and other eGFR equations cannot be used interchangeably to estimate kidney function [16].

The findings from this study are consistent with the work done by Stevens et al., which showed that CKD-EPIcr was better than MDRD even in estimating GFR > 60 ml/min/1.73 m^2 [17]. Particularly in subgroup of >65 years old, CKD-EPIcr has lower bias throughout all CKD stages. We reported that CKD-EPIcr is more accurate with reasonably low bias, greater precision, accuracy, and lower limits of agreement as compared with the measured GFR.

It is unlikely that one single eGFR equation will work equally well in different cohort of patients. In particular, the use of eGFR equations in the elderly is more challenging as it can be affected by physiological change of aging process. It is worth to note that both the MDRD and CKD-EPI study were performed in a much younger population. The mean age of patients in MDRD and CKD-EPI study was 52 and 47 years, respectively [6, 18]. The elderly were underrepresented in both studies, hence leaving a gap in the evidence.

We have also explored the practicality of using cystatin-C as an endogenous marker alternative to serum creatinine. It is mainly filtered by the kidney and achieved 94% of renal clearance calculated using ^{51}Cr-EDTA in previous literatures [9, 19–21]. Although it can be affected by renal tubular catabolism, reabsorption, use of systemic glucocorticoids, and thyroid dysfunction, cystatin-C was proposed to be better in comparison to serum creatinine as an endogenous marker of GFR [9].

Comparison between creatinine based and cystatin-C based equation using iohexol as exogenous marker of GFR in elderly patients was studied by Kilbride et al. [22]. In a cohort of 394 elderly patients with median age of 80 years, CKD-EPIcr equation was less biased and more accurate than the MDRD. None of the equations including CKD-EPI using cystatin-C alone or in combination with creatinine concentration achieved an ideal accuracy within 30% in the overall population of that study. Similarly, this present study also failed to document the advantage of using cystatin-C based equation over creatinine based equation in estimating GFR in the elderly. By right, incorporation of cystatin-C in eGFR equations is supposed to have better performance due to its unique properties as outlined before. Nevertheless, our study population was too small to draw any strong conclusion with regard to the utility of cystatin-C based equation.

5. Limitations of the Study

The authors would like to emphasize that this is a small uni-centre cohort of CKD patients, predominantly male and mainly consisted of CKD stages 3 and 4. A balanced number of patients in different GFR groups could not be controlled due to the continuous sampling method used in this study. We recommend a larger and more robust study to ascertain the validity of this study results specifically in our multiethnic

cohort of South East Asian population. Although this study has the above-mentioned limitations, this is the first study to be conducted in Malaysia using ^{51}Cr-EDTA as reference GFR and cystatin-C among the elderly patients.

6. Conclusion

We conclude that CKD-EPIcr formula appeared to be more accurate and correlates better with measured GFR in this cohort of Malaysian elderly. The expected advantage of cystatin-C based equation was not observed in this present study possibly because of the limitations stated before. The use of commonly available eGFR equations, namely, 4-MDRD and CKD-EPIcr, should be encouraged for better kidney function assessment. Cockcroft-Gault equation in the elderly leads to overestimation of GFR and may pose significant adverse situations. Further studies should be done to ascertain the best GFR estimation formula in our multiethnic elderly population especially looking at the potential role of cystatin-C for kidney function assessment.

Abbreviations

CKD:	Chronic kidney disease
GFR:	Glomerular filtration rate
CGBSA:	Cockcroft-Gault corrected for body surface area
4-MDRD:	Modification of diet in renal disease
CKD-EPI:	Chronic Kidney Disease Epidemiology Collaboration
^{51}Cr EDTA:	51-chromium ethylenediamine tetraacetic acid
mGFR:	Measured glomerular filtration rate
BSA:	Body surface area
CKD-EPIcr:	CKD-EPI creatinine
CKD-EPIcys:	CKD-EPI cystatin.

Ethical Approval

The study was approved by UMMC Medical Ethics Committee (UMEC) in accordance with the Helsinki Declaration under MECID number 20145-324.

Authors' Contributions

Maisarah Jalalonmuhali and Salma Mohamed Abouzriba Elagel are the main investigators responsible for executing the study, collected and analyzed the data, and drafted the manuscript. Maw Pin Tan and Soo Kun Lim helped in patient's recruitment and provided critical opinion on the overall process. Kok Peng Ng coordinated study administration and provided administrative support. All authors critically revised the manuscript for important intellectual content and approved the final manuscript.

Acknowledgments

The authors would like to express their sincere thanks to the dedicated staff of Nuclear Medicine Unit of Department of Biomedical Imaging, University of Malaya Medical Centre, for their contribution in performing the GFR measurement for the subjects. This study was financially supported by the University of Malaya Research Grant (UMRG) under Grant ID RG35211HTM.

References

[1] M. Mallappallil, E. A. Friedman, B. G. Delano, S. I. McFarlane, and M. O. Salifu, "Chronic kidney disease in the elderly: evaluation and management," *Clinical Practice*, vol. 11, no. 5, pp. 525–535, 2014.

[2] https://www.dosm.gov.my.

[3] P. J. Swedko, H. D. Clark, K. Paramsothy, and A. Akbari, "Serum creatinine is an inadequate screening test for renal failure in elderly patients," *JAMA Internal Medicine*, vol. 163, no. 3, pp. 356–360, 2003.

[4] A. S. Levey, J. P. Bosch, J. B. Lewis, T. Greene, N. Rogers, and D. Roth, "A more accurate method to estimate glomerular filtration rate from serum creatinine: a new prediction equation. Modification of Diet in Renal Disease Study Group," *Annals of Internal Medicine*, vol. 130, no. 6, pp. 461–470, 1999.

[5] E. D. Poggio, X. Wang, T. Greene, F. Van Lente, and P. M. Hall, "Performance of the modification of diet in renal disease and Cockcroft-Gault equations in the estimation of GFR in health and in chronic kidney disease," *Journal of the American Society of Nephrology*, vol. 16, no. 2, pp. 459–466, 2005.

[6] A. S. Levey, L. A. Stevens, C. H. Schmid et al., "A new equation to estimate glomerular filtration rate," *Annals of Internal Medicine*, vol. 150, no. 9, pp. 604–612, 2009.

[7] E. Randers, J. H. Kristensen, E. J. Erlandsen, and H. Danielsen, "Serum cystatin C as a marker of the renal function," *Scandinavian Journal of Clinical & Laboratory Investigation*, vol. 58, no. 7, pp. 585–592, 1998.

[8] J. Westhuyzen, "Cystatin C: a promising marker and predictor of impaired renal function," *Annals of Clinical & Laboratory Science*, vol. 36, no. 4, pp. 387–394, 2006.

[9] V. R. Dharnidharka, C. Kwon, and G. Stevens, "Serum cystatin C is superior to serum creatinine as a marker of kidney function: a meta-analysis," *American Journal of Kidney Diseases*, vol. 40, no. 2, pp. 221–226, 2002.

[10] P. Fossati, L. Prencipe, and G. Berti, "Enzymic creatinine assay: A new colorimetric method based on hydrogen peroxide measurement," *Clinical Chemistry*, vol. 29, no. 8, pp. 1494–1496, 1983.

[11] F. J. Hoek, F. A. W. Kemperman, and R. T. Krediet, "A comparison between cystatin C, plasma creatinine and the Cockcroft and Gault formula for the estimation of glomerular filtration rate," *Nephrology Dialysis Transplantation*, vol. 18, no. 10, pp. 2024–2031, 2003.

[12] G. Van Pottelbergh, B. Vaes, J. Morelle, M. Jadoul, P. Wallemacq, and J. Degryse, "Estimating GFR in the oldest old: does it matter what equation we use?" *Age and Ageing*, vol. 40, no. 3, pp. 401–405, 2011.

[13] G. Van Pottelbergh, L. Van Heden, C. Matheï, and J. Degryse, "Methods to evaluate renal function in elderly patients: a systematic literature review," *Age and Ageing*, vol. 39, no. 5, pp. 542–548, 2010.

[14] P. P. Reese, A. R. Cappola, J. Shults et al., "Physical performance and frailty in chronic kidney disease," *American Journal of Nephrology*, vol. 38, no. 4, pp. 307–315, 2013.

[15] A. S. Buchman, R. S. Wilson, J. L. Bienias, and D. A. Bennett, "Change in frailty and risk of death in older persons," *Experimental Aging Research*, vol. 35, no. 1, pp. 61–82, 2009.

[16] C. Pedone, A. Corsonello, and R. A. Incalzi, "Estimating renal function in older people: A comparison of three formulas," *Age and Ageing*, vol. 35, no. 2, pp. 121–126, 2006.

[17] L. A. Stevens, C. H. Schmid, T. Greene et al., "Comparative performance of the CKD Epidemiology Collaboration (CKD-EPI) and the Modification of Diet in Renal Disease (MDRD) Study equations for estimating GFR levels above 60 mL/min/1.73 m2," *American Journal of Kidney Diseases*, vol. 56, no. 3, pp. 486–495, 2010.

[18] S. Klahr, A. S. Levey, G. J. Beck et al., "The effects of dietary protein restriction and blood-pressure control on the progression of chronic renal disease," *The New England Journal of Medicine*, vol. 330, no. 13, pp. 877–884, 1994.

[19] A. O. Grubb, "Cystatin C—properties and use as diagnostic marker," *Advances in Clinical Chemistry*, vol. 35, pp. 63–99, 2000.

[20] O. Tenstad, A. B. Roald, A. Grubb, and K. Aukland, "Renal handling of radiolabelled human cystatin C in the rat," *Scandinavian Journal of Clinical & Laboratory Investigation*, vol. 56, no. 5, pp. 409–414, 1996.

[21] B. Jacobsson, H. Lignelid, and U. S. R. Bergerheim, "Transthyretin and cystatin C are catabolized in proximal tubular epithelial cells and the proteins are not useful as markers for renal cell carcinomas," *Histopathology*, vol. 26, no. 6, pp. 559–564, 1995.

[22] H. S. Kilbride, P. E. Stevens, G. Eaglestone et al., "Accuracy of the MDRD (Modification of Diet in Renal Disease) study and CKD-EPI (CKD Epidemiology Collaboration) equations for estimation of GFR in the elderly," *American Journal of Kidney Diseases*, vol. 61, no. 1, pp. 57–66, 2013.

13

Cost-Utility Analysis of Mycophenolate Mofetil versus Azathioprine Based Regimens for Maintenance Therapy of Proliferative Lupus Nephritis

Robert Nee, Ian Rivera, Dustin J. Little, Christina M. Yuan, and Kevin C. Abbott

Department of Nephrology, Walter Reed National Military Medical Center, 8901 Wisconsin Avenue, Bethesda, MD 20889-5600, USA

Correspondence should be addressed to Robert Nee; robert.nee.civ@mail.mil

Academic Editor: Kazunari Kaneko

Background/Aims. We aimed to examine the cost-effectiveness of mycophenolate mofetil (MMF) and azathioprine (AZA) as maintenance therapy for patients with Class III and Class IV lupus nephritis (LN), from a United States (US) perspective. *Methods.* Using a Markov model, we conducted a cost-utility analysis from a societal perspective over a lifetime horizon. The modeled population comprised patients with proliferative LN who received maintenance therapy with MMF (2 gm/day) versus AZA (150 mg/day) for 3 years. Risk estimates of clinical events were based on a Cochrane meta-analysis while costs and utilities were retrieved from other published sources. Outcome measures included costs, quality-adjusted life-years (QALY), incremental cost-effectiveness ratios (ICER), and net monetary benefit. *Results.* The base-case model showed that, compared with AZA strategy, the ICER for MMF was $2,630,592/QALY at 3 years. Over the patients' lifetime, however, the ICER of MMF compared to AZA was $6,454/QALY. Overall, the ICER results from various sensitivity and subgroup analyses did not alter the conclusions of the model simulation. *Conclusions.* In the short term, an AZA-based regimen confers greater value than MMF for the maintenance therapy of proliferative LN. From a lifelong perspective, however, MMF is cost-effective compared to AZA.

1. Introduction

Lupus nephritis (LN) is a serious and costly cause of kidney disease worldwide [1]. An analysis of United States (US) medical expenditures found that the annual costs per patient among those with LN exceeded $46,000 (USD) versus matched controls and $42,000 versus systemic lupus erythematosus (SLE) patients without nephritis [2]. These findings suggest that LN is a key driver of economic burden in the SLE population.

The Kidney Disease Improving Global Outcomes (KDIGO) practice guidelines for initial or induction therapy for LN are well accepted [3]; however, they do not indicate a preference for maintenance therapy with azathioprine- (AZA-) or mycophenolate mofetil- (MMF-) based regimens. The Task Force Panel of the American College of Rheumatology recommended that either AZA or MMF be used for maintenance [4]. These recommendations were based, in large part, on two randomized controlled trials of long-term

maintenance therapies for LN. In the MAINTAIN Nephritis Trial, a predominantly Caucasian cohort was randomized to MMF 2 gm/day or AZA 2 mg/kg/day as maintenance therapy after induction with a fixed, low dose intravenous (IV) cyclophosphamide (CYC) regimen [5]. After a mean follow-up of 4 years, this European-based study found that MMF was not superior to AZA in preventing renal flares, without significant differences in adverse events except for higher rate of cytopenias in the AZA group. In the larger Aspreva Lupus Management Study (ALMS) trial, a multinational population was randomized to MMF 2 gm/day or AZA 2 mg/kg/day after response to initial induction therapy [6]. After 3 years, MMF was superior to AZA as maintenance therapy, based on the primary composite end point of death, end stage renal disease (ESRD), doubling of the serum creatinine, renal flare, or requirement for rescue therapy.

To our knowledge, a cost-effectiveness analysis of maintenance therapy for proliferative LN from a US perspective has not been reported. We conducted a cost-utility analysis

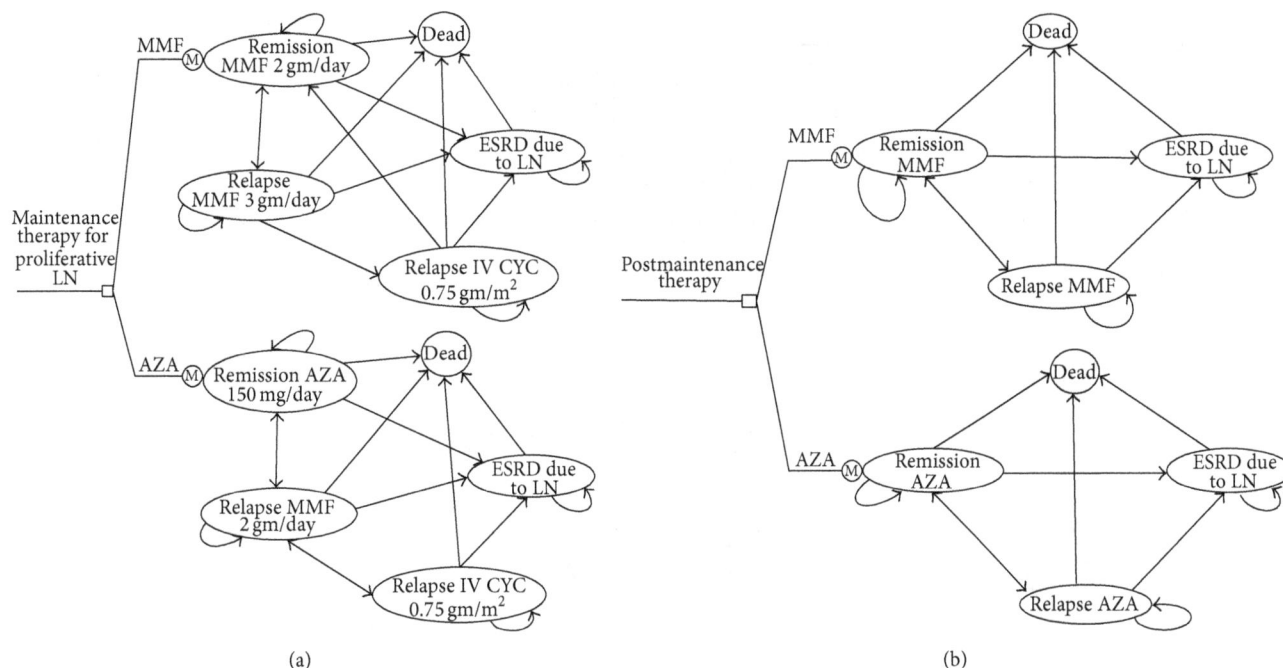

(a)   (b)

FIGURE 1: (a) Markov state transition diagram illustrating the health states and transitions for each treatment strategy for the initial 3 years. The lifetime model consists of the initial 3-year period of maintenance therapy followed by a posttreatment phase as shown in (b). (b) Markov state transition diagram illustrating the health states and transitions for each treatment strategy for the posttreatment phase (after 3 years). LN: lupus nephritis; AZA: azathioprine; MMF: mycophenolate mofetil; IV CYC: intravenous cyclophosphamide; ESRD: end stage renal disease.

from a societal perspective to evaluate the cost-effectiveness of the 3-year maintenance regimens (MMF versus AZA) for proliferative LN over a lifetime horizon.

2. Methods

2.1. Study Design. We constructed a Markov state transition model to estimate the quality-adjusted life-years (QALY) and costs associated with maintenance therapy with MMF versus AZA. Markov models analyze uncertain events over time and are suited to decisions where the timing of events is important and when events are recursive in nature [7]. While decision trees model uncertain events at chance nodes, Markov models analyze these events as transitions between health states. Markov models are suited to modelling chronic conditions, where costs and outcomes (QALY) are spread over a long period of time.

Our model encompasses an initial 3-year treatment phase after which simulated patients are no longer on immunosuppressive agents and followed long term (Tables 1(a) and 2(a); Supplemental Data Sources) (see Supplementary Material available online at http://dx.doi.org/10.1155/2015/917567). The time horizon in Markov models is divided into discrete time periods, called cycles. Each cycle length in our model is 6 months for the first 3 years and 12 months thereafter, reflecting the natural history of renal flares and remissions in LN. Analyses were performed using TreeAge Pro 2012 (TreeAge Software, Williamstown, MA) and Microsoft Excel 2010 (Microsoft Corp., Redmond, WA). Institutional review

board approval was not required for this study. We adhered to the CHEERS (Consolidated Health Economic Evaluation Reporting Standards) reporting guidelines in our study [8].

2.2. Target Population. The modeled population is a hypothetical cohort of 1,000 patients with proliferative LN receiving maintenance therapy, having responded to their induction regimen. The starting age ranges from 20 to 40 years old, and various racial/ethnic groups are represented in the model, reflecting the demographic characteristics of study participants in the clinical trials.

2.3. Model Structure. The general structure of the model is shown as a state transition diagram in Figures 1(a) and 1(b) and Markov cycle trees (Supplemental Model Structure, Model Assumptions, and Supplemental Figures 1 and 2). We did not include the costs and QALY with *induction* therapy for proliferative LN given that this was a study of the differences between two maintenance treatment strategies and inclusion would not alter the conclusion of the analysis. We attempt to simulate patient-oriented outcomes and treatment strategies that are typically utilized in "real-world" clinical practice. For both strategies, after model entry each patient would progress through five potential health states, in 6-month cycles:

(1) Remission state on MMF or AZA as maintenance therapy;

(2) relapse of LN requiring MMF rescue therapy (escalation of MMF dose if maintained on MMF);

TABLE 1: (a) Base-case three-year model inputs of probability parameters (Cochrane data). (b) Three-year model inputs of direct and indirect costs. (c) Three-year model inputs of utility parameters.

(a)

Probability parameters (over 6-month period or one cycle)[a]	Mean	Range (95% CI)	Probability distribution[b]	Sources
Remission AZA				
Probability of lupus-related death during remission	0.0025	0.0004–0.0157	Beta (24.3, 9830.3)	Cochrane 2012 [13]
Probability of major infection during remission	0.0138	0.0047–0.0430	Beta (751.2, 53,686.0)	Cochrane 2012 [13]
Probability of ESRD during remission	0.0030	0.0006–0.0160	Beta (35.9, 11,927.1)	Cochrane 2012 [13]
Probability of relapse during remission	0.0364	0.0234–0.0587	Beta (5106, 135,192.3)	Cochrane 2012 [13]
Remission MMF				
Probability of lupus-related death during remission	0.0043	0.0007–0.0285	Beta (4.2, 963.5)	Cochrane 2012 [13]
Probability of major infection during remission	0.0160	0.0055–0.0510	Beta (3.9, 241.1)	Cochrane 2012 [13]
Probability of ESRD during remission	0.0012	0.0002–0.0063	Beta (3.9, 3269.0)	Cochrane 2012 [13]
Probability of relapse during remission	0.0185	0.0122–0.0286	Beta (4.1, 219.5)	Cochrane 2012 [13]
Relapse MMF (2 gm/d or 3 gm/d)				
Probability of lupus-related death during relapse	0.0410	0.0210–0.0790	Beta (64.4, 1507.3)	Cochrane 2012 [13]
Probability of major infection during relapse	0.1210	0.0810–0.1830	Beta (514.6, 3738.7)	Cochrane 2012 [13]
Probability of ESRD during relapse	0.0610	0.0230–0.1580	Beta (139.7, 2150.5)	Cochrane 2012 [13]
Probability of complete and partial remissions	0.5900	0.4180–0.7380	Beta (56.5, 39.3)	Cochrane 2012 [13]
Relapse CYC				
Probability of lupus-related death during relapse	0.0400	0.0200–0.0780	Beta (61.4, 1473.6)	Cochrane 2012 [13]
Probability of major infection during relapse	0.1090	0.0730–0.1650	Beta (105.8, 864.4)	Cochrane 2012 [13]
Probability of ESRD during relapse	0.0855	0.0320–0.2220	Beta (66.8, 714.1)	Cochrane 2012 [13]
Probability of complete and partial remissions	0.5220	0.3920–0.6520	Beta (51.6, 47.2)	Cochrane 2012 [13]
ESRD due to lupus nephritis				
Probability of death due to lupus nephritis ESRD	0.0513	0.0481–0.0548	Beta (99.8, 1845.9)	Costenbader et al. 2011 [14]

AZA: azathioprine; MMF: mycophenolate mofetil; CYC: cyclophosphamide; ESRD: end stage renal disease; CI: confidence interval.

[a]Probabilities from the data sources were reported over various follow-up durations. *Probabilities were converted to* rates *and then to 6-month probabilities* [15]. First, the probabilities were converted to yearly rates (event per patient per year) using the equation $r = -(1/t)\ln(1 - P)$, where r = rate; t = time in years; P = probability of an event occurring during time t. These annual rates were then converted to 6-month probabilities using the equation $P = 1 - e^{-rt}$, where r = one-year rate; t = time in years; P = probability of an event occurring during time t.

[b]Beta distributions are characterized by (α, β).

(b)

Cost parameters (over 6-month period)	Mean costs ($)	Range ($)	Probability distribution[g]	Sources/Comments
AZA 150 mg/day × 6 months[a]	769.86	343.98–2626.26	Gamma (59.1, 0.08)	Red Book 2013 [12]
MMF 2000 mg/day × 6 months[b]	4833.92	1135.68–5773.04	Gamma (23.4, 0.005)	Red Book 2013 [12]
MMF 3000 mg/day × 6 months[b]	7250.88	1703.52–8659.56	Gamma (52.6, 0.007)	Red Book 2013 [12]
Monthly infusion of CYC 0.75 gm/m² × 6 months to treat LN relapse[d]	6233.52[c]	4675.14–7791.90	Gamma (42.1, 0.006)	Red Book 2013 [12], CMS 2013 [16]; range assumed to be ±25% mean

(b) Continued.

Cost parameters (over 6-month period)	Mean costs ($)	Range ($)	Probability distribution[g]	Sources/Comments
Direct costs × 6 months (nonpharmaceuticals)[e]				
Remission	1684.17	1263.13–2105.21	Gamma (31.5, 0.019)	Clarke et al. 2008 [17]; Clarke et al. 2004 [18]; range assumed to be ±25% mean
Relapse	3243.43	2432.57–4054.29	Gamma (29.2, 0.009)	Clarke et al. 2008 [17]; Clarke et al. 2004 [18]; range assumed to be ±25% mean
Indirect costs × 6 months[f]				
Remission	8033.19	6024.89–10041.49	Gamma (16.1, 0.002)	Clarke et al. 2008 [17]; Panopalis et al. 2007 [19]; range assumed to be ±25% mean
Relapse	8564.07	6423.05–10705.09	Gamma (18.3, 0.002)	Clarke et al. 2008 [17]; Panopalis et al. 2007 [19]; range assumed to be ±25% mean
ESRD/dialysis: mean cost per person × 6 months	43,304	n/a	Gamma (75.0, 0.002)	USRDS 2012 [20]
Major infection (inpatient cost for septicemia, ICD9 code 038.9)	17,183	16,849–17,517	Gamma (32.8, 0.002)	Healthcare Cost and Utilization Project [21]

AZA: azathioprine. MMF: mycophenolate mofetil; CYC: cyclophosphamide (intravenous); ESRD: end stage renal disease; USRDS: United States Renal Data System; LN: lupus nephritis.

[a]Based on unit cost of AZA 50 mg tablet = $1.41 (range 0.63–4.81) [12].

[b]Based on unit cost of MMF 500 mg tablet = $6.64 (range 1.56–7.93) [12].

[c]Based on monthly cost of intravenous CYC 0.75 gm/m^2 = $1038.92 [12, 16].

[d]See Supplemental Table 6: costs of individual components of intravenous cyclophosphamide infusion.

[e]Components of direct costs included care provided by specialists, nonspecialists, nonphysician healthcare professionals, laboratory studies, imaging studies, emergency room visits, outpatient surgery, and hospitalizations [18].

[f]Indirect costs included time lost from labor and nonlabor (i.e., household work) market activity as well as time that a caregiver spent helping the patient receiving healthcare services and the time the caregiver spent doing housework [19].

[g]Gamma distributions are characterized by (α, λ); $\alpha = \mu^2/s^2$, $\lambda = \mu/s^2$, where μ = mean; s^2 = variance.

(c)

Utility parameters	Base-case mean	Range[b]	Probability distribution[c]	Sources/Comments
Utility of ESRD on dialysis	0.67	0.54–0.85	Beta (14.1, 6.9)	Liem et al. 2008 [22], based on TTO method
Utility of remission, on MMF or AZA	0.70	0.65–0.80	Beta (14.0, 6.0)	Grootscholten et al. 2007 [23], Clarke et al. 2008 [17], based on VAS method
Utility of relapse, requiring MMF rescue therapy	0.60	0.50–0.70	Beta (13.8, 9.2)	Grootscholten et al. 2007 [23], Clarke et al. 2008 [17], based on VAS method
Utility of relapse, requiring CYC rescue therapy	0.50	0.40–0.60	Beta (12.0, 12, 0)	Tse et al. 2006 [24]; requiring CYC after failing MMF rescue therapy
Disutility[a] of major infection (sepsis)	0.31	0.20–0.56	Fixed	Cost-Effectiveness Analysis Registry 2013 [25]
Utility of death	0.00	n/a	n/a	Drummond et al. 2005 [26]

AZA: azathioprine; MMF: mycophenolate mofetil; CYC: cyclophosphamide (intravenous); ESRD: end stage renal disease; TTO: time trade-off; VAS: visual analog scale.

[a]Disutility = 1 − utility weight.

[b]Based on 95% confidence interval or standard deviation.

[c]Beta distributions are characterized by (α, β).

TABLE 2: (a) Base-case inputs of probability parameters in lifetime model (Cochrane data). (b) Lifetime model inputs of direct and indirect costs. (c) Lifetime model inputs of utility parameters.

(a)

Probability parameters (1-year cycle)[a]	Base-case value	Range (95% CI)	Probability distribution[b]	Sources
Remission in AZA group				
Probability of lupus-related death during remission	Age-dependent[g]	n/a	n/a	Bernatsky et al. 2006 [27]; Arias 2011 [28]; Cochrane 2012 [13]
Probability of ESRD during remission	0.0061	0.0012–0.0317	Beta (35.9, 11,927.1)	Cochrane 2012 [13]
Probability of relapse during remission	0.0716	0.0463–0.1140	Beta (5106.9, 135,192.3)	Cochrane 2012 [13]
Remission in MMF group				
Probability of lupus-related death during remission	Age-dependent[f]	n/a	n/a	Bernatsky et al. 2006 [27]; Arias 2011 [28]; Cochrane 2012 [13]
Probability of ESRD during remission	0.0025	0.0005–0.0125	Beta (16.6, 6771.3)	Cochrane 2012 [13]
Probability of relapse during remission	0.0367	0.0244–0.0564	Beta (16.0, 419.5)	Cochrane 2012 [13]
Relapse in MMF group				
Probability of lupus-related death during relapse	Age-dependent[e]	n/a	n/a	Bernatsky et al. 2006 [27]; Arias 2011 [28]
Probability of ESRD during relapse	0.1183	0.0455–0.2910	Beta (491.1, 3670.9)	Cochrane 2012 [13]
Probability of complete and partial remissions	0.8319	0.6613–0.9313	Beta (45.7, 9.2)	Cochrane 2012 [13]
Relapse in AZA group				
Probability of lupus-related death during relapse	Age-dependent[e]	n/a	n/a	Bernatsky et al. 2006 [27]; Arias 2011 [28]
Probability of ESRD during relapse	0.1183[c]	0.0455–0.2910	Beta (491.1, 3670.9)	Cochrane 2012 [13]
Probability of complete and partial remissions	0.8319[c]	0.6613–0.9313	Beta (45.7, 9.2)	Cochrane 2012 [13]
ESRD due to lupus nephritis				
Probability of death due to lupus nephritis ESRD	Age-dependent[d]	n/a	n/a	USRDS 2012 [20]; Sule et al. 2011 [29]

AZA: azathioprine; MMF: mycophenolate mofetil; CYC: cyclophosphamide; ESRD: end stage renal disease; CI: confidence interval.

[a]Probabilities from the data sources were reported over various follow-up durations. Probabilities were converted to rates and then to 6-month probabilities [15]. First, the probabilities were converted to yearly rates (event per patient per year) using the equation $r = -(1/t)\ln(1 - P)$, where r = rate; t = time in years; P = probability of an event occurring during time t.

These annual rates were then converted to 6-month probabilities using the equation $P = 1 - e^{-rt}$, where r = one-year rate; t = time in years; P = probability of an event occurring during time t.

[b]Beta distributions are characterized by (α, β).

[c]Probability based on MMF for relapse in either AZA- or MMF-based regimen.

[d]The age-specific annual mortality rate for the general dialysis population in 2011 [20] is multiplied by hazard ratio (HR) 1.7. In a USRDS study, Sule et al. found that adult patients with ESRD secondary to SLE were at increased risk of death compared with other adult patients (HR 1.7; 95% CI 1.2–2.7) [29]. Conversion between rates and probabilities as noted above.

[e]In the relapse state for both MMF and AZA strategies, the rate of lupus-related death is derived from age-specific annual mortality rate in the general population [28] multiplied by a standardized mortality ratio (SMR) 7.9. In a cohort of 9,547 SLE patients, Bernatsky et al. estimated an SMR 7.9 in those with nephritis [27]. Conversion between rates and probabilities as noted above.

[f]Values in (e) divided by 9.3, given that the relative risk of lupus-related death during relapse versus remission on MMF treatment is 9.3 [13].

[g]Values in (f) × 0.58, given that the relative risk of lupus-related death during remission on AZA versus MMF is 0.58 [13].

(b)

Cost parameters (over 1-year period)	Mean costs ($)	Range ($)	Probability distribution[c]	Sources/Comments
Direct costs × 1 year (nonpharmaceuticals)[a]				
Remission	3,368.34	1263.13–2105.21	Gamma (31.5, 0.019)	Clarke et al. 2004 [18]; Clarke et al. 2008 [17]; range assumed to be ±25% mean
Relapse	6,486.85	2432.57–4054.29	Gamma (29.2, 0.009)	Clarke et al. 2004 [18]; Clarke et al. 2008 [17]; range assumed to be ±25% mean

(b) Continued.

Cost parameters (over 1-year period)	Mean costs ($)	Range ($)	Probability distribution[c]	Sources/Comments
Indirect costs × 1 year[b]				
Remission	16,066.38	6024.89–10041.49	Gamma (16.1, 0.002)	Panopalis et al. 2007 [19]; Clarke et al. 2008 [17]; range assumed to be ±25% mean
Relapse	17,128.13	6423.05–10705.09	Gamma (18.3, 0.002)	Panopalis et al. 2007 [19]; Clarke et al. 2008 [17]; range assumed to be ±25% mean
ESRD/dialysis: mean cost per person × 1 year	86,608	n/a	Gamma (75.0, 0.002)	USRDS 2012 [20]

ESRD: end stage renal disease; USRDS: United States Renal Data System.

[a] Direct costs included care provided by specialists, nonspecialists, nonphysician healthcare professionals, laboratory studies, imaging studies, emergency room visits, and outpatient surgery and hospitalizations [18].

[b] Indirect costs included time lost from labor and nonlabor (i.e., household work) market activity as well as time that a caregiver spent helping the patient receiving healthcare services and the time the caregiver spent doing housework [19].

[c] Gamma distributions are characterized by (α, λ); $\alpha = \mu^2/s^2$, $\lambda = \mu/s^2$, where $\mu =$ mean; $s^2 =$ variance.

(c)

Utility parameters	Base-case mean	Range[a]	Probability distribution[b]	Sources/Comments
Utility of ESRD on dialysis	0.67	0.54–0.85	Beta (14.1, 6.9)	Liem et al. 2008 [22], based on TTO method
Utility of remission, on MMF or AZA	0.70	0.65–0.80	Beta (14.0, 6.0)	Grootscholten et al. 2007 [23], Clarke et al. 2008 [17], based on VAS method
Utility of relapse, on MMF or AZA	0.60	0.50–0.70	Beta (13.8, 9.2)	Grootscholten et al. 2007 [23], Clarke et al. 2008 [17], based on VAS method
Utility of death	0.00	n/a	n/a	Drummond et al. 2005 [26]

AZA: azathioprine; MMF: mycophenolate mofetil; ESRD: end stage renal disease; TTO: time trade-off; VAS: visual analog scale.

[a] Based on 95% confidence interval or standard deviation.

[b] Beta distributions are characterized by (α, β).

(3) relapse of LN despite MMF rescue therapy, requiring monotherapy with IV CYC;

(4) ESRD due to LN;

(5) death.

Upon completing the 3-year maintenance therapy, patients in each arm are assumed to be off the immunosuppressive medications and would progress through four potential health states in the lifetime model, in 12-month cycles:

(1) Remission;

(2) relapse of LN;

(3) ESRD due to LN;

(4) death.

2.4. Interventions. We evaluated MMF (2 gm/day) and AZA (150 mg/day) as maintenance therapy for LN. The model accounted for sequential rescue therapy during 3 years of maintenance therapy. There is a paucity of clinical trial data on the treatment of LN flares. Therefore, the treatment approach in our model reflects the current recommendations of national and international experts [9, 10].

2.5. Costs. Costs of healthcare products and services were undertaken from a societal perspective. All costs were adjusted for inflation to 2013 US dollars by using the Consumer Price Index for Medical Care [11]. Drug costs are based on average wholesale prices (AWP) [12]; other cost items were obtained from previous literature and public sources. Tables 1(b) and 2(b) show the components of *direct* and *indirect* costs incurred during the 3-year maintenance therapy with either MMF or AZA and thereafter in the lifetime model (Supplemental Costs). As noted above, patients are assumed to be off immunosuppressive therapy after 3 years; therefore, costs of MMF, AZA, and CYC are not included in the lifetime model.

2.6. Utilities (QALY). QALY is the product of the utility score and the number of years spent in a particular health state. A utility score reflects preference of a surveyed sample of individuals for a particular health state; a preference score of 1.0 represents perfect health, whereas a 0 score represents death. Tables 1(c) and 2(c) show the various utility weights of the health states in the model, obtained from previous literature (Supplemental Utilities).

2.7. Outcome Measures. The first outcome measure is the incremental cost-effectiveness ratios (ICER) which is the difference in costs between two strategies divided by the difference in effectiveness [7]:

$$\text{ICER} = \frac{\Delta C}{\Delta E} = \frac{(C_1 - C_2)}{(E_1 - E_2)}, \tag{1}$$

where C_1 is the cost of strategy 1, C_2 is the cost of strategy 2, E_1 is the QALY of strategy 1, and E_2 is the QALY of strategy 2.

The second outcome measure is the net monetary benefit (NMB) which represents the difference between the monetary value of an incremental QALY and the cost of achieving the benefit. The strategy with the highest NMB is the most cost-effective given a WTP parameter [7]

$$\text{NMB} = (E \times \lambda) - C, \tag{2}$$

where E is effectiveness (QALY), λ is WTP, and C is cost.

WTP is the amount society that is willing to pay for an additional QALY. We used a WTP of \$50,000–\$100,000 per QALY gained, often cited as the cost-effectiveness threshold in the literature [30].

2.8. Data Analysis. Our model is based on Reference Case analysis, a standard set of methodological practices for cost-effectiveness analysis [31]. We conducted a two-dimensional simulation via a combination of probabilistic sensitivity analysis (PSA) and microsimulation [32] (Supplemental Data Analysis). We conducted sensitivity analyses to assess uncertainty in our model (Supplemental Sensitivity Analysis). We also conducted value of information analyses, using NMB calculations from the 3-year base-case model, to estimate the expected benefit of future research [32] (Supplemental Expected Value of Perfect Information). Total costs and QALY were calculated after six 1/2-year cycles in the 3-year model and after forty 1-year cycles in the base-case lifetime model.

3. Results

3.1. Model Validation. In assessing *external validity*, we compared predicted outputs from the 3-year model with observed data, which were generally comparable and within standard deviations (Supplemental Model Validation, Assessment of External Validity, and Supplemental Table 7). We also compared simulated 10-year and 15-year survival rates from the lifetime model with actual event data [33, 34]. Overall, the predicted outcomes from the lifetime model approximated observed data from these studies (Supplemental Assessment of External Validity).

3.2. 3-Year Model

3.2.1. Base-Case Analysis (Cochrane Data)

(i) Cost-Effectiveness. Compared with an AZA-based regimen, MMF had an incremental cost of \$17,611 and gain of 0.0067 QALY, with an ICER of \$2,630,592 per QALY (Table 3(a)).

(ii) Sensitivity Analyses. In a one-way sensitivity analysis, the MMF-based regimen was the favored strategy if the 6-month cost of MMF 2 gm/day was <\$954.13 at WTP \$50,000/QALY (Supplemental Figure 3). This is equivalent to \$1.33 per 500 mg MMF tablet and represents 20.0% of the actual AWP. As shown in Table 3(b), we conducted other sensitivity analyses by excluding indirect costs, varying utility weights or changing model assumptions; the ICER (MMF

TABLE 3: (a) Costs, effectiveness, and incremental cost effectiveness ratios (ICER) of the base-case and individual clinical trials in three-year model. (b) Sensitivity analysis of three-year model using Cochrane data.

(a)

Scenarios	Total cost ($)	Total effectiveness (QALY)	Incremental costs ($)	Incremental effectiveness (QALY)	ICER ($/QALY)
Cochrane (base-case)					
AZA	54,249.98	1.6367			
MMF	71,861.21	1.6434	17,611.23	0.0067	2,630,591.76
Subgroups					
ALMS					
AZA	55,959.12	1.6125			
MMF	72,619.05	1.6363	16,659.92	0.0238	700,001.12
MAINTAIN					
AZA	54,527.62	1.6318			
MMF	72,511.65	1.6148	17,984.04	−0.0170	Dominated

QALY: quality-adjusted life-years; AZA: azathioprine; MMF: mycophenolate mofetil.

(b)

Scenarios	ICER MMF versus AZA (US$)
Base-case	2,630,591.76
Excludes indirect costs in both strategies	2,529,609.93
Utility	
Remission = 0.8 (versus base-case 0.7)	1,476,631.93
Relapse requiring MMF = 0.5 (versus base-case 0.6)	1,654,369.09
Utility of relapse requiring CYC = utility of relapse requiring MMF rescue	2,555,137.00
Conditions biased against AZA-based strategy	
Indirect costs × 6 months during remission ($10,041.49) [higher indirect costs for AZA group]	2,410,632.95
Indirect costs × 6 months during remission ($10,041.49) + utility of remission state (0.8) [higher indirect costs for AZA group + higher utility during remission]	1,380,997.67
Indirect costs × 6 months during remission ($10,041.49) + utility of remission state (0.8) + drug costs of AZA × 6 months ($2626) [higher indirect costs for AZA group + higher utility during remission + higher drug costs of AZA]	709,870.18
Revised assumptions	
AZA group receives 3 gm/day of MMF as rescue (base-case 2 gm/day MMF)	1,900,694.28
Patients in the AZA group who remit on CYC rescue therapy are treated with AZA maintenance therapy (base-case MMF 2 gm/day)	2,273,422.51

ICER: incremental cost effectiveness ratio; AZA: azathioprine; MMF: mycophenolate mofetil.

versus AZA) of these analyses far exceeded the standard WTP $50,000–$100,000/QALY thresholds.

(iii) Tornado Analysis. At a WTP $50,000/QALY, the model was most sensitive to (1) indirect costs during remission; (2) utility weight of the remission state; (3) drug price of AZA 150 mg/day (Figure 2). These three parameters accounted for 82.4% of the total model uncertainty.

(iv) Scenario Analysis. Despite simulated conditions biased against AZA, the MMF-based regimen remained cost ineffective compared to its alternative at 3 years, with an ICER $709,870 per QALY (Table 3(b)).

(v) Probabilistic Sensitivity Analyses. The incremental cost-effectiveness (ICE) scatterplot and the cost-effectiveness acceptability curve (CEAC) showed that an AZA-based regimen had a near 100% probability of being cost-effective over a 3-year time frame, at WTP thresholds of $50,000 and $100,000/QALY (Figure 3(a), Supplemental Figure 4).

(vi) Expected Value of Perfect Information (EVPI). The *population* EVPI represents the upper bound on the expected gain on investment on further data collection, which we calculated to be $2,058,206 at WTP $100,000/QALY in the US population, assuming a period of 10 years with 3% discount rate (Supplemental Expected Value of Perfect Information).

Tornado analysis (WTP $50,000)

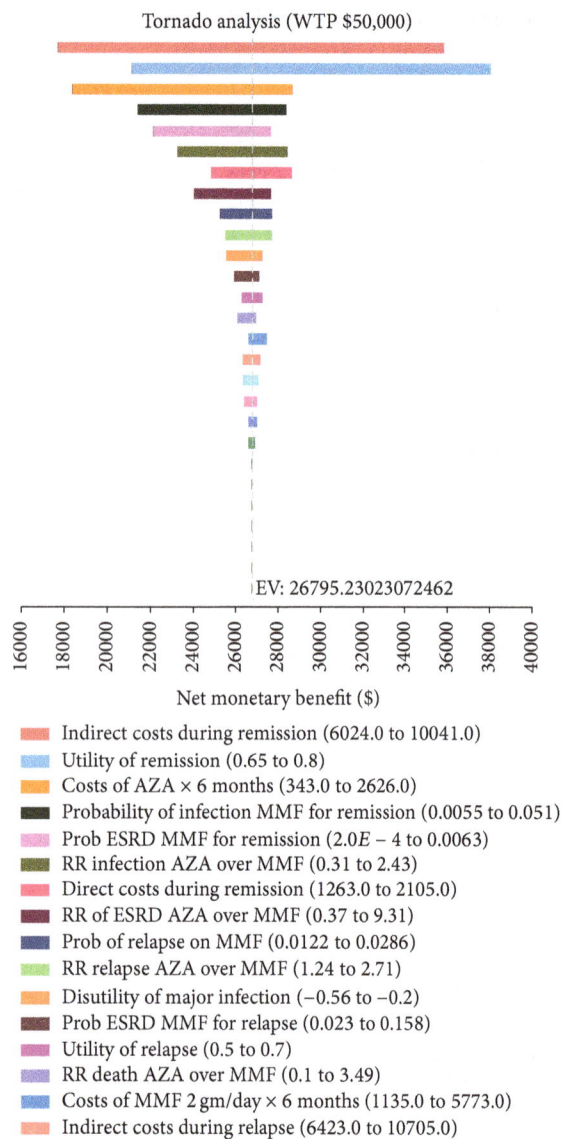

EV: 26795.23023072462

Net monetary benefit ($)

- Indirect costs during remission (6024.0 to 10041.0)
- Utility of remission (0.65 to 0.8)
- Costs of AZA × 6 months (343.0 to 2626.0)
- Probability of infection MMF for remission (0.0055 to 0.051)
- Prob ESRD MMF for remission (2.0E − 4 to 0.0063)
- RR infection AZA over MMF (0.31 to 2.43)
- Direct costs during remission (1263.0 to 2105.0)
- RR of ESRD AZA over MMF (0.37 to 9.31)
- Prob of relapse on MMF (0.0122 to 0.0286)
- RR relapse AZA over MMF (1.24 to 2.71)
- Disutility of major infection (−0.56 to −0.2)
- Prob ESRD MMF for relapse (0.023 to 0.158)
- Utility of relapse (0.5 to 0.7)
- RR death AZA over MMF (0.1 to 3.49)
- Costs of MMF 2 gm/day × 6 months (1135.0 to 5773.0)
- Indirect costs during relapse (6423.0 to 10705.0)

FIGURE 2: Tornado diagram of the 3-year base-case model, demonstrating one-way sensitivity analysis of each variable in the model. Each bar represents a range of expected values (EV), expressed as net monetary benefit in US dollars, over plausible estimates for an individual variable. The dotted vertical line indicates the base-case expected value. WTP: willingness-to-pay.

3.2.2. Subgroup Analysis. Based on ALMS data, MMF had an ICER of $700,001 per QALY compared with an AZA-based regimen (Table 3(a)). Furthermore, AZA was both cost-saving and more effective than MMF using data from the MAINTAIN trial (Table 3(a)).

3.3. Lifetime Model (40 Years)

3.3.1. Base-Case Analysis (Cochrane Data)

(i) Cost-Effectiveness. Compared with an AZA-based regimen, MMF had an incremental cost of $5,976 and gain of 0.9260 QALY, with an ICER of $6,454 per QALY (Table 4(a)).

(ii) Probabilistic Sensitivity Analyses. The CEAC showed that an MMF-based regimen had a near 100% probability of being cost-effective over a 40-year time frame, at WTP thresholds of $50,000 and $100,000/QALY (Supplemental Figure 5).

(iii) Sensitivity Analyses. As shown in Table 4(b), the ICER (MMF versus AZA) decreased over time such that MMF became cost-effective compared to AZA at 10 years postmaintenance therapy (Figures 3(b) and 3(c)). We also conducted sensitivity analyses by varying the probability of ESRD in the relapse state, demonstrating that the higher the risk of ESRD, the greater the cost-effectiveness of MMF versus AZA. Given the higher baseline risk of ESRD on AZA maintenance therapy, any incremental increase in this risk would disproportionately affect AZA (higher costs and lower QALY) as compared to MMF, resulting in a lower ICER (MMF versus AZA). We conducted other sensitivity analyses by excluding indirect costs, varying utility weights or discount rates, with the ICER (MMF versus AZA) well below the WTP $50,000/QALY threshold (Table 4(b)).

(iv) Scenario Analysis. The ICER of the base-case ($6,454/QALY) was based on the assumption that the treatment effect of MMF and AZA during the trial phase would persist over a lifetime. As shown in Table 4(b), MMF remained cost-effective over lifetime even if the treatment effect of both therapies diminished by 1% or 2% per year. However, assuming no treatment benefit after 3 years of maintenance therapy with either agent, MMF was not cost-effective compared to AZA ($428,894/QALY).

3.3.2. Subgroup Analysis. MMF had favorable ICER compared to AZA over lifetime using ALMS ($4,394/QALY) and MAINTAIN data ($54,891/QALY), below the WTP $50,000–$100,000/QALY (Table 4(a)).

4. Discussion

MMF and AZA are the most widely used therapeutic agents for long-term maintenance therapy of proliferative LN [35]. However, there is no consensus on the agent of choice, reflected by current clinical practice guideline recommendations [3, 4]. To evaluate the cost-effectiveness of MMF versus AZA-based regimens, we developed a Markov model to simulate patient-oriented outcomes, both from short-term and from lifetime horizon.

We found poor cost-effectiveness of MMF versus AZA-based therapy at 3 years, with an ICER $2,630,592/QALY. The ICER of MMF versus AZA remained substantially elevated in sensitivity analyses, even in conditions biased against AZA. Over a lifetime, however, our base-case analysis demonstrated MMF to be cost-effective compared to AZA, with an ICER $6,454/QALY. Overall, the ICER results from various sensitivity analyses did not alter the conclusions of the lifetime model, except in an unlikely scenario where the treatment effect was nil after 3 years of maintenance therapy. In contrast to the initial 3-year time period, subgroup analysis of ALMS and MAINTAIN trials showed that the MMF-based

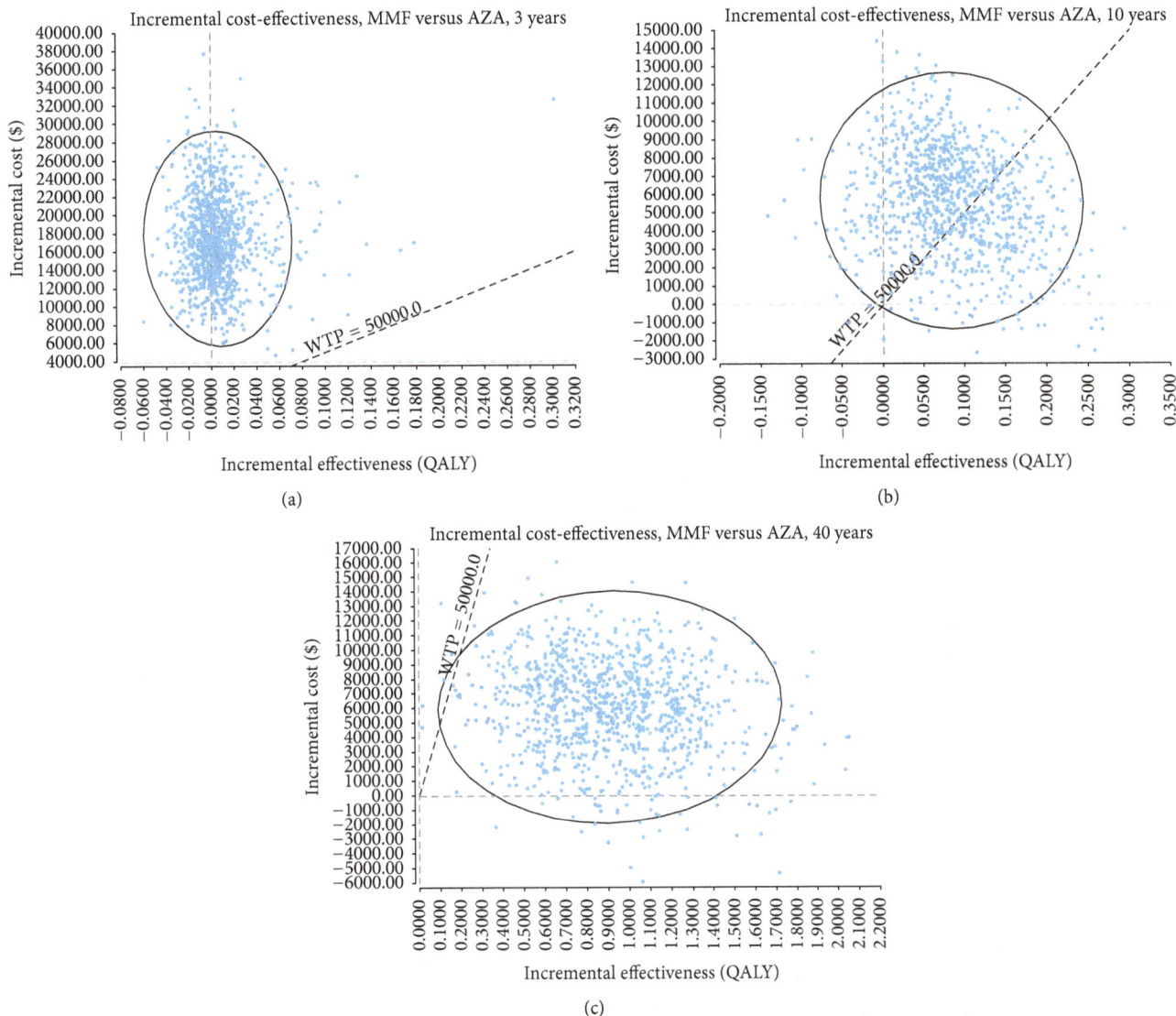

FIGURE 3: Incremental cost-effectiveness scatter plots of the base-case model. (a) 3 years; (b) 10 years after completing 3-year maintenance therapy; (c) 40 years after completing 3-year maintenance therapy. Each single point represents pairs of incremental cost and effectiveness values from probabilistic sensitivity analyses via second-order Monte Carlo simulation of 1,000 iterations. The ellipsis represents the 95% confidence interval. The dotted diagonal line represents the WTP threshold of $50,000/QALY. AZA: azathioprine; MMF: mycophenolate mofetil; WTP: willingness-to-pay; QALY: quality-adjusted life-years.

strategy was cost-effective compared to AZA from a lifetime perspective, at WTP $50,000–$100,000/QALY.

To our knowledge, there are only two published cost-effectiveness analyses of LN treatment. Wilson et al. estimated the cost-utility of MMF versus IV CYC as induction therapy for 6 months from the perspective of the National Health Service in the United Kingdom (UK) [36]. Their analysis suggested that MMF was likely to result in better quality of life and be less expensive than IV CYC as induction therapy. More recently, Mohara et al. conducted a lifetime cost-utility analysis of four different immunosuppressive regimens for LN patients in Thailand [37]. The study demonstrated that, from a Thai perspective, induction with IV CYC followed by AZA was the most cost-effective regimen of all

the alternatives. Our study reached different conclusions due to notable mutual differences in the model structure and assumptions, setting (US versus Thailand), target population, cost and utility parameters, and transition probabilities; and the Cochrane meta-analysis was not used as data source in Mohara's study.

Our study has certain limitations. First, lifetime modeling required extrapolation of data beyond the period observed in clinical trials which could lead to inconsistent results. We therefore assessed the uncertainty of future treatment benefit by conducting sensitivity analyses based on established guidelines [38]. Second, we assume that patients in our model receive immunosuppressive maintenance therapy for 3 years based on published clinical trials [13]. Due to lack of data from

TABLE 4: (a) Costs, effectiveness, and incremental cost effectiveness ratios (ICER) of the base-case and individual clinical trials in lifetime model (40 years). (b) Sensitivity analysis of lifetime model using Cochrane data.

(a)

Scenarios	Total cost ($)	Total effectiveness (QALY)	Incremental costs ($)	Incremental effectiveness (QALY)	ICER ($/QALY)
Cochrane (base-case)					
AZA	478,333.42	14.1623			
MMF	484,309.78	15.0882	5976.36	0.9260	6454.24
Subgroups					
ALMS					
AZA	485,791.18	13.5979			
MMF	493,953.07	15.4554	8161.89	1.8575	4393.90
MAINTAIN					
AZA	469,825.11	14.0140			
MMF	486,758.11	14.3225	16,933.00	0.3085	54,891.42

QALY: quality-adjusted life-years; AZA: azathioprine; MMF: mycophenolate mofetil.

(b)

Scenarios	ICER MMF versus AZA (US$)
Base-case (40-year time horizon)	$6,454.24
Excluding indirect costs	Dominant[a]
Utility	
Remission 0.8 (versus base-case 0.7)	$4067.55
Relapse 0.5 (versus base-case 0.6)	$5,808.27
Relapse 0.7 (versus base-case 0.6)	$7,695.58
Increase in probability of ESRD with relapse	
0.5% per year	$4590.37
1.0% per year	$3112.96
2.0% per year	$2717.08
Extrapolated treatment effect after 3-year maintenance therapy	
Same as during treatment phase (base-case)	$6,454.24
No treatment effect from both MMF and AZA during extrapolated phase[b]	$428,894.16
Treatment effect from both MMF and AZA decreases 1% per year[c]	$15,096.38
Treatment effect from both MMF and AZA decreases 2% per year[c]	$25,713.36
Time horizon (number of years after maintenance therapy)	
5 years	$513,712.88
10 years	$67,203.94
20 years	Dominant[a]
30 years	$5,232.11
Discount rate (base-case 3% for costs and utility)	
0%	$5,830.11
5%	$10,230.91
7%	$14,374.62

ICER: incremental cost effectiveness ratio; AZA: azathioprine; MMF: mycophenolate mofetil; ESRD: end stage renal disease.
[a]MMF is less costly and more effective than AZA-based regimen.
[b]Assuming 100% probability of relapse during remission on either MMF or AZA after completing 3-year maintenance therapy.
[c]Assuming 1% or 2% per year increase in relapse during remission on either MMF or AZA after completing 3-year maintenance therapy.

long-term randomized studies of maintenance therapy in patients with proliferative lupus nephritis, we did not model scenarios whereby patients are kept on maintenance therapy for >3 years. Modeling such scenarios based on incomplete medical evidence would compromise face validity. Furthermore, we would not be able to test the model for external validity (comparing predicted results from the model with actual event data) [39]. Third, the *total* costs of each strategy are likely underestimated since cost data are based on the Tri-Nation Study which included lupus patients from the US, Canada, and UK [18, 19]. This study estimated that direct and indirect costs in the US are 20% and 29% higher, respectively, than Canada. However, this underestimation of total costs does not change the conclusions of our analysis which is based on incremental calculations. Fourth, our model included utility scores that were measured by VAS [17, 23] which does not involve a trade-off that a subject must choose between the health states, in contrast to the standard gamble and time trade-off techniques. However, VAS was demonstrated to be a valid and reliable measure of health related quality of life in a SLE cohort [40]. Lastly, we incorporated major infection in the model as the most severe side effect of immunosuppressive therapy but did not consider gastrointestinal disturbance, leukopenia, alopecia, or infertility.

Acknowledging these limitations, our study does suggest that, from a cost-effectiveness standpoint, an AZA-based regimen confers greater value than MMF for the maintenance therapy of proliferative LN in the short term. Value of information analysis suggests a population EVPI of $2,058,206 at WTP $100,000/QALY which represents the expected maximum gain on investment on further research. The implication is that spending more than this amount on additional data collection would represent a poor investment of limited research funds. In contrast to the short-term perspective, MMF is cost-effective compared to AZA at the standard WTP threshold in the US over the patients' lifetime. Despite the relatively higher upfront costs of MMF during the 3-year maintenance phase, its salutary effects (lower risk of LN relapse and progression to ESRD compared to AZA) make MMF a cost-effective option over the long term. Our analysis is consistent with the general notion that the time frame of a model should be sufficiently long to capture future differences in costs and health outcomes between treatment strategies.

Given the substantial economic burden of LN in our healthcare system, the findings of this study should be an important factor in selecting the optimal maintenance regimen for patients with proliferative LN. Furthermore, these findings may provide useful information to support more individualized therapy.

Disclaimer

The views expressed in this paper are those of the authors and do not necessarily reflect the official policy or position of the Department of the Army, the Department of the Navy, the Department of Defense, or the United States government.

Acknowledgment

The authors would like to acknowledge Annie Nguyen, PharmD, for her assistance in obtaining data for drug costs.

References

[1] K. A. Slawsky, A. W. Fernandes, L. Fusfeld, S. Manzi, and T. F. Goss, "A structured literature review of the direct costs of adult systemic lupus erythematosus in the US," *Arthritis Care & Research*, vol. 63, no. 9, pp. 1224–1232, 2011.

[2] G. Carls, T. Li, P. Panopalis et al., "Direct and indirect costs to employers of patients with systemic lupus erythematosus with and without nephritis," *Journal of Occupational and Environmental Medicine*, vol. 51, no. 1, pp. 66–79, 2009.

[3] Kidney Disease: Improving Global Outcomes (KDIGO) Glomerulonephritis Work Group, "KDIGO clinical practice guideline for glomerulonephritis," *Kidney International Supplements*, vol. 2, no. 2, pp. 139–274, 2012.

[4] B. H. Hahn, M. A. McMahon, A. Wilkinson et al., "American College of Rheumatology guidelines for screening, treatment, and management of lupus nephritis," *Arthritis Care and Research*, vol. 64, no. 6, pp. 797–808, 2012.

[5] F. A. Houssiau, D. D'Cruz, S. Sangle et al., "Azathioprine versus mycophenolate mofetil for long-term immunosuppression in lupus nephritis: results from the MAINTAIN Nephritis Trial," *Annals of the Rheumatic Diseases*, vol. 69, no. 12, pp. 2083–2089, 2010.

[6] M. A. Dooley, D. Jayne, E. M. Ginzler et al., "Mycophenolate versus azathioprine as maintenance therapy for lupus nephritis," *The New England Journal of Medicine*, vol. 365, no. 20, pp. 1886–1895, 2011.

[7] A. M. Gray, P. M. Clarke, J. L. Wolstenholme, and S. Wordsworth, *Applied Methods of Cost-Effectiveness Analysis in Health Care*, Oxford University Press, New York, NY, USA, 2011.

[8] D. Husereau, M. Drummond, S. Petrou et al., "Consolidated health economic evaluation reporting standards (CHEERS)—explanation and elaboration: a report of the ISPOR health economic evaluation publication guidelines good reporting practices task force," *Value in Health*, vol. 16, no. 2, pp. 231–250, 2013.

[9] B. Sprangers, M. Monahan, and G. B. Appel, "Diagnosis and treatment of lupus nephritis flares—an update," *Nature Reviews Nephrology*, vol. 8, no. 12, pp. 709–717, 2012.

[10] R. J. Falk, P. H. Schur, and G. B. Appel, "Therapy of resistant or relapsing diffuse or focal proliferative lupus nephritis," UpTo-Date, May 2013, http://www.uptodate.com/.

[11] Bureau of Labor Statistics, "Consumer Price Index," December 2013, http://www.bls.gov/cpi/home.htm.

[12] Red Book Online, June 2013, http://www.redbook.com/redbook/online/.

[13] L. Henderson, P. Masson, J. C. Craig et al., "Treatment for lupus nephritis," *Cochrane Database of Systematic Reviews*, vol. 12, Article ID CD002922, 2012.

[14] K. H. Costenbader, A. Desai, G. S. Alarcón et al., "Trends in the incidence, demographics, and outcomes of end-stage renal disease due to lupus nephritis in the US from 1995 to 2006," *Arthritis & Rheumatism*, vol. 63, no. 6, pp. 1681–1688, 2011.

[15] F. A. Sonnenberg and J. R. Beck, "Markov models in medical decision making: a practical guide," *Medical Decision Making*, vol. 13, no. 4, pp. 322–338, 1993.

[16] Centers for Medicare & Medicaid Services, December 2013, http://www.cms.gov/Medicare/Medicare-Fee-for-Service-Payment/HospitalOutpatientPPS/Addendum-A-and-Addendum-B-Updates.html.

[17] A. E. Clarke, P. Panopalis, M. Petri et al., "SLE patients with renal damage incur higher health care costs," *Rheumatology*, vol. 47, no. 3, pp. 329–333, 2008.

[18] A. E. Clarke, M. Petri, S. Manzi et al., "The systemic lupus erythematosus tri-nation study: absence of a link between health resource use and health outcome," *Rheumatology*, vol. 43, no. 8, pp. 1016–1024, 2004.

[19] P. Panopalis, M. Petri, S. Manzi et al., "The systemic lupus erythematosus tri-nation study: cumulative indirect costs," *Arthritis Care and Research*, vol. 57, no. 1, pp. 64–70, 2007.

[20] US Renal Data System, *USRDS 2012 Annual Data Report: Atlas of Chronic Kidney Disease and End-Stage Renal Disease in the United States*, National Institutes of Health, National Institute of Diabetes and Digestive and Kidney Diseases, Bethesda, Md, USA, 2012.

[21] Healthcare Cost and Utilization Project and Agency for Healthcare Research and Quality, 2013, http://hcupnet.ahrq.gov/HCUPnet.jsp?Id=5452BD185046B6A8&Form=DispTab&JS=Y&Action=%3E%3ENext%3E%3E&GoTo=MAINSEL.

[22] Y. S. Liem, J. L. Bosch, and M. G. M. Hunink, "Preference-based quality of life of patients on renal replacement therapy: a systematic review and meta-analysis," *Value in Health*, vol. 11, no. 4, pp. 733–741, 2008.

[23] C. Grootscholten, F. J. Snoek, M. Bijl et al., "Health-related quality of life and treatment burden in patients with proliferative lupus nephritis treated with cyclophosphamide or azathioprine/methylprednisolone in a randomized controlled trial," *Journal of Rheumatology*, vol. 34, no. 8, pp. 1699–1707, 2007.

[24] K. C. Tse, C. S. O. Tang, W. I. Lio, M. F. Lam, and T. M. Chan, "Quality of life comparison between corticosteroid-and-mycofenolate mofetil and corticosteroid-and-oral cyclophosphamide in the treatment of severe lupus nephritis," *Lupus*, vol. 15, no. 6, pp. 371–379, 2006.

[25] Tufts' Cost-Effectiveness Analysis Registry, December 2013, https://research.tufts-nemc.org/cear4/Home.aspx.

[26] M. F. Drummond, M. J. Sculpher, G. W. Torrance, B. J. O'Brien, and G. L. Stoddart, *Methods for the Economic Evaluation of Health Care Programmes*, Oxford University Press, New York, NY, USA, 3rd edition, 2005.

[27] S. Bernatsky, J.-F. Boivin, L. Joseph et al., "Mortality in systemic lupus erythematosus," *Arthritis & Rheumatism*, vol. 54, no. 8, pp. 2550–2557, 2006.

[28] E. Arias, "United States life tables, 2007," *National Vital Statistics Reports*, vol. 59, pp. 1–60, 2011.

[29] S. Sule, B. Fivush, A. Neu, and S. Furth, "Increased risk of death in pediatric and adult patients with ESRD secondary to lupus," *Pediatric Nephrology*, vol. 26, no. 1, pp. 93–98, 2011.

[30] R. S. Braithwaite, D. O. Meltzer, J. T. King Jr., D. Leslie, and M. S. Roberts, "What does the value of modern medicine say about the $50,000 per quality-adjusted life-year decision rule?" *Medical Care*, vol. 46, no. 4, pp. 349–356, 2008.

[31] M. C. Weinstein, J. E. Siegel, M. R. Gold, M. S. Kamlet, and L. B. Russell, "Recommendations of the panel on cost-effectiveness in health and medicine," *Journal of the American Medical Association*, vol. 276, no. 15, pp. 1253–1258, 1996.

[32] B. Groot Koerkamp, M. C. Weinstein, T. Stijnen, M. H. Heijenbrok-Kal, and M. G. M. Hunink, "Uncertainty and patient heterogeneity in medical decision models," *Medical Decision Making*, vol. 30, no. 2, pp. 194–205, 2010.

[33] F. A. Houssiau, C. Vasconcelos, D. D'Cruz et al., "The 10-year follow-up data of the Euro-Lupus Nephritis Trial comparing low-dose and high-dose intravenous cyclophosphamide," *Annals of the Rheumatic Diseases*, vol. 69, no. 1, pp. 61–64, 2010.

[34] C. C. Mok, R. C. L. Kwok, and P. S. F. Yip, "Effect of renal disease on the standardized mortality ratio and life expectancy of patients with systemic lupus erythematosus," *Arthritis and Rheumatism*, vol. 65, no. 8, pp. 2154–2160, 2013.

[35] O. Lenz, A. A. Waheed, A. Baig, A. Pop, and G. Contreras, "Lupus nephritis: maintenance therapy for lupus nephritis—do we now have a plan?" *Clinical Journal of the American Society of Nephrology*, vol. 8, no. 1, pp. 162–171, 2013.

[36] E. C. F. Wilson, D. R. W. Jayne, E. Dellow, and R. J. Fordham, "The cost-effectiveness of mycophenolate mofetil as firstline therapy in active lupus nephritis," *Rheumatology*, vol. 46, no. 7, pp. 1096–1101, 2007.

[37] A. Mohara, R. P. Velasco, N. Praditsitthikorn, Y. Avihingsanon, and Y. Teerawattananon, "A cost-utility analysis of alternative drug regimens for newly diagnosed severe lupus nephritis patients in Thailand," *Rheumatology*, vol. 53, no. 1, Article ID ket304, pp. 138–144, 2014.

[38] NICE guide to the methods of technology appraisal 2013, 2014, http://www.nice.org.uk/article/PMG9/chapter/5-The-reference-case.

[39] D. M. Eddy, W. Hollingworth, J. J. Caro, J. Tsevat, K. M. McDonald, and J. B. Wong, "Model transparency and validation: a report of the ISPOR-SMDM modeling good research practices task force-7," *Medical Decision Making*, vol. 32, no. 5, pp. 733–743, 2012.

[40] A. D. Moore, A. E. Clarke, D. S. Danoff et al., "Can health utility measures be used in lupus research? A comparative validation and reliability study of 4 utility indices," *Journal of Rheumatology*, vol. 26, no. 6, pp. 1285–1290, 1999.

14

Primary Hyperoxaluria Type 1 in 18 Children: Genotyping and Outcome

Mohamed S. Al Riyami, Badria Al Ghaithi, Nadia Al Hashmi, and Naifain Al Kalbani

Pediatric Nephrology Unit, Department of Child Health, Royal Hospital, P.O. Box 1331, 111 Muscat, Oman

Correspondence should be addressed to Mohamed S. Al Riyami; alriyamimohamed@gmail.com

Academic Editor: Alessandro Amore

Background. Primary hyperoxaluria belongs to a group of rare metabolic disorders with autosomal recessive inheritance. It results from genetic mutations of the *AGXT* gene, which is more common due to higher consanguinity rates in the developing countries. Clinical features at presentation are heterogeneous even in children from the same family; this study was conducted to determine the clinical characteristics, type of *AGXT* mutation, and outcome in children diagnosed with PH1 at a tertiary referral center in Oman. *Method*. Retrospective review of children diagnosed with PH1 at a tertiary hospital in Oman from 2000 to 2013. *Result*. Total of 18 children were identified. Females composed 61% of the children with median presentation age of 7 months. Severe renal failure was initial presentation in 39% and 22% presented with nephrocalcinosis and/or renal calculi. Family screening diagnosed 39% of patients. Fifty percent of the children underwent hemodialysis. 28% of children underwent organ transplantation. The most common mutation found in Omani children was c.33-34insC mutation in the *AGXT* gene. *Conclusion*. Due to consanguinity, PH1 is a common cause of ESRD in Omani children. Genetic testing is recommended to help in family counseling and helps in decreasing the incidence and disease burden; it also could be utilized for premarital screening.

1. Introduction

Primary hyperoxaluria (PH) belongs to a group of rare metabolic disorders with autosomal recessive inheritance [1]. Type-1 PH (PH1) results from genetic mutations of the *AGXT* gene, which encodes the hepatic peroxisomal enzyme, alanine:glyoxylate-aminotransferase (AGT). *AGXT* is the only gene known to encode AGT and, thus far, approximately 146 mutations have been associated with PH1 [2–4]. In the absence of AGT activity, glyoxylate is converted to oxalate, and increased urinary oxalate excretion results in progressive intrarenal crystal deposition and kidney function deterioration [1]. The end result is systemic oxalosis [1]. The estimated prevalence of PH1 in Europe is 1–3 cases per million people [1, 5, 6], and the median age at initial presentation is 4 to 7 years old but ranges from the early neonatal period to the sixth decade of life [1, 6, 7]. Clinical features at presentation are heterogeneous and include recurrent hematuria, abdominal pain and urinary tract infections, nephrocalcinosis, nephrolithiasis, and even end-stage renal disease (ESRD), which hastens systemic oxalosis development [8]. However, PH1 can be a silent disease that is detected only during family screening [9]. The combination of a positive family history among siblings and cousins, ultrasonographic findings of nephrocalcinosis or nephrolithiasis, and suggestive laboratory features should alert nephrologists to the diagnosis. Conservative treatment measures should be initiated as soon as PH1 is suspected to prevent intrarenal crystal deposition and to slow progression to ESRD. These measures include high fluid intake, pyridoxine, and inhibitors of urinary crystallization such as citrate [1, 10].

This study was conducted to determine the clinical characteristics, type *AGXT* mutation, and outcome in children who were diagnosed to have PH1 at a tertiary referral center in Oman.

2. Methods

This study was a retrospective analysis of all Omani children <13 years old who were diagnosed with PH1 at the Royal

TABLE 1: Demographic data and clinical features.

Number	Sex	Age at presentation (months)	Type of presentation	Age at onset of ESRD (years)
Ia	Male	18	NC, distal RTA, renal stone	11
Ib	Female	18	Family screening, NC	6
Ic	Male	2	ESRD	At presentation
IIa	Female	12	NC, RTA, renal stone	11
IIb	Female	7	ESRD	At presentation
IIc	Female	2	Family screening, NC	8
IId	Male	2	Family screening, NC, CKD	4
IIIa	Female	60	ESRD	At presentation
IIIb	Female	36	ESRD	At presentation
IIIC	Male	24	Family screening, NC	Normal RFT
IIId	Male	7	ESRD	At presentation
IVa	Female	6	NC, renal stone, UTI	7
IVb	Female	1	Family screening, NC	Below 1 year
IVc	Male	48	NC, polyuria	CKD
IVd	Female	1	Family screening, NC	CKD
IVe	Male	4	ESRD, NC	At presentation
IVf	Female	3	Family screening, NC	CKD
IVg	Female	2	ESRD, NC	At presentation

Family number 1 (I), family number 2 (II), family number 3 (III), and family number 4 (IV).
ESRD: end-stage renal disease, NC: nephrocalcinosis, RTA: renal tubular acidosis, RFT: renal function test, CKD: chronic kidney disease, and UTI: urinary tract infection.

Hospital, Muscat, Oman, from January 2000 to December 2013. Royal Hospital is the main tertiary referral center for children with kidney disease in Oman. Children included in this study were diagnosed with PH1 based on clinical features, family history, high urine oxalate, liver enzyme assay of AGT, or mutation analysis of the *AGXT* gene. The study was approved by the Royal Hospital Ethical Committee and written informed consent was obtained from a legal guardian.

Data collected from electronic medical records included sex, age, type of presentation, urinary oxalate findings, AGT activity results, *AGXT* gene analysis (if performed), type of conservative management received, age at ESRD development, type of dialysis received, and outcome (i.e., chronic kidney disease (CKD), transplant, or death).

Children with nephrocalcinosis or renal calculi that were suspected to have PH or were siblings of PH1 patients had blood investigations for renal function, renal ultrasound, and 24-hour urinary oxalate.

Hyperoxaluria was defined as urine oxalate >0.5 mmol/ 1.73 m^2/day [11]. In children who presented with severe renal failure and had low urine oxalate level, plasma oxalate level was obtained.

To confirm the PH diagnosis and type, frozen liver samples from one patient in each family were evaluated for AGT activity at University College London Hospital, London, UK. Among the four families, *AGXT* mutation

was analyzed in 7 patients at Center for Nephrology and Metabolic Disorder, Weisswasser, Germany.

Descriptive statistics were presented as percentages, means, and median.

3. Results

A total of 18 children from 4 different families were diagnosed with PH1 during the study period from January 2000 to December 2013. Table 1 summarizes the main patient demographics. There were 61% females (11 out of 18 patients). Median age at presentation was 7 months (range 1–60 months). All children were below 5 years of age and 61% (11 out of 18 patients) were below 1 year of age at presentation. Nephrocalcinosis and/or renal calculi were common at presentation in 22% of our cohort (4 out of 18). Thirty-nine percent (7 out of 18) of patients presented with severe renal failure; majority were below the age of 1 year. In 4 out of these 18 children, the initial diagnosis of PH1 was not clear. Two patients were initially diagnosed to have renal tubular acidosis with nephrocalcinosis, but they later developed recurrent renal calculi and stone workup revealed elevated 24-hour urinary oxalate. The other two patients were initially diagnosed clinically as having autosomal recessive polycystic kidney disease. The first child presented with ESRD, started on peritoneal dialysis, and was only retrospectively diagnosed

TABLE 2: Management and outcome.

Number	Supportive therapy	Follow-up period (year)	RRT	Transplant	Outcome
Ia	C, F, P, ESWL	13	HD	—	Alive
Ib	C, F, P	7.5	HD	LUL	Alive
Ic	C, P	3.5	HD	—	Died
IIa	C, F, P, ESWL	13	HD	LRL and 2 LRK	Alive
IIb	C, P	2	PD	—	Died
IIc	C, F, P	9	HD	LRL and LRK	Alive
IId	C, F, P	3	—	—	Died
IIIa	C, P	4.5	HD	—	Died
IIIb	C, P	3.5	HD	—	Died
IIIc	C, F, P	4	—	LRL	Alive
IIId	C, P	2.5	HD	—	Alive
IVa	C, F, P, ESWL	9	HD	LUL	Died
IVb	C, P	1.5	—	—	Died
IVc	C, F, P	9	Supportive	—	*47
IVd	C, F, P	1.5	Supportive	—	*16
IVe	C, P	1	PD	—	Died
IVf	C, F, P	4	Supportive	—	*64
IVg	C, P	2	PD	—	Died

Family number 1 (I), family number 2 (II), family number 3 (III), and family number 4 (IV). ESRD: end-stage renal disease, C: citrate, F: fluid, P: pyridoxine, ESWL: electric shock wave lithotripsy, CKD: chronic kidney disease, HD: hemodialysis, PD: peritoneal dialysis, LRL: living-related liver transplant, LRK: living-related kidney transplant, LUL: living-unrelated liver transplant, and *estimated glomerular filtration rate (eGFR mL/min/m^2).

with PH1 after other siblings were diagnosed with PH1. The second child's diagnosis was reevaluated after developing recurrent renal calculi; stone workup showed high 24-hour urinary oxalate levels. 39% (7 out of 18) of the patients were diagnosed after family screening of confirmed PH1 siblings.

Supportive therapy such as citrate and pyridoxine was initiated in all patients (Table 2). High fluid intake was advised to patients who did not reach ESRD. Three children were at different stages of chronic kidney disease with current estimated GFR as shown in Table 2 under close follow-up. Renal replacement therapy in the form of intermittent hemodialysis (HD) was required for 50% of the children (9 out of 18). Peritoneal dialysis was performed in 3 infants who presented with renal failure and all of them died during follow-up. Two patients did not receive renal replacement therapy due to family refusal and later died due to systemic oxalosis. Three patients received liver transplantation only, while 2 patients received both liver and kidney transplantation. Patient IIa underwent renal transplantation twice; first renal graft was lost due to disease recurrence although liver transplant was working well. Fifty percent of patients with PH1 included in the study died.

Regarding liver biopsy result, AGT immunoreactivity was negative in two patients and AGT enzyme activity was low in all children who underwent liver biopsies (Table 3). Genetic testing after administrative approval was done in 7 patients among the 4 families. Five patients from 3 families had a c.33-34insC homozygous frame shift mutation in the AGXT gene. Two children from family IV had a C.346 G>A mutation in the AGXT gene as shown in Table 3. Consanguinity was confirmed in all four families.

4. Discussion

This is the first report of PH1 in Omani children. We identified 18 affected children from 4 different families, with each family having more than one affected child. Thus, the PH1 consanguinity rate in this study was 100%. There are many similar reports from different Middle East countries that showed elevated PH1 rates associated with increased consanguinity [12–15]. Mbarek et al. reported on 57 patients with PH1 from 40 different families. In their cohort, more than one family member was affected and the reported consanguinity rate was 75% [15]. In our study, all patients diagnosed with PH1 were <5 years old and the median age at initial PH1 symptom onset was 7 months. This age is lower compared to other reports. In the Netherlands, the median age at initial PH1 symptom onset is 6 years (range 0–50 years) [5], and in Japan the median age of onset was 13 years [16]. However, Mbarek et al. reported that the median age at presentation for patients carrying the 33-34insC mutation in Tunisian children was 3 years (range 5 months–61 years), while those children carrying the 1244T mutation were older, median age of 13 years (range 3 months–38 years) [15].

The clinical features at presentation in Omani PH1 patients were similar to those described in previous reports [5, 15, 17]. We found early-onset ESRD in our study; 39% (7 out of 18) presented with severe infantile PH1 and developed ESRD in the first year of life. Overall, the median age at ESRD development was about 4 years. In a study by van Woerden et al. [5] with a 7.7-year median follow-up, 33% of Dutch adult and child PH1 patients had ESRD at presentation and 16% developed ESRD during follow-up. While nine infants had

TABLE 3: 24-hour urinary oxalate, plasma oxalate, *AGXT* mutations and AGT activity.

Patient number	Urinary oxalate, mmol/24 h	Plasma oxalate, μmol/L	*AGXT* mutation	AGT activity, μmol/h/mg protein
Ia*	2.440	65	—	—
Ib	—	—	c.33-34insC	4.7
Ic*	0.228	—	—	—
IIa*	1.309	41	C.33-34insC	2.8
IIb	—	—	—	—
IIc*	0.331	27.7	C.33-34insC	—
IId*	0.224	58	—	—
IIIa	0.164	202	—	—
IIIb	0.052	109	—	2.4
IIIc*	1.567	—	C.33-34insC	—
IIId	0.076	27.0	C.33-34insC	—
IVa*	0.889	40	—	4.7
IVb*	0.526	—	c.346 G>A	—
IVc*	1.538	—	c.346 G>A	—
IVd*	0.165	—	—	—
IVe	0.021	127.0	—	—
IVf*	0.479	—	—	—
IVg	0.072	—	—	—

Family number 1 (I), family number 2 (II), family number 3 (III), and familynumber 4 (IV). *24-hour oxalate >0.5 mmol/1.73 m^2. Lab reference range for plasma oxalate <33 μmol/L. AGT activity reference range (19.1–47.9 μmol/h/mg); —: not done.

infantile PH1, five of these patients developed ESRD, four out of these nine children were sensitive to pyridoxine, during follow-up three of them showed improved renal function or decreased nephrocalcinosis, and one had preserved renal function after pyridoxine administration.

A cohort of 222 PH1 patients from the Rare Kidney Stone Consortium (RKSC) registry showed renal survival rates of 89% at 10 years of age and 75% at 20 years of age [18]. We found two *AGXT* gene mutations in our patients: c.33-34insC in Families I, II, and III and a C.346 G>A mutation in Family IV. The 33-34insC mutation has been described before in many studies [15, 19, 20]; it is due to microinsertion on the major or minor alleles of the *AGXT* gene [21]. Children with this mutation in a homozygous state display no immunoreactive protein and no catalytic activity [22] compared to other mutations due to peroxisome-to-mitochondrial mistargeting. For example, *AGXT* mutations such as Gly170Arg and phe15Ile confer different degrees of catalytic activity and better outcomes because patients retain good responsiveness to pyridoxine [23, 24], whereas the previously reported 33-34insC mutation may retain only some responsiveness to pyridoxine [24, 25]. The C.346 G>A mutation is a missense mutation of *AGXT* gene; it was also described previously [20, 26]. However it is uncommon compared to 33-34insC mutation. In genetic analysis of 55 patients from USA using complete sequencing of the whole *AGXT* coding region, Monico et al. reported that the most common mutation in this cohort was G170R and then c.33-34inC but C.346 G>A was only found in one patient [20]. In our study, all children were very young at presentation and majority progressed rapidly to ESRD despite supportive measures including pyridoxine administration. However,

confounding factors were therapy compliance issues and failure to regularly assess pyridoxine response.

van Woerden et al. [5, 19] previously conducted mutation analysis of 33 PH1 patients from a cohort of 57 patients and reported that the 33insC mutation was the third most common mutation and children who had this *AGXT* mutation in a homozygous state developed ESRD during early infancy with high mortality rate [19], similar to our findings. The results of the study by Mbarek et al. [15] are also in line with our findings. They identified the 33-34insC mutation as the second most common *AGXT* mutation, and children with this mutation display a severe form of PH1 with a high mortality rate. We noted no genotype-phenotype correlation between the two mutations in our cohort in view of similarities on severe early presentation and poor outcome. Our patients had severe disease with early presentation and genetic mutation was identified in at least one patient from each family. Therefore PHII is unlikely diagnosis among our cohort.

Regarding ESRD treatment, most of our patients received HD and a few were administered peritoneal dialysis. Many patients developed systemic oxalosis and this is attributed to multiple factors including the following. First, our patients had specific mutations that are associated with poor outcomes with multiple siblings affected within the family. However, previous reports [27, 28] showed poor correlation between genotype and phenotype, and even siblings with the same mutation can display different clinical features and have varied prognosis. Some studies have shown good outcomes with the homozygous 508G>A mutation compared to the 33insC mutation [19, 25]. Second, more intensive dialysis approaches such as daily HD or a combination of high flux

HD and peritoneal dialysis were not routinely practiced in our institution. These more intensive dialysis approaches have better results compared to conventional dialysis, due to improved oxalate removal [7, 29]. The third and perhaps most important reason for the high mortality rate observed might be due to limited access to organ transplantation for both kidney and liver in our country; this observation is noted in other developing countries [15].

Five children in our study underwent organ transplantation. Two patients had living-related dual liver-kidney transplantation, two children with ESRD had living-unrelated liver transplants, and one patient with normal renal function had a preemptive living-related liver transplant. On follow-up, one patient died and the second child developed disease recurrence and required a second renal transplant. Hence, the overall survival rate in our cohort who underwent organs transplantation was 80%. European and American studies indicate that combined liver and kidney transplantation is the best currently available therapy for PH1 patients [29, 30]. The European registry reported that 1-, 5-, and 10-year patient survival rates were 86%, 80%, and 69%, respectively [30]. The US Renal Data System reported PH1 patient survival >80% at 5 years and a death-censored graft survival of 76% at 8 years after transplant [31]. We elected to do a preemptive liver transplant for one patient even though he displayed only nephrocalcinosis with normal renal function. This was decided with strong family support because he had confirmed genetic mutation and history of 2 siblings who died with the same disease. Preemptive isolated liver transplantation can be considered in selected cases but can raise ethical issues in view of PH1 heterogeneity in the progression of the disease and improvement on the conservative management of these patients in the last decade [7, 29].

5. Conclusion

PH1 is a common cause of ESRD in Omani children due to the high consanguinity rate. PH1 screening should be done in any child that presents with ESRD with unexplained reason. Genetic testing is recommended to determine the gene mutation which helps in family counseling and ultimately decreasing the incidence of this disease. Conservative measurements should be started immediately as they may delay the progression, with regular close monitoring for response. Children who progress to ESRD should have more aggressive dialysis and plan for early liver-kidney transplantation. This report is limited by being a retrospective study with a small sample size. Further studies are recommended to identify local gene mutations and help tailor therapies accordingly. In conclusion, this report is the first from Oman and the gulf region; it highlights the huge disease burden of an autosomal recessive mutation and importance of family screening and genetic counseling.

Acknowledgments

The authors would like to thank Dr. Mato Nagel, Center for Nephrology and Metabolic disorder, Weisswasser, Germany, for genetic analysis, Dr. Gill Rumsby, Department of Clinical Biochemistry, University College London Hospital, London, UK, for AGT activity assessment, and Dr. Anisa Al Maskary and Dr. Lekha Hrishikesan for helping in patients evaluation and management.

References

[1] J. Harambat, S. Fargue, J. Bacchetta, C. Acquaviva, and P. Cochat, "Primary hyperoxaluria," *International Journal of Nephrology*, vol. 2011, Article ID 864580, 11 pages, 2011.

[2] M. B. Coulter-Mackie, C. T. White, R. M. Hurley, B. H. Chew, and D. Lange, "Primary hyperoxaluria type 1," in *Gene Reviews*, R. A. Pagon, T. D. Bird, C. R. Dolan, K. Stephens, and M. P. Adam, Eds., University of Washington, Seattle, Wash, USA, 1993.

[3] A. Robbiano, G. Mandrile, M. de Marchi et al., "Novel human pathological mutations. Gene symbol: AGXT. Disease: hyperoxaluria.," *Human genetics*, vol. 127, no. 4, pp. 463–468, 2010.

[4] E. L. Williams, C. Acquaviva, A. Amoroso et al., "Primary hyperoxaluria type 1: update and additional mutation analysis of the AGXT gene," *Human Mutation*, vol. 30, no. 6, pp. 910–917, 2009.

[5] C. S. van Woerden, J. W. Groothoff, R. J. A. Wanders, J.-C. Davin, and F. A. Wijburg, "Primary hyperoxaluria type 1 in The Netherlands: prevalence and outcome," *Nephrology Dialysis Transplantation*, vol. 18, no. 2, pp. 273–279, 2003.

[6] P. Cochat, A. Deloraine, M. Rotily, F. Olive, I. Liponski, and N. Deries, "Epidemiology of primary hyperoxaluria type 1," *Nephrology Dialysis Transplantation*, vol. 10, no. 8, pp. 3–7, 1995.

[7] P. Cochat, A. Liutkus, S. Fargue, O. Basmaison, B. Ranchin, and M.-O. Rolland, "Primary hyperoxaluria type 1: still challenging!," *Pediatric Nephrology*, vol. 21, no. 8, pp. 1075–1081, 2006.

[8] B. Hoppe, B. B. Beck, and D. S. Milliner, "The primary hyperoxalurias," *Kidney International*, vol. 75, no. 12, pp. 1264–1271, 2009.

[9] B. Hoppe, "Evidence of true genotype-phenotype correlation in primary hyperoxaluria type 1," *Kidney International*, vol. 77, no. 5, pp. 383–385, 2010.

[10] L. Borghi, T. Meschi, F. Amato, A. Briganti, A. Novarini, and A. Giannini, "Urinary volume, water and recurrences in idiopathic calcium nephrolithiasis: a 5-year randomized prospective study," *The Journal of Urology*, vol. 155, no. 3, pp. 839–843, 1996.

[11] P. Cochat, S.-A. Hulton, C. Acquaviva et al., "Primary hyperoxaluria Type 1: indications for screening and guidance for diagnosis and treatment," *Nephrology, Dialysis, Transplantation*, vol. 27, no. 5, pp. 1729–1736, 2012.

[12] K. Madani, H. Otoukesh, A. Rastegar, and S. Van Why, "Chronic renal failure in Iranian children," *Pediatric Nephrology*, vol. 16, no. 2, pp. 140–144, 2001.

[13] A. Kamoun and R. Lakhoua, "End-stage renal disease of the Tunisian child: epidemiology, etiologies, and outcome," *Pediatric Nephrology*, vol. 10, no. 4, pp. 479–482, 1996.

[14] A. Al-Eisa, M. Naseef, N. Al-Hamad, R. Pinto, N. Al-Shimeri, and M. Tahmaz, "Chronic renal failure in Kuwaiti children: an

eight-year experience," *Pediatric Nephrology*, vol. 20, no. 12, pp. 1781–1785, 2005.

[15] I. B. Mbarek, S. Abroug, A. Omezzine et al., "Selected *AGXT* gene mutations analysis provides a genetic diagnosis in28% of Tunisian patients with primary Hyperoxaluria," *BMC Nephrology*, vol. 12, article 25, 2011.

[16] T. Takayam, M. Nagata, I. Ichiyama, and S. Ozono, "Primary hyperoxaluria in Japan," *American Journal of Nephrology*, vol. 25, pp. 297–302, 2005.

[17] B. Hoppe and C. B. Langman, "A United States survey on diagnosis, treatment, and outcome of primary hyperoxaluria," *Pediatric Nephrology*, vol. 18, no. 10, pp. 986–991, 2003.

[18] V. O. Edvardsson, D. S. Goldfarb, J. C. Lieske et al., "Hereditary causes of kidney stones and chronic kidney disease," *Pediatric Nephrology*, vol. 28, no. 10, pp. 1923–1942, 2013.

[19] C. S. Van Woerden, J. W. Groothoff, F. A. Wijburg, C. Annink, R. J. A. Wanders, and H. R. Waterham, "Clinical implication of mutation analysis in primary hyperoxaluria type1," *Kidney International*, vol. 66, no. 2, pp. 746–752, 2004.

[20] C. G. Monico, S. Rossetti, H. A. Schwanz et al., "Comprehensive mutation screening in 55 probands with type 1 primary hyperoxaluria shows feasibility of a gene-based diagnosis," *Journal of the American Society of Nephrology*, vol. 18, no. 6, pp. 1905–1914, 2007.

[21] M. B. Coulter-Mackie, D. Applegarth, J. R. Toone, and H. Henderson, "The major allele of the alanine:glyoxylate aminotransferase gene: seven novel mutations causing primary hyperoxaluria type 1," *Molecular Genetics and Metabolism*, vol. 82, no. 1, pp. 64–68, 2004.

[22] M. B. Coulter-Mackie and G. Rumsby, "Genetic heterogeneity in primary hyperoxaluria type 1: impact on diagnosis," *Molecular Genetics and Metabolism*, vol. 83, no. 1-2, pp. 38–46, 2004.

[23] P. Cochat and G. Rumsby, "Primary hyperoxaluria," *The New England Journal of Medicine*, vol. 369, no. 7, pp. 649–658, 2013.

[24] C. G. Monico, S. Rossetti, J. B. Olson, and D. S. Milliner, "Pyridoxine effect in type I primary hyperoxaluria is associated with the most common mutant allele," *Kidney International*, vol. 67, no. 5, pp. 1704–1709, 2005.

[25] A. Amoroso, D. Pirulli, F. Florian et al., "AGXT gene mutations and their influence on clinical heterogeneity of type 1 primary hyperoxaluria," *Journal of the American Society of Nephrology*, vol. 12, no. 10, pp. 2072–2079, 2001.

[26] A. Amoroso, D. Pirulli, D. Puzzer et al., "Gene symbol: AGXT. Disease: primary hyperoxaluria type I," *Human Genetics*, vol. 104, no. 5, p. 441, 1999.

[27] B. Hoppe, C. J. Danpure, G. Rumsby et al., "A vertical (pseudodominant) pattern of inheritance in the autosomal recessive disease primary hyperoxaluria type 1: lack of relationship between genotype, enzymic phenotype, and disease severity," *American Journal of Kidney Diseases*, vol. 29, no. 1, pp. 36–44, 1997.

[28] E. Leumann and B. Hoppe, "Primary hyperoxaluria type 1: is genotyping clinically helpful?" *Pediatric Nephrology*, vol. 20, no. 5, pp. 555–557, 2005.

[29] P. Cochat and J. Groothoff, "Primary hyperoxaluria type 1: practical and ethical issues," *Pediatric Nephrology*, vol. 28, no. 12, pp. 2273–2281, 2013.

[30] N. V. Jamieson, "A 20-year experience of combined liver/kidney transplantation for primary hyperoxaluria (PH1): the European PH1 transplant registry experience 1984–2004," *The American Journal of Nephrology*, vol. 25, no. 3, pp. 282–289, 2005.

[31] D. M. Cibrik, B. Kaplan, J. A. Arndorfer, and H.-U. Meier-Kriesche, "Renal allograft survival in patients with oxalosis," *Transplantation*, vol. 74, no. 5, pp. 707–710, 2002.

15

Single Nucleotide Polymorphisms in Pediatric Idiopathic Nephrotic Syndrome

Maija Suvanto,[1] Timo Jahnukainen,[1] Marjo Kestilä,[2] and Hannu Jalanko[1]

[1]*Children's Hospital, University of Helsinki and Helsinki University Hospital, 00290 Helsinki, Finland*
[2]*Department of Chronic Disease Prevention, National Institute for Health and Welfare, 00271 Helsinki, Finland*

Correspondence should be addressed to Maija Suvanto; maija.suvanto@helsinki.fi

Academic Editor: Kazunari Kaneko

Polymorphic variants in several molecules involved in the glomerular function and drug metabolism have been implicated in the pathophysiology of pediatric idiopathic nephrotic syndrome (INS), but the results remain inconsistent. We analyzed the association of eleven allelic variants in eight genes *(angiopoietin-like 4 (ANGPTL4), glypican 5 (GPC5), interleukin-13 (IL-13), macrophage migration inhibitory factor (MIF), neural nitric oxide synthetase (nNOS), multidrug resistance-1 (MDR1), glucocorticoid-induced transcript-1 (GLCCI1), and nuclear receptor subfamily-3 (NR3C1))* in 100 INS patients followed up till adulthood. We genotyped variants using PCR and direct sequencing and evaluated estimated haplotypes of MDR1 variants. The analysis revealed few differences in SNP genotype frequencies between patients and controls, or in clinical parameters among the patients. Genotype distribution of MDR1 SNPs rs1236, rs2677, and rs3435 showed significant ($p < 0.05$) association with different medication regimes (glucocorticoids only versus glucocorticoids plus additional immunosuppressives). Some marginal association was detected between *ANGPTL4, GPC5, GLCCI1,* and *NR3C1* variants and different medication regimes, number of relapses, and age of onset. *Conclusion.* While *MDR1* variant genotype distribution associated with different medication regimes, the other analyzed gene variants showed only little or marginal clinical relevance in INS.

1. Introduction

Childhood-onset idiopathic nephrotic syndrome (INS) is a common kidney disease in children. It is characterized by minimal glomerular changes in light microscopy and podocyte foot process effacement in electron microscopy. The great majority (80–90%) of INS patients show good responsiveness to steroid treatment, but recurrent episodes occur in at least 70% of the patients. Development of renal failure occurs rarely.

The pathophysiology of INS is still unknown. During the past few years, polymorphic variants of several molecules involved in the glomerular function have been analyzed in INS patients and animal models of proteinuria to discover genetic components that would participate in the development of disease or modify its phenotype. These include angiopoietin-like 4 *(Angptl4)*, glycoprotein, which is upregulated in rats with steroid sensitive proteinuria [1, 2],

interleukin-13 *(IL-13)*, a cytokine that alters podocyte function and is reported to be upregulated in patients with active INS [3, 4], macrophage migration inhibitory factor *(MIF)*, a proinflammatory cytokine and counter regulator of the immunosuppressive effects of glucocorticoids [5, 6], glypican-5 gene *(GPC5)*, which encodes a podocyte cell surface proteoglycan whose variants are associated with a podocyte injury and proteinuria [7], and neural nitric oxide synthetase *(nNOS)* that plays a role in glomerular hyperpermeability [8].

In addition to the five functional molecules, there are reports on the association of INS with polymorphic variants of molecules involved in the glucocorticoid metabolism. These include multidrug resistance-1 gene *(MDR1)* encoding P-glycoprotein-170 (P-gp), which transports steroids across the cell membranes [9–12], nuclear receptor subfamily-3 gene *(NR3C1)* that encodes cytosolic glucocorticoid receptor (GR) [13, 14], and glucocorticoid-induced transcript 1 gene

TABLE 1: Primer sequences. T_m, annealing temperature.

Gene	SNP	Forward 5'-3'	Reverse 5'-3'	T_m (°C)
Angptl4	rs1044250 (c.797C>T)	CTACAAGGCGGGGTTTGGGGAT	AAGTGGAGAAGGGTACGGAGAGGCC	62
GPC5	rs16946160 (c.325+1026376G>A)	AGAGTTGACAAGAGTTAAACAGCA	GTCATCTCTGACTCCGCAGTAT	58
IL-13	rs848 (c.*526C>A)	GTTTGTCACCGTTGGGGATTGG	CAATGTCCCCTCCCCCAGTGTT	62
MIF	rs755622 (c.-270G>C)	CTAAGAAAGACCCGAGGCGA	GGCACGTTGGTGTTTACGAT	58
nNOS	rs2662826 (c.*276C>T)	ACTCCTTGAGTTTTCCTGCTGCGA	CCATGTTCCAGTGGTTTCATGCACCC	62
MDR1	rs1128503 (c.1236C>T)	TATCCTGTGTCTGTGAATTGCC	CTGACTCACCACACCAATG	62
	rs2032582 (c.2677G>T/A)	TGCAGGCTATAGGTTCCAGG	TTTAGTTTGACTCACCTTCCCG	60
	rs1045642 (c.3435C>T)	TGTTTTCAGCTGCTTGATGG	AAGGCATGTATGTTGGCCTC	58
GLCCI1	rs37972 (c.-1473T>C)	GACCCCTGCATATAGTGCCT	AATGAAACTGAAAGCGTACAAAGA	58
	rs37973 (c.-1106G>A)	AATTCCTTGTTGACCCCTGC	AGCTGAGTTTTCGTGACCAG	62
NR3C1	rs41423247 (c.1184+646C>G)	AAATTGAAGCTTAACAATTTTGGC	GCAGTGAACAGTGTACCAGACC	58

(*GLCCI1*) that encodes Glcci1 protein that associated with glucocorticoid (GC) responsiveness and development of proteinuria in animal models [15, 16].

In this study, we genotyped eleven single nucleotide polymorphisms (SNPs) from the above mentioned eight genes from DNA samples obtained from a unique cohort of INS patients followed up over 30 years. The results show that the variants in the genes coding for functional kidney proteins have little clinical relevance in INS while variants in genes involved in glucocorticoid metabolism show marginal association with INS. The genotype distribution of MDR1 SNPs shows significant association with medication regime as the minor alleles of the SNPs are more frequent in patients who receive immunosuppressive medication in addition to glucocorticoids.

2. Materials and Methods

2.1. Patients. The study cohort included 100 INS patients of whom 83 were diagnosed within 1965–1981 at the Hospital for Children and Adolescents, University of Helsinki. These 83 patients were enrolled in the International Study of Kidney Disease in Children (ISKDC) and were treated by protocols still used in pediatric nephrology. The mean age at the last follow-up was 35.0 years (range 25.1–44.1 years). Clinical data were carefully recorded from the patient records as was previously reported in detail [17]. The remaining 17 patients were diagnosed more recently at the Hospital for Children and Adolescents, University of Helsinki, and were still children or adolescents; of them SNP genotypes were used in statistical comparison between INS patients and controls. A blood sample for DNA extraction was gathered from all.

The controls included a cohort of 101 subjects who were either healthy adults or suffered from nonkidney related condition.

2.2. SNPs and PCR Analysis. We selected eleven SNPs from eight genes to this study based on previous reports in literature on their association with INS. The genes and SNPs were *Angptl4* SNP rs1044250 (c.797C>T), *GPC5* SNP rs16946160 (c.325+102637G>A), *IL-13* SNP rs848 (c.*526C>A), *MIF* rs755622 (c.-270G>C), *nNOS* rs2682826 (c.*276C>T), *MDR1* SNPs rs1128503 (c.1236C>T), rs2032582 (c.2677G>T/A), rs1045642 (c.3435C>T), *GLCCI1* SNPs rs37972 (c.-1473C>T), and rs37973 (c.-1106A>G) and *NR3C1* rs41423247 (c.1184+646G>C). Analysis was carried out using direct sequencing. Exons were amplified by PCR with flanking intronic primers, and the reactions were performed in total volumes of $25\,\mu$L as previously described [18]. Occasionally, the denaturation temperature was raised up to 98°C, or betaine was added to the reaction mixture. PCR products were genotyped using automated sequence analysis by BigDye-terminator chemistry (v.3.1) on Genetic Analyzer 3730 (Applied Biosystems). The sequences were analyzed with GeneComposer version 1.1.0.1051 (http://www.GeneComposer.com/). The genotypes were compared between patients and controls and among various clinical variables that include age of onset (<3 yr versus >3 yr), number of relapses (<5 versus >5), frequent relapses (no versus yes), response to GC (normal versus slow/no response), treatment (only GC versus GC together with immunosuppressive (IS) drugs), and GC dependence (no versus yes).

The genotypes of the three *MDR1* variants (rs1236, rs2677, and rs3435) were used to carry out a haplotype analysis. Twelve haplotypes were derived from the genotype data using the program PHASE (v2.1) [19, 20]. The estimated *MDR1* haplotype frequencies were compared between patients and controls and among various clinical variables.

All primers are presented in Table 1. Most of the primer sequences are gathered from literature: *Angptl4* rs1044250 [21], *IL-13* rs848 [4], *MIF* rs755622 [22], *nNOS* rs2682826 [8], *MDR1* rs1128503, rs2032582, rs1045642 [9], and *NR3C1* rs41423247 [23]. Primers for *GLCCI1* (NM_138426), rs37972 and rs37973, and *GPC5* (NM_004466) rs16946160 were designed using primer3 program (http://www.ncbi.nlm.nih.gov/tools/primer-blast/).

2.3. Statistics. The statistical analysis was carried out using statistical software JMP 10 (http://www.jmp.com/, SAS institute Inc., Cary, NC, USA). Logistic regression analysis was used to calculate odds ratios (OD) and 95% confidence intervals (CI) for the association between genotypes and the risk of INS. The difference between selected clinical variables and genotypes was determined by Fisher's exact test. Statistical significance was defined as $p < 0.05$.

2.4. Ethics. All patients or their parents were informed of the content of the study and they signed a form of consent. The Ethics Committee of the Children's Hospital, University of Helsinki, approved the study (IRB: HUS509/E7/05).

3. Results

Eleven SNPs from eight genes encoding proteins related to kidney function and steroid metabolism (*Angptl4*, *GPC5*, *MIF*, *nNOS*, *IL-13*, *MDR1*, and *NR3C1 GLCCl1*) were analyzed from 100 INS patients. The distribution of observed genotypes was consistent with those expected under the assumptions of the Hardy-Weinberg Equilibrium ($p \geq 0.05$) (Table 2).

Comparison of the frequencies of the 11 SNPs between INS patients and controls was made and is presented in Table 3. No association between variants and disease status was observed except in rs848 variant in *IL-13* gene, where heterozygotic genotype showed difference in frequency between patients and controls (53% versus 38%, OR 2.025, CI 1.095–3.785, and $p = 0.0243$).

Comparison of the SNP genotype frequencies among INS patients with various clinical parameters is presented in Tables 4 and 5. These variables included age of onset (<3 yr versus >3 yr), number of relapses (<5 versus >5), frequent relapses (no versus yes), response to GC (normal versus slow/no response), treatment (only GC versus GC together with immunosuppressive (IS) drugs), and GC dependence (no versus yes).

Few clinically relevant correlations were found in relation to the SNPs in genes *IL13*, *MIF*, and *nNOS*. *Angptl4* SNP rs1044250 allele C was more frequent in patients who received IS medication in addition to GCs compared to those who only received GCs (72 versus 56%, $p = 0.0228$). In *GPC5*, SNP rs16946160 A allele was more frequent in patients with disease onset less than three years of age than in those with disease onset more than three years of age (16 versus 5%, $p = 0.0421$).

The genotype distribution in *MDR1* SNPs showed difference in patients who received only GCs compared to those who also received IS medication as allele T frequency was higher in the latter group in rs1128503 (70.6 versus 28.6%, $p = 0.0012$), in rs2032582 (67.9 versus 42.9%, $p = 0.0028$) and in rs1045642 (73.1 versus, 52.4%, $p = 0.0092$). Similarly, in *GLCCI1* SNP rs37973 A allele was more frequent in patients who received IS medication (67 versus 50%, $p = 0.0387$). Patients with more than five relapses also had *GLCCI1* SNP rs37973 A allele more frequently than those with fewer relapses (70 versus 52%, $p = 0.0377$). A curious finding was that *NR3C1* SNP rs41423247 heterozygous GC genotype was more frequent in patients with more than five relapses

(68 versus 32.7%) and in patients with frequent relapses (60 versus 34%).

Haplotype analysis of the three MDR1 variants (rs1236, rs2677, and rs3435) revealed twelve estimated haplotypes among cases and controls. These data are presented in Table 6. Curiously, the patient samples were less varied, as the allele frequency of the two most common haplotypes, TTT and CGC, was 70% (42.2 and 27.5%, resp.) while in the control samples it took the four most common haplotypes, TTT, CGC, CTT, and TGT, to achieve the same (23.4, 18.6, 15.6 and 12.6%, resp.). Most of the haplotypes had $p < 0.05$. The distribution of the allele frequencies of the haplotypes among clinical variables showed no significant difference between groups with the exception of the comparison between patients with less than five relapses and patients with more than five relapses, as is seen in Table 6. In other variants, only TTT and CGC haplotypes had allele frequency higher than 10% in any of the variables and the combined allele frequency of these two varied between 71 and 86.7%.

4. Discussion

The discovery of causative or disease modifying genetic factors underlying INS is of great interest and could have a profound clinical impact. In this study, we genotyped eleven SNPs from eight genes that had previously been studied in relation to INS and proteinuric animal models. We compared the SNP frequencies in INS patients and controls as well as in the subgroups of INS patients. Very little alteration was detected in the distribution of SNPs between patients and controls, and only marginal differences were observed among the INS subgroups in the *Angptl4*, *GPC5*, *MDR1*, and *NR3C1* genes. An exception is the genotype distribution of *MDR1* SNPs in patients who receive GC medication and those who also receive IS as the T alleles are more frequent in the latter group. Summation of the findings of this study and a comparison to other recent studies can be found in Table 7.

Angptl4 is a secretory protein involved in lipid metabolism and its increased expression has been observed in podocytes and circulation in human and experimental INS [24, 25]. The genetic variant SNP rs1044250 in exon 6 leads to amino acid change p.T266M and the homozygous C genotype of this variant has been associated with lower plasma *Angptl4* levels [26]. Recently, Clement et al. [2] discovered that increases in circulating *Angptl4* reduced proteinuria but at the cost of inducing hypertriglyceridemia. In our analysis p.T266M genotype was not associated with the occurrence of INS disease or clinical severity of the disorder. However, the C allele was more frequent [72 versus 54%] in patients who received IS drug medication instead of GCs only.

Recently, Okamoto et al. [7] identified an association between variants of glypican-5 (*GPC5*) gene and acquired NS (focal segmental glomerulosclerosis, proteinuric IgA nephropathy) through a genome wide association study and replication analysis. They showed that glypican-5 is localized on podocyte cell surface membranes and that the risk genotype (AA) of the *GPC5* SNP rs16946160 was associated with higher expression. In our study, we observed an association

TABLE 2: The distribution of observed and expected genotypes. p values of 0.05 or above signal consistency with the assumptions of the Hardy-Weinberg Equilibrium.

Gene	SNP	Genotype	Patients				Controls			
			Observed	Expected	χ^2	p	Observed	Expected	χ^2	p
Angptl4	rs1044250 (c.797C>T)	CC	35	33.6	0.31	>0.05	30	22.3	0.14	>0.05
		CT	46	48.7			39	42.0		
		TT	19	17.6			15	19.7		
GPC5	rs16946160 (c.325+1026376G>A)	GG	88	88.4	0.41	>0.05	86	85.6	0.25	>0.05
		GA	12	11.3			14	14.7		
		AA	0	0.4			1	0.6		
IL13	rs848 (c.*526C>A)	CC	31	33.1	0.71	>0.05	45	40.6	3.63	>0.05
		CA	53	48.9			38	46.9		
		AA	16	18.1			18	13.6		
MIF	rs755622 (c.-270G>C)	GG	61	60.8	0.01	>0.05	63	59.5	3.88	$p = 0.05$
		GC	34	34.3			29	36.1		
		CC	5	4.8			9	5.5		
nNOS	rs2662826 (c.*276C>T)	CC	49	49.0	0.0	>0.05	52	48.8	2.38	>0.05
		CT	42	42.0			35	41.4		
		TT	9	9.0			12	8.8		
MDR1	rs1128503 (c.1236C>T)	CC	22	23.5	0.37	>0.05	23	21.1	0.58	>0.05
		CT	53	50.0			45	48.8		
		TT	25	26.5			30	28.1		
	rs2032582 (c.2677G>T/A)	GG	17	19.4	1.66	>0.05	24	23.5	0.36	>0.05
		GT	49	45.8			45	46.5		
		TT	26	27.0			24	23.0		
		TA	3	4.2			2	2.4		
		GA	5	3.5			3	2.4		
		AA	0	0.2			0	0.1		
	rs1045642 (c.3435C>T)	CC	13	14.1	0.21	>0.05	10	13.6	2.41	>0.05
		CT	49	46.9			53	45.8		
		TT	38	39.1			35	38.6		
GLCCI1	rs37972 (c.-1473T>C)	CC	35	35.4	0.03	>0.05	25	29.0	2.63	>0.05
		CT	49	48.2			56	48.1		
		TT	16	16.4			16	20.0		
	rs37973 (c.-1106G>A)	AA	33	33.6	0.07	>0.05	24	27.8	2.60	>0.05
		GA	50	48.7			52	44.4		
		GG	17	17.6			14	17.8		
NR3C1	rs41423247 (c.1184+646C>G)	GG	32	30.8	0.24	>0.05	37	34.2	1.53	>0.05
		GC	47	49.4			37	42.6		
		CC	21	19.8			16	13.2		

between rs16946160 A allele and early disease onset (16 versus 5%) but we did not find an association between this SNP and INS in general. It is, however, notable that none of our patients and only one of the controls carried the AA genotype. Okamoto et al. found the A allele frequency of controls to be 0.168 and dbSNP (http://www.ncbi.nlm.nih.gov/snp/) puts it at 0.161. In our study, it was only 0.08. Thus, it is possible that due to the frequency differences between populations the association between the risk genotype and INS is not visible in our patients.

Alasehirli et al. [8] found that, in *nNOS* gene polymorphism rs2682826, the TT genotype was associated with INS but not with GC responsiveness. NO attenuates many functions in the kidney and all forms of *NOS* are expressed in the kidney but the role of NO in renal disease is unclear. In our study, we did not find an association of rs2682826 genotypes with INS or with any clinical features of the disease.

Our results of the two cytokines, *IL-13* and *MIF*, whose genetic variants have been associated with NS, were also negative. While Wei et al. [4] reported that 3'UTR SNPs

TABLE 3: Comparison of patient and control genotype distribution. OR, odds ratio. CI, confidence interval. *p* values lower than 0.05 are marked with ∗.

Gene	SNP	Genotype	Patients (%)	Controls (%)	OR (95% CI)	*p*
			n = 100	*n* = 84		
		CC	35 (35)	30 (36)	Reference	
		CT	46 (46)	39 (46)	1.01 (0.53–1.93)	*0.974*
Angptl4	rs1044250 (c.797C>T)	TT	19 (19)	15 (18)	1.09 (0.47–2.53)	*0.847*
		C	116 (58)	99 (58.9)	Reference	
		T	84 (42)	69 (41.1)	1.04 (0.69–1.58)	*0.857*
			n = 100	*n* = 101		
		GG	88 (88)	86 (85)	Reference	
		GA	12 (12)	14 (14)	0.84 (0.36–1.92)	*0.674*
GPC5	rs16946160 (c.325+1026376G>A)	AA	0 (0)	1 (1)	6×10^{-7} (0–5.75)	*0.236*
		G	188 (94)	186 (92.1)	Reference	
		A	12 (6)	16 (7.9)	0.74 (0.34–1.60)	*0.449*
			n = 100	*n* = 101		
		CC	31 (31)	45 (45)	Reference	
		CA	53 (53)	38 (38)	2.03 (1.10–3.79)	**0.024**∗
IL13	rs848 (c.∗526C>A)	AA	16 (16)	18 (18)	1.29 (0.57–2.92)	*0.540*
		C	115 (57.5)	126 (63)	Reference	
		A	85 (42.5)	74 (37)	1.26 (0.84–1.89)	*0.261*
			n = 100	*n* = 101		
		GG	61 (61)	63 (62)	Reference	
		GC	34 (34)	29 (29)	1.21 (0.66–2.23)	*0.537*
MIF	rs755622 (c.-270G>C)	CC	5 (5)	9 (9)	0.57 (0.17–1.76)	*0.335*
		G	156 (78)	155 (76.7)	Reference	
		C	44 (22)	47 (23.3)	0.93 (0.58–1.49)	*0.761*
			n = 100	*n* = 99		
		CC	49 (49)	52 (53)	Reference	
		CT	42 (42)	35 (35)	1.27 (0.70–2.32)	*0.425*
nNOS	rs2662826 (c.∗276C>T)	TT	9 (9)	12 (12)	0.80 (0.30–2.05)	*0.636*
		C	140 (70)	139 (70.2)	Reference	
		T	60 (30)	59 (29.8)	1.01 (0.66–1.55)	*0.965*
			n = 100	*n* = 98		
		CC	22 (22)	23 (23)	Reference	
		CT	53 (53)	45 (46)	1.60 (0.82–3.19)	*0.169*
	rs1128503 (c.1236C>T)	TT	25 (25)	30 (31)	1.48 (0.68–3.29)	*0.328*
		C	97 (48.5)	91 (46.4)	Reference	
		T	103 (51.5)	105 (53.6)	0.92 (0.62–1.37)	*0.680*
			n = 100	*n* = 98		
		GG	17 (17)	24 (24)	Reference	
		GT	49 (49)	45 (45)	1.54 (0.74–3.26)	*0.253*
		TT	26 (26)	24 (24)	1.53 (0.67–3.55)	*0.316*
MDR1	rs2032582 (c.2677G>T/A)	TA	3 (3)	2 (2)	2.12 (0.32–17.42)	*0.432*
		GA	5 (5)	3 (3)	2.35 (0.51–12.75)	*0.274*
		G	88 (44)	96 (49)	Reference	
		T	104 (52)	95 (48.5)	1.19 (0.80–1.79)	*0.386*
		A	8 (4)	5 (2.6)	1.75 (0.56–5.96)	*0.338*
			n = 100	*n* = 98		
		CC	13 (13)	10 (10)	Reference	
		CT	49 (49)	53 (54)	0.711 (0.28–1.76)	*0.462*
	rs1045642 (c.3435C>T)	TT	38 (38)	35 (36)	0.84 (0.32–2.14)	*0.708*
		C	75 (37.5)	73 (37.2)	Reference	
		T	125 (62.5)	123 (62.8)	0.99 (0.66–1.49)	*0.958*

TABLE 3: Continued.

Gene	SNP	Genotype	Patients (%)	Controls (%)	OR (95% CI)	p
			$n = 100$	$n = 97$		
		CC	35 (35)	25 (26)	Reference	
		CT	49 (49)	56 (58)	0.63 (0.38–1.18)	0.149
	rs37972 (c.-1473T>C)	TT	16 (16)	16 (16)	0.71 (0.30–2.70)	0.444
		C	119 (59)	106 (54.6)	Reference	
		T	81 (41)	88 (45.4)	0.82 (0.55–1.22)	0.330
GLCCI1			$n = 100$	$n = 90$		
		AA	33 (33)	24 (27)	Reference	
		GA	50 (50)	52 (58)	0.70 (0.36–1.34)	0.282
	rs37973 (c.-1106G>A)	GG	17 (17)	14 (16)	0.88 (0.37–2.15)	0.782
		A	116 (58)	100 (55.6)		
		G	84 (42)	80 (44.4)	0.91 (0.60–1.36)	0.631
			$n = 100$	$n = 90$		
		GG	32 (32)	37 (41)	Reference	
		GC	47 (47)	37 (41)	1.47 (0.78–2.80)	0.238
NR3C1	rs41423247 (c.1184+646C>G)	CC	21 (21)	16 (18)	1.52 (0.68–3.43)	0.308
		G	111 (55.5)	111 (61.7)	Reference	
		C	89 (44.5)	69 (38.3)	1.29 (0.86–1.95)	0.223

of the *IL-13* gene correlate with long term outcome of INS, we did not see any association between the analyzed SNP and the number of relapses, response to medication, or any other feature. *MIF* is counterregulated by glucocorticoids and the rs755622 SNPs have been studied in association with NS. Vivarelli et al. [6] found that the frequency of C allele was higher in Italian patients than in controls and higher in steroid resistant NS (SRNS) than in steroid sensitive NS (SSNS). Similarly, Berdeli et al. [5] found that GC genotype and C allele were higher in patients than in controls and CC genotype was more frequent in patients with SRNS than in those with SSNS. On the other hand, Choi et al. [22] did not see this association in Korean patients. Similarly, our study did not reveal any association between rs755622 SNP and INS or any of the clinical parameters.

MDR-1 gene codes for a membranous P-gp, which is a multidrug transporter expressed in the proximal tubule cells. Certain SNPs in *MDR1* gene are believed to affect the expression of the gene or activity of the protein it codes. The common SNP rs1045642 in exon 26 has garnered a lot of attention. It is synonymously variant and it has been suggested that it is not causal itself but linked with another polymorphism or has an effect on DNA structure or RNA stability [12]. Of the other two common SNPs included in this study rs2032582 does lead to amino acid change, Ala899Ser/Thr. This change could possibly increase the drug resistance of the cell [27, 28]. The data on the significance of these SNPs from different studies are contradictory. The distribution of rs2032582 genotypes was found to be significantly different in healthy controls compared to patients in Indian and Egyptian populations [11, 12] while studies in Polish and Korean subjects did not find the association [9, 22].

We did not find any difference in the Finnish patients and controls in rs2032582 genotypes. Wasilewska et al. [9],

Jafar et al. [11], and Youssef et al. [12] found an association between rs1045642 and NS (allele T and genotype TT were higher in patients) while Choi et al. [22] did not. All the subjects in these studies come from different populations; thus it is possible that the difference in results is due to genetic heterogeneity among populations. Youssef et al. [12] compared rs1045642 allele frequencies in their Egyptian control subjects and found that the frequencies (C 66.4%, T 33.6%) were consistent with frequencies previously reported in African populations but different from frequencies found in Caucasian, Asian, and Indian populations [11, 29]. In our study, these frequencies were nearly the opposite (C 37.2%, T 62.8%) of those determined by Youssef et al. [12]. This may affect the association between rs1045642 genotypes and NS that was observed in Egyptian population but not in Finnish population. Also, in our study population, *MDR1* SNP rs1045642 CC genotype showed association with higher age of onset (20 versus 0%). Youssef et al. reported similar association for SNPS rs2032582 as well as rs1045642. Other studies did not show this association [9, 22].

In our study, all three *MDR1* SNPs showed association with treatment choices, T allele and TT genotype being more common in patients who needed IS drugs compared to those who were only medicated with GCs, which indicates that T and TT are associated with more complicated form of the disease. Surprisingly, only rs1045642 showed significant association between genotype distribution and GC responsiveness (T allele was more frequent in poor responders), although it must be noted that only ten of our patients were not responsive to GCs; this small cohort size may affect these results.

We carried out haplotype analysis of the three *MDR1* variants. In previous studies, Wasilewska et al. [9] reported significant association of haplotype frequencies with steroid

TABLE 4: Comparison of genotype and allele frequencies of functional kidney gene variants and selected clinical features. p values lower than 0.05 are marked with *.

Gene	SNP	Genotype	Relapses			Frequent relapser (%)			Age of onset (%)			Response to steroids			Treatment		
			<5 $n=52$	>5 $n=25$	p	No $n=41$	Yes $n=40$	p	<3 $n=16$	>3 $n=65$	p	Normal $n=67$	Slow/NR $n=13$	p	Only GC $n=42$	IS $n=39$	p
Angptl4	rs1044250 (c.797C>T)	CC	20 (38)	11 (44)	0.9426	14 (34)	18 (44)	0.4133	8 (50)	24 (37)	0.3311	25 (37)	6 (46)	0.8494	12 (29)	20 (51)	0.0679
		CT	25 (48)	11 (44)		19 (46)	18 (44)		6 (38)	31 (48)		32 (48)	5 (38)		21 (50)	16 (41)	
		TT	7 (13)	3 (12)		8 (20)	4 (10)		2 (13)	10 (15)		10 (15)	2 (15)		9 (21)	3 (8)	
		C	65 (62.5)	33 (66)	0.7230	47 (57)	54 (68)	0.1977	22 (69)	79 (61)	0.5416	82 (61)	17 (65)	0.8094	45 (54)	56 (72)	0.0228*
		T	39 (37.5)	17 (34)		35 (43)	26 (33)		10 (31)	51 (39)		52 (39)	9 (35)		39 (46)	22 (28)	
GPC5	rs16946160 (c.325+1026376G>A)	GG	47 (90)	20 (80)	0.2789	37 (90)	33 (83)	0.3493	11 (69)	59 (91)	0.0359*	58 (87)	11 (85)	1.000	38 (90)	32 (82)	0.3389
		GA	5 (10)	5 (20)		4 (10)	7 (18)		5 (31)	6 (9)		9 (13)	2 (15)		4 (10)	7 (18)	
		AA	0 (0)	0 (0)		0 (0)	0 (0)		0 (0)	0 (0)		0 (0)	0 (0)		0 (0)	0 (0)	
		G	99 (95)	45 (90)	0.2951	78 (95)	73 (91)	0.3663	27 (84)	124 (95)	0.0421*	125 (93)	24 (92)	0.6322	80 (95)	71 (91)	0.3567
		A	5 (5)	5 (10)		4 (5)	7 (9)		5 (16)	6 (5)		9 (7)	2 (8)		4 (5)	7 (9)	
IL13	rs848 (c.*526C>A)	CC	18 (35)	8 (32)	0.8456	10 (24)	16 (40)	0.3114	7 (44)	19 (29)	0.6420	24 (36)	2 (15)	0.3703	15 (36)	11 (28)	0.7568
		CA	25 (48)	14 (56)		24 (59)	19 (48)		7 (44)	35 (54)		33 (49)	9 (69)		21 (50)	21 (54)	
		AA	9 (17)	3 (12)		7 (17)	5 (13)		2 (13)	11 (17)		10 (15)	2 (15)		6 (14)	7 (18)	
		C	61 (59)	30 (60)	1.000	44 (54)	51 (64)	0.2056	21 (66)	73 (56)	0.4246	81 (60)	13 (50)	1.000	51 (61)	43 (55)	0.5253
		A	43 (41)	20 (40)		38 (46)	29 (36)		11 (34)	57 (44)		53 (40)	13 (50)		33 (39)	35 (45)	
MIF	rs755622 (c.-270G>C)	GG	31 (60)	16 (64)	1.000	26 (63)	24 (60)	0.9284	9 (56)	40 (62)	0.0634	40 (60)	8 (62)	1.000	25 (60)	24 (62)	0.7481
		GC	18 (35)	8 (32)		13 (32)	14 (35)		7 (44)	21 (32)		23 (34)	5 (38)		14 (33)	14 (36)	
		CC	3 (6)	1 (4)		2 (5)	2 (5)		0 (0)	4 (6)		4 (6)	0 (0)		3 (7)	1 (3)	
		G	80 (77)	40 (80)	0.8359	65 (79)	62 (78)	0.8497	25 (78)	101 (78)	1.000	103 (77)	21 (81)	1.000	64 (76)	62 (79)	0.7063
		C	24 (23)	10 (20)		17 (21)	18 (23)		7 (22)	29 (22)		31 (23)	5 (19)		20 (24)	16 (21)	
nNOS	rs2682826 (c.*276C>T)	CC	24 (46)	10 (4)	0.7393	19 (46)	17 (43)	0.2027	5 (31)	31 (48)	0.4080	29 (43)	7 (54)	0.6178	19 (45)	17 (44)	0.5406
		CT	23 (44)	11 (44)		20 (49)	16 (40)		8 (50)	28 (43)		31 (46)	4 (31)		20 (48)	16 (41)	
		TT	5 (10)	4 (16)		2 (5)	7 (18)		3 (19)	6 (9)		7 (10)	2 (15)		3 (7)	6 (15)	
		C	71 (68)	31 (62)	0.4702	58 (71)	50 (63)	0.4075	18 (56)	90 (69)	0.2089	89 (66)	18 (69)	0.458	58 (69)	50 (64)	0.5103
		T	33 (32)	19 (38)		24 (29)	30 (38)		14 (44)	40 (31)		45 (34)	8 (31)		26 (31)	28 (36)	

TABLE 5: Comparison of genotype and allele frequencies of glucocorticoid metabolism gene variants and selected clinical features. GC, glucocorticoid medication. NR, no response. IS, immunosuppressive drugs. p values lower than 0.05 are marked with *.

Gene	SNP	Genotype	Relapses			Frequent relapser (%)			Age of onset (%)			Response to GC			Treatment		
			<5 n=52	>5 n=25	p	No n=41	Yes n=40	p	<3 n=16	>3 n=65	p	Normal n=67	Slow/NR n=13	p	Only GCs n=42	IS n=39	p
	rs1128503 (c.1236C>T)	CC	12 (23)	4 (16)	0.2330	9 (22)	8 (20)	0.4526	1 (6)	16 (25)	0.2863	14 (21)	3 (23)	1.000	12 (29)	5 (17)	0.01*
		CT	29 (56)	11 (44)		23 (56)	18 (45)		10 (63)	31 (48)		34 (51)	6 (46)		24 (57)	7 (24)	
		TT	11 (21)	10 (40)		9 (22)	14 (35)		5 (31)	18 (28)		19 (28)	4 (31)		6 (14)	17 (59)	
		C	53 (51)	19 (38)	0.1678	41 (50)	34 (43)	0.3496	12 (38)	63 (48)	0.3240	62 (46)	12 (46)	0.0566	48 (57)	17 (29)	0.0012*
		T	51 (49)	31 (62)		41 (50)	46 (58)		20 (63)	67 (52)		72 (54)	14 (54)		36 (43)	41 (71)	
MDR1	rs2032582 (c.2677G>T/A)	GG	9 (17)	4 (16)	0.5655	6 (15)	7 (18.5)	0.3793	1 (6)	12 (18)	0.3311	12 (18)	1 (8)	0.4136	10 (24)	3 (8)	0.0067*
		GT	25 (48)	11 (44)		22 (54)	17 (43.5)		7 (44)	32 (49)		32 (48)	6 (46)		22 (53)	17 (44)	
		TT	13 (25)	10 (40)		9 (22)	15 (38.5)		7 (44)	17 (26)		20 (30)	4 (31)		6 (14)	18 (46)	
		TA	2 (4)	0 (0)		2 (5)	0 (0)		1 (6)	1 (2)		1 (1)	1 (8)		2 (5)	0 (0)	
		GA	3 (6)	0 (0)		2 (5)	1 (3.5)		0	3 (5)		2 (3)	1 (8)		2 (5)	1 (3)	
		G	46 (44)	19 (38)	0.1985	36 (44)	32 (40)	0.3448	9 (28)	59 (45)	0.1642	58 (43)	9 (35)	0.0529	44 (52)	24 (31)	0.0028*
		T	53 (51)	31 (62)		42 (51)	47 (59)		22 (69)	67 (52)		73 (54)	15 (58)		36 (43)	53 (68)	
		A	5 (6)	0 (0)		4 (5)	1 (1)		1 (3)	4 (3)		3 (3)	2 (8)		4 (5)	1 (1)	
	rs1045642 (c.3435C>T)	CC	9 (17)	4 (16)	1.000	8 (20)	5 (12)	0.4179	0 (0)	13 (20)	0.0315*	12 (18)	1 (8)	0.8447	10 (24)	3 (8)	0.0389*
		CT	23 (44)	11 (44)		19 (46)	16 (39)		11 (69)	24 (37)		28 (42)	6 (46)		20 (48)	15 (38)	
		TT	20 (38)	10 (40)		14 (34)	19 (46)		5 (31)	28 (43)		27 (40)	6 (46)		12 (29)	21 (54)	
		C	41 (39)	19 (38)	1.000	35 (43)	26 (33)	1.1977	11 (34)	50 (38)	0.8389	52 (39)	8 (31)	0.0113*	40 (48)	21 (27)	0.0092*
		T	63 (61)	31 (62)		47 (57)	54 (68)		21 (66)	80 (62)		82 (61)	18 (69)		44 (52)	57 (73)	
GLCCI1	rs37972 (c.-1473T>C)	CC	16 (31)	11 (44)	0.4931	13 (32)	15 (38)	0.8291	8 (50)	20 (31)	0.2289	24 (36)	4 (31)	1.000	11 (26)	17 (44)	0.2726
		CT	26 (50)	11 (44)		21 (51)	20 (50)		5 (31)	35 (54)		33 (49)	7 (54)		23 (55)	17 (44)	
		TT	10 (19)	3 (12)		7 (17)	5 (13)		3 (19)	10 (15)		10 (15)	2 (15)		8 (19)	5 (13)	
		C	58 (56)	33 (66)	0.2938	47 (57)	50 (63)	0.525	21 (66)	75 (58)	0.5473	81 (60)	15 (58)	1.000	45 (54)	51 (65)	0.1506
		T	46 (44)	17 (34)		35 (43)	30 (38)		11 (34)	55 (42)		53 (40)	11 (42)		39 (46)	27 (35)	
	rs37973 (c.-1106G>A)	AA	14 (27)	12 (48)	0.1197	12 (29)	15 (38)	0.6024	8 (50)	19 (29)	0.1861	22 (33)	5 (38)	0.8423	9 (21)	18 (46)	0.0623
		GA	26 (50)	11 (44)		21 (51)	20 (50)		5 (31)	35 (54)		33 (49)	7 (54)		24 (57)	16 (41)	
		GG	12 (23)	2 (8)		8 (20)	5 (13)		3 (19)	11 (17)		12 (18)	1 (8)		9 (21)	5 (13)	
		A	54 (52)	35 (70)	0.0377*	45 (55)	50 (63)	0.3427	21 (66)	73 (56)	0.4246	77 (57)	17 (65)	0.6321	42 (50)	52 (67)	0.0387*
		G	50 (48)	15 (30)		37 (45)	30 (38)		11 (34)	57 (44)		57 (43)	9 (35)		42 (50)	26 (33)	
NR3C1	rs41423247 (c.1184+646C>G)	GG	20 (38)	5 (20)	0.0173*	14 (34)	11 (28)	0.0442*	5 (31)	21 (32)	0.5928	23 (34)	2 (15)	0.2363	16 (38)	10 (26)	0.0655
		GC	17 (33)	17 (68)		14 (34)	24 (60)		6 (38)	31 (48)		31 (46)	6 (46)		14 (33)	23 (59)	
		CC	15 (29)	3 (12)		13 (32)	5 (13)		5 (31)	13 (20)		13 (19)	5 (38)		12 (29)	6 (15)	
		G	57 (55)	27 (54)	1.000	42 (51)	46 (58)	0.4352	16 (50)	73 (56)	0.5571	77 (57)	10 (38)	0.3479	46 (55)	43 (55)	1.000
		C	47 (45)	23 (46)		40 (49)	34 (43)		16 (50)	57 (44)		57 (43)	16 (62)		38 (45)	35 (45)	

TABLE 6: Comparison of haplotype distributions of the MDR1 loci in patients and controls as well as in patients with less than 5 relapses and patients with five or more relapses. Variants in order rs1128503, rs2032582, and rs1045642. p values lower than 0.05 are marked with *.

Haplotype	Patients ($n = 82$)		Controls ($n = 98$)		OR (95% CI)	p
	N	%	N	%		
CTC	69	42.2	46	23.4	0.42 (0.27–0.66)	**0.002**
TGT	45	27.5	36	18.6	0.60 (0.36–0.98)	**0.0412**
TTC	13	8.1	31	15.6	2.18 (1.10–4.33)	**0.0254**
CGC	7	4.5	25	12.6	3.28 (1.38–7.79)	**0.0072**
TGC	11	6.5	20	10.0	1.58 (0.73–3.40)	*0.242*
CGT	7	4.2	15	7.8	1.86 (0.74–4.67)	*0.1877*
TTT	2	1.3	15	7.7	6.71 (1.51–29.80)	**0.0123**
Other	9	5.7	8	4.3	0.73 (0.28–1.94)	*0.5425*
Haplotype	Relapses <5 ($n = 52$)		Relapses >5 ($n = 25$)		OR (95% CI)	p
	N	%	N	%		
CTC	42	40.6	28	55.3	1.88 (0.95–3.71)	**0.07**
TGT	32	30.4	16	31.4	1.06 (0.51–2.91)	*0.88*
TGC	10	9.5	1	2.4	0.19 (0.02–1.54)	*0.1205*
TTC	6	6.2	2	4.2	0.68 (0.13–3.50)	*0.64*
CGT	2	2.0	2	4.0	2.13 (0.29–15.54)	*0.4578*
CTT	3	3.2	1	2.6	0.69 (0.07–6.78)	*0.7479*
Other	8	8.1	0	0.0	0.11 (0.01–1.99)	*0.1359*

response time. Similar association was observed by Choi et al. [22] and Youssef et al. [12], although, interestingly, the major haplotype linked with this property varies between studies. Our study did not find this association and Cizmarikova et al. [30] reached similar conclusion. The two major haplotypes found in our study were TTT and CGC. These two were predominant in patient samples with combined allele frequency of 70%. The remaining 30% was distributed between eight other haplotypes, none of them reaching 10% frequency. In control patients TTT and CGC were also the most common haplotypes but the distribution was more diverse, as five haplotypes had higher than 10% frequency. Previous studies have also shown that TTT and CGC are prevalent haplotypes both in patients and in control subjects [9, 12, 22, 30]. Interestingly Choi et al. [22] and Youssef et al. [12] found haplotype TGC to have a frequency equal to TTT and CGC and have association to steroid responsiveness while Cizmarikova et al. [30] found the frequency of TGC to be under 3% in patients and in controls and have no association to any clinical attribute. Our results are similar to the latter study as TGC frequency reaches just 10% in control samples and 6.5% in patients. It is possible that the differences are caused by haplotype frequency differences between populations.

NR3C1 codes for glucocorticoid receptor (GR) that can affect the regulation of many biological functions, including responsiveness to GC, and its functional variability may play a role in the therapeutic response to GC. In this study, we analyzed NR3C1 SNP rs41423247 and curiously found that patients with more than five relapses carried more frequently heterozygous GC genotype than those with less than five relapses (68 versus 33%). The amount of both CC and GG homozygotes was diminished in these frequent relapsers. The allele distribution between groups with over and under five relapses showed no difference. In some previous studies, G allele (especially as a part of the intron B three-SNP haplotype) has been associated with increased GC sensitivity [31, 32] while others could not confirm the association [14]. It is still unclear how our findings fit in with these studies. Similar increased portion of heterozygous genotype was seen in patients with severe course of the disease compared to those with milder course (63 versus 34%).

An interesting new gene in the context of INS is GLCCI1. Tantisira et al. [33] first showed that SNPs rs37973 and rs37972, which are in linkage disequilibrium, associated with poor responsiveness to GCs in asthmatic patients. Soon afterwards, Nishibori et al. [15] showed that Glcci1-protein is highly expressed in glomerular podocytes and its deficiency leads to proteinuria. Based on these findings, Cheong et al. [16] looked to see if these SNPs were playing a role in GC responsiveness in NS but could find no association. Similarly our results show no direct association between the alleles and/or genotypes of either SNP or GC responsiveness. However, while rs37972 showed no significant association with any clinical feature, the frequency of the rs37973 A allele was higher in patients with more than five relapses (70 versus 52%) and in patients who received IS drugs compared to those who received only GC medication (67 versus 50%). To our knowledge this association has not been looked into in other studies.

TABLE 7: Comparison between the found associations of the analyzed SNPs in this study and in previous studies.

Gene	Found association	Current study	Referenced study
GPC5	*rs16946160 (c.325+1026376G>A)*		
	Association of AA genotype with NS	No	Yes [7]
	Association of A allele with disease onset	Yes	
	A allele frequency	0,168	0,08 [7]
IL13	*rs848 (c.*526C>A)*		
	Association of genotype distribution with long term outcome	No	Yes [4]
MIF	*rs755622 (c.-270G>C)*		
	Association of C allele and/or GC genotype with NS	No	Yes [5], yes [6], no [22]
	Association of CC genotype with GC resistance	No	Yes [5], yes [6], no [22]
nNOS	*rs2662826 (c.*276C>T)*		
	Association of TT genotype with NS	No	Yes [8]
	Association of TT genotype with GC responsiveness	No	No [8]
MDR1	*rs1128503 (c.1236C>T)*		
	Association of T allele and/or TT genotypes with IS medication need	Yes	
	rs2032582 (c.2677G>T/A)		
	Association of genotype distribution with NS	No	No [9], yes [11], yes [12], no [22]
	Association of CC genotype with age of onset	No	No [9], no [11], yes [12], no [22]
	Association of T allele and/or TT genotype with GC responsiveness	Yes	
	Association of T allele and/or TT genotypes with IS medication need	Yes	
	rs1045642 (c.3435C>T)		
	Association of T allele and/or TT genotype with NS	No	Yes [9], yes [11], yes [12], no [22]
	Allele frequencies of controls (C/T, %)	37.2/62.8	45,2/54,8 [9], 66.4/33.6 [11], 58.5/41.5 [12], 42.0/58.0 [22], 42.4/57.6 [30]
	Association of CC genotype with age of onset	Yes	No [9], no [11], yes [12], no [22]
	Association of T allele and/or TT genotypes with IS medication need	Yes	
	Haplo type		
	Association with GC responsiveness	No	Yes [9], yes [12], yes [22], no [30]
	Frequency of TGC haplotype (case/control, %)	6.5.2010	1.1* [9], 8.3/6.5 [11], 21,7/18.6 [12], 21.2/18 [22], 1.1/2.3 [30]
GLCCI1	*rs37972 (c.-1473T>C)*		
	Association of genotype distribution with GC responsiveness	No	No [16]
	rs37973 (c.-1106G>A)		
	Association of genotype distribution with GC responsiveness	No	No [16]
	Association of A allele with patients with more than five relapses	Yes	
	Association of A allele with IS medication need	Yes	

*Only control.

5. Conclusion

The studied genetic variants have little role in the course of NS in Finnish patients. A notable exception to this is MDR1 SNPs whose genotype and allele distribution show significant association to different medication regimes. The genetic background to GC sensitivity is very heterogenic and varies between ethnic groups, which may have to be considered when drawing up treatment strategies for individual patients. More work needs to be done to discover other contributing molecules before the genetics of steroid responsiveness in NS can be understood.

References

[1] L. C. Clement, C. Avila-Casado, C. Macé et al., "Podocyte-secreted angiopoietin-like-4 mediates proteinuria in glucocorticoid-sensitive nephrotic syndrome," *Nature Medicine*, vol. 17, no. 1, pp. 117–122, 2011.

[2] L. C. Clement, C. Macé, C. Avila-Casado, J. A. Joles, S. Kersten, and S. S. Chugh, "Circulating angiopoietin-like 4 links proteinuria with hypertriglyceridemia in nephrotic syndrome," *Nature Medicine*, vol. 20, no. 1, pp. 37–46, 2014.

[3] B. Acharya, T. Shirakawa, A. Pungky et al., "Polymorphism of the interleukin-4, interleukin-13, and signal transducer and activator of transcription 6 genes in Indonesian children with minimal change nephrotic syndrome," *American Journal of Nephrology*, vol. 25, no. 1, pp. 30–35, 2005.

[4] C.-L. Wei, W. Cheung, C.-K. Heng et al., "Interleukin-13 genetic polymorphisms in Singapore Chinese children correlate with long-term outcome of minimal-change disease," *Nephrology Dialysis Transplantation*, vol. 20, no. 4, pp. 728–734, 2005.

[5] A. Berdeli, S. Mir, N. Ozkayin, E. Serdaroglu, Y. Tabel, and A. Cura, "Association of macrophage migration inhibitory factor -173C allele polymorphism with steroid resistance in children with nephrotic syndrome," *Pediatric Nephrology*, vol. 20, no. 11, pp. 1566–1571, 2005.

[6] M. Vivarelli, L. E. D'Urbano, G. Stringini et al., "Association of the macrophage migration inhibitory factor -173*C allele with childhood nephrotic syndrome," *Pediatric Nephrology*, vol. 23, no. 5, pp. 743–748, 2008.

[7] K. Okamoto, K. Tokunaga, K. Doi et al., "Common variation in GPC5 is associated with acquired nephrotic syndrome," *Nature Genetics*, vol. 43, no. 5, pp. 459–463, 2011.

[8] B. Alasehirli, A. Balat, O. Barlas, and A. Kont, "Nitric oxide synthase gene polymorphisms in children with minimal change nephrotic syndrome," *Pediatrics International*, vol. 51, no. 1, pp. 75–78, 2009.

[9] A. Wasilewska, G. Zalewski, L. Chyczewski, and W. Zoch-Zwierz, "MDR-1 gene polymorphisms and clinical course of steroid-responsive nephrotic syndrome in children," *Pediatric Nephrology*, vol. 22, no. 1, pp. 44–51, 2007.

[10] S. Funaki, S. Takahashi, N. Wada, H. Murakami, and K. Harada, "Multiple drug-resistant gene 1 in children with steroid-sensitive nephrotic syndrome," *Pediatrics International*, vol. 50, no. 2, pp. 159–161, 2008.

[11] T. Jafar, N. Prasad, V. Agarwal et al., "MDR-1 gene polymorphisms in steroid-responsive versus steroid-resistant nephrotic syndrome in children," *Nephrology Dialysis Transplantation*, vol. 26, no. 12, pp. 3968–3974, 2011.

[12] D. M. Youssef, T. A. Attia, A. S. El-Shal, and F. A. Abduelometty, "Multi-drug resistance-1 gene polymorphisms in nephrotic syndrome: impact on susceptibility and response to steroids," *Gene*, vol. 530, no. 2, pp. 201–207, 2013.

[13] J. Ye, Z. Yu, J. Ding et al., "Genetic variations of the NR3C1 gene in children with sporadic nephrotic syndrome," *Biochemical and Biophysical Research Communications*, vol. 348, no. 2, pp. 507–513, 2006.

[14] N. Teeninga, J. E. Kist-van Holthe, E. L. T. van den Akker et al., "Genetic and in vivo determinants of glucocorticoid sensitivity in relation to clinical outcome of childhood nephrotic syndrome," *Kidney International*, vol. 85, no. 6, pp. 1444–1453, 2014.

[15] Y. Nishibori, K. Katayama, M. Parikka et al., "Glcci1 deficiency leads to proteinuria," *Journal of the American Society of Nephrology*, vol. 22, no. 11, pp. 2037–2046, 2011.

[16] H. I. Cheong, H. G. Kang, and J. Schlondorff, "GLCCI1 single nucleotide polymorphisms in pediatric nephrotic syndrome," *Pediatric Nephrology*, vol. 27, no. 9, pp. 1595–1599, 2012.

[17] A.-T. Lahdenkari, M. Suvanto, E. Kajantie, O. Koskimies, M. Kestilä, and H. Jalanko, "Clinical features and outcome of childhood minimal change nephrotic syndrome: is genetics involved?" *Pediatric Nephrology*, vol. 20, no. 8, pp. 1073–1080, 2005.

[18] U. Lenkkeri, M. Männikkö, P. McCready et al., "Structure of the gene for congenital nephrotic syndrome of the finnish type (NPHS1) and characterization of mutations," *The American Journal of Human Genetics*, vol. 64, no. 1, pp. 51–61, 1999.

[19] M. Stephens, N. J. Smith, and P. Donnelly, "A new statistical method for haplotype reconstruction from population data," *American Journal of Human Genetics*, vol. 68, no. 4, pp. 978–989, 2001.

[20] M. Stephens and P. Scheet, "Accounting for decay of linkage disequilibrium in haplotype inference and missing-data imputation," *American Journal of Human Genetics*, vol. 76, no. 3, pp. 449–462, 2005.

[21] N. E. Buroker, X.-H. Ning, Z.-N. Zhou et al., "AKT3, ANGPTL4, eNOS3, and VEGFA associations with high altitude sickness in Han and Tibetan Chinese at the Qinghai-Tibetan plateau," *International Journal of Hematology*, vol. 96, no. 2, pp. 200–213, 2012.

[22] H. J. Choi, H. Y. Cho, H. Ro et al., "Polymorphisms of the MDR1 and MIF genes in children with nephrotic syndrome," *Pediatric Nephrology*, vol. 26, no. 11, pp. 1981–1988, 2011.

[23] I. Fleury, P. Beaulieu, M. Primeau, D. Labuda, D. Sinnett, and M. Krajinovic, "Characterization of the BclI polymorphism in the glucocorticoid receptor gene," *Clinical Chemistry*, vol. 49, no. 9, pp. 1528–1531, 2003.

[24] K. Yoshida, T. Shimizugawa, M. Ono, and H. Furukawa, "Angiopoietin-like protein 4 is a potent hyperlipidemia-inducing factor in mice and inhibitor of lipoprotein lipase," *Journal of Lipid Research*, vol. 43, no. 11, pp. 1770–1772, 2002.

[25] S. S. Chugh, L. C. Clement, and C. Macé, "New insights into human minimal change disease: lessons from animal models," *American Journal of Kidney Diseases*, vol. 59, no. 2, pp. 284–292, 2012.

[26] M. C. Smart-Halajko, M. R. Robciuc, J. A. Cooper et al., "The relationship between plasma angiopoietin-like protein 4 levels, angiopoietin-like protein 4 genotype, and coronary heart disease risk," *Arteriosclerosis, Thrombosis, and Vascular Biology*, vol. 30, no. 11, pp. 2277–2282, 2010.

[27] R. B. Kim, B. F. Leake, E. F. Choo et al., "Identification of functionally variant MDR1 alleles among European Americans and African Americans," *Clinical Pharmacology and Therapeutics*, vol. 70, no. 2, pp. 189–199, 2001.

[28] D. Anglicheau, M. Flamant, M. H. Schlageter et al., "Pharmacokinetic interaction between corticosteroids and tacrolimus after renal transplantation," *Nephrology Dialysis Transplantation*, vol. 18, no. 11, pp. 2409–2414, 2003.

[29] M.-M. Ameyaw, F. Regateiro, T. Li et al., "MDR1 pharmacogenetics: frequency of the C3435T mutation in exon 26 is significantly influenced by ethnicity," *Pharmacogenetics*, vol. 11, no. 3, pp. 217–221, 2001.

[30] M. Cizmarikova, L. Podracka, L. Klimcakova et al., "MDR1 polymorphisms and idiopathic nephrotic syndrome in Slovak children: preliminary results," *Medical Science Monitor*, vol. 21, pp. 59S–68S, 2015.

16

Causes for Withdrawal in an Urban Peritoneal Dialysis Program

Biruh Workeneh,[1] **Danielle Guffey,**[2] **Charles G. Minard,**[2] **and William E. Mitch**[1]

[1]*Division of Nephrology, Baylor College of Medicine, Houston, TX 77030, USA*
[2]*Dan L. Duncan Institute for Clinical & Translational Research, Baylor College of Medicine, Houston, TX 77030, USA*

Correspondence should be addressed to Biruh Workeneh; bworkene@bcm.edu

Academic Editor: Francesca Mallamaci

Background. Peritoneal dialysis (PD) is an underutilized dialysis modality in the United States, especially in urban areas with diverse patient populations. Technique retention is a major concern of dialysis providers and might influence their approach to patients ready to begin dialysis therapy. *Methods.* Records from January 2009 to March 2014 were abstracted for demographic information, technique duration, and the reasons for withdrawal. *Results.* The median technique survival of the 128 incident patients during the study window was 781 days (2.1 years). The principle reasons for PD withdrawal were repeated peritonitis (30%); catheter dysfunction (18%); ultrafiltration failure (16%); patient choice or lack of support (16%); or hernia, leak, or other surgical complications (6%); and a total of 6 patients died during this period. Of the patients who did not expire and were not transplanted, most transferred to in-center hemodialysis and 8% transitioned to home-hemodialysis. *Conclusions.* Our findings suggest measures to ensure proper catheter placement and limiting infectious complications should be primary areas of focus in order to promote technique retention. Lastly, more focused education about home-hemodialysis as an option may allow those on PD who are beginning to demonstrate signs of technique failure to stay on home therapy.

1. Introduction

Peritoneal dialysis (PD) is an underutilized dialysis modality in the United States, especially in urban centers with diverse patient populations. Overall, excluding patients who may have difficulty performing the procedure (e.g., stroke, poor vision, and previous abdominal surgery), as many as 85% of stage 5 chronic kidney disease (CKD) patients are medically eligible for peritoneal dialysis [1]. However, patients on PD comprise only 10% of the entire end-stage renal disease (ESRD) population and the percentage of African-American and Hispanic ESRD patients treated with peritoneal dialysis has been consistently lower than that of White dialysis patients [2]. Surveys show that only two-thirds of ESRD patients beginning maintenance dialysis are presented with peritoneal dialysis as an option. African-Americans comprise 37% of the ESRD population but comprise only 25% of the patients receiving PD. Hispanic patients comprise 17% of

the total ESRD population but only 13% of PD patients [3]. The reasons for this disparity are complex and are the subject of ongoing study.

Several studies have identified the physician's role in dialysis choice; however physician bias is difficult to gauge [4, 5]. One reason that is clear from the data is that if the physician does not believe that patients have sufficient family or social support then they are referred to PD at significantly lower rates [6]. This suggests that the physician's assessment of the probability of technique retention is a major factor in encouraging one modality over another, and presumably this disproportionately affects patients who are resource-poor in urban settings.

When technique failure does occur in PD, it does so at a rate over 40% in the first year [7]. Unfortunately, there have been only a handful of dated reports that have examined this issue in-depth. Previous reports suggest that age, gender, comorbid diabetes, and low socioeconomic factors are independently associated with technique failure [8, 9]. We sought to examine technique survival and the particular reasons for PD withdrawal among incident patients in an urban, racially diverse practice setting near downtown Houston, Texas.

2. Methods

Approval from the Human Subjects IRB at Baylor College of Medicine and authorization from the dialysis center (Satellite Health/Wellbound of Houston) were obtained prior to the conduct of this study. Records of all adult patients from January 2009 (when the unit began to recruit patients) to March 2014 were abstracted for demographic information, technique duration, and the reasons for withdrawal. Patients were classified as African-American, Hispanic-Latino, White, Asian, and Native American based on what was indicated on Center for Medicare and Medicaid Services (CMS) reporting forms. ESRD diagnosis was also abstracted from reporting forms. Catheter malfunction, peritonitis, and exit site infection were assessed as well as kidney transplantation. Technique failure was defined as discontinuation of PD for more than 6 weeks, but this did not include patients who were transplanted or recovered renal function.

Patient characteristics are summarized using mean and standard deviation or frequency and percentage. Patients who expired, were transplanted or recovered kidney function were censored in the analysis and all others were considered as treatment failure (events). Kaplan-Meier plots were generated to indicate time to treatment failure, log-rank test was used to compare time to event between groups, and Cox proportional hazards regression was used to evaluate associations between age, race, and gender with risk of treatment failure. Death and transplant were explored as competing risks but did not change the results and were not included in the analysis.

3. Results

There were 128 incident ESRD patients included in the study and their characteristics are listed in Table 1 and the reasons for PD withdrawal in Figure 1. The principle reasons for PD withdrawal were repeated peritonitis (30%); catheter dysfunction (18%); ultrafiltration failure (16%); patient choice or lack of support (16%); or hernia, leak, or other surgical complications (6%); and a total of 6 patients died during this period. Of the patients who did not expire and were not transplanted, 51% transferred to in-center hemodialysis and 8% to home-hemodialysis at the same center. Not included in the calculation were 12 patients (17% of discharges) who were transplanted and 8 patients (12% of discharges) who changed PD units.

The median technique survival was 781 days (2.1 years) during the study window. Figure 2 shows the aggregate Kaplan-Meier time to technique failure among all the patients analyzed. Of the 128 patients, a total of 54 patients were classified as technique failure (excluding transplant, renal recovery, and death) during the study window and the mean

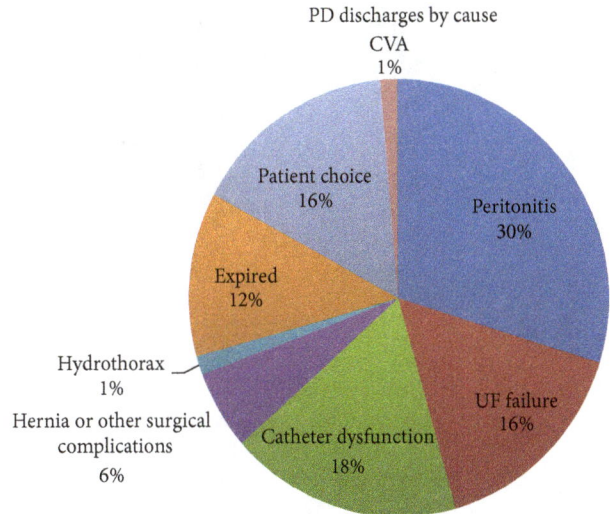

FIGURE 1

TABLE 1: Description of subjects.

All patients	$N = 128$
Age, mean (SD)	52.0 (13.4)
BMI, mean (SD)	28.0 (5.9)
Race, N (%)	
African-American	54 (42%)
Asian	7 (5%)
Hispanic-Latino	53 (41%)
Native American	1 (1%)
White	13 (10%)
Male, N (%)	81 (63%)
Diagnosis, N (%)	
Failed transplant	2 (2%)
GN	13 (10%)
HIVAN	3 (2%)
HTN	39 (30%)
Nephrotoxicity	1 (1%)
Obstructive nephropathy	2 (2%)
PCKD	2 (2%)
RCC nephrectomy	1 (1%)
Type 1 DM	4 (3%)
Type 2 DM	54 (42%)
Unknown	7 (5%)

length of technique survival in this group who withdrew from PD was 344 days.

Several factors that may have influenced technique survival were examined. Gender was not associated with time to technique failure ($p = 0.951$). Race is not associated with time to technique failure ($p = 0.548$) when race has 5 categories (African-American, Asian, Hispanic, Native American, and White). When grouping Asian and Native American together race still was not associated with time to technique failure ($p = 0.7233$) (Figure 3). Categories of age by quartiles were not associated with technique failure

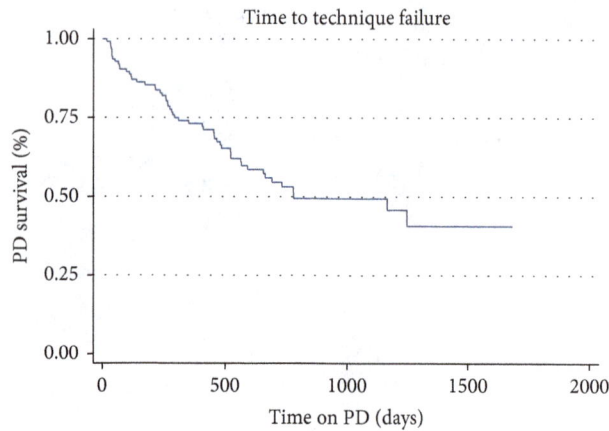

FIGURE 2

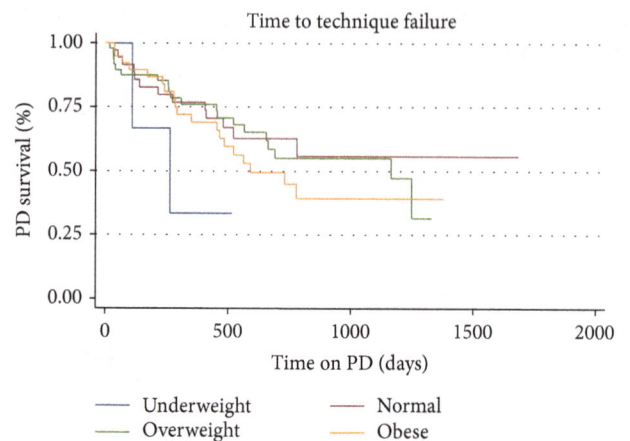

FIGURE 4

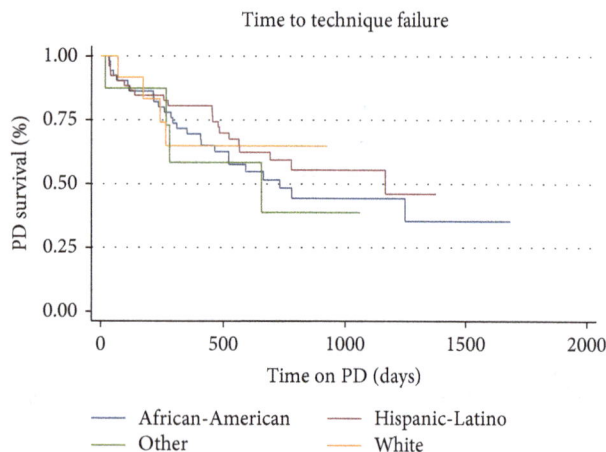

FIGURE 3

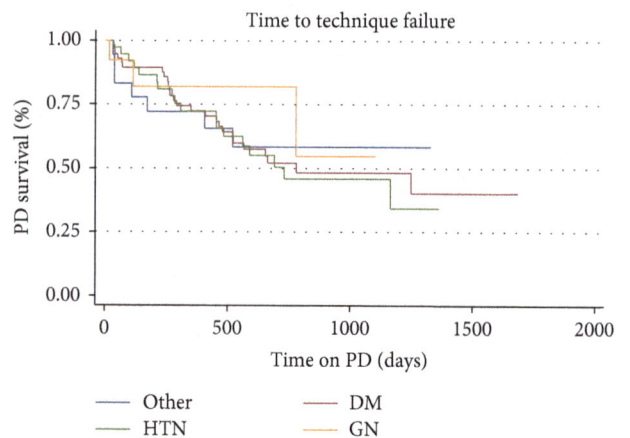

FIGURE 5

($p = 0.904$). BMI by quartiles was also not associated with time to technique failure ($p = 0.974$). When BMI was defined by weight categories (underweight: BMI < 18.5; normal: 18.5–25; overweight: 25–30; obese: >30), it was also not associated with time to technique failure ($p = 0.3794$) (Figure 4). When limited to 3 major categories and "other," there was no significant difference in survival by cause of ESRD ($p = 0.885$) (Figure 5). From the Cox proportional hazards model individual or combined, none of the variables examined were significantly associated with hazard of technique failure.

4. Discussion

In our analysis, peritonitis is the primary cause of transfer from PD, and we acknowledge that although peritonitis is a leading precipitating event for transfer, we speculate that the genuine reason may be patient burn-out, noncompliance, inadequate dialysis, a request based on lifestyle, or a persistent exit site infection. Although our sample size may be too small to make definitive conclusions, factors such as gender, BMI, and ESRD diagnosis did not make a difference in technique survival and African-American and Hispanic patients compare favorably to other groups.

The merits of peritoneal dialysis are apparent, including safety, cost, and quality of life. There are no differences in peritoneal transport characteristics and likelihood of achieving adequacy among varying racial groups [10]. Furthermore, technique survival and the reasons for technique failure are not appreciably different in this population comprised of mostly African-American and Hispanic patients in prior surveys that have been performed [11]. A report by Korbet et al. and Tanna et al. found that PD may be associated with better long-term patient survival in African-Americans [12, 13]. Still other studies found that sociodemographic factors, such as fewer years of education, employment, and US minority status, are associated with lower technique survival [14]. More updated studies with more rigorous methodologies outcomes are needed.

An analysis by DePasquale et al. suggests that there may be differences in the way patients and families of different backgrounds make informed treatment choices, and a better understanding of these differences can help dialysis providers more effectively facilitate decisions related to dialysis choice [15]. In light of the present study and the ones that have been reported previously PD as technique should be supported in all eligible populations.

This study does have its limitations including a relatively small sample size and lack of "exit" surveys in the methodology, which may have enhanced understanding of the results. A regional analysis of incident and prevalent patients in urban PD programs that have a critical mass of patients and that collected center specific data (e.g., physician, nursing experience, etc.) would be an ideal design.

5. Conclusions

Our findings suggest that there are a number of causes of PD failure and measures to limit peritonitis should be a primary focus in order to promote technique retention. Other measures such as ensuring patient support to avoid burn-out and coordinating with surgeons to ensure proper catheter function and limiting surgical complications may also contribute to technique retention. More focused education about home-hemodialysis as an option, 8% in our analysis, may present an opportunity for those on PD who are beginning to demonstrate signs of technique failure to stay on home therapy. Lastly, concentrated efforts to educate and offer peritoneal dialysis to Hispanic and African-American could result in a higher proportion choosing PD as a treatment option.

References

[1] M. B. Rivara and R. Mehrotra, "The changing landscape of home dialysis in the United States," *Current Opinion in Nephrology and Hypertension*, vol. 23, no. 6, pp. 586–591, 2014.

[2] F. Martino, Z. Adibelli, G. Mason et al., "Home visit program improves technique survival in peritoneal dialysis," *Blood Purification*, vol. 37, no. 4, pp. 286–290, 2014.

[3] U.S. Renal Data System, *USRDS 2013 Annual Data Report: Atlas of Chronic Kidney Disease and End Stage Renal Disease in the United States*, National Institutes of Health, National Institute of Diabetes and Digestive and Kidney Diseases, Bethesda, Md, USA, 2013.

[4] J. Little, A. Irwin, T. Marshall, H. Rayner, and S. Smith, "Predicting a patient's choice of dialysis modality: experience in a United Kingdom renal department," *American Journal of Kidney Diseases*, vol. 37, no. 5, pp. 981–986, 2001.

[5] D. C. Mendelssohn, S. R. Mullaney, B. Jung, P. G. Blake, and R. L. Mehta, "What do American nephrologists think about dialysis modality selection?" *American Journal of Kidney Diseases*, vol. 37, no. 1, pp. 22–29, 2001.

[6] K. J. Jager, J. C. Korevaar, F. W. Dekker, R. T. Krediet, E. W. Boeschoten, and NECOSAD Study Group, "The effect of contraindications and patient preference on dialysis modality selection in ESRD patients in the Netherlands," *American Journal of Kidney Diseases*, vol. 43, no. 5, pp. 891–899, 2004.

[7] M. Chidambaram, J. M. Bargman, R. R. Quinn, P. C. Austin, J. E. Hux, and A. Laupacis, "Patient and physician predictors of peritoneal dialysis technique failure: a population based,

retrospective cohort study," *Peritoneal Dialysis International*, vol. 31, no. 5, pp. 565–573, 2011.

[8] J. Pulliam, N.-C. Li, F. Maddux, R. Hakim, F. O. Finkelstein, and E. Lacson Jr., "First-year outcomes of incident peritoneal dialysis patients in the United States," *American Journal of Kidney Diseases*, vol. 64, no. 5, pp. 761–769, 2014.

[9] U. Joshi, Q. Guo, C. Yi et al., "Clinical outcomes in elderly patients on chronicperitoneal dialysis: a retrospective study from a single center in China," *Peritoneal Dialysis International*, vol. 34, no. 3, pp. 299–307, 2014.

[10] P. H. Juergensen, N. Gorban-Brennan, L. Troidle, and F. O. Finkelstein, "Racial differences and peritonitis in an urban peritoneal dialysis center," *Advances in Peritoneal Dialysis*, vol. 18, pp. 117–118, 2002.

[11] D. S. C. Raj, J. Roscoe, A. Manuel, K. Abreo, S. S. Dominic, and J. Work, "Is peritoneal dialysis a good option for black patients?" *American Journal of Kidney Diseases*, vol. 33, no. 2, pp. 325–333, 1999.

[12] S. M. Korbet, D. Shih, K. N. Cline, and E. F. Vonesh, "Racial differences in survival in an urban peritoneal dialysis program," *American Journal of Kidney Diseases*, vol. 34, no. 4, pp. 713–720, 1999.

[13] M. M. Tanna, E. F. Vonesh, and S. M. Korbet, "Patient survival among incident peritoneal dialysis and hemodialysis patients in an urban setting," *The American Journal of Kidney Diseases*, vol. 36, no. 6, pp. 1175–1182, 2000.

[14] J. I. Shen, A. A. Mitani, A. B. Saxena, B. A. Goldstein, and W. C. Winkelmayer, "Determinants of peritoneal dialysis technique failure in incident us patients," *Peritoneal Dialysis International*, vol. 33, no. 2, pp. 155–166, 2013.

[15] N. DePasquale, P. L. Ephraim, J. Ameling et al., "Selecting renal replacement therapies: what do African American and non-African American patients and their families think others should know? A mixed methods study," *BMC Nephrology*, vol. 14, article 9, 2013.

17

Mortality and Recovery of Renal Function in Acute Kidney Injury Patients Treated with Prolonged Intermittent Hemodialysis Sessions Lasting 10 versus 6 Hours: Results of a Randomized Clinical Trial

Bianca Ballarin Albino ⓘ,[1] **Mariele Gobo-Oliveira,**[1]
André Luís Balbi ⓘ,[1] **and Daniela Ponce** ⓘ[1,2]

[1]*Botucatu School of Medicine, University of São Paulo State (UNESP), Brazil*
[2]*Course of Medicine, University of São Paulo (USP), Bauru, Brazil*

Correspondence should be addressed to Daniela Ponce; dponce@fmb.unesp.br

Academic Editor: Laszlo Rosivall

Purpose. This trial aimed to compare mortality and recovery of renal function in acute kidney injury (AKI) patients treated with different durations of prolonged hemodialysis (PHD) sessions (6 h versus 10 h). *Methodology*. We included patients with sepsis-associated AKI, >18 years, who are in use of a norepinephrine (lower than 0.7 ucg/kg/min). *Results*. One hundred and ninety-four patients were treated with 531 sessions of PHD (G1=104 and G2=90 patients). The two groups were similar in age and SOFA. There was no significant difference in hypotension, hypokalemia, and anticoagulation during PHD sessions. The two groups showed differences in filter clotting, hypophosphatemia, and treatment discontinuation (12.3 versus 23.1%, p=0.002; 15.5 versus 25.8%, p=0.005; and 7.9 versus 15.6%, p=0.008, respectively). There was no difference in fluid balance (FB) before and after PHD sessions. Death and complete recovery of renal function were similar (81.3 versus 82.2%, p=0.87 and 21 versus 31.2%, p=0.7, respectively). At logistic regression, the positive FB before and after dialysis was identified as risk factor for death, while volume overload after three PHD sessions and predialysis creatinine were negatively associated with recovery of renal function in 28 days. *Conclusion*. There was no difference in the mortality and recovery of renal function of AKI patients submitted to different durations of PHD and sessions lasting 10 h presented higher filter clotting, hypophosphatemia, and treatment discontinuation. ISRCTN Registry number is ISRCTN33774458.

1. Introduction

Acute kidney injury (AKI) is a complex and frequent syndrome in septic patients admitted to intensive care units (34%). Despite the reduction of its mortality rate in recent years, it still remains high, reaching 62% in critical patients and 80% in those who require dialysis [1–5].

Peritoneal dialysis (PD) and hemodialysis (HD) are options for acute kidney injury support. Depending on their duration and flow of blood and dialysate they can be classified as conventional intermittent hemodialysis (IHD), prolonged intermittent hemodialysis (PHD), and continuous renal replacement therapy (CRRT) [6, 7]. So far there has been no evidence of one method being superior to the others.

PHD consists of a hybrid method with IHD characteristics, such as the use of machines and filters similar to those used in the treatment of chronic dialysis patients. It also has CRRT characteristics, such as smaller flow of blood and dialysate, between 70-250 ml/min and 70-300 ml/min, respectively [8–10]. The duration of PHD therapy varies between 6 and 18 hours [7, 9–11]. This method is considered to be as effective as conventional IHD and CRRT in regard to metabolic and volume control. It also has advantages when compared to CRRT, such as a lower cost, a reduced need for anticoagulation, and time optimization, with the possibility of having the patient undergo exams and procedures away from the ICU [12–14].

At the moment the literature does not include any studies that have evaluated and compared mortality rates and recovery of renal function in patients with AKI treated with PHD sessions of different durations.

This clinical trial was designed to evaluate and compare the recovery of renal function, mortality, and intra- and postdialysis complications in critically ill AKI patients undergoing PHD sessions lasting 6 or 10 h. We hypothesized that PHD sessions lasting 10 hours would cause less hypotension than PHD sessions lasting 6 hours, leading to faster partial recovery of renal function.

2. Methods

2.1. Studied Population. This is a randomized clinical trial conducted from January 2012 to March 2016 in patients enrolled in the Brazilian University Hospital. The protocol was approved by the Institutional Ethical Committee (CAAE Protocol: 28146714.6.0000.5411). Written informed consent was obtained from patients or their next of kin. The study also was registered in the ISRCTN Registry under the number ISRCTN33774458.

Patients were eligible for enrolment if they were 18 years of age or older, with AKI associated with sepsis and on a noradrenaline dose lower than $0.7 \mu g/kg/min$. AKI was defined according to of KDIGO [15]. Exclusion criteria were chronic kidney disease stages 4 and 5, previous chronic dialysis, kidney transplantation, patients previously treated with any acute dialysis during ICU stay, pregnancy, and taking noradrenaline dose higher than $0.7 \mu g/kg/min$. These last patients were excluded because they could not tolerate actual ultrafiltration (UF) of 300–500 mL/h and because of that, they were treated with CRRT.

2.2. Criteria for Initiating and Stopping PHD. The indications for dialysis were uraemic symptoms, BUN level > 100 mg/dL (azotaemia), volume overload, electrolyte imbalance (potassium > 6 mEq/L after clinical treatment), or acid-base refractory disturbances (bicarbonate < 10 mEq/L after reposition).

A patient was considered for enrolment if the judgment of the treating nephrologists was that he or she required dialysis and the mean arterial blood pressure (BP) was higher than 80 mmHg, with a noradrenaline dose lower than $0.7 \mu g/kg/min$ in the 8 hours preceding randomization.

The patients were randomly assigned to two groups, according to the treatment duration prescribed. The randomization was computerized by the randomization.com website.

Group 1: Patients treated with PHD sessions lasting 6 hours

Group 2: Patients treated with PHD sessions lasting 10 hours

The hemodialysis sessions were accompanied by the same research team until the patient's final clinical outcome (recovery of renal function, change of dialysis method, or death).

After diagnosing the sepsis-associated AKI and indicating PHD for dialysis, the central venous catheter was implanted to initiate treatment. The PHD session lasted 6 or 10 hours according to randomization and, for practical reasons, it was decided that PHD would be carried out 6 days a week (Monday–Saturday).

We used proportion machines (Fresenius 4008) and capillary polysulfone membranes (surface areas of 1.0 and $1.2 m^2$) for the sessions.

The PHD sessions were performed with blood and dialysate flows of 200 and 300 mL/min, respectively. For Group 1 we used FX 80 capillary dialyzers, while for Group 2 we used FX 60 capillary dialyzers in order to minimize the difference between the dialysis doses provided. During the sessions, the patients were anticoagulated with a 50 to 100 IU/kg bolus dose of heparin, and then with 500 to 1000 IU/hour in the following hours. In cases of contraindication to anticoagulation, the system was washed with 50 ml of 0.9% sodium chloride every 30 minutes, throughout the entire procedure. The concentrations of bicarbonate (26-36 mEq/L), potassium (1-3 mEq/L), sodium (140-145 mEq/L), and calcium (2.5 to 3.5 mEq/L) of the dialysis bath were adjusted according to the exams and individual needs of the patients. The ultrafiltration rate (UF) did not exceed 500 ml/hour and the bath temperature ranged from 35 to 35.5°C.

We evaluated hypotension and filter clotting as intradialytic complications. Hypotension was defined as systolic blood pressure (BP) below 90 mmHg, or as a sudden BP drop of 20 mmHg. Filter clotting was defined as the presence of blood clots in the circuit, composed of a dialyzer and lines, precluding the continuation of therapy. As preventive measures to hypotension we used UF rates not exceeding 500 ml/h, dialysate temperature between 35 and 35.5°C, and high dialysate sodium concentration (140-145 mEq/L). When we observed the presence of thrombi and blood clots in the system, we conducted saline flushes or administered an extra dose of heparin to prevent coagulation, according to medical prescription. As postdialysis complications we evaluated the presence of hypokalemia and hypophosphatemia, characterized by serum levels below 3.5 mEq/l and 3.5 mg/dl, respectively.

We evaluated the outcomes of death and recovery of renal function in 28 days. The recovery of renal function was assessed using the relationship between the reference creatinine level and the creatinine level at 28 days after hospital discharge (reference Cr/Cr at 28 days) and classified the recovery as complete if above 0.9, partial if between 0.5 and 0.9, and as nonrecovery if below 0.5. [16]

We collected the following clinical data: name, gender, age, race, presence of comorbidities (diabetes, chronic kidney disease, and hypertension), primary diagnosis, sepsis etiology, and AKI specific prognostic score (ATN-ISS) [17], Sequential Organ Failure Assessment (SOFA) [18], date of hospitalization, PHD starting date, concentration of vasoactive drug before and after PHD. We quantified urea, creatinine, sodium, potassium, phosphorus, calcium, and venous gas every day, before and after HD. Posttreatment BUN levels were measured by the slow flow method (with blood pump speed reduced to 50 mL/min). Blood samples were obtained from the arterial sampling port before the blood reached the dialyzer. HD adequacy was determined by using urea kinetic modelling based on Kt/V [19]. The delivered dose was determined by the single-pool Kt/V value, corrected for actual UF but not for the reappearance of urea nitrogen [19].

As dialytic therapy data we evaluated the number of sessions performed and of filters used, blood and dialysate flows, volume of UF prescribed and obtained, urea removal rate, BP every 30 minutes, and the presence of hypotension and filter clotting as previously defined. To solve hypotension during PHD, we applied protocols which included saline infusion, decreasing or discontinuing UF and increasing the vasoactive drug, according to the clinical and volume conditions of the patient. Therapy was interrupted when, despite taking these measures, hemodynamic instability persisted and presented risks to the patient.

Dialysis was interrupted when there was partial recovery of renal function (dialysis-independent) defined as restoration of urine output higher than 1000 mL/24 h associated with a progressive fall in serum values for creatinine (<4 mg/100 mL) and BUN (<50 mg/dL), a need to change dialysis method because of infectious, mechanical, or haemodynamic complications, more than 30 days of follow-up, or death.

2.3. Statistical Analysis. Considering alpha error as 5%, beta error as 20%, statistical power of the test as 80%, and detecting a 15% mortality rate difference between groups, the sample size for each group was calculated as 94 patients.

We described the variables with normal distribution as mean value ± standard deviation and the variables with nonnormal distribution as mean value and interquartile range.

We performed comparisons of the continuous variables between the two groups using Student's t-test for data with normal distribution and the Mann–Whitney test for nonnormal data. For the comparative analysis of categorical variables we used the Chi-squared tests. For comparing variables by session between the groups we used the mixed model of repeated measures over time with an adjustment for Tukey's test. We used univariate and multivariate linear regression for the association of risk factors for death and nonrecovery of renal function in 28 days.

We considered a 5% significance level in all of the tests performed.

For data analysis we used the SAS program for Windows, version 9.2 (developed in 2009, in Cary, North Carolina, USA).

3. Results

A hundred and ninety-four patients with sepsis-associated AKI received 531 PHD sessions. The mean age was 60.8 ± 14.9 years, and 69.5% of the patients were male. The main infection focus was pulmonary (41.2%) and hypertension was the most prevalent of the comorbidities (52.5%). The specific prognosis index for AKI, the ATN-ISS, was 0.77 ± 0.1 and the mean SOFA score was 14.2 ± 2.9.

G1 was composed of 104 patients, treated for 276 sessions. G2 was composed of 90 patients, treated for 255 sessions. When comparing clinical characteristics, both groups were similar in relation to the predominance of males (70.1% in G1 and 68.8% in G2, p=0.84), mean age of 61.4 ± 14.4 years in G1 and 60.5 ± 15.5 years in G2 (p=0.55), presence of comorbidities such as hypertension and diabetes (55.7% versus 48.8%, p=0.33 and 27.8% versus 26.6%, p=0.84, respectively), specific prognosis for ATN (ATN-ISS), and SOFA (0.76 ± 0.1 versus 0.77 ± 0.2, p=0.87 and 14.1 ± 3 versus 14.4 ± 2.9 p=0.47, respectively). In Group 1, pulmonary infection focus was prevalent (41.3%), while in Group 2, the main focus was abdominal (42.2%, p = 0.07). Most patients were on mechanical ventilation, 94.2% in Group 1, compared to 93.3% in Group 2 (p = 0.96). The groups were similar regarding initial and final doses of vasoactive drug (0.56 versus 0.55, p = 0.97 and 0.69 versus 0.7, p = 0.91, respectively) as shown in Table 1.

Table 2 shows the presence of dialysis complications during hemodialysis sessions, in general and divided by groups. The main complication among them was hypotension (50%), followed by filter clotting, hypophosphatemia, and hypokalemia, which happened in 17.5%, 20.5%, and 11.2% of the sessions, respectively. There was a significant difference between the groups in relation to filter clotting (12.3 versus 23.1%, p = 0.002), hypophosphatemia (15.5 versus 25.8%, p = 0.005), and hemodialysis session interruption due to the presence of persistent hypotension after refractory measures (7.9 versus 15.6%, p = 0.008). Both groups were similar in relation to hypotension (46.7 versus 53.7%, p = 0.13), hypokalemia (11.5 versus 10.9%, p = 0.93), and the use of anticoagulation in the PHD sessions (45.2 versus 36.8%, p = 0.06).

The main outcome was death, present in 81.7% of the general population. Recovery of renal function (RF) was assessed among the survivors: 25.7% presented complete recovery, 68.5% presented partial recovery, and 5.7% presented nonrecovery. There was no difference between the groups in relation to outcomes (death: 81.3 versus 82.2%, p = 0.87; complete recovery of FR: 21 versus 31.2%, p = 0.7; partial recovery of RF: 68.4 versus 68.7%, p = 0.7; nonrecovery of RF: 10.5 versus 0%, p = 0.48), as shown in Table 3.

The metabolic and volume controls of the AKI patients treated with PHD sessions lasting 6 and 10 hours were assessed after the first three sessions and are presented in Table 4. The target metabolic and volume control was reached in both groups we studied with urea lower than 120 mg/dl, pH above 7.3, minimum weekly Kt/v of 3.9, and cumulative fluid balance close to zero after 3 sessions. The groups showed differences in the values of urea reduction ratio (URR) on the first and third sessions (S1: 0.6 ± 0.1 versus 0.68 ± 0.1; p < 0.001, S3: 0.56 ± 0.1 versus 0.62 ± 0.1; p = 0.03), being higher in G2. Potassium and phosphorous serum values were (4.3 ± 0.8 versus 3.9 ± 0.6, p = 0.04; 5.8 ± 2.2 versus 4.1 ± 1.6, p = 0.009, respectively), being lower in G2. The rate of ultrafiltration (UF) prescribed in the first three sessions was (S1: 2064 ± 927 versus 2580 ± 1000, p= 0.0002; S2: 2262 ± 852 versus 2626 ± 1123, p=0.02, and S3: 2217 ± 755 versus 2656 ± 1004, p=0.03) and real UF in the first session was (1791±963 versus 2345 ± 1017, p = 0.0006), which were higher in G2. However, the UF in ml/h was lower in G2 in all sessions we studied. The other parameters assessed were similar between the groups.

TABLE 1: Clinical and laboratory characteristics of patients with AKI treated with PHD.

Parameters	General (n = 194)	G1 (n = 104)	G2 (n = 90)	p value
Age (in years)	60.8 ± 14.9	61.4 ± 14.4	60.2 ± 15.5	0.55
Males, n (%)	135 (69.5)	73 (70.1)	62 (68.8)	0.84
Weight	74.8 ± 22.5	74.1 ± 24	75.6 ± 20.8	0.63
Infectious focus n (%)				
Pulmonary	80 (41.2)	43 (41.3)	37 (41.2)	0.97
Abdominal	69 (35.5)	31 (29.8)	38 (42.2)	0.07
Comorbidities, n (%)				
(i) SAH	102 (52.5)	58 (55.7)	44 (48.8)	0.33
(ii) DM	53 (27.2)	29 (27.8)	24 (26.6)	0.84
(iii) CKD	19 (9.7)	12 (11.5)	7 (7.7)	0.37
ATN-ISS	0.77 ± 0.1	0.76 ± 0.1	0.77 ± 0.2	0.87
SOFA	14.2 ± 2.9	14.1 ± 3	14,4 ± 2,9	0.47
Pre-dialysis FB (l)	3.36 ± 1.8	3.27 ± 1.9	3.47 ± 1.7	0.47
Ur (mg/dl)	155.3 ± 105.7	158.6 ± 59.5	151.6 ± 141.2	0.64
Cr (mg/dl)	3.7 ± 1.5	3.7 ± 1.4	3.6 ± 1.7	0.64
K (mEq/L)	4.7 ± 1	4.7 ± 1	4.8 ± 1	0.48
Bic (mEq/L)	19.1 ± 4.6	18.8 ± 4.7	19.5 ± 4.6	0.39
Mechanical Ventilation	182 (93.8)	98 (94.2)	84 (93.3)	0.96
Initial vasoactive drug dose	0.55 ± 0.18	0.55 ± 0.17	0.56 ± 0.19	0.97
Final vasoactive drug dose	0.69 ± 0.19	0.69 ± 0.16	0.70 ± 0.20	0.91

Values are presented in frequency, mean values and standard deviation, median, and proportions.
AKI: acute renal injury, PHD: prolonged hemodialysis, SAH: systemic arterial hypertension, DM: diabetes mellitus, CKD: chronic kidney disease, ATN-ISS: acute tubular necrosis individual severity score, SOFA: sequential organ failure assessment score, FB: fluid balance, Ur: urea, Cr: creatinine, K: potassium, Bic: bicarbonate, and UF: ultrafiltration.

TABLE 2: Dialysis complications by PHD sessions according to the groups studied.

Complications	General (n = 531)	G1 (n = 276)	G2 (n = 255)	p value
Hypotension, n (%)	266 (50)	129 (46.7)	137 (53.7)	0.13
Filter clotting, n (%)	93 (17.5)	34 (12.3)	59 (23.1)	0.002
Hypokalemia, n (%)	60 (11.2)	32 (11.5)	28 (10.9)	0.93
Hypophosphataemia, n (%)	109 (20.5)	43 (15.5)	66 (25.8)	0.005
Use of anticoagulation, n (%)	219 (41.2)	125 (45.2)	94 (36.8)	0.06
Treatment discontinuation, n (%)	62 (11.6)	22 (7.9)	40 (15.6)	0.008

Values are presented in proportions.
PHD: prolonged hemodialysis.

Fluid balance was assessed before the first and third sessions of PHD, and there was no difference between the groups (S1: 3.27 ± 1.9 versus 3.47 ± 1.7, p = 0.47 and S3: 1.33 ± 2.6 versus 0.47 ± 2.4, p = 0.09).

A logistic regression was conducted for the death outcomes and the variables of weight, SOFA, fluid balance before and after 3 sessions, presession potassium, and the presence of hypokalemia were identified as risk factors. After the multivariate analysis, the association remained only for fluid balance before and after 3 sessions. This data is included in Tables 5 and 6.

Similarly, the logistic regression was carried out for the recovery of renal function in 28 days, and the values of fluid balance before and after 3 sessions and creatinine presession presented significant negative association, which remained

after the multivariate analysis. This data is shown in Tables 7 and 8.

4. Discussion

This clinical trial study aimed to assess and compare the mortality rate and recovery of renal function in critical patients with AKI, treated with PHD sessions of different durations (6 and 10 hours). There are very few studies on PHD in the literature and, until now, none of them compared the clinical evolution of patients in PHD of different durations.

Hypotension was the most common complication and occurred in 50% of the sessions, despite the use of precautionary measures, such as low dialysate temperature, high sodium concentrations, and UF rate not exceeding 500 ml/h. Similar

TABLE 3: Main outcomes of patients with AKI treated with PHD according to the duration of the PHD sessions.

Outcomes	General (n = 194)	G1 (n = 104)	G2 (n = 90)	p value
Death, n (%)	157 (81.7)	83 (81.3)	74 (82.2)	0.87
Complete recovery of RF, n (%)	9 (25.7)	4 (21)	5 (31.2)	0.7
Partial recovery of RN, n (%)	24 (68.5)	13 (68.4)	11 (68.7)	0.7
Non-recovery of RF, n (%)	2 (5.7)	2 (10.5)	0	0.48

Values are presented in proportions.
AKI: acute renal injury, PHD: prolonged hemodialysis, and RF: renal function.

results were reported by Fieghen et al. [20], Ponce et al. [21], And Albino et al. [22].

However, there was no difference between the groups treated in our study. The longest session duration time in Group 2 resulted in a lower ultrafiltration rate (ml/hour), though it did not prevent and/or improve the frequency of hypotension. The dose of the vasoactive substance was higher at the end of the PHD sessions, when compared to the dose at the beginning, in an attempt to keep arterial pressure steady during therapy, and it was similar between the groups.

The second most frequent dialysis complication in our study was filter clotting, which occurred in 11.2% sessions, similar to the data reported in the literature [3, 12, 21, 22]. The use of anticoagulation in the PHD sessions was carried out according to the comorbidities and bleeding risk related to the patient. Anticoagulation occurred in 41.2% of the sessions and there was no difference between the groups.

The prevalence of filter clotting was different between the groups as was treatment discontinuation. These facts may be related to the longer duration of treatment of Group 2 patients, making them more susceptible to the persistence of intradialytic complications.

Hypokalemia and hypophosphatemia are postdialysis complications that are rarely addressed in the previous studies conducted on PHD, which complicates the analysis and comparison of the results obtained in our study. Marshall et al. [23] analyzed 145 PHD sessions in 37 patients and found hypokalemia and hypophosphatemia in 7 (4.8%) and 18 (12.4%) occurrences, respectively, and these results are similar to those found in our study. Similarly, Palevsky et al. [24] found a prevalence of hypophosphatemia in 12.4% of the patients treated with PHD in their ATN study.

There was a difference between the groups we studied in relation to hypophosphatemia, probably associated with the longer therapy duration and consequently greater removal of solutes, and the groups were similar in relation to hypokalemia.

The target metabolic and volume control was reached in both groups we studied. However, there was difference between the groups regarding the URR and Kt/V, which were higher in group 2. Despite the use of capillaries with a smaller area for Group 2, due to the 10-hour treatment duration, these patients received a slightly higher Kt/v.

Although the Kt/V was higher in Group 2, the mortality rate was similar between the groups, in accordance with

previous studies that showed that more intensive dialysis is not associated with better outcomes [25, 26].

The ultrafiltration value was prescribed according to the fluid balance of the patient, and it ranged between 1500 and 3000 ml per session. There was a difference between the groups. Group 2 had higher prescribed and actual UF. However, the fluid balance was similar between the studied populations after 3 sessions of therapy. There was no difference in cumulative fluid balance before and after 3 dialysis sessions between the groups.

Death occurred in 81.7% of the general population and there was no difference between the groups. The mortality rate we found was higher than those reported in previous studies carried out in European countries and in North America, such as in a study conducted in Toronto by Kitchlu et al., who observed death in 54% of patients treated with PHD [12]. Our mortality rate, however, was similar to those observed in critical patients with AKI in developing countries. In Brazilian studies, mortality of AKI patients that underwent dialysis ranged from 67 to 85% [3, 22, 27, 28]. This data is similar to that described by George et al., who performed a study in India and obtained mortality over 75% in patients with AKI [29].

Considering we included patients with sepsis-associated AKI and elevated prognostic indexes (ATN-ISS and SOFA of 0.77 ± 0.1 and 14.2 ± 2.9, respectively), the patients studied were in severe conditions, which justifies the unfavorable outcomes. It is important to emphasize that we only evaluated septic patients, which was not made in other studies.

We identified cumulative fluid balance before dialysis and after 3 sessions of PHD as the only death-associated factor. These results are in agreement with previous studies that reported low urine output, fluid overload, and sepsis are associated with worse prognostic of AKI patients [21, 26, 30, 31]. Clinical data show that positive fluid balance and oliguria can contribute negatively to prognosis lung, leading to increased time of invasive mechanical ventilation, durations of hospitalization, and mortality [30, 31].

In our study, we could not identify dialysis dose as a risk factor for death, in agreement with Palevsky et al. [25] and Bellomo et al. [26] in the trials ATN and RENAL, respectively.

Recovery of renal function was assessed among the survivors: 25.7% had complete recovery and 68.5% had partial recovery. Similar results reported that a quarter of the patients obtained complete recovery of renal function after 30 days. In our study, the predialysis creatinine value and fluid balance

TABLE 4: Metabolic and volume control of the studied groups in the first three sessions of PHD.

	G1 = 6 h (n = sessions)			G2 = 10 h (n = sessions)			p value*
	S1 (n = 104)	S2 (n = 70)	S3 (n = 38)	S1 (n = 90)	S2 (n = 63)	S3 (n = 44)	
Predialysis Ur (mg/dl)	158 ± 59	123 ± 48	119 ± 44	137 ± 6[a]	102 ± 140[b]	89 ± 43[c]	NS
URR	0.6 ± 0.1	0.6 ± 0.1	0.56 ± 0.1	0.68 ± 0.1[d]	0.58 ± 0.1[b]	0.62 ± 0.1[f]	<.0001
Kt/V	1.05 ± 0.05	1.06 ± 0.05	1.03 ± 0.05	1.23 ± 0.06[d]	1.04 ± 0.05	1.18 ± 0.06[f]	0.01
Cr (mg/dl)	3.7 ± 1.4	2.8 ± 1.2	2.9 ± 1.1	3.6 ± 1.7[a]	2.5 ± 1[b]	2.4 ± 1.2[c]	NS
K (mEq/L)	4.7 ± 1	4.4 ± 0.9	4.3 ± 0.8	4.8 ± 1[a]	4.3 ± 0.8[b]	3.9 ± 0.6[f]	0.04
P (mEq/L)	6.5 ± 2.6	5.5 ± 2.1	5.8 ± 2.2	6 ± 2.5[a]	5.5 ± 3.2[b]	4.1 ± 1.6[f]	0.009
Bic (mEq/L)	18.3 ± 4.3	20.3 ± 4	20.3 ± 4	19.2 ± 4.3[a]	20.9 ± 5.5[b]	22.1 ± 3.5[c]	NS
pH	7.2 ± 0.1	8.4 ± 8.8	7.2 ± 0.09	7.2 ± 0.1[a]	7.2 ± 0.1[b]	7.2 ± 0.1[f]	0.03
Presc. UF (ml)	2064 ± 927	2262 ± 852	2217 ± 755	2580 ± 1000[d]	2626 ± 1123[e]	2656 ± 1004[f]	0.0002
Real UF (ml)	1791 ± 963	2032 ± 930	1940 ± 931	2345 ± 1017[d]	2097 ± 1494[b]	2240 ± 1295[c]	0.0006
Real UF (ml/h)	298 ± 160	338 ± 156	331 ± 149	234 ± 98	209 ± 147	224 ± 129	0.003
FB (l)	3.27 ± 1.9	-	1.33 ± 2.6	3.47 ± 1.7	-	0.47 ± 2.4	NS

Values are presented in mean and standard deviation.

PHD: prolonged hemodialysis, Ur: urea, URR: urea reduction ratio, Cr: creatinine, K: potassium, P: phosphorus, Bic: bicarbonate, UF: ultrafiltration, and Presc.: prescribed.

a: similar to S1 of G1, b: similar to S2 of G1, and c: similar to S3 of G1.

d: different from S1 of G1, e: different from S2 of G1, and f: different from S3 of G1.

NS: not significant (p >:0.05).

TABLE 5: Univariate logistic regression of clinical and laboratory characteristics, and dialysis complications associated with the death of patients with AKI treated with PHD.

Parameter	OR	Confidence Interval	p value
Age	1.01	0.99 – 1.03	0.24
Gender	0.60	0.28 – 1.28	0.19
Weight	1.01	1.00 – 1.03	0.04
Infectious focus	0.95	0.33 – 2.70	0.87
SAH	0.84	0.40 – 1.75	0.64
DM	0.73	0.31 – 1.74	0.48
CKD	0.22	0.02 – 1.76	0.15
ATN-ISS	0.94	0.11- 7.98	0.95
SOFA	1.22	1.06 – 1.40	0.004
Pre FB	1.47	1.12 – 1.93	0.004
Post FB	1.38	1.11 – 1.72	0.003
Pre Ur	0.99	0.99 – 1.0	0.15
Post Ur	1.00	0.99 – 1.01	0.67
Pre Cr	1.01	0.80 – 1.28	0.88
CR post	0.94	0.60 – 1.47	0.78
Pre K	1.79	1.18 – 2.73	0.006
Post K	1.82	0.82 – 4.00	0.13
Pre Bic	0.93	0.85 – 1.01	0.11
Post Bic	0.90	0.75 – 1.08	0.27
Pre UF	0.93	0.78 – 1.12	0.49
Post UF	0.86	0.67 – 1.12	0.28
RF outcome	1.0	<0,001 - >999,999	0.85
Hypotension	0.50	0.23 – 1.09	0.008
Coagulation	0.76	0.34 – 1.70	0.5
Hypokalemia	3.7	1.62 – 8.83	0.002
Hypophosphataemia	1.48	0.66 - 3.31	0.33

Or: odds ratio.
AKI: acute renal injury, PHD: prolonged hemodialysis, SAH: systemic arterial hypertension, DM: diabetes mellitus, CKD: chronic kidney disease, ATN-ISS: acute tubular necrosis individual severity score, SOFA: sequential organ failure assessment score, FB: fluid balance, Ur: urea, Cr: creatinine, K: potassium, Bic: bicarbonate, UF: ultrafiltration, and RF: renal function. Pre = 1st session, post = 3rd session of PHD.

TABLE 6: Multivariate logistic regression of clinical and laboratory characteristics and dialysis complications associated with the death of patients with AKI treated with PHD.

Parameter	OR	Confidence Interval	p value
Weight	1.01	0.98 – 1.04	0.51
SOFA	1.08	0.34 – 1.38	0.52
Pre FB	1.60	1.04 – 2.47	0.03
Post FB	1.54	1.16 – 2.04	0.002
Hypokalemia	1.69	0.39 – 7.22	0.47

Or: odds ratio.
AKI: acute kidney injury, HDP: prolonged hemodialysis, SOFA: sequential organ failure assessment score, and FB: fluid balance.

after 3 sessions were identified as risk factors for the recovery of renal function. Hamzić-Mehmedbašić et al. identified that the female gender, comorbidities, and sepsis were risk factors for a worse evolution of renal function [32].

Our study presents several limitations, such as the small number of studied patients and its execution in a single center. Due to the different duration of treatment between the groups, we were not able to perform the randomization blindly. The assessment of long-term survival was also not performed. Despite these limitations, this was the first study to assess the clinical evolution of patients with AKI treated with different durations of PHD [33].

In conclusion, our results show that mortality and recovery of renal function are similar between the groups treated with PHD lasting 6 and 10 h. However, Group 2 showed higher incidence of dialysis complications, such as filter clotting and hypophosphatemia, probably related to the

TABLE 7: Univariate logistic regression of clinical and laboratory characteristics and dialysis complications associated with the recovery of renal function in patients with AKI treated with PHD.

Parameter	OR	Confidence Interval	p value
Age	1.01	0.99 – 1.03	0.17
Gender	0.74	0.37 – 1.50	0.41
Weight	0.99	0.97 – 1.00	0.27
Infectious focus			
SAH	0.66	0.34 – 1.27	0.21
DM	0.98	0.48 – 1.97	0.95
CKD	1.9	0.52 – 7.2	0.32
ATN-ISS	1.17	0.15 – 9.18	0.87
SOFA	0.92	0.81 – 1.04	0.19
Pre FB	0.93	0.78 -1.10	0.41
Post FB	0.83	0.69 – 0.99	0.04
Pre Ur	1.00	0.99 – 1.00	0.71
Post Ur	0.99	0.98 – 1.00	0.65
Pre Cr	0.88	0.57 – 0.96	0.03
Post Cr	1.00	0.97- 1.03	0.57
Pre K	0.77	0.56 – 1.05	0.10
Post K	0.68	0.34 – 1.38	0,29
Pre Bic	1.07	0.99 – 1.15	0.08
Post Bic	1.00	0.85 – 1.18	0.92
Pre UF	1.09	0.94 – 1.27	0,24
Post UF	0.94	0.72 – 1.23	0,67
Hypotension	1.8	0.92 – 3.67	0,08
Coagulation	0.86	0.44 – 1.69	0.67
Hypokalemia	0.74	0.33 – 1.67	0.47
Hypophosphataemia	1.10	0.53 – 2.29	0.78

OR: odds ratio.
AKI: acute renal injury, PHD: prolonged hemodialysis, SAH: systemic arterial hypertension, DM: diabetes mellitus, CKD: chronic kidney disease, ATN-ISS: acute tubular necrosis individual severity score, SOFA: sequential organ failure assessment score, FB: fluid balance, Ur: urea, Cr: creatinine, K: potassium, Bic: bicarbonate, UF: ultrafiltration, and RF: renal function. Pre = 1st session, post = 3rd session of PHD.

TABLE 8: Multivariate logistic regression of clinical and laboratory characteristics and dialysis complications associated with the recovery of renal function in patients with AKI treated with PHD.

Parameter	OR	Confidence Interval	p value
SOFA	0.86	0.68-1.12	0.48
Pre FB	0.94	0.72-1.08	0.08
Post FB	0.98	0.65-0.97	0.009
Pre Cr	0.82	0.59-0.91	0.04

OR: odds ratio.
AKI: acute kidney injury, HDP: prolonged hemodialysis, SOFA: sequential organ failure assessment score, FB: fluid balance, and Pre Cr: creatinine at 1st PHD session.

extended duration of therapy. Therefore, there is no benefit in treating patients with 10-hour sessions.

Future work in this area should aim to clarify factors that inform decision-making around time of PHD modality. Larger and trial studies will need to clarify the impact of PHD on patient survival and recovery of renal function.

Disclosure

All authors have agreed to the submission to the journal and that the manuscript is not currently under submission in any other journal.

References

[1] R. L. Mehta, J. A. Kellum, S. V. Shah et al., "Acute Kidney Injury Network: report of an initiative to improve outcomes in acute kidney injury," *Critical Care*, vol. 11, no. 2, article R31, 2007.

[2] C. H. Chang, P. C. Fan, M. Y. Chang et al., "Acute kidney injury enhances outcome prediction ability of sequential organ failure assessment score in critically ill patients," *PLoS ONE*, vol. 9, no. 10, 2014.

[3] R. A. Caires, R. C. R. M. Abdulkader, V. T. Costa e Silva et al., "Sustained low-efficiency extended dialysis (SLED) with single-pass batch system in critically-ill patients with acute kidney injury (AKI)," *Journal of Nephrology*, vol. 29, no. 3, pp. 401–409, 2016.

[4] J. Himmelfarb and T. A. Ikizler, "Acute kidney injury: changing lexicography, definitions, and epidemiology," *Kidney International*, vol. 71, no. 10, pp. 971–976, 2007.

[5] S. Uchino, J. A. Kellum, R. Bellomo et al., "Acute renal failure in critically ill patients: a multinational, multicenter study," *The Journal of the American Medical Association*, vol. 294, no. 7, pp. 813–818, 2005.

[6] N. Pannu, S. Klarenbach, N. Wiebe, B. Manns, and M. Tonelli, "Renal replacement therapy in patients with acute renal failure: a systematic review," *Journal of the American Medical Association*, vol. 299, no. 7, pp. 793–805, 2008.

[7] J. T. Kielstein, M. Schiffer, and C. Hafer, "Back to the future: extended dialysis for treatment of acute kidney injury in the intensive care unit," *Journal of Nephrology*, vol. 23, no. 5, pp. 494–501, 2010.

[8] R. Shingarev, K. Wille, and A. Tolwani, "Management of complications in renal replacement therapy," *Seminars in Dialysis*, vol. 24, no. 2, pp. 164–168, 2011.

[9] W. Sulowicz and A. Radziszewski, "Pathogenesis and treatment of dialysis hypotension," *Kidney International*, vol. 70, no. 104, pp. S36–S39, 2006.

[10] R. A. Sherman, J. T. Daugirdas, and T. S. Ing, "Complications during hemodialysis," in *Handbook of Dialysis*, J. T. Daugirdas, P. G. Blake, and T. S. Ing, Eds., pp. 158–164, Lippincott Williams & Wilkins, Philadelphia, PA, USA, 4th edition, 2007.

[11] M. Doshi and P. T. Murray, "Approach to intradialytic hypotension in intensive care unit patients with acute renal failure," *Artificial Organs*, vol. 27, no. 9, pp. 772–780, 2003.

[12] A. Kitchlu, N. Adhikari, K. E. Burns et al., "Outcomes of sustained low efficiency dialysis versus continuous renal replacement therapy in critically ill adults with acute kidney injury: a cohort study," *BMC Nephrology*, vol. 16, no. 1, 2015.

[13] L. Zhang, J. Yang, G. M. Eastwood, G. Zhu, A. Tanaka, and R. Bellomo, "Extended daily dialysis versus continuous renal replacement therapy for acute kidney injury: a meta-analysis," *American Journal of Kidney Diseases*, vol. 66, no. 2, pp. 322–330, 2015.

[14] M. M. Levy, R. P. Delinger, S. R. Townsend et al., "Surviving sepsis campaign: results of an international guideline-based performance improvement program targeting severe sepsis," *Critical Care Medicine*, vol. 38, pp. 367–374, 2010.

[15] Kidney Disease: Improving Global Outcomes (KDIGO) CKD Work Group, "KDIGO 2012 clinical practice guideline for the evaluation and management of chronic kidney disease," *Kidney International Supplements*, vol. 3, pp. 1–150, 2013.

[16] J.-P. Lafrance and D. R. Miller, "Acute kidney injury associates with increased long-term mortality," *Journal of the American Society of Nephrology*, vol. 21, no. 2, pp. 345–352, 2010.

[17] F. Liano, A. Gallego, J. Pascual et al., "Prognosis of acute tubular necrosis: an extended prospectively contrasted study," *Nephron*, vol. 63, no. 1, pp. 21–31, 1993.

[18] F. Lopes Ferreira, D. Peres Bota, A. Bross, C. Mélot, and J.-L. Vincent, "Serial evaluation of the SOFA score to predict outcome in critically ill patients," *Journal of the American Medical Association*, vol. 286, no. 14, pp. 1754–1758, 2001.

[19] J. T. Daugirdas, "Physiologic principles and urea kinetic modeling," in *Handbook of Dialysis*, J. T. Daugirdas, P. G. Blake, and T. S. Ing, Eds., pp. 23–53, Lippincott Williams & Wilkins, Philadelphia, PA, USA, 4th edition, 2007.

[20] H. E. Fieghen, J. O. Friedrich, K. E. Burns et al., "The hemodynamic tolerability and feasibility of sustained low efficiency dialysis in the management of critically ill patients with acute kidney injury," *BMC Nephrology*, vol. 11, no. 1, article 32, 2010.

[21] D. Ponce, J. M. Abrão, B. B. Albino, A. L. Balbi, and J. I. Salluh, "Extended daily dialysis in acute kidney injury patients: metabolic and fluid control and risk factors for death," *PLoS ONE*, vol. 8, no. 12, 2013.

[22] B. B. Albino, A. L. Balbi, J. M. G. Abrão, and D. Ponce, "Dialysis complications in acute kidney injury patients treated with prolonged intermittent renal replacement therapy sessions lasting 10 versus 6 hours: results of a randomized clinical trial," *Artificial Organs*, vol. 39, no. 5, pp. 423–431, 2015.

[23] M. R. Marshall, T. A. Golper, M. J. Shaver, M. G. Alam, and D. K. Chatoth, "Sustained low-efficiency dialysis for critically ill patients requiring renal replacement therapy," *Kidney International*, vol. 60, no. 2, pp. 777–785, 2001.

[24] P. M. Palevsky, J. H. Zhang, T. Z. O'Connor et al., "Intensity of renal support in critically ill patients with acute kidney injury," *The New England Journal of Medicine*, vol. 359, no. 1, pp. 7–20, 2008.

[25] R. Bellomo, A. Cass, L. Cole et al., "Intensity of continuous renal-replacement therapy in critically ill patients," *The New England Journal of Medicine*, vol. 361, no. 17, pp. 1627–1638, 2009.

[26] J. A. Silversides, R. Pinto, R. Kuint et al., "Fluid balance, intradialytic hypotension, and outcomes in critically ill patients undergoing renal replacement therapy: a cohort study," *Critical Care*, vol. 18, no. 6, pp. 624–628, 2014.

[27] V. T. Costa e Silva, F. Liaño, A. Muriel, R. Díez, I. de Castro, and L. Yu, "Nephrology referral and outcomes in critically Ill acute kidney injury patients," *PLoS ONE*, vol. 8, no. 8, 2013.

[28] E. Q. Lima, D. M. T. Zanetta, I. Castro, and L. Yu, "Mortality risk factors and validation of severity scoring systems in critically ill patients with acute renal failure," *Renal Failure*, vol. 27, no. 5, pp. 547–556, 2005.

[29] J. George, S. Varma, S. Kumar, J. Thomas, S. Gopi, and R. Pisharody, "Comparing continuous venovenous hemodiafiltration and peritoneal dialysis in critically ill patients with acute kidney injury: a pilot study," *Peritoneal Dialysis International*, vol. 31, no. 4, pp. 422–429, 2011.

[30] D. Payen, A. C. de Pont, Y. Sakr, C. Spies, K. Reinhart, and J. L. Vincent, "A positive fluid balance is associated with a worse outcome in patients with acute renal failure," *Critical Care*, vol. 12, no. 3, article R74, 2008.

[31] D. Ponce, M. B. Buffarah, C. Goes, and A. Balbi, "Peritoneal dialysis in acute kidney injury: Trends in the outcome across time periods," *PLoS ONE*, vol. 10, no. 5, 2015.

18

The Role of Sodium Bicarbonate in the Management of Some Toxic Ingestions

Aibek E. Mirrakhimov,[1] **Taha Ayach,**[1] **Aram Barbaryan,**[2] **Goutham Talari,**[1] **Romil Chadha,**[1] **and Adam Gray**[1]

[1]*Department of Medicine, University of Kentucky College of Medicine, Lexington, KY, USA*
[2]*University of Kansas Medical Center, Kansas City, KS, USA*

Correspondence should be addressed to Aibek E. Mirrakhimov; amirrakhimov1@gmail.com

Academic Editor: Anil K. Agarwal

Adverse reactions to commonly prescribed medications and to substances of abuse may result in severe toxicity associated with increased morbidity and mortality. According to the Center for Disease Control, in 2013, at least 2113 human fatalities attributed to poisonings occurred in the United States of America. In this article, we review the data regarding the impact of systemic sodium bicarbonate administration in the management of certain poisonings including sodium channel blocker toxicities, salicylate overdose, and ingestion of some toxic alcohols and in various pharmacological toxicities. Based on the available literature and empiric experience, the administration of sodium bicarbonate appears to be beneficial in the management of a patient with the above-mentioned toxidromes. However, most of the available evidence originates from case reports, case series, and expert consensus recommendations. The potential mechanisms of sodium bicarbonate include high sodium load and the development of metabolic alkalosis with resultant decreased tissue penetration of the toxic substance with subsequent increased urinary excretion. While receiving sodium bicarbonate, patients must be monitored for the development of associated side effects including electrolyte abnormalities, the progression of metabolic alkalosis, volume overload, worsening respiratory status, and/or worsening metabolic acidosis. Patients with oliguric/anuric renal failure and advanced decompensated heart failure should not receive sodium bicarbonate.

1. Introduction

In the USA, at least 34% of the population regularly takes at least one prescription medication [1]. In the vast majority of cases the use of such prescribed medications provides clinical benefit to patients. However, in some cases, these medications may result in harm including a severe illness and death due to intentional or unintentional overdose or as a result of idiosyncratic drug reaction.

The goal of this article is to review the data and evidence on the use of sodium bicarbonate in the management of some pharmacological overdoses. We will first briefly review the mechanisms of metabolic acidosis related biochemical derangements since some of the overdoses are associated with metabolic acidosis. Second, we will discuss the mechanism of action, potential side effects, and typical dosing of sodium bicarbonate. Third, we will review the literature on the role of sodium bicarbonate in the management of sodium channel blocker toxicities. Fourth, the data on the role of sodium bicarbonate in the management of salicylate poisoning will be provided. Finally, we will discuss the place of sodium bicarbonate in the management of toxic alcohol ingestions.

The management of the toxicities mentioned above is complicated, requiring additional measures than sodium bicarbonate alone. Additional information on other aspects of management can be obtained elsewhere and is not the goal of this article.

2. Mechanism of Action and Potential Complications of Sodium Bicarbonate Therapy

Bicarbonate is an essential chemical regulating the acid-base balance acting as a buffer [2]. Carbon dioxide (CO_2) is a

TABLE 1: Constituents and characteristics of commonly used crystalloids and plasma.

Solution	Ph	Na^+ (mmol/l)	Cl^- (mmol/l)	K^+ (mmol/l)	Osmolality (mOsmol/kg)
Plasma	7.35–7.45	136–145	95–105	3.5–5.0	275–295
Lactated Ringer	6.6	130	109	4	273
3% sodium chloride	5.0	513	513	0	1027
Normal saline (0.9%)	5.7	154	154	0	308
Half-normal saline (0.45%)	5.6	77	77	0	154
Dextrose 5% in water (D5W)	4.5	0	0	0	253
Bicarbonate (8.4%)*	8	1000	0	0	2000

*1 ampule contains 50 milliliters with 50 mEq of sodium bicarbonate.

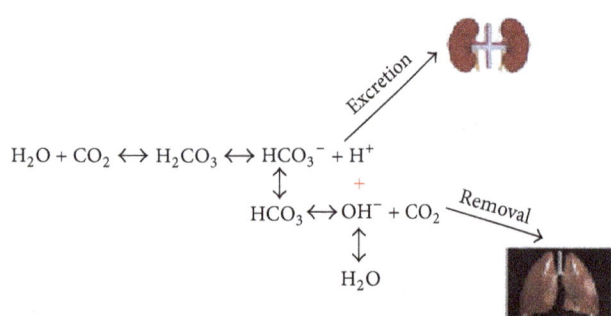

$$H_2O + CO_2 \leftrightarrow H_2CO_3 \leftrightarrow HCO_3^- + H^+$$

$$HCO_3 \leftrightarrow OH^- + CO_2$$

$$H_2O$$

FIGURE 1: An overview of the endogenous bicarbonate metabolism.

major byproduct of energy metabolism in living organisms and a conjugate acid. Carbonic anhydrase enzyme facilitates the chemical interaction between CO_2 and water producing carbonic acid (H_2CO_3). Carbonic acid in turn dissociates into bicarbonate (HCO_3^-) and hydrogen ion (H^+) with the latter being removed via kidneys. HCO_3^- can also bind extra H^+ producing carbonic acid. Indeed, all the reactions are reversible and can go in any direction.

Sodium bicarbonate ($NaHCO_3$) is one of the few pharmacological agents aiming to mimic the endogenous effects of HCO_3^-. Sodium bicarbonate is widely used in many clinical situations including cardiac arrest [3, 4] and prevention of contrast-induced renal failure [5] and in patients with different types of metabolic acidosis (such as lactic acidosis and diabetic ketoacidosis) [6], despite limited and controversial evidence of its benefits. A simplified view on the bicarbonate chemistry is provided in Figure 1. An overview of chemical characteristics of commonly used crystalloids is presented in Table 1.

The potential benefits of exogenous intravenous sodium bicarbonate include the correction of metabolic acidosis with its associated detrimental effects. However, the role of sodium bicarbonate in the management of acute acidosis remains controversial and may even be associated with potential side effects and complications such as volume overload, metabolic alkalosis, hypercapnia, hypokalemia, hypernatremia and hyperosmolality, and ionized hypocalcemia [6, 7].

When administered, sodium bicarbonate dissociates into a molecule of sodium and bicarbonate. The molecule of

bicarbonate in turn binds hydrogen converting into carbonic acid with its subsequent dissociation into carbon dioxide and water.

Carbon dioxide under normal conditions (intact lung perfusion and ventilation) is exhaled, maintaining delicate acid-base equilibrium. Under extreme conditions such as shock states and impaired ventilation, carbon dioxide may accumulate, leading to worsening acidosis [8, 9]. CO_2 penetrates cellular membranes easily, and through this ability may exacerbate intracellular acidosis. Furthermore, by correcting the systemic acidosis, sodium bicarbonate administration may reduce respiratory drive leading to accumulation of CO_2 in the central nervous system and associated adverse neurological sequelae [10]. Serum potassium may decrease as a result of potassium shift into the cells in the patient with metabolic acidosis treated with sodium bicarbonate. Other potential adverse effects of administered sodium bicarbonate may be related to its chemical features such as supraphysiologic sodium content and osmolality and alkaline pH (comparative chemical features of sodium bicarbonate and commonly used crystalloid solutions to plasma is presented in Table 1). Ionized calcium may be decreased, such as in metabolic alkalosis [11], which may cause tetany, decrease cardiac contractility, and potentially predispose to cardiac arrhythmias via prolongation of QT interval [12]. Serum sodium and osmolality tend to increase which may lead to cellular dehydration and systemic hypervolemia [13]. Lactic acid production may be increased in certain situations via alkalosis dependent activation of 6-phosphofructokinase enzyme [11, 14], and ketone bodies production may be enhanced [15]. Decreased cardiac oxygen supply and arterial vasoconstriction may also occur secondary to metabolic alkalosis [16, 17]. Lastly, serious skin injuries can occur in the setting of extravasation of hypertonic bicarbonate solutions, and whenever possible it should be administered through large bore intravenous lines or central venous lines.

Nevertheless, these adverse effects of sodium bicarbonate such as an increase in systemic pH and high sodium load may be useful in the management of certain pharmacological toxicities and overdoses. Below we will review the utility and likely mechanisms of sodium bicarbonate in the management of certain pharmacological toxicities: sodium channel blockers, salicylates, methanol and ethylene glycol poisonings, and, finally, miscellaneous pharmacological toxicities.

TABLE 2: List of some drugs with sodium channel blocking properties.

Class	Representative medications
Class Ia antiarrhythmics	Quinidine, Procainamide
Class Ib antiarrhythmics	Lidocaine, Phenytoin
Class Ic antiarrhythmics	Propafenone, Flecainide
Class III antiarrhythmics	Amiodarone, Sotalol
Tricyclic antidepressants	Amitriptyline, Doxepin
Antiepileptic medications	Carbamazepine, Lamotrigine, Zonisamide, Lacosamide
Selective serotonin reuptake inhibitors	Citalopram, Venlafaxine, Fluoxetine
Antihistamines	Diphenhydramine
Miscellaneous	Cocaine, local anesthetics, Thioridazine, Propranolol, Amantadine, Chloroquine, Hydroxychloroquine, Cyclobenzaprine

3. The Role of Sodium Bicarbonate in the Management of Sodium Channel Blocker Toxicities

Sodium channels are essential ion channels responsible for transcellular sodium influx, primarily in cardiac and neurological tissue [18]. Pharmacological agents targeting sodium channels are used in cardiac electrophysiology and neurology (particularly in the areas of pain management and epilepsy) [19, 20], as well as depression [21]. However, in cases of excessive administration (intentional or not), sodium channel blockade may lead to serious cardiac dysfunction. A list of some of the commonly used medications possessing sodium channel blocking activities is presented in Table 2.

Tricyclic antidepressants (TCAs) are among the oldest antidepressant medications that may also be used in the management of mood disorders, generalized anxiety disorder, panic disorder, and neuropathic pain [21]. Despite being an effective class, it is notorious for its narrow therapeutic index and major side effect profile in cases of overdose. TCAs were responsible for approximately 58% of all antidepressant medications related fatal toxicities in 2013 [22]. The pathogenesis of TCA toxicity in regard to sodium channel blockade is fundamental to the understanding of other sodium channel toxicities, as is the therapeutic role of intravenous (IV) sodium bicarbonate. It is important to remember that the pharmacopathogenesis of TCA toxicities is more complex than just sodium channel blockade and also includes inhibition of muscarinic, alpha-1 adrenergic, and antihistamine receptors [23]. Inhibition of cardiac sodium channels may manifest on the electrocardiogram (ECG) as the prolongation of QRS interval, new onset right axis deviation, deep S wave in lead AVL, tall R wave, and increased R wave to S wave ration in lead AVR and Brugada-like pattern [24–28]. Clinically the effects of sodium channel blockade may present as cardiac arrhythmias and hemodynamic instability [29]. Metabolic acidosis that occurs in cases of hemodynamic deterioration potentiates the sodium blocking activity of TCA medications by increasing the binding to sodium channels [29–31]. Furthermore, TCA toxicity can cause seizures resulting in persistence of metabolic acidosis

and propagation of detrimental metabolic disturbances. TCA toxicity may be delayed and patients may initially appear clinically well until decompensation occurs.

The scientific data on the use of sodium bicarbonate in the management of TCA toxicity is predominantly originated from animal studies, case reports, and case series [32, 33]. Sodium bicarbonate is commonly administered as 8.4% solution 1-2 mEq/kg (see Table 1) in cases of TCA associated ECG abnormalities (such as QRS prolongation > 100 msec), hemodynamic compromise, and malignant ventricular arrhythmias [34–36]. The benefit of sodium bicarbonate in the setting of TCA overdose is probably due to both an increase in serum pH and the increase in extracellular sodium. Alkalization favors the neutral form of the drug and reducing the amount of active cyclic antidepressants. The high sodium load increases the electrochemical gradient across cardiac cell membranes, potentially attenuating the TCA-induced blockade of sodium channels [29, 30].

Based on clinical experience and available literature, the majority of patients tend to respond via improvement in hemodynamic and ECG parameters. 12-lead ECG of sodium channel blocker toxicity before and after administration of sodium bicarbonate is presented in Figures 2(a) and 2(b).

It may be necessary to continue sodium bicarbonate after bolus doses in the form of IV infusion by diluting 2-3 ampules in 1 liter of dextrose 5% solution that is nearly isotonic to plasma to decrease the risk of potential rebound deterioration, while, on IV sodium bicarbonate, patients should be monitored for evidence of fluid overload, respiratory status with advanced airway management when indicated, electrolyte abnormalities (hypernatremia, hypokalemia, hypocalcemia), and metabolic alkalosis (potential target pH of 7.5). It is important to keep in mind that because of its anticholinergic properties, the absorption of the TCA may be delayed (due to delayed gastrointestinal motility); these patients should be closely monitored, and, in cases of reemerging symptoms, sodium bicarbonate and other therapies must be timely administered. Patients treated with sodium bicarbonate should be monitored in the intensive care setting with continuous monitoring and reassessment. Frequency of laboratory testing and electrocardiographic

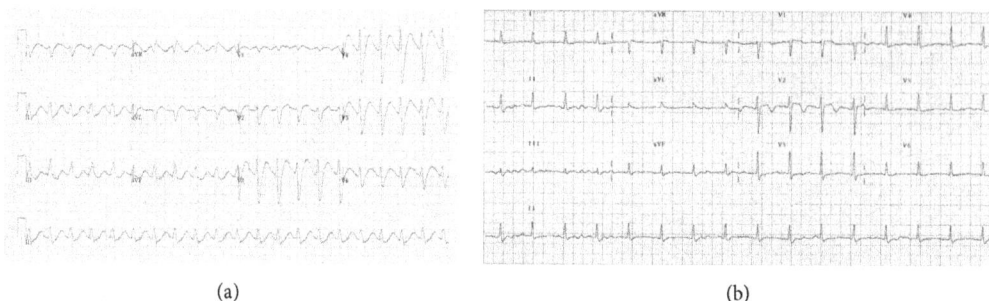

(a)   (b)

FIGURE 2: (a) *Sodium channel toxicity on 12-lead ECG (taken from https://lifeinthefastlane.com).* On this 12-lead ECG you can see regular wide QRS tachycardia with no clear P waves, right axis deviation, tall R wave in AVR, and poor R wave progression in precordial leads. (b) *Sodium channel toxicity on 12-lead ECG after administration of sodium bicarbonate (taken from https://lifeinthefastlane.com).* On this 12-lead ECG after administration of sodium bicarbonate you can see atrioventricular dissociation with normal QRS, normal axis, and resolution of tall R wave in AVR.

monitoring should be individualized. Blood gas analysis (arterial or venous) and chemistry tests should be monitored at least every 4 hours or more frequently if clinically indicated in patients treated with sodium bicarbonate. It is important to keep calcium and potassium within normal range and replete them if low to decrease the risk of cardiac arrhythmias.

Other medications such as antiarrhythmics [36–38], non-TCA antidepressants [39, 40], antiepileptic medications [41–43], cyclobenzaprine [43, 44], propranolol [45], cocaine [46], and certain antihistamines [47] may produce similar ECG and clinical manifestations with favorable response to similarly administered IV sodium bicarbonate. Amantadine overdose may result in a similar cardiac sodium channel toxicity though IV sodium bicarbonate was not specifically used in the reported cases because of concomitant hypokalemia [48]. Animal research supports the beneficial effects of sodium bicarbonate in case of thioridazine toxicity [49].

In conclusion, the literature on the use of sodium bicarbonate in the management of sodium channel blocker toxicities is limited to animal research and case series; randomized trials are precluded due to ethical reasons. IV sodium bicarbonate should be considered in the cases of suspected sodium channel blocker toxicity associated with hemodynamic and ECG abnormalities, given the very high risk of adverse outcome without aggressive treatment [50]. Nevertheless, it is important to keep in mind that IV sodium bicarbonate represents only a single tool in the management of these toxicities and additional mechanisms of toxicity may account for protean clinical manifestations of these poisonings.

4. The Role of Sodium Bicarbonate in the Management of Salicylate Toxicity

Salicylates are a group of pharmacological agents that include aspirin, bismuth salicylate, and local skin preparations such as salicylic acid and methyl salicylate (topical preparations that rarely cause toxicity if used in an excessive amount or in patients with skin damage leading to increased absorption) [51, 52]. Aspirin, which is a major representative of the class,

has myriad of indications including cardiovascular diseases, rheumatic diseases, and analgesia [53].

Analgesics, including aspirin, were the most common etiology of all drug poisonings in the USA, with salicylate poisoning leading to a fatal outcome in 34 patients out of 2113 deaths reported in 2013 [54]. The major mechanism of action of aspirin is mediated via inhibition of cyclooxygenase enzyme, resulting in decreased production of thromboxane A2 and various prostaglandins [53]. However, with higher dosages, other biochemical alterations may occur such as uncoupling of oxidative phosphorylation in the electron transport chain, resulting in heat release and stimulation of respiratory center in the medulla [23]. The decrease in the blood pH will favor formation of lipid soluble salicylic acid which easily penetrates blood-brain barrier and undergoes renal reabsorption [55].

Patients with salicylate toxicity typically present with tinnitus, gastrointestinal complications (nausea, vomiting, bleeding, and liver toxicity), hyperthermia (via uncoupling of oxidative phosphorylation), pulmonary edema, and mixed acid-base disorder (high anion gap metabolic acidosis and respiratory alkalosis via stimulation of respiratory center in the brain stem) [55].

Alkalinization with sodium bicarbonate is an essential component of management of the aspirin-poisoned patient. The first report in the English language medical literature of the positive effect of sodium bicarbonate in the management of salicylate-poisoned patient originates in 1948 [55].

Salicylic acid (HS) is a weak acid that exists in a charged (deprotonated, sal^-) and uncharged (protonated, H^+) form: $H^+ + sal^- \Leftrightarrow HS$. Uncharged molecules (HS), unlike charged molecules (sal^-), can move easily across cellular barriers, including the blood-brain barrier and the epithelium of the renal tubule. Metabolic acidosis drives the above reaction to the right and increases the plasma concentration of HS, thereby promoting diffusion across the blood-brain barrier into the CNS. In patients with salicylate intoxication, the beneficial effects of sodium bicarbonate are mediated by the production of metabolic alkalosis that decreases the amount of lipid soluble salicylate and driving the above reaction to the left resulting in decreased penetration into central

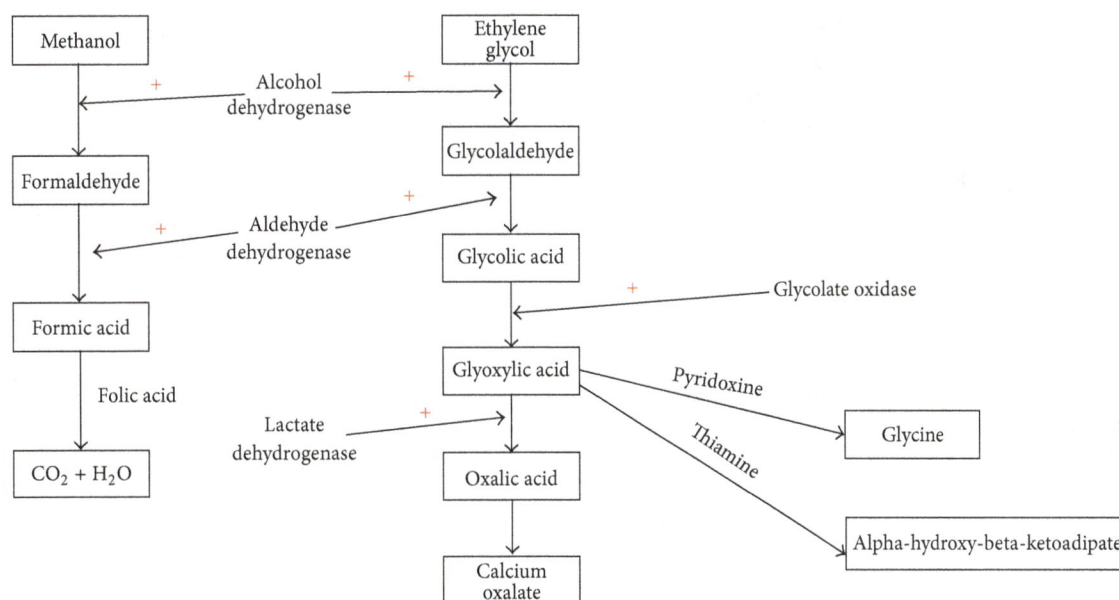

FIGURE 3: An overview of in vivo methanol and ethylene glycol metabolism.

nervous system and in increased urinary clearance [56]. As was discussed above, IV sodium bicarbonate may have serious undesired effects including hypokalemia. The development of hypokalemia is particularly detrimental to the patients with salicylate-mediated toxicity because of increase in hydrogen ion urinary excretion resulting in more acidic urine and greater salicylate reabsorption and thus, should be aggressively corrected [55, 56]. It is important to note that mild alkalemia from a respiratory alkalosis (arterial pH < 7.55) is not a contraindication to sodium bicarbonate therapy in salicylate poisoning. There is no scientifically validated dosing of IV sodium bicarbonate (as in the management of sodium channel blocker toxicities) but it is typically dosed as 1-2 mEq/kg initially administered in bolus doses (see Table 1) and then may be administered as a continuous IV infusion after dilution in dextrose 5% solution [56]. The infusion rate should be titrated to target a urine pH 7.5–8. Blood gas analysis every two hours is indicated for monitoring to prevent severe alkalemia (arterial pH > 7.60) [55, 56]. Patients with anuric renal failure should not receive IV sodium bicarbonate but rather be evaluated for renal replacement therapy [55].

5. The Role of Sodium Bicarbonate in the Management of Methanol and Ethylene Glycol Poisoning

Methanol and ethylene glycol are alcohols commonly used in household solutions such as various cleaners, solvents, machine fluids, and antifreeze solutions [57]. There were 52430 exposures to alcohols resulting in 174 fatalities in 2013 [55]. The majority of toxicities arise either as a result of a suicidal attempt or after drinking the toxic alcohol as a substitute for ethanol [57].

To understand the basic pathogenesis of methanol and ethylene glycol toxicity, it is important to review briefly the metabolism in vivo. When ingested, both methanol and ethylene glycol undergo an initial biochemical reaction catalyzed by alcohol dehydrogenase (the same enzyme metabolizing ethanol) converting the parent alcohol into formaldehyde and glycolaldehyde, respectively. The metabolism of methanol and ethylene glycol disrupts cellular energy metabolism leading to cellular damage [58, 59]. The final products of methanol and ethylene glycol metabolism are formic acid and oxalic acid, respectively [57]. These end products result in classic features of toxicity such as retinal toxicity caused by methanol and renal injury mediated by oxalic acid. A brief sketch of the in vivo methanol and ethylene glycol metabolism is presented in Figure 3.

Clinical presentations of methanol and ethylene glycol overlap, including central nervous system (CNS) symptoms such as headache, altered mental status, and seizures. Retinal toxicity and blindness are more specific for methanol; acute kidney injury and hypocalcemia are more typical for ethylene glycol intoxication. Laboratory testing and diagnosis are based on the presence of high anion gap metabolic acidosis, the presence of a serum osmolal gap (the difference between measured and calculated osmolality > 10), and measuring the levels of toxic alcohols (used for confirmation; typically, this testing is not time sensitive, and the treatment should not be withheld in any patient suspected of having toxic alcohol ingestion).

As in the management of other discussed toxidromes, the literature on the benefits of IV sodium bicarbonate originates from case reports and consensus guidelines [58, 59]. Beneficial effects of sodium bicarbonate in the management of methanol and ethylene glycol poisoning are believed to be secondary to the formation and enhanced urinary clearance of less toxic metabolites (formate) [59]. Acidemia leads to protonation of methanol and ethylene glycol metabolites to uncharged molecules (e.g., formic acid and oxalic acid), making them more likely to penetrate end-organ tissues (such as the retina) and more likely to be reabsorbed across the renal epithelium from the urine [58]. The suggested regimen for IV sodium bicarbonate is similar to the above-discussed indications. However, according to the consensus guidelines, the therapy with IV sodium bicarbonate should be strongly considered when pH falls below 7.3 with the therapeutic aim of pH normalization. As is the case with any treatment involving IV sodium bicarbonate, administration necessitates frequent monitoring of metabolic parameters (serum electrolytes and renal function), cardiopulmonary, and renal status of the patient. Administration of sodium bicarbonate should be used with caution in a patient with oliguric/anuric renal failure (which is classically seen in severe ethylene glycol toxicity). It is important to note that symptomatic hypocalcemia should be corrected (the routine correction of asymptomatic hypocalcemia is discouraged because of the possible increase in the formation of calcium oxalate crystals in ethylene glycol toxicity).

6. The Role of Sodium Bicarbonate in the Management of Miscellaneous Drug Toxicities

IV administration of sodium bicarbonate may result in enhanced urinary excretion of certain chemicals through urinary alkalinization [56]. The urinary clearance of methotrexate, phenobarbital, chlorpropamide, and fluoride is increased after reaching urinary pH levels of 7.5–8.0 via formation of lipid insoluble metabolite of the parent drug.

Metformin toxicity is another instance where sodium bicarbonate may be used [60]. In rare circumstances (such as acute illness and worsening renal function), metformin administration may result in the development of lactic acidosis that is believed to be secondary to mitochondrial dysfunction, with a shift towards anaerobic glycolysis [60–62]. Though the literature on the role of systemic bicarbonate administration in cases of metformin poisoning is very scant, the use of IV sodium bicarbonate should be probably limited to nonanuric patients with metformin-associated advanced metabolic acidosis and pH < 7.1, given the questionable efficacy and potential for adverse effects.

In conclusion, the data on the role of sodium bicarbonate in the management of the above-listed medications is even more limited and cannot be recommended as a first line.

7. Conclusion

Based on the available literature and empiric experience, the IV administration of sodium bicarbonate appears to be beneficial in the management of certain pharmacological toxicities such as sodium channel blockers poisonings, salicylate intoxication, and ingestion of methanol and ethylene glycol. However, most of the data originates from case reports, case series, and expert consensus recommendations. The data on the management of metformin-associated lactic acidosis, chlorpropamide, methotrexate, and phenobarbital is even more limited. However, it seems very unlikely that randomized controlled trials assessing the impact of sodium bicarbonate will be performed due to ethical concerns.

The potential mechanisms of sodium bicarbonate administration include high sodium load, development of metabolic alkalosis with resultant decreased tissue penetration of the toxic substance, and its increased urinary excretion, while, on IV sodium bicarbonate, the patients must be monitored for the development of associated side effects including electrolyte abnormalities (hypokalemia, hypocalcemia, and hypernatremia), progression of metabolic alkalosis volume overload, worsening respiratory status (volume overload and increased CO_2 production), and worsening metabolic acidosis (paradoxical increase in lactic acid production secondary to the activation of glycolytic enzymes). Frequency of laboratory testing should be individualized. Blood gas analysis (arterial or venous) and chemistry tests should be monitored at least every 4 hours or more frequently if clinically indicated in patients treated with sodium bicarbonate. It is important to keep calcium and potassium within normal range to decrease the risk of cardiac arrhythmias.

Patients with oliguric/anuric renal failure and advanced decompensated heart failure should not receive IV sodium bicarbonate. IV administration of sodium bicarbonate represents only one aspect of the complex management of medication and chemical toxicities, and, for a thorough discussion of the management of these toxicities, the reader is referred to focused reviews.

Abbreviations

CNS: Central nervous system
ECG: Electrocardiogram
IV: Intravenous
TCA: Tricyclic antidepressant
USA: United States of America.

References

[1] http://www.cdc.gov/nchs/data/hus/hus14.pdf#085, 2015.

[2] K. Alka and J. R. Casey, "Bicarbonate transport in health and disease," *IUBMB Life*, vol. 66, no. 9, pp. 596–615, 2014.

[3] T. Dybvik, T. Strand, and P. A. Steen, "Buffer therapy during out-of-hospital cardiopulmonary resuscitation," *Resuscitation*, vol. 29, no. 2, pp. 89–95, 1995.

[4] R. B. Vukmir and L. Katz, "Sodium bicarbonate improves outcome in prolonged prehospital cardiac arrest," *American Journal of Emergency Medicine*, vol. 24, no. 2, pp. 156–161, 2006.

[5] S. S. Brar, A. Y.-J. Shen, M. B. Jorgensen et al., "Sodium bicarbonate vs sodium chloride for the prevention of contrast medium-induced nephropathy in patients undergoing coronary angiography: a randomized trial," *JAMA—Journal of the*

American Medical Association, vol. 300, no. 9, pp. 1038–1046, 2008.

[6] S. M. Forsythe and G. A. Schmidt, "Sodium bicarbonate for the treatment of lactic acidosis," *Chest*, vol. 117, no. 1, pp. 260–267, 2000.

[7] A. Viallon, F. Zeni, P. Lafond et al., "Does bicarbonate therapy improve the management of severe diabetic ketoacidosis?" *Critical Care Medicine*, vol. 27, no. 12, pp. 2690–2693, 1999.

[8] M. H. Weil, E. C. Rackow, R. Trevino, W. Grundler, J. L. Falk, and M. I. Griffel, "Difference in acid-base state between venous and arterial blood during cardiopulmonary resuscitation," *The New England Journal of Medicine*, vol. 315, no. 3, pp. 153–156, 1986.

[9] H. J. Adrogue, N. Rashad, A. B. Gorin, J. Yacoub, and N. E. Madias, "Assessing acid-base status in circulatory failure. Differences between arterial and central venous blood," *Survey of anesthesiology*, vol. 33, no. 6, article 320, 1989.

[10] J. B. Posner and F. Plum, "Spinal-fluid pH and neurologic symptoms in systemic acidosis," *The New England Journal of Medicine*, vol. 277, no. 12, pp. 605–613, 1967.

[11] M. Peacock, "Calcium metabolism in health and disease," *Clinical Journal of the American Society of Nephrology*, vol. 5, supplement 1, pp. S23–S30, 2010.

[12] R. M. Lang, S. K. Fellner, A. Neumann, D. A. Bushinsky, and K. M. Borow, "Left ventricular contractility varies directly with blood ionized calcium," *Annals of Internal Medicine*, vol. 108, no. 4, pp. 524–529, 1988.

[13] C. Overgaard-Steensen and T. Ring, "Clinical review: practical approach to hyponatraemia and hypernatraemia in critically ill patients," *Critical Care*, vol. 17, no. 1, article 206, 2013.

[14] V. L. Hood and R. L. Tannen, "Mechanisms of disease: Protection of acid-base balance by pH regulation of acid production," *New England Journal of Medicine*, vol. 339, no. 12, pp. 819–826, 1998.

[15] Y. Okuda, H. J. Adrogue, J. B. Field, H. Nohara, and K. Yamashita, "Counterproductive effects of sodium bicarbonate in diabetic ketoacidosis," *Journal of Clinical Endocrinology and Metabolism*, vol. 81, no. 1, pp. 314–320, 1996.

[16] W. A. Neill and M. Hattenhauer, "Impairment of myocardial O2 supply due to hyperventilation," *Circulation*, vol. 52, no. 5, pp. 854–858, 1975.

[17] J. R. Wilson, S. Goldberg, J. W. Hirshfeld, and A. H. Harken, "Effects of respiratory alkalosis on coronary vascular dynamics and myocardial energetics in patients with coronary artery disease," *American Heart Journal*, vol. 102, no. 2, pp. 202–205, 1981.

[18] C. H. Peters and P. C. Ruben, "Introduction to sodium channels.," *Handbook of experimental pharmacology*, vol. 221, pp. 1–6, 2014.

[19] M. R. Rosen and P. J. Schwartz, "The Sicilian gambit. A new approach to the classification of antiarrhythmic drugs based on their actions on arrhythmogenic mechanisms," *Circulation*, vol. 84, no. 4, pp. 1831–1851, 1991.

[20] C. E. Stafstrom, "Mechanisms of action of antiepileptic drugs: the search for synergy," *Current Opinion in Neurology*, vol. 23, no. 2, pp. 157–163, 2010.

[21] J. M. Dupuy, M. J. Ostacher, J. Huffman, R. H. Perlis, and A. A. Nierenberg, "A critical review of pharmacotherapy for major depressive disorder," *International Journal of Neuropsychopharmacology*, vol. 14, no. 10, pp. 1417–1431, 2011.

[22] W. A. Watson, T. L. Litovitz, G. C. Rodgers Jr. et al., "2004 Annual report of the American Association of Poison Control Centers Toxic Exposure Surveillance System," *American Journal of Emergency Medicine*, vol. 23, no. 5, pp. 589–666, 2005.

[23] P. K. Gillman, "Tricyclic antidepressant pharmacology and therapeutic drug interactions updated," *British Journal of Pharmacology*, vol. 151, no. 6, pp. 737–748, 2007.

[24] K. H. Choi and K.-U. Lee, "Serial monitoring of lead aVR in patients with prolonged unconsciousness following tricyclic antidepressant overdose," *Psychiatry Investigation*, vol. 5, no. 4, pp. 247–250, 2008.

[25] F. Eyer, J. Stenzel, T. Schuster et al., "Risk assessment of severe tricyclic antidepressant overdose," *Human and Experimental Toxicology*, vol. 28, no. 8, pp. 511–519, 2009.

[26] J. Veris-van Dieren, L. Valk, I. Van Geijlswijk, D. Tjan, and A. Van Zanten, "Coma with ECG abnormalities: consider tricyclic antidepressant intoxication," *Netherlands Journal of Medicine*, vol. 65, no. 4, pp. 142–146, 2007.

[27] A. Meert, N. Vermeersch, R. Beckers, W. Hoste, P. Brugada, and I. Hubloue, "Brugada-like ECG pattern induced by tricyclic antidepressants," *European Journal of Emergency Medicine*, vol. 17, no. 6, pp. 325–327, 2010.

[28] R. A. Harrigan and W. J. Brady, "ECG abnormalities in tricyclic antidepressant ingestion," *American Journal of Emergency Medicine*, vol. 17, no. 4, pp. 387–393, 1999.

[29] A. H. Glassman, "Cardiovascular effects of tricyclic antidepressants," *Annual Review of Medicine*, vol. 35, pp. 503–511, 1984.

[30] B. I. Sasyniuk and V. Jhamandas, "Mechanism of reversal of toxic effects of amitriptyline on cardiac Purkinje fibers by sodium bicarbonate," *Journal of Pharmacology and Experimental Therapeutics*, vol. 231, no. 2, pp. 387–394, 1984.

[31] P. Pentel and N. Benowitz, "Efficacy and mechanism of action of sodium bicarbonate in the treatment of desipramine toxicity in rats," *The Journal of Pharmacology and Experimental Therapeutics*, vol. 230, pp. 12–19, 1984.

[32] J. R. Hoffman, S. R. Votey, M. Bayer, and L. Silver, "Effect of hypertonic sodium bicarbonate in the treatment of moderate-to-severe cyclic antidepressant overdose," *American Journal of Emergency Medicine*, vol. 11, no. 4, pp. 336–341, 1993.

[33] S. M. Bradberry, H. K. R. Thanacoody, B. E. Watt, S. H. L. Thomas, and J. A. Vale, "Management of the cardiovascular complications of tricyclic antidepressant: poisoning role of sodium bicarbonate," *Toxicological Reviews*, vol. 24, no. 3, pp. 195–204, 2005.

[34] H. Sanaei-Zadeh and A. Ghassemi Toussi, "Resolution of wide complex tachycardia after administration of hypertonic sodium bicarbonate in a patient with severe tricyclic antidepressant poisoning," *Resuscitation*, vol. 82, no. 6, pp. 792–793, 2011.

[35] K. Blackman, S. G. A. Brown, and G. J. Wilkes, "Plasma alkalinization for tricyclic antidepressant toxicity: a systematic review," *Emergency Medicine*, vol. 13, no. 2, pp. 204–210, 2001.

[36] C. Köppel, U. Oberdisse, and G. Heinemeyer, "Clinical course and outcome in class ic antiarrhythmic overdose," *Clinical Toxicology*, vol. 28, no. 4, pp. 433–444, 1990.

[37] E. Bou-Abboud and S. Nattel, "Relative role of alkalosis and sodium ions in reversal of class I antiarrhythmic drug-induced sodium channel blockade by sodium bicarbonate," *Circulation*, vol. 94, no. 8, pp. 1954–1961, 1996.

[38] P.-Y. Courand, F. Sibellas, S. Ranc, A. Mullier, G. Kirkorian, and E. Bonnefoy, "Arrhythmogenic effect of flecainide toxicity," *Cardiology Journal*, vol. 20, no. 2, pp. 203–205, 2013.

[39] D. D. Lung, A. H. B. Wu, and R. R. Gerona, "Cardiotoxicity in a citalopram and olanzapine overdose," *Journal of Emergency Medicine*, vol. 45, no. 4, pp. 554–558, 2013.

[40] A. Graudins, C. Vossler, and R. Wang, "Fluoxetine-induced cardiotoxicity with response to bicarbonate therapy," *American Journal of Emergency Medicine*, vol. 15, no. 5, pp. 501–503, 1997.

[41] T. J. S. Herold, "Lamotrigine as a possible cause of QRS prolongation in a patient with known seizure disorder," *Canadian Journal of Emergency Medicine*, vol. 8, no. 5, pp. 361–364, 2006.

[42] N. Venkatraman, D. O'Neil, and A. Hall, "Life-threatening overdose with lamotrigine, citalopram, and chlorpheniramine," *Journal of Postgraduate Medicine*, vol. 54, no. 4, pp. 316-317, 2008.

[43] J. L. Chua-Tuan, D. Cao, J. L. Iwanicki, and C. O. Hoyte, "Cardiac sodium channel blockade after an intentional ingestion of lacosamide, cyclobenzaprine, and levetiracetam: case report," *Clinical Toxicology*, vol. 53, no. 6, pp. 565–568, 2015.

[44] V. S. Bebarta, J. Maddry, D. J. Borys, and D. L. Morgan, "Incidence of tricyclic antidepressant-like complications after cyclobenzaprine overdose," *American Journal of Emergency Medicine*, vol. 29, no. 6, pp. 645–649, 2011.

[45] U. R. Shanker, J. Webb, and A. Kotze, "Sodium bicarbonate to treat massive β blocker overdose," *Emergency Medicine Journal*, vol. 20, no. 4, p. 393, 2003.

[46] E. A. Kalimullah and S. M. Bryant, "Case files of the medical toxicology fellowship at the toxikon consortium in Chicago: cocaine-associated wide-complex dysrhythmias and cardiac arrest—treatment nuances and controversies," *Journal of Medical Toxicology*, vol. 4, no. 4, pp. 277–283, 2008.

[47] D. H. Jang, A. F. Manini, N. S. Trueger et al., "Status epilepticus and wide-complex tachycardia secondary to diphenhydramine overdose," *Clinical Toxicology*, vol. 48, no. 9, pp. 945–948, 2010.

[48] M. D. Schwartz, M. M. Patel, Z. N. Kazzi, and B. W. Morgan, "Cardiotoxicity after massive amantadine overdose," *Journal of Medical Toxicology*, vol. 4, no. 3, pp. 173–179, 2008.

[49] R. Y. Wang and R. M. Raymond, "The effects of sodium bicarbonate on thioridazine-induced cardiac dysfunction in the isolated perfused rat heart," *Veterinary and Human Toxicology*, vol. 43, pp. 73–77, 2001.

[50] R. E. Bruccoleri and M. M. Burns, "A literature review of the use of sodium bicarbonate for the treatment of QRS widening," *Journal of Medical Toxicology*, vol. 12, no. 1, pp. 121–129, 2016.

[51] J. E. Davis, "Are one or two dangerous? Methyl salicylate exposure in toddlers," *Journal of Emergency Medicine*, vol. 32, no. 1, pp. 63–69, 2007.

[52] J. Herres, D. Ryan, and M. Salzman, "Delayed salicylate toxicity with undetectable initial levels after large-dose aspirin ingestion," *American Journal of Emergency Medicine*, vol. 27, no. 9, pp. 1173-e1, 2009.

[53] J. Y. Wick, "Aspirin: a history, a love story," *Consultant Pharmacist*, vol. 27, no. 5, pp. 322–329, 2012.

[54] J. B. Mowry, D. A. Spyker, L. R. Cantilena Jr., N. McMillan, and M. Ford, "2013 annual report of the American Association of Poison Control Centers' National Poison Data System (NPDS): 31st annual report," *Clinical Toxicology*, vol. 52, no. 10, pp. 1032–1283, 2014.

[55] G. F. O'Malley, "Emergency department management of the salicylate-poisoned patient," *Emergency Medicine Clinics of North America*, vol. 25, no. 2, pp. 333–346, 2007.

[56] A. T. Proudfoot, E. P. Krenzelok, and J. A. Vale, "Position Paper on Urine Alkalinization," *Journal of Toxicology - Clinical Toxicology*, vol. 42, no. 1, pp. 1–26, 2004.

[57] J. A. Kraut, "Diagnosis of toxic alcohols: limitations of present methods," *Clinical Toxicology*, vol. 53, no. 7, pp. 589–595, 2015.

[58] D. G. Barceloux, E. P. Krenzelok, K. Olson, W. Watson, and H. Miller, "American academy of clinical toxicology practice guidelines on the treatment of ethylene glycol poisoning. Ad Hoc committee," *Journal of Toxicology—Clinical Toxicology*, vol. 37, no. 5, pp. 537–560, 1999.

[59] D. G. Barceloux, G. R. Bond, E. P. Krenzelok, H. Cooper, and J. A. Vale, "American Academy of Clinical Toxicology practice guidelines on the treatment of methanol poisoning," *Journal of Toxicology—Clinical Toxicology*, vol. 40, no. 4, pp. 415–446, 2002.

[60] A. Protti, A. Lecchi, F. Fortunato et al., "Metformin overdose causes platelet mitochondrial dysfunction in humans," *Critical Care*, vol. 16, no. 5, article R180, 2012.

[61] J.-C. Orban, E. Fontaine, and C. Ichai, "Metformin overdose: time to move on," *Critical Care*, vol. 16, no. 5, article 164, 2012.

[62] B. A. Kriegsman and B. G. Hanna, "Metformin-associated lactic acidosis in a patient with normal renal function," *Clinical Diabetes*, vol. 33, no. 4, pp. 193-194, 2015.

19

Assessing the Association between Serum Ferritin, Transferrin Saturation, and C-Reactive Protein in Northern Territory Indigenous Australian Patients with High Serum Ferritin on Maintenance Haemodialysis

Sandawana William Majoni,[1,2,3] **Paul D. Lawton,**[3] **Federica Barzi,**[3] **Alan Cass,**[3] **and Jaquelyne T. Hughes**[1,3]

[1]*Royal Darwin Hospital, Department of Nephrology, Division of Medicine, Tiwi, Darwin, NT, Australia*
[2]*Northern Territory Medical Programme, Flinders University School of Medicine, Tiwi, Darwin, NT, Australia*
[3]*Wellbeing and Preventable Chronic Disease Division, Menzies School of Health Research, Charles Darwin University, Casuarina, NT, Australia*

Correspondence should be addressed to Sandawana William Majoni; sandawanaw@aol.com

Academic Editor: Jaime Uribarri

Objective. To determine the significance of high serum ferritin observed in Indigenous Australian patients on maintenance haemodialysis in the Northern Territory, we assessed the relationship between ferritin and transferrin saturation (TSAT) as measures of iron status and ferritin and C-reactive protein (CRP) as markers of inflammation. *Methods.* We performed a retrospective cohort analysis of data from adult patients ($\geq$18 years) on maintenance haemodialysis (>3 months) from 2004 to 2011. *Results.* There were 1568 patients. The mean age was 53.9 (11.9) years. 1244 (79.3%) were Indigenous. 44.2% (n = 693) were male. Indigenous patients were younger (mean age [52.3 (11.1) versus 57.4 (15.2), p < 0.001]) and had higher CRP [14.7 mg/l (7–35) versus 5.9 mg/l (1.9–17.5), p < 0.001], higher median serum ferritin [1069 μg/l (668–1522) versus 794.9 μg/l (558.5–1252.0), p < 0.001], but similar transferrin saturation [26% (19–37) versus 28% (20–38), p = 0.516]. We observed a small positive correlation between ferritin and TSAT (r^2 = 0.11, p < 0.001), no correlation between ferritin and CRP (r^2 = 0.001, p < 0.001), and positive association between high serum ferritin and TSAT (p < 0.001), Indigenous ethnicity (p < 0.001), urea reduction ratio (p = 0.001), and gender (p < 0.001) after adjustment in mixed regression analysis. *Conclusion.* Serum ferritin and TSAT may inadequately reflect iron status in this population. The high ferritin was poorly explained by inflammation.

1. Introduction

The effective treatment of anaemia in patients on maintenance haemodialysis (MHD) includes identification and correction of iron deficiency [1], use of erythropoiesis stimulating agents (ESA) as necessary, and achieving dialysis adequacy. Interpretation of iron status from most guidelines on anaemia management in people on MHD has been mainly based on transferrin saturation [the ratio of serum iron to the total iron binding capacity (TIBC) as a percentage, TSAT] and serum ferritin. Other measures of iron status have also been examined and include percentage hypochromic red cells (PHRC), reticulocyte haemoglobin content, and soluble transferrin receptor [2–4]. The accurate determination of iron status is critical in patients dependent on maintenance haemodialysis in order to avoid overtreatment resulting in iron overload and minimising continuing anaemia from undertreatment of iron deficiency.

The combination of serum ferritin levels and TSAT are commonly used worldwide in Renal Anaemia Management guidelines [2, 5]. Low TSAT and low ferritin are indicative of iron deficiency. However, recent published evidence suggests

TABLE 1: Guidelines on target levels of markers of iron status in people with CKD.

Guidelines	Continent	Ferritin (μg/l)	TSAT (%)
Canadian Renal Guidelines	Canada	100–500	>20
KDIGO	Worldwide	100–500	>20
ERA-EDTA	Europe	200–300	30–50
CARI	Australia & New Zealand	200–500	30–40
KDOQI	United States	200–500	30–50
UK Renal Association/NICE	United Kingdom	250–500	>20

CARI: Caring for Australasians with Renal Insufficiency, KDOQI: Kidney Disease Outcome Quality Initiative, UK Renal Association: United Kingdom Renal Association, NICE: National Institute for Health and Care Excellence, ERA-EDTA: European Renal Association-European Dialysis and Transplant Association, and KDIGO: Kidney Disease: Improving Global Outcomes [1, 7].

that TSAT is a better marker of iron status than ferritin and is more predictive of the response to treatment of anaemia in MHD patients [6]. Therapeutic supplementation of iron is provided to MHD patients until predetermined targets of these measures are achieved. Internationally, the target levels vary (Table 1). In our analysis, we used the ferritin and TSAT target levels in the Kidney Disease: Improving Global Outcomes (KDIGO) and Caring for Australasians with Renal Insufficiency (CARI) guidelines and their modifications to suit our local needs developed using the results from the DRIVE studies because these guidelines encompass international consensus and apply to our region, respectively.

We recently reported excessive serum ferritin concentrations among Indigenous Australian patients on MHD [7]. However, anaemia management guidelines worldwide presently do not guide iron supplementation in settings of high ferritin, including when high ferritin, an acute phase reactant, occurs in the setting of inflammation. The use of either measure alone has significant problems with lack of accuracy and has been discouraged in a recent special report from the United Kingdom National Institute for Health and Care Excellence (NICE) [8]. There is accumulating evidence that high serum ferritin concentrations are associated with high rates of hospitalisations, cardiovascular disease, and mortality. Given the concerns of high dose iron supplementation in ESKD among populations with high background serum ferritin levels and high comorbid cardiovascular disease, in this study, we examined the relationship between serum ferritin levels and TSAT as measures of iron status and serum ferritin levels and C-reactive protein (CRP) as markers of inflammation among Indigenous Australian patients dependent on MHD [7]. The analysis tested the hypothesis that (1) the high serum ferritin levels and TSAT may be inadequate as measures of iron status and (2) the high serum ferritin levels had no association with CRP as an inflammatory marker in Indigenous Australian patients from the Northern Territory who were on MHD.

2. Materials and Methods

2.1. Study Design and Participant Selection. We performed a retrospective cohort analysis of prospectively collected data for the 8-year period from 2004 to 2011 from the renal units serving a majority of Indigenous Australian population of Northern Australia. Adult patients over 18 years of age who

had been on maintenance haemodialysis for at least 3 months were included in the analysis.

2.2. Data Source and Selection. Deidentified data were extracted from the Renal Anaemia Management (RAM) database which contained data collected prospectively every month from all renal units. The RAM database is a system developed by ©Syreon Corporation: Vancouver, BC, Canada, and was maintained by Janssen-Cilag© Pty Limited from all the renal units.

The data from the RAM database was imported into Stata for exploration for errors and consistence. Data quality checks for data integrity was performed that no significant information was lost during the transfer. Only variables relevant to the aims of the analysis were included in the final dataset.

2.3. Statistical Analysis. Exploratory analysis was performed for each variable summarising the data as means and their standard deviations (SD) for continuous normally distributed variables and medians and interquartile ranges (IR) for variables with skewed distributions. A summary analysis was also performed by ethnicity. Pearson's product-moment correlation was run to assess the relationship between (1) ferritin and TSAT as measures of iron status and (2) ferritin and CRP as markers of inflammation.

As part of building a statistical model to assess the relationship between ferritin and TSAT and CRP, a bivariate analysis of the relationship between ferritin and each of the variables was first performed. As the data was longitudinal with multiple observations for each variable and some of them unequally balanced, analyses were carried out using mixed models approach including a random intercept and a random effect to take account of intercorrelation between measurements taken over time for the same patient. Associations of ferritin with the variables were therefore assessed by (1) mixed regression analysis with ferritin as a continuous dependent variable and TSAT as the primary predictor variable and the rest of the variables as covariates and (2) mixed multinomial logistic regression analysis for categorical data with ferritin as a categorical variable as outlined below.

For fitting a regression model to assess the association between ferritin and TSAT with ferritin as a continuous dependent variable, a square root transformation of the ferritin levels was required as the distribution of ferritin was

TABLE 2: Differences in variables by ethnicity.

Variable	Whole sample	Indigenous	Non-Indigenous	p value (by ethnicity)
Ferritin (μg/l)	1022 (590–1491)	1069.5 (668–1522)	558.5 (199–1252)	<0.001
Transferrin saturation (%)	26 (19–37)	26 (19–37)	28 (20–38)	0.516
Haemoglobin (g/l)	107.6 (18.2)	106.6 (18.8)	113.2 (19.0)	<0.001
Potassium (mmol/l)	4.66 (0.86)	4.7 (0.9)	4.6 (0.8)	0.398
BMI (kg/m^2)	26.8 (5.9)	26.3 (6.0)	26.4 (5.2)	0.259
CRP (mg/l)	13.9 (6.0–33.1)	14.7 (7–35)	5.9 (1.9–17.5)	<0.001
Corrected calcium (mmol/l)	2.27 (0.22)	2.26 (0.22)	2.32 (0.19)	<0.001
Albumin (g/l)	37.8 (5.5)	37.7 (5.5)	38.6 (5.4)	<0.001
Magnesium (mmol/l)	0.80 (0.14)	0.79 (0.13)	0.83 (0.16)	<0.001
Bicarbonate (mmol/l)	23.7 (4.6)	23.6 (4.7)	24.0 (4.1)	<0.001
Calcium phosphate product	3.67 (1.40)	3.66 (1.41)	3.75 (1.43)	0.163
Phosphate (mmol/l)	1.63 (0.65)	1.63 (0.65)	1.63 (0.63)	0.163
KT/V	1.61 (0.25)	1.61 (0.26)	1.61 (0.23)	0.171
URR (%)	74.6 (9.3)	74.8 (9.1)	73.2 (11.1)	0.010
ESA dose (IU per week)	11517 (8350)	11691 (8286)	9945 (8757)	<0.001

Data are median (IR) or mean (SD) as indicated.

positively skewed. A variance component model was performed to assess if there was sufficient variance represented at a higher level in the data to justify the use of the mixed model approach. The currently accepted rule is that at least 10% of the total variance needs to be represented at a given level [9]. We used the level of the RAMID (level 2) and the level of the observations (level 1) to determine the total variance. Using only ferritin with no predictors, an empty model was created giving the variance component model estimates at level 2 (i.e., RAMID) and at level 1 (i.e., observations). Estimates from the variance components model were used to calculate the Intraclass Correlation Coefficient (ICC) which was determined as level 2 (RAMID) variance divided by level 2 (RAMID) variance + level 1 (observations) variance. The ICC was $444.3577^2/(444.3577^2 + 521.7812^2) = 0.42037432$. This means that approximately 42% of the total variance in the ferritin levels was represented at the level of the RAMID which is well above the 10% expected to justify using the mixed model. TSAT was then added to the model as the primary predictor followed by the other covariates to build a final multivariable model. Interaction between variables was also assessed, particularly the interaction between ethnicity and the other variables, using product terms to determine any potential interaction among the predictor variables.

For the second part of the assessment ferritin was categorized into 4 categories as low (less than 100 μg/l), "within treated range" (100–800 μg/l), high (800–1200 μg/l), and very high (>1200 μg/l) according to our local guidelines [7] to assess if there were any associations between the different categories of ferritin and TSAT, CRP, and the other variables. TSAT was also categorized as low (<20%), "within treated range" ($\geq$20% to $\leq$30%), high (>30% to <50%), and very high ($\geq$50%) and CRP as low (<10 mg/l) and high ($\geq$10 mg/l).

We also performed complementary sensitivity analyses splitting the sample by ethnicity into Indigenous patients versus non-Indigenous patients in order to examine the association between ferritin and CRP and ferritin and infused iron dose in participants where the infused dose of iron was available.

All analyses were performed using Stata (R) version 13.1 (SE Copyright 1985–2013).

3. Results

There were 1568 adult patients in the study with a mean age of 53.9 (11.9) years; 79.3% ($n = 1244$) were Indigenous Australian patients; and 44.2% were male ($n = 693$). Indigenous patients were younger than non-Indigenous [52.3 (11.1) years versus 57.4 (15.2) years, $p < 0.001$]. The commonest comorbidities in Indigenous patients were hypertension (61.9%), diabetes mellitus (66.6%), and coronary artery disease (61.6%).

Compared with non-Indigenous patients, Indigenous Australian patients had lower haemoglobin ($p < 0.001$), higher serum ferritin levels ($p < 0.001$), CRP ($p < 0.001$), URR ($p = 0.010$), and ESA weekly dose ($p < 0.001$). There were no differences for phosphate ($p = 0.163$), calcium and phosphate product ($p = 0.173$), BMI ($p = 0.259$), TSAT ($p = 0.516$), and KT/V ($p = 0.171$) (Table 2).

3.1. Correlation between Ferritin and TSAT, CRP, and Other Covariates. Ferritin was positively correlated with TSAT ($r^2 = 0.11$, $p < 0.001$) and had a significant association with URR ($p < 0.001$) and KT/V ($p = 0.024$). Ferritin was inversely associated with non-Indigenous ethnicity compared to Indigenous ($p < 0.001$), older age ($p < 0.001$), and higher BMI ($p = 0.009$). There was no correlation observed between ferritin and CRP ($r^2 = 0.001$, $p < 0.001$) (Table 3 and Figures 1 and 2).

3.2. Mixed Regression Model of Serum Ferritin with TSAT as Predictor Variable. A final model developed by stepwise

TABLE 3: Bivariate association of ferritin and other factors using mixed methods.

Variable	Coefficient	p value	95% confidence interval
Male*	0.05	0.590	−0.36–1.12
Non-Indigenous**	−50.70	<0.001	−65.60−−37.95
Haemoglobin	0.00	0.069	0.00–0.00
Potassium	0.10	0.115	−0.03–0.23
Albumin	0.00	0.981	−0.02–0.02
Corrected calcium	−0.09	0.768	−0.69–0.51
Phosphate	0.17	0.085	−0.02–0.37
Calcium phosphate product	0.09	0.068	−0.01–0.18
Parathyroid hormone	0.001	0.800	−0.01–0.01
CRP	0.001	0.546	−0.001–0.003
Urea reduction ratio	0.06	<0.001	0.03–0.09
KTV	2.38	0.024	0.31–4.46
Age at the last review date	−0.06	<0.001	−0.09−−0.03
Body mass index	−0.08	0.009	−0.14−−0.02
Weekly darbepoetin dose	0.00	0.989	−0.01–0.01
Weekly epoetin alfa dose	0.00	0.891	0.00–0.00

*Female is the baseline. **Indigenous is the baseline.

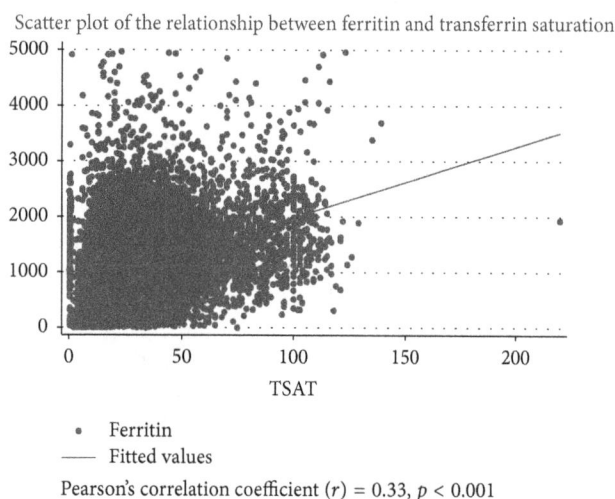

Scatter plot of the relationship between ferritin and transferrin saturation

- Ferritin
—— Fitted values

Pearson's correlation coefficient $(r) = 0.33$, $p < 0.001$

FIGURE 1: Scatter plot of the relationship between serum ferritin concentration and TSAT.

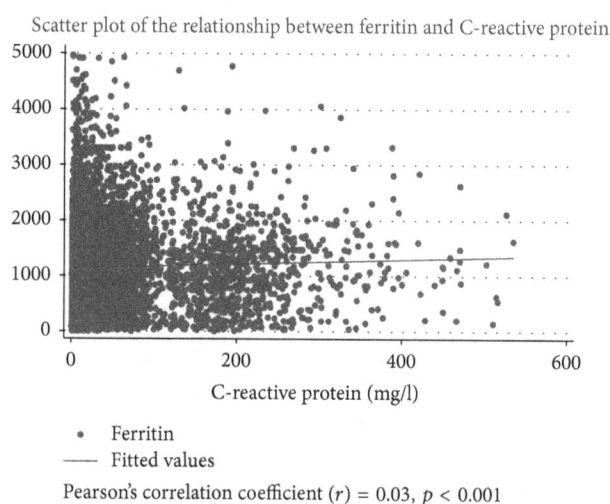

Scatter plot of the relationship between ferritin and C-reactive protein

- Ferritin
—— Fitted values

Pearson's correlation coefficient $(r) = 0.03$, $p < 0.001$

FIGURE 2: Scatter plot of the relationship between serum ferritin concentration and CRP.

sequential selection and addition of variables with a significance level of $p < 0.25$ from the bivariate analysis included no interaction terms as there was no significant interaction between the different covariates. After adjusting for all the covariates, there remained a statistically significant association between ferritin and TSAT ($p < 0.001$), ethnicity ($p < 0.001$), and URR ($p = 0.001$) (Table 4). There was no significant association with CRP.

On mixed multinomial logistic regression, categories of ferritin were positively associated with "within treated range" and higher categories of TSAT ($p < 0.001$), Indigenous ethnicity ($p < 0.001$), and male gender ($p < 0.001$). There was no association between ferritin categories and all CRP categories (Table 5).

We found that although ferritin levels and CRP were higher in Indigenous Australian patients, the sensitivity analyses of the examination of the association between ferritin and CRP and ferritin and infused iron dose in participants where the infused dose of iron was available did not alter the findings observed in the combined cohort.

4. Discussion

Indigenous MHD patients in this study had lower haemoglobin, higher ferritin, CRP, and ESA weekly dose, despite similar concentration of TSAT and similar degree of measures of dialysis adequacy than non-Indigenous patients. Two key findings in this analysis were as follows: (1) the high ferritin levels in our patients are only partly explained by iron

TABLE 4: The final model after stepwise sequential fitting of the model.

Variable	Change in square root of ferritin level[*]	p value	95% confidence intervals
TSAT (%)	0.04	<0.001	0.04–0.05
Indigenous	(1.00)	—	—
Non-Indigenous	−13.47	<0.001	−29.16–3.80
URR	0.04	0.001	0.02–0.07

[*]Change in the square root of ferritin per unit change in the independent variables.

TABLE 5: Results of two-level (multilevel) multinomial logistic regression: final model.

Predictor	Ferritin (μg/l) categories[*]		
	Category 2 ≥ 100 < 800	Category 3 ≥ 800 < 1200	Category 4 ≥ 1200
	1.58	2.31	2.35
TSAT ≥ 20% and ≤30%	<0.001	<0.001	<0.001
	1.39–1.77	2.12–2.51	2.15–2.54
	2.28	3.33	3.67
TSAT > 30% and ≥50%	<0.001	<0.001	<0.001
	1.98–2.57	3.03–3.63	3.37–3.96
	2.67	4.15	4.99
TSAT > 50%	<0.001	<0.001	<0.001
	2.02–3.32	3.50–4.80	4.34–5.64
	−2.46	−3.43	−3.53
Non-Indigenous ethnicity	<0.001	<0.001	<0.001
	−2.88––2.04	−3.85––3.00	−3.96––3.11
	1.49	1.33	1.19
Male gender	<0.001	<0.001	<0.001
	1.13–1.86	0.96–1.70	0.82–1.56
	−0.04	−0.07	−0.09
CRP ≥ 10 mg/l	0.693	0.513	0.375
	−0.24–0.16	−0.28–0.14	−0.30–0.11

Data are coefficient, p value, and 95% confidence interval. Reference groups for categorical variables are TSAT < 20%, female gender, Indigenous ethnicity, and CRP < 10 mg. [*]Compared to base outcome of ferritin category 1 (serum ferritin < 100 μg/l).

levels (TSAT) and (2) high ferritin levels in our patients are likely to be poorly explained by inflammation given the poor association between ferritin and CRP.

Recent evidence has shown that TSAT (compared with serum ferritin) was a better predictor of iron status and response to treatment with ESA in dialysis patients [6]. Our data revealed that only 11% of the variation in ferritin levels could be explained by the TSAT with 89% bearing no relationship. Although there was a statistically significant association between ferritin and TSAT on mixed regression analysis, a unit rise in TSAT was associated with a very small rise in ferritin which supports the correlation findings. This suggests that the high ferritin levels in our patients are only partly explained by iron levels. Our local iron management protocols have focussed on serum measures of TSAT and ferritin and are thus in accordance with other international anaemia management guidelines (Table 1). Yet we have shown that TSAT and ferritin are in fact likely to insufficiently direct optimal iron replacement, given the lower achieved haemoglobin among Indigenous clients in this cohort. Consequently, there is a clear need to explore

other measures of iron status in addition to the ferritin and TSAT.

We recently reported that our patients, who have high serum ferritin concentrations, are also exposed to higher than usual levels of therapeutic iron doses [7], which is one consequence of a persisting evidence gap to guide management of iron deficiency in dialysis patients with high ferritin. In our patients, high serum ferritin concentrations, in combination with low TSAT, are observed prior to haemodialysis initiation. In contrast, data from the United States has shown that, with reductions in ESA use and increased iron supplementation, a rise in serum ferritin concentration among MHD patients is observed [10]. In the mixed regression analysis, we also showed no association between ferritin and ESA weekly dose, even though Indigenous patients required significantly higher doses of ESA.

We investigated the effect of inflammation, using CRP, as an alternate differential of high serum ferritin. Dialysis patients are known to have high vulnerability to bacterial infections [11], in our region, melioidosis bacteraemia [12], and staphylococcal bacteraemia [13]. In spite of this, our data showed that CRP was not associated with serum ferritin levels in maintenance haemodialysis patients. This suggests as yet unexplained causes of high serum ferritin, beyond infection in this population. This data was reported from a retrospective clinical dialysis database. Therefore, we did not have other more specific or novel measures of inflammation. We acknowledge that other markers of infectious and noninfectious inflammation may have been better surrogates of relationship between ferritin and inflammation. These may include more specific inflammatory markers such as interleukin-6 (IL-6) and tumour necrosis factor-a (TNF-a) [14].

Although the possibility of iron overload as a potential explanation for the lack of association between the high ferritin and CRP was considered, an analysis of the available data supported what we found in our other recent study that the administered iron did not explain the lack of association between the high ferritin and the CRP [7].

Although we performed sensitivity analyses which showed no difference in the association between ferritin and CRP and ferritin and infused iron dose in participants where the infused dose of iron was available compared to the findings observed in the combined cohort, the lack of association between ferritin and infused iron dose and ferritin and CRP may be explained by the low data for infused iron dose available in the dataset.

There is a significant potential risk of iatrogenic iron overload generated by the administration of iron in our dialysis patients with high ferritin where guidelines are lacking on the appropriate dosing in those with other evidence of iron deficiency. Although we have adjusted our local guidelines [7] in line with the findings in the Ferric Gluconate Is Highly Efficacious in Anaemic Haemodialysis Patients with High Serum Ferritin and Low Transferrin Saturation: Results of the Dialysis Patients' Response to IV Iron with Elevated Ferritin (DRIVE) studies [15, 16], a significant number of patients have the high ferritin levels above those used in these studies. Therefore, this needs further evaluation. A cross-sectional study assessing the best markers of iron stores in this population will be informative in helping to determine the best measures of the iron stores. However, the appropriate dosing of iron will need to be evaluated by a clinical trial comparing outcomes between the dosing of iron among different levels of high ferritin.

Dialysis adequacy as measured by URR was highly significantly associated with higher ferritin. This may reflect either better utilisation of iron in those patients who are dialysing well compared to those with poor dialysis or an indication that those who attend adequate dialysis receive iron treatment. This will need further assessment, including a prospective study as the question was beyond the scope of this study.

The lack of correlation with ferritin and TSAT suggests the need to examine the role of regulatory and functional markers of iron such as hepcidin [17–21] and other measures of iron stores, particularly soluble transferrin receptor which has been shown to be a better marker of iron status than ferritin in Indigenous children [22]. Other measures of iron stores such as low MCV and hypochromic, microcytic RBCs on blood film, percentage hypochromic red cells (PHRC), and reticulocyte haemoglobin content will need further exploration in prospective studies in this population. Although the PHRC produces comparable or somewhat better results than reticulocyte haemoglobin content, the blood sample needs to be analyzed on site, which makes its widespread adoption difficult in our setting [23].

Causes of very high serum ferritin concentrations (>10,000 μg/l) include genetic causes, transfusional iron overload, juvenile idiopathic arthritis, lupus, and haemophagocytic lymphohistiocytosis. Iron overload may be another differential of high serum ferritin in this cohort, although our data did not support this among our patients, since the TSAT was not elevated. Direct assessments of iron status such as measuring liver iron levels could be considered [24]. The traditional invasive methods to determine body iron levels such as bone marrow biopsy [25] and liver biopsy are associated with increased mortality and morbidity [26]. However, the recent increase in the use of noninvasive but accurate methods such as the magnetic resonance imaging- (MRI-) based technique spin-density projection-assisted (SDPA) R2-MRI (FerriScan®) provides an opportunity to determine the relationship between the high ferritin and liver iron status to exclude iron overload [27–29].

Almost 20 years ago, Moirand et al. identified the relationship between unexplained high serum ferritin (median values > 500 μg/l) and normal transferrin saturation [30]. They reported that the majority of participants with unexplained high serum ferritin had numerous clinical indicators of the metabolic syndrome [30]. This has also been supported more recently [31], with ferritin having strong association with insulin and c-peptide, which unfortunately were not routinely available in all our patients. It is reported that insulin increases externalisation of the transferrin receptor, thereby stimulating cellular iron uptake. Type 2 diabetes is a leading cause of end stage kidney disease in Indigenous Australians [32] and reflected in 66.6% of our participants. Hyperinsulinaemia and metabolic syndrome are also highly prevalent among the general population of Indigenous Australians in our region [33, 34]; hyperferritinaemia in the absence of acute infection may potentially reflect sustained hyperinsulinaemia among our patients. We therefore plan to investigate the association between high serum ferritin and markers of the metabolic syndrome in our MHD patients.

The study had several limitations including the retrospective design which is associated with potential bias due to reliance on data collected for a different aim to the study. However, there was enough information in the datasets to confidently assess the relationship between ferritin and the other variables to answer the question. Some important information on essential variables to this analysis was incomplete; for example, total dose of iron per annum had too few observations in the first few years of the data collection to be included in the analysis. This may have affected the levels of ferritin. However, this would not have affected the relationship between ferritin and TSAT as both are expected to rise with iron therapy. One of the limitations of the study as a retrospective analysis was that the data collection for iron infusion was not complete. In the earlier years covered by the study, the data entry was limited to whether iron infusion was given or not without specifying the dose. It was only in the last 12 months that the dose was included in the entry. Most of the analysis was performed on the whole sample and then by ethnicity. However, detail could not be provided on iron infusion and ferritin by ethnicity due to the limited available data.

A prospective study is also required to further comprehensively explore the potential causes of the high ferritin and the clinical outcomes that may be associated with the high ferritin in this patient group. Future studies to clarify these unanswered questions include a prospective study which combines assessing the association of ferritin with measures of regulatory and functional markers of iron status such as hepcidin, markers of inflammation mentioned above, and other surrogate methods of assessing iron status such as soluble transferrin receptor will provide a clear method of assessing iron status in our patients. Hepcidin is particularly increasingly recognised as a key player in iron metabolism and will need exploration in this population especially with respect to functional iron deficiency [17, 35]. An assessment of the relationship between ferritin and other clinical correlates such as hepatitis B infections, hospitalisations, cardiovascular disease, other infections, and conditions such as diabetes mellitus will also need further studies.

The implication of this study is that it raises questions on the veracity of using ferritin and transferrin saturation as the main determination of iron requirements and therapy in Indigenous patients on haemodialysis. The study clearly raises the need to further explore the use of other measures of iron stores. It also raises the need to conduct a clinical trial assessing the safety and efficacy of administering iron in patients with higher ferritin levels than in the DRIVE studies [15, 16].

5. Conclusion

We report a population of MHD clients with high ESA usage, hyperferritinaemia, and low-normal TSAT. Our data has revealed the limited utility of using only ferritin and TSAT to guide Renal Anaemia Management protocols in our region. We suggest exploring the utility of additional markers of iron status to guide our clinical practice. We have further shown the lack of correlation of ferritin with serum CRP, as a marker inflammation. There is clear need for further evaluation of the causes of this high ferritin and the possible associated detrimental clinical outcomes in these patients. Unlike populations without severe renal disease, we suspect that there may be an association between hyperferritinaemia and metabolic syndrome which could explain some of the variance in high serum ferritin concentrations in our patients. Should this be confirmed in future studies in our patients, then interventions targeting metabolic syndrome may also be incorporated into our local anaemia management guidelines.

Abbreviations

TSAT: Transferrin saturation
NT: Northern Territory
MHD: Maintenance haemodialysis
CRP: C-reactive protein

TIBC: Total iron binding capacity
ESA: Erythropoiesis stimulating agents
PHRC: Percentage hypochromic red cells
CARI: Caring for Australasians with Renal Insufficiency
KDOQI: Kidney Disease Outcome Quality Initiative
NICE: National Institute for Health and Clinical Excellence
ERA-EDTA: European Renal Association-European Dialysis and Transplant Association
KDIGO: Kidney Disease: Improving Global Outcomes
ESKD: End stage kidney disease
HREC: Human Research Ethics Committee
RAM: Renal Anaemia Management
BMI: Body mass index
URR: Urea reduction ratio
TNF: Tumour necrosis factor.

Ethical Approval

The study was approved by the Human Research Ethics Committee of the Northern Territory Department of Health and Menzies School of Health Research (HREC 11-1567) and the Central Australian Human Research Ethics Committee.

Acknowledgments

The authors would like to acknowledge members of the renal team in both Central Australia and Top End of the Northern Australia. The authors would like to acknowledge the pathology departments in the Northern Territory for the pathology results, the renal unit staff, and Janssen-Cilag for maintaining the RAM database. The authors also acknowledge the anaemia coordinators from all units in the Northern Territory for the data entry into the RAM database.

References

[1] F. Locatelli, P. Bárány, A. Covic et al., "Kidney Disease: Improving Global Outcomes guidelines on anaemia management in chronic kidney disease: a European Renal Best Practice position statement," *Nephrology Dialysis Transplantation*, vol. 28, no. 6, pp. 1346–1359, 2013.

[2] J. B. Wish, "Assessing iron status: beyond serum ferritin and transferrin saturation," *Clinical Journal of the American Society of Nephrology*, vol. 1, supplement 1, pp. S4–S8, 2006.

[3] F. J. Baillie, A. E. Morrison, and I. Fergus, "Soluble transferrin receptor: a discriminating assay for iron deficiency," *Clinical and Laboratory Haematology*, vol. 25, no. 6, pp. 353–357, 2003.

[4] T. Berlin, A. Meyer, P. Rotman-Pikielny, A. Natur, and Y. Levy, "Soluble transferrin receptor as a diagnostic laboratory test for detection of iron deficiency anemia in acute illness of

hospitalized patients," *Israel Medical Association Journal*, vol. 13, no. 2, pp. 96–98, 2011.

[5] R. MacGinley, R. Walker, and M. Irving, "KHA-CARI guideline: use of iron in chronic kidney disease patients," *Nephrology*, vol. 18, no. 12, pp. 747–749, 2013.

[6] A. E. Gaweda, P. Bhat, G. A. Maglinte et al., "TSAT is a better predictor than ferritin of hemoglobin response to Epoetin alfa in US dialysis patients," *Hemodialysis International*, vol. 18, no. 1, pp. 38–46, 2014.

[7] S. W. Majoni, J.-A. Ellis, H. Hall, A. Abeyaratne, and P. D. Lawton, "Inflammation, high ferritin, and erythropoietin resistance in indigenous maintenance hemodialysis patients from the Top End of Northern Australia," *Hemodialysis International*, vol. 18, no. 4, pp. 740–750, 2014.

[8] L. E. K. Ratcliffe, W. Thomas, J. Glen et al., "Diagnosis and management of iron deficiency in CKD: a summary of the NICE guideline recommendations and their rationale," *American Journal of Kidney Diseases*, vol. 67, no. 4, pp. 548–558, 2016.

[9] S. Rabe-Hesketh and A. Skrondal, *Multilevel and Longitudinal Modeling Using Stata, Volumes I and II, Third Edition: Multilevel and Longitudinal Modeling Using Stata, Volume II ... Counts, and Survival, Third Edition*, Stata Press, 2012.

[10] A. Karaboyas, J. Zee, H. Morgenstern et al., "Understanding the recent increase in ferritin levels in united states dialysis patients: Potential impact of changes in intravenous iron and erythropoiesis-stimulating agent dosing," *Clinical Journal of the American Society of Nephrology*, vol. 10, no. 10, pp. 1814–1821, 2015.

[11] R. Vanholder and S. Ringoir, "Infectious morbidity and defects of phagocytic function in end-stage renal disease: a review," *Journal of the American Society of Nephrology*, vol. 3, no. 9, pp. 1541–1554, 1993.

[12] R. M. S. Chalmers, S. W. Majoni, L. Ward, G. J. Perry, Z. Jabbar, and B. J. Currie, "Melioidosis and end-stage renal disease in tropical northern Australia," *Kidney International*, vol. 86, no. 5, pp. 867–870, 2014.

[13] B. J. Stewart, T. Gardiner, G. J. Perry, and S. Y. C. Tong, "Reduction in *Staphylococcus aureus* bacteraemia rates in patients receiving haemodialysis following alteration of skin antisepsis procedures," *Journal of Hospital Infection*, vol. 92, no. 2, pp. 191–193, 2016.

[14] P. M. Ridker, C. H. Hennekens, J. E. Buring, and N. Rifai, "C-reactive protein and other markers of inflammation in the prediction of cardiovascular disease in women," *New England Journal of Medicine*, vol. 342, no. 12, pp. 836–843, 2000.

[15] D. W. Coyne, T. Kapoian, W. Suki et al., "Ferric gluconate is highly efficacious in anemic hemodialysis patients with high serum ferritin and low transferrin saturation: results of the Dialysis Patients' Response to IV Iron with Elevated Ferritin (DRIVE) study," *Journal of the American Society of Nephrology*, vol. 18, no. 3, pp. 975–984, 2007.

[16] T. Kapoian, N. B. O'Mara, A. K. Singh et al., "Ferric gluconate reduces epoetin requirements in hemodialysis patients with elevated ferritin," *Journal of the American Society of Nephrology*, vol. 19, no. 2, pp. 372–379, 2008.

[17] D. W. Coyne, "Hepcidin: clinical utility as a diagnostic tool and therapeutic target," *Kidney International*, vol. 80, no. 3, pp. 240–244, 2011.

[18] D. S. Larson and D. W. Coyne, "Understanding and exploiting hepcidin as an indicator of anemia due to chronic kidney disease," *Kidney Research and Clinical Practice*, vol. 32, no. 1, pp. 11–15, 2013.

[19] E. Rossi, "Hepcidin-the iron regulatory hormone," *The Clinical biochemist. Reviews*, vol. 26, no. 3, pp. 47–49, 2005.

[20] C.-Y. Wang and J. L. Babitt, "Hepcidin regulation in the anemia of inflammation," *Current Opinion in Hematology*, vol. 23, no. 3, pp. 189–197, 2016.

[21] G. Weiss, "Anemia of chronic disorders: new diagnostic tools and new treatment strategies," *Seminars in Hematology*, vol. 52, no. 4, pp. 313–320, 2015.

[22] B. Ritchie, Y. McNeil, and D. R. Brewster, "Soluble transferrin receptor in Aboriginal children with a high prevalence of iron deficiency and infection," *Tropical Medicine and International Health*, vol. 9, no. 1, pp. 96–105, 2004.

[23] S. Fishbane, W. Shapiro, P. Dutka, O. F. Valenzuela, and J. Faubert, "A randomized trial of iron deficiency testing strategies in hemodialysis patients," *Kidney International*, vol. 60, no. 6, pp. 2406–2411, 2001.

[24] J. C. Wood, "Diagnosis and management of transfusion iron overload: the role of imaging," *American Journal of Hematology*, vol. 82, supplement 12, pp. 1132–1135, 2007.

[25] S. Stancu, A. Stanciu, A. Zugravu et al., "Bone marrow iron, iron indices, and the response to intravenous iron in patients with non—dialysis-dependent CKD," *American Journal of Kidney Diseases*, vol. 55, no. 4, pp. 639–647, 2013.

[26] R. Fischer and P. R. Harmatz, "Non-invasive assessment of tissue iron overload," *Hematology American Society of Hematology. Education Program*, pp. 215–221, 2009.

[27] P. Ferrari, H. Kulkarni, S. Dheda et al., "Serum iron markers are inadequate for guiding iron repletion in chronic kidney disease," *Clinical Journal of the American Society of Nephrology*, vol. 6, no. 1, pp. 77–83, 2011.

[28] G. Rostoker, M. Griuncelli, C. Loridon et al., "Reassessment of iron biomarkers for prediction of dialysis iron overload: an MRI study," *PLoS ONE*, vol. 10, no. 7, Article ID e0132006, 2015.

[29] T. G. St. Pierre, A. El-Beshlawy, M. Elalfy et al., "Multicenter validation of spin-density projection-assisted R2-MRI for the noninvasive measurement of liver iron concentration," *Magnetic Resonance in Medicine*, vol. 71, no. 6, pp. 2215–2223, 2014.

[30] R. Moirand, A. M. Mortaji, O. Loréal, F. Paillard, P. Brissot, and Y. Deugnier, "A new syndrome of liver iron overload with normal transferrin saturation," *The Lancet*, vol. 349, no. 9045, pp. 95–97, 1997.

[31] R. Brudevold, T. Hole, and J. Hammerstrøm, "Hyperferritinemia is associated with insulin resistance and fatty liver in patients without iron overload," *PLoS ONE*, vol. 3, no. 10, Article ID e3547, 2008.

[32] S. McDonald, "Incidence and treatment of esrd among indigenous peoples of australasia," *Clinical Nephrology*, vol. 74, no. 1, pp. S28–S31, 2010.

[33] K. O'Dea, J. Cunningham, L. Maple-Brown et al., "Diabetes and cardiovascular risk factors in urban Indigenous adults: results from the DRUID study," *Diabetes Research and Clinical Practice*, vol. 80, no. 3, pp. 483–489, 2008.

[34] K. O'Dea, R. J. Lion, A. Lee, K. Traianedes, J. L. Hopper, and C. Rae, "Diabetes, hyperinsulinemia, and hyperlipidemia in small aboriginal community in northern Australia," *Diabetes Care*, vol. 13, no. 8, pp. 830–835, 1990.

[35] Y. Hamada and M. Fukagawa, "Is hepcidin the star player in iron metabolism in chronic kidney disease," *Kidney International*, vol. 75, no. 9, pp. 873–874, 2009.

20

Cancer in ANCA-Associated Glomerulonephritis: A Registry-Based Cohort Study

Sanjeevan Sriskandarajah,[1] Leif Bostad,[1,2] Tor Åge Myklebust,[3] Bjørn Møller,[3] Steinar Skrede,[4,5] and Rune Bjørneklett[1,6]

[1]Department of Clinical Medicine, University of Bergen, Bergen, Norway
[2]Department of Pathology, Haukeland University Hospital, Bergen, Norway
[3]Department of Clinical and Registry-Based Research, Cancer Registry of Norway, Institute of Population-Based Cancer Research, Oslo, Norway
[4]Department of Clinical Science, University of Bergen, Bergen, Norway
[5]Department of Medicine, Haukeland University Hospital, Bergen, Norway
[6]Emergency Care Clinic, Haukeland University Hospital, Bergen, Norway

Correspondence should be addressed to Sanjeevan Sriskandarajah; sanjeevan87@hotmail.com

Academic Editor: Tibor Nadasdy

Background. Immunosuppressive therapy for antineutrophil cytoplasmic antibody-associated vasculitis has been associated with increased malignancy risk. *Objectives.* To quantify the cancer risk associated with contemporary cyclophosphamide-sparing protocols. *Methods.* Patients from the Norwegian Kidney Biopsy Registry between 1988 and 2012 who had biopsy-verified pauci-immune glomerulonephritis and positive antineutrophil cytoplasmic antibody (ANCA) serology were included. Standardised incidence ratios (SIRs) were calculated to compare the study cohort with the general population. *Results.* The study cohort included 419 patients. During 3010 person-years, cancer developed in 41 patients (9.79%); the expected number of cancer cases was 37.5 (8.95%). The cohort had SIRs as follows: 1.09, all cancer types (95% CI, 0.81 to 1.49); 0.96, all types except nonmelanoma skin cancer (95% CI, 0.69 to 1.34); 3.40, nonmelanoma skin cancer (95% CI, 1.62 to 7.14); 3.52, hematologic cancer (95% CI, 1.32 to 9.37); 2.12, posttransplant cancer (95% CI, 1.01 to 4.44); and 1.53, during the 1–5-year follow-up after diagnosis (95% CI, 1.01 to 2.32). *Conclusions.* Cancer risk did not increase significantly in this cohort with ANCA-associated glomerulonephritis. However, increased risk of nonmelanoma skin cancer, posttransplant cancer, and hematologic cancer indicates an association between immunosuppression and malignancy.

1. Introduction

Historically, antineutrophil cytoplasmic antibody- (ANCA-) associated vasculitis (AAV) was a fatal disease. The introduction of cyclophosphamide (CYC) treatment in the 1960s improved the prognosis and made long-term survival possible for patients with AAV [1, 2]. However, evidence soon emerged that the long-term survival of patients with AAV was associated with significant morbidity including a substantially increased cancer risk [3–7]. Immunosuppressive therapy using CYC was particularly associated with malignancy. Although the severe adverse effects have elicited a search for

less toxic treatment regimens, CYC still remains the first-line drug [8].

High occurrence of cancer has been demonstrated in patients with AAV treated with cumulative CYC doses exceeding 36 g [9–11] or when the treatment duration lasted for more than a year [4, 12–14]. In the current clinical practice, cumulative CYC doses and treatment duration rarely exceed these limits [15–18], which questions the relevance of previous CYC-associated increased cancer risk observations in patients with AAV. There is a relative paucity of data regarding cancer risk in AAV patients treated with current therapy protocols, and, to our knowledge, only 4 studies have published such data [5, 11, 13, 19]. In these studies, increased incidence of malignancy was observed. After excluding nonmelanoma skin cancer (NMSC) from the analyses, the incidence of malignancy no longer significantly increased in any of these investigations. However, these 4 studies were relatively small, with a limited statistical power to detect small- to medium-range associations between cancer and AAV. Furthermore, most of these reports are single-center studies, which limits their generalizability.

Interestingly, in the most recent study, the standardised incidence ratio (SIR) of all cancer types treated with CYC was 4.61 (95% confidence interval (CI) 1.16 to 39.38) times higher than that with rituximab-based therapy. However, after excluding NMSC from their analysis, the risk was only 1.30 (95% CI not reported) times higher with CYC compared with rituximab-based therapy [19].

To further investigate the association of cancer and AAV, we analysed data from the Norwegian Kidney Biopsy Registry (NKBR) and the Norwegian Cancer Registry. Additionally, we merged data from the present and the 4 recent studies on this topic and investigated the cancer risk in a total of 1532 patients with AAV diagnosed after 1988.

2. Materials and Methods

The study was approved by the Regional Committees for Medical and Health Research Ethics (REC South-East 2013/1083).

2.1. Study Population and Registries. The NKBR was established in 1988. We estimate that ~90% of all kidney biopsies are registered. The registry contains morphological, laboratory, and clinical data collected when the biopsy was performed. The Norwegian Cancer Registry was established in 1953. Reporting to this registry is mandatory and based on reports from clinical and pathological departments and death certificates. A near complete registration (98-99%) of solid tumors, except for basal skin cell carcinomas, is documented [20]. Annual sex-specific incidence rates for cancer and cancer subtypes are available for age groups and time periods in 5-year intervals. These data allow for an accurate calculation of the expected cancer case numbers in the study cohort. The Norwegian Cause of Death Registry is part of Statistics Norway and based on the mandatory Norwegian death certificate. The Norwegian Renal Registry was established in 1980 and has registered all patients with end-stage renal disease, defined by the commencement of maintenance dialysis or receiving kidney transplantation.

2.2. Data Collection and Definitions. We included patients registered in the NKBR and diagnosed from 1988 to 2012, with a pauci-immune necrotising glomerulonephritis and a positive ANCA serology. Patients with cancer prior to the AAV diagnosis were excluded. Baseline clinical data, including sex, age, ANCA specificity, and estimated glomerular filtration rate (eGFR) (determined by the Modification of Diet in Renal Disease equation) [21] were obtained from the NKBR. The primary study end-point was incidence of cancer. By using the unique 11-digit Norwegian personal number, the study

cohort was linked with the Norwegian Cancer Registry to identify the cancer incidence. Causes of deaths in the study cohort were identified through linkage with the Norwegian Cause of Death Registry and classified as vascular, malignant, infectious, or active inflammation and other causes. The observation period was from the kidney biopsy date to incident cancer, end of 2013, or death, whichever came first. Patients with end-stage renal disease and those receiving kidney transplants were identified through record linkage with the Norwegian Renal Registry. When we calculated the cancer risk in transplanted patients, the observation period started from the kidney transplantation date.

2.3. SIR Calculation. We calculated the SIR as the ratio between the observed and expected cancer case numbers in the cohort. The expected cancer case number was calculated as follows: first, the number of person-years was calculated in the cohort, stratified by 5-year age groups and 1-year time periods. Second, this person-time was multiplied with the corresponding incidence rate in the general population to get the expected number of cases in each age group and 1-year period. The total number of expected cancer cases was then calculated as the sum of expected cases across age groups and time periods. The observed cancer case number was determined by record linkage of the study cohort and the Norwegian Cancer Registry using the 11-digit unique Norwegian personal number. A Poisson distribution of cancer incidence was assumed when 95% CIs were calculated. We calculated the SIR throughout the study period and stratified in accordance with disease duration periods (0-1, 1-5, 5-10, and >10 years after kidney biopsy), sex, ANCA specificity [cytoplasmic ANCA (C-ANCA)/proteinase 3 ANCA (PR3-ANCA) or perinuclear ANCA (P-ANCA)/myeloperoxidase ANCA (MPO-ANCA)], time periods (1988-2002 and 2003-2012), and posttransplantation observation period.

2.4. Pooled Analysis. A systematic PubMed search was conducted to identify previous studies reporting the cancer risk in patients with AAV diagnosed after 1988. The search was restricted to papers published in English language. Studies who do not report SIR data were excluded. The SIRs were calculated as the sum of the observed cancer cases divided by that of the expected cancer cases in all studies.

2.5. Treatment. Information regarding cumulative CYC doses administered to the patients is not available in the NKBR. In a previous Norwegian study including patients with Wegener's granulomatosis diagnosed between 1988 and 1998, the majority of patients received intravenous CYC with a median cumulative dose of 17 g. In patients receiving oral CYC, the median cumulative dose was 48 g [22]. Most centers since approximately 2003 have substituted CYC with azathioprine for maintenance treatment, substantially lowering the exposure to CYC [23]. In some patients, rituximab has been used for induction and maintenance treatment. Some patients have also received plasma exchange treatments [24].

2.6. Statistical Analyses. Continuous variables were expressed as medians with 25th and 75th percentiles and

TABLE 1: Baseline demographics of 419 Norwegian patients with AAV.

Characteristic	Total	Nonmalignancy	Malignancy	p value
Age (median, IQR)	62 (49–72)	61 (48–72)	65 (56–73)	0.04
Male sex (%)	229 (55%)	200 (53%)	29 (71%)	0.03
eGFR (median, IQR)	23 (11–46)	24 (11–47)	19 (9–39)	0.29
C-ANCA/PR3-ANCA	237 (57%)	213 (56%)	24 (59%)	0.89

AAV, ANCA-associated vasculitis; IQR, interquartile range; eGFR, estimated glomerular filtration rate, mL/min/1.73 m^2; C-ANCA, cytoplasmic ANCA; PR3-ANCA, proteinase 3 ANCA.

categorical variables as numbers (%). Comparisons of continuous and categorical variables in the baseline characteristics were calculated using the Mann–Whitney U test and the X^2 or Fisher's exact test, respectively. A two-tailed p value of ≤0.05 and 95% CI was considered statistically significant. All statistical analyses were performed using the SPSS software, V.23, and STATA software, V.14.

3. Results

3.1. Baseline Characteristics. Between 1988 and 2012, 454 patients diagnosed with AAV and glomerulonephritis were identified. Of these, 35 were excluded as a result of cancer diagnosis prior to the observation period. Thus, 419 patients were included in the study cohort. As shown in Table 1, the median age in the cohort was 62 years [interquartile range, 48 to 72 years], and 229 (55%) were men. The median eGFR at the time of kidney biopsy was 23 mL/min/1.73 m^2 (interquartile range, 11 to 46). A positive C-ANCA/PR3-ANCA was found in 237 (57%) and P-ANCA/MPO-ANCA in 183 (43%) patients.

The median length of follow-up was 5.7 years (interquartile range, 2.8 to 11.3). The mean length of follow-up was 7.2 years (standard deviation, 5.8), and the total number of person-years of observation was 3010. A total of 148 (35%) patients died during the observation period. Causes of deaths are registered for 138 patients, of which 69 (50%) died from infectious disease or active inflammation/vasculitis, 36 (26%) cardiovascular disease, 12 (9%) malignancy, and 21 (15%) from other causes. Kidney transplantation was performed in 60 (14%) patients.

3.2. Observed Cancer Cases. During follow-up, 46 cancer cases were reported in 41 (9.5%) patients. The first occurring cancer cases were as follows: NMSC (7 cases), lung (7), prostate (5), hematologic (4), urinary bladder and ureter (3), rectum (3), colon (2), uterus (2), central nerve system (2), unknown primary site (2), thyroid (1), ovary (1), lymphoma (1), and pancreas (1). Five patients had 2 distinct cancer diagnoses; the second occurring cancer cases were as follows: lung (1), NMSC (1), prostate (1), hematologic (1), and stomach (1). Seven patients who received transplants were diagnosed with cancer; the first occurring cancer cases were as follows: lung (4), prostate (1), lymphoma (1), and NMSC (1). Two of the 5 patients with 2 distinct cancers underwent transplant, with the cases of secondary cancer involving the prostate and lungs.

3.3. Comparison of Patients with and without Cancer. The comparison of the patients with and without cancer during follow-up is shown in Table 1. The patients with cancer were significantly older [65 years versus 61 years (p = 0.04)] at the time of AAV diagnosis, and a significantly higher percentage were men (71% versus 53% (p = 0.03)). There were no significant differences in eGFR and ANCA specificity between those with cancer and those without cancer during follow-up. A higher percentage of patients with cancer died during follow-up [25 (61%) versus 123 (33%) (p < 0.001)].

3.4. Comparison with the General Population. As shown in Table 2(a), the SIR of overall malignancy was 1.09 (95% CI 0.81 to 1.49). The SIR of all cancer types, except NMSC, was 0.96 (95% CI 0.69 to 1.34). In the 1–5-year period after AAV diagnosis, the cancer risk in the study cohort significantly increased compared to that in the general population (SIR, 1.53; 95% CI 1.01 to 2.32). The SIR did not increase in the first year or >5 years of follow-up after AAV diagnosis. In gender-, ANCA-, and time period specificity-stratified analyses, SIR of cancer was not significantly increased for males of 1.27 (95% CI 0.88 to 1.83), in the C-ANCA/PR3-ANCA positive group of 1.17 (95% CI 0.78 to 1.74) and in the 1988–2002 time period of 1.14 (95% CI 0.78 to 1.68). Compared to the general population, the transplanted patients in the study cohort had a significantly increased malignancy risk (SIR, 2.12; 95% CI 1.01 to 4.44), whereas the nontransplanted patients had no increased risk (SIR, 0.99; 95% CI 0.71 to 1.39).

The SIR calculation for the most common site-specific cancer cases showed significantly increased risks of NMSC (SIR, 3.40; 95% CI 1.62 to 7.14) and hematologic malignancies (SIR, 3.52; 95% CI 1.32 to 9.37). The SIR did not significantly increase in any other site-specific cancer type (Table 2(b)).

3.5. Pooled Analysis of the 5 Cohort Studies. The separate and merged SIRs of all cancer types in the present and the 4 previously reported studies are shown in Table 3 and Figure 1. This analysis included a total of 1532 patients, 8801 patient-years of observation, and 236 cancer cases. The merged SIR of all cancer types was 1.72 (95% CI 1.51 to 1.95) and that of all cancer types, except NMSC, was 1.21 (95% CI 1.01 to 1.45).

4. Discussion

In the present study, there was no statistically significant increase in the cancer incidence in the patients with AAV and glomerulonephritis compared to the age- and sex-matched

TABLE 2

(a) Standardised incidence ratios for cancers in all sites in the study population

Characteristic	Observed	Expected	SIR	95% CI
All	41	37.5	1.09	0.81 to 1.49
Non-NMSC	34	35.4	0.96	0.69 to 1.34
Sex				
Male	29	22.9	1.27	0.88 to 1.83
Female	12	14.6	0.82	0.47 to 1.44
Follow-up period				
0–1 year	3	4.3	0.70	0.22 to 2.16
1–5 years	22	14.4	1.53	1.01 to 2.32
5–10 years	11	11.1	0.99	0.55 to 1.78
>10 years	5	7.6	0.66	0.27 to 1.57
Transplantation				
Yes	7	3.3	2.12	1.01 to 4.44
No	34	34.2	0.99	0.71 to 1.39
ANCA serology				
C-ANCA/PR3-ANCA	24	20.6	1.17	0.78 to 1.74
P-ANCA/MPO-ANCA	17	16.9	1.01	0.63 to 1.62
Study period				
1988–2002	26	22.7	1.14	0.78–1.68
2003–2012	15	14.8	1.02	0.61–1.68

SIR, standardised incidence ratio; 95% CI, 95% confidence interval; NMSC, nonmelanoma skin cancer; C-ANCA, cytoplasmic ANCA; PR3-ANCA, proteinase 3 ANCA; P-ANCA, perinuclear ANCA; MPO-ANCA, myeloperoxidase ANCA.

(b) Standardised incidence ratios for the most common organ-specific cancers in the study population

Organs	Observed	Expected	SIR	95% CI
NMSC	7	2.1	3.40	1.62 to 7.14
Hematologic	4	1.1	3.52	1.32 to 9.37
Lung	7	4.0	1.73	0.83 to 3.63
Colon	2	1.2	1.73	0.43 to 6.93
Urothelium	3	2.0	1.48	0.47 to 4.59
Prostate	5	7.0	0.72	0.30 to 1.73
NHL	1	1.2	0.86	0.12 to 6.12

SIR, standardised incidence ratio; 95% CI, 95% confidence interval; NMSC, nonmelanoma skin cancer; NHL, non-Hodgkin lymphoma.

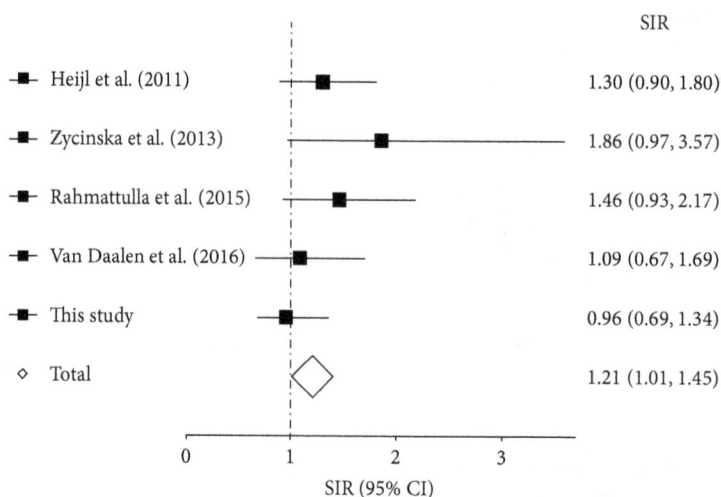

FIGURE 1: Forest plot showing the risk of malignancy except for nonmelanoma skin cancer in observational studies of patients with ANCA-associated vasculitis. SIR, standardised incidence ratio; 95% CI, 95% confidence interval.

TABLE 3: Studies on cancer incidence in patients with AAV.

Characteristic	Heijl et al. (2011)	Zycinska et al. (2013)	Rahmattulla et al. (2015)	Van Daalen et al. (2016)	This study	Total
Study period	1995–2007	1990–2008	1991–2013	2000–2014	1988–2012	
Number of patients	535	117	138	323	419	1532
Cumulative person-years	2650	NR	1339	1802	3010	8801
Number of observed cancers	50	15	85	45	41	236
Number of expected cancers	31.7	6[a]	38.5[a]	23.8	37.5	137.5
SIR (95% CI)	1.58 (1.17 to 2.08)	2.50 (1.20 to 2.90)	2.21 (1.64 to 2.92)	1.89 (1.38 to 2.53)	1.09 (0.81 to 1.49)	1.72 (1.51 to 1.95)
All non-NMSC sites						
Number of observed cancers	35	9[a]	24	20	34	122
Number of expected cancers	25.9	4.8[a]	16.4[a]	18.33	35.4	100.8
SIR (95% CI)	1.30 (0.90 to 1.80)	1.86[a] (0.97 to 3.57)	1.46 (0.93 to 2.17)	1.09 (0.67 to 1.69)	0.96 (0.69 to 1.34)	1.21 (1.01 to 1.45)

[a]Not reported; calculated by the authors of this study; SIR, standardised incidence ratio; 95% CI, 95% confidence interval; NR, not reported; NMSC, nonmelanoma skin cancer.

general population (SIR, 1.09; 95% CI 0.89 to 1.49). Excluding the study by Holle et al. that reported an SIR of 0.82 (95% CI 0.45 to 1.38) [25], most previous studies, including those investigating patients with AAV diagnosed after 1988, have reported a significantly increased cancer risk [3–5, 9, 11, 13, 14, 19]. A couple of methodological discrepancies might partially explain the contrasting findings between the present and the majority of previous studies. First, basal skin cell carcinomas are not registered in the Norwegian Cancer Registry and were thus excluded in our analysis. Second, among patients with diagnoses of several cancers, we only included the primary cancer when calculating the SIRs. In contrast, other studies have included subsequent cancer cases, particularly NMSC, in their SIR estimates.

The studies investigating cancer incidences in patients with AAV diagnosed after 1988 reflect contemporary treatment regimens, in which NMSC accounts for the majority of the observed increased malignancy risk [5, 11, 13, 19]. In the present study, the SIR decreased from 1.09 to 0.96 (95% CI 0.69 to 1.34) when NMSC cases were excluded. Further, in the pooled analysis (Table 3), the SIR decreased from 1.72 (95% CI 1.51 to 1.95) to 1.21 (95% CI 1.01 to 1.45) after excluding NMSC. Moreover, part of the residual cancer risk after excluding NMSC can be attributed to posttransplant malignancies, with the SIR posttransplant of 2.12 (95% CI 1.01 to 4.44) in the present study and 4.31 (95% CI 1.17 to 11.04) in that by Van Daalen et al. [19].

In the organ-specific subanalysis, the SIR of NMSC was 3.40 (95% CI 1.62 to 7.14), which is consistent with that of previous studies [5, 9, 11, 13, 14, 19]. An increased risk of NMSC is observed in immunocompromised patients and associated with both environmental factors as chronic human papillomavirus infection [26–29] and a direct effect of individual immunosuppressant, for example, azathioprine [19, 30]. A significantly increased hematologic cancer risk was also found (SIR, 3.52; 95% CI 1.32 to 9.37). Traditionally, CYC use was associated with a very high risk of acute myelogenous leukemia [9, 14, 31]. Interestingly, no case of this cancer form was observed in our cohort, and the increased hematologic malignancy risk was caused by 2 cases of myelodysplastic syndrome and 2 cases of chronic lymphocytic leukemia. To what extent these cases are related to CYC-based therapy or immunosuppression specifically is unclear [32]. In comparison, Zycinska et al. found an increased risk of acute myelogenous leukemia in their study (SIR, 4.3; 95% CI 2.1 to 11.7). Notably, oral CYC was used in the majority of their patients, and 22% received >36 g of cumulative CYC dosage. In addition, a significantly increased urothelial cancer risk was also found in their study, in contrast to those of other recent groups (SIR, 3.4; 95% CI 1.6 to 5.2) [11].

Some previous groups have indicated that the cancer risk, perhaps caused by a higher tendency of relapses and thus higher cumulative immunosuppressive drug doses, is higher in C-ANCA/PR3-ANCA than in P-ANCA/MPO-ANCA positive patients [5, 13]. In contrast, we observed no significantly increased risk in these subgroups compared to the general population.

An important measure to reduce cancer risk in patients with AAV has been replacing CYC with azathioprine for maintenance treatment. This practice change occurred around 2003 concurrent with the publication of the CYCAZAREM study [23, 33]. In the present study cohort, SIR of cancer was not significantly increased, neither in the 1988–2002 nor in the 2003–2012 time periods. Of notice, in a study including a subgroup of the 1988–2002 cohort, cumulative doses of CYC were found fairly low, median 17 grams in intravenous CYC-treated patients [34].

The findings by Van Daalen et al. indicate that rituximab use is associated with a substantially lower risk of malignancy. However, this difference was primarily related to excess NMSC cases. The calculated SIR of cancer, except NMSC, was 1.14 (95% CI 0.49 to 2.25) with CYC and 0.88 (95% CI 0.11 to 3.19) with rituximab treatment. Thus, the SIR of cancer, except NMSC, was only 1.30-fold higher (CI not reported by Van Daalen et al.) in the CYC group than in the rituximab group. Further, the SIR of cancer, except NMSC, was only marginally higher in the present CYC-treated study cohort than in the rituximab group in their study, estimated SIR of 0.96 (95% CI 0.69 to 1.34) and 0.88 (95% CI 0.11 to 3.19), respectively. Finally, no adjustment for posttransplantation malignancies has been performed when comparing CYC- and rituximab-treated patients [19]. In summary, whether replacing low-dose CYC regimens with rituximab would have a beneficial effect on non-NMSC malignancy risk remains uncertain.

NMSC occurrence is still substantially increased in patients with AAV. Although NMSC by no means should be considered as an inconsequential morbidity, deaths caused by these tumors are rare [35]. A number of measures can be taken to reduce the risk and morbidity related to NMSC in immunosuppressed patients; the most important measures include limiting sun exposure of the skin and vigilant monitoring with early NMSC detection and treatment when they appear. Interestingly, Van Daalen et al. observed that rituximab use is associated with a lower NMSC risk than CYC use, which represents a new possible solution to such complication in patients with AAV [19]. However, the decision to replace CYC with rituximab as the first-line treatment in patients with AAV must also include considerations, such as efficacy, treatment-related complications, and cost-benefit.

The major strengths of the present study include its population-based approach and identification of patients with AAV from quality registries with histologic and serologic data. Information on expected and observed cancer cases was retrieved from the same registry, the Norwegian Cancer Registry, which limits potential information biases in the SIR calculation. This registry also has high accuracy and only few missing cases owing to mandatory reporting of cancer cases. Moreover, the pooled analysis strengthens the statistical power and increases the detection rate of significant differences. Some weaknesses of our study must be admitted. Most importantly, we could not correlate our findings to the cumulative CYC doses administered. Treatment data were unavailable in the NKBR. However, we have shown from previous reports of this cohort that these patients have received therapy according to international recommendations [22–24]. Another weakness is the lack of information regarding extrarenal and relapsing disease. Relapsing disease in particular is associated with increased treatment length and cumulative doses of immunosuppressive drugs that might affect risk of cancer development. Also, owing to a lack of sufficient data, we could not calculate pooled SIRs for single-site cancers or for malignancy after excluding posttransplant cancers.

In summary, we have demonstrated that the risk of malignancy in patients with AAV and glomerulonephritis is not significantly increased. However, significantly increased NMSC, hematologic malignancy, and posttransplantation cancer risks were found. These findings indicate the presence of associations, although relatively weak, between immunosuppression and cancer development. However, recently published data suggest that substituting CYC with rituximab could eliminate the risk of developing NMSC. Our findings confirm that the long-term international efforts of developing CYC-minimizing strategies had an important beneficial effect on cancer morbidity in patients with AAV.

Authors' Contributions

All authors contributed to the generation of hypotheses. Tor Åge Myklebust and Bjørn Møller performed statistical analyses; Sanjeevan Sriskandarajah and Rune Bjørneklett drafted the manuscript. All of the authors contributed to revisions and approved the final version of the manuscript.

Acknowledgments

The authors thank all nephrologists and pathologists in Norway who reported important data to the Norwegian Kidney Biopsy Registry. They also thank Torbjørn Leivestad for data linkage of the study cohort with the Norwegian Renal Registry.

References

[1] J. C. Jennette and R. J. Falk, "Small-vessel vasculitis," The New England Journal of Medicine, vol. 337, no. 21, pp. 1512–1523, 1997.

[2] A. S. Fauci, B. F. Haynes, P. Katz, and S. M. Wolff, "Wegener's granulomatosis: prospective clinical and therapeutic experience with 85 patients for 21 years," Annals of Internal Medicine, vol. 98, no. 1, pp. 76–85, 1983.

[3] G. S. Hoffman, G. S. Kerr, R. Y. Leavitt et al., "Wegener granulomatosis: an analysis of 158 patients," Annals of Internal Medicine, vol. 116, no. 6, pp. 488–498, 1992.

[4] K. W. A. Westman, P. G. Bygren, H. Olsson, J. Ranstam, and J. Wieslander, "Relapse rate, renal survival, and cancer morbidity in patients with Wegener's granulomatosis or microscopic polyangiitis with renal involvement," Journal of the American Society of Nephrology, vol. 9, no. 5, pp. 842–852, 1998.

[5] C. Heijl, L. Harper, O. Flossmann et al., "Incidence of malignancy in patients treated for antineutrophil cytoplasm antibody-associated vasculitis: Follow-up data from European Vasculitis Study Group clinical trials," Annals of the Rheumatic Diseases, vol. 70, no. 8, pp. 1415–1421, 2011.

[6] C. Talar-Williams, Y. M. Hijazi, M. McClellan et al., "Cyclophosphamide-induced cystitis and bladder cancer in patients with Wegener granulomatosis," Annals of Internal Medicine, vol. 124, no. 5, pp. 477–484, 1996.

[7] J. Robson, H. Doll, R. Suppiah et al., "Damage in the ANCA-associated vasculitides: Long-term data from the European Vasculitis Study Group (EUVAS) therapeutic trials," Annals of the Rheumatic Diseases, vol. 74, no. 1, pp. 177–184, 2015.

[8] C. Mukhtyar, "SP0095 EULAR/ERA-EDTA Recommendations for The Management of ANCA-Associated Vasculitis," Annals of the Rheumatic Diseases, vol. 75, no. Suppl 2, pp. 24.1-24, 2016.

[9] M. Faurschou, I. J. Sorensen, L. Mellemkjaer et al., "Malignancies in wegener's granulomatosis: incidence and relation to cyclophosphamide therapy in a cohort of 293 patients," The Journal of Rheumatology, vol. 35, no. 1, pp. 100–105, 2008.

[10] M. Faurschou, L. Mellemkjaer, A. Voss, K. K. Keller, I. T. Hansen, and B. Baslund, "Prolonged risk of specific malignancies following cyclophosphamide therapy among patients with granulomatosis with polyangiitis," Rheumatology, vol. 54, no. 8, pp. 1345–1350, 2015.

[11] K. Zycinska, J. Kostrzewa-Janicka, A. Nitsch-Osuch, and K. Wardyn, "Cancer Incidence in Pulmonary Vasculitis," in Neurobiology of Respiration, vol. 788 of Advances in Experimental Medicine and Biology, pp. 349–353, Springer, Dordrecht, Netherlands, 2013.

[12] A. Knight, J. Askling, F. Granath, P. Sparen, and A. Ekbom, "Urinary bladder cancer in Wegener's granulomatosis: risks and relation to cyclophosphamide," Annals of the Rheumatic Diseases, vol. 63, no. 10, pp. 1307–1311, 2004.

[13] C. Rahmattulla, A. E. Berden, S.-C. Wakker et al., "Incidence of malignancies in patients with antineutrophil cytoplasmic antibody-associated vasculitis diagnosed between 1991 and 2013," Arthritis & Rheumatology, vol. 67, no. 12, pp. 3270–3278, 2015.

[14] A. Knight, J. Askling, and A. Ekbom, "Cancer incidence in a population-based cohort of patients with Wegener's granulomatosis," International Journal of Cancer, vol. 100, no. 1, pp. 82–85, 2002.

[15] M. Walsh, M. Faurschou, A. Berden et al., "Long-term follow-up of cyclophosphamide compared with azathioprine for initial maintenance therapy in anca-associated vasculitis," Clinical Journal of the American Society of Nephrology, vol. 9, no. 9, pp. 1571–1576, 2014.

[16] R. M. Smith, "Update on the treatment of ANCA associated vasculitis," La Presse Médicale, vol. 44, no. 6, pp. e241–e249, 2015.

[17] R. L. Rhee, S. L. Hogan, C. J. Poulton et al., "Trends in Long-Term Outcomes Among Patients With Antineutrophil Cytoplasmic Antibody–Associated Vasculitis With Renal Disease," Arthritis & Rheumatology, vol. 68, no. 7, pp. 1711–1720, 2016.

[18] K. De Groot, L. Harper, D. R. W. Jayne et al., "Pulse versus daily oral cyclophosphamide for induction of remission in antineutrophil cytoplasmic antibody-associated vasculitis: a randomized trial," Annals of Internal Medicine, vol. 150, no. 10, pp. 670–680, 2009.

[19] E. E. Van Daalen, R. Rizzo, A. Kronbichler et al., "Effect of rituximab on malignancy risk in patients with ANCA-Associated vasculitis," Annals of the Rheumatic Diseases, vol. 76, no. 6, pp. 1064–1069, 2016.

[20] I. K. Larsen, M. Småstuen, T. B. Johannesen et al., "Data quality at the Cancer Registry of Norway: An overview of comparability, completeness, validity and timeliness," European Journal of Cancer, vol. 45, no. 7, pp. 1218–1231, 2009.

[21] A. S. Levey, J. Coresh, T. Greene et al., "Expressing the modification of diet in renal disease study equation for estimating glomerular filtration rate with standardized serum creatinine values," *Clinical Chemistry*, vol. 53, no. 4, pp. 766–772, 2007.

[22] K. Aasarod, "Renal histopathology and clinical course in 94 patients with Wegener's granulomatosis," *Nephrology Dialysis Transplantation* , vol. 16, no. 5, pp. 953–960.

[23] S. Sriskandarajah, K. Aasarød, S. Skrede, T. Knoop, A. V. Reisæter, and R. Bjørneklett, "Improved prognosis in Norwegian patients with glomerulonephritis associated with anti-neutrophil cytoplasmic antibodies," *Nephrology Dialysis Transplantation* , vol. 30, pp. i67–i75, 2015.

[24] E. Besada, W. Koldingsnes, and J. C. Nossent, "Long-term efficacy and safety of pre-emptive maintenance therapy with rituximab in granulomatosis with polyangiitis: results from a single centre," *Rheumatology*, vol. 52, no. 11, Article ID ket257, pp. 2041–2047, 2013.

[25] J. U. Holle, W. L. Gross, U. Latza et al., "Improved outcome in 445 patients with Wegener's granulomatosis in a German vasculitis center over four decades," *Arthritis & Rheumatology*, vol. 63, no. 1, pp. 257–266, 2011.

[26] N. Reusser, C. Downing, J. Guidry, and S. Tyring, "HPV Carcinomas in Immunocompromised Patients," *Journal of Clinical Medicine*, vol. 4, no. 2, pp. 260–281, 2015.

[27] A. E. Grulich, M. T. van Leeuwen, M. O. Falster, and C. M. Vajdic, "Incidence of cancers in people with HIV/AIDS compared with immunosuppressed transplant recipients: a meta-analysis," *The Lancet*, vol. 370, no. 9581, pp. 59–67, 2007.

[28] E. N. Pritchett, A. Doyle, C. M. Shaver et al., "Nonmelanoma skin cancer in nonwhite organ transplant recipients," *JAMA Dermatology*, vol. 152, no. 12, pp. 1348–1353, 2016.

[29] S. Euvrard, J. Kanitakis, and A. Claudy, "Skin cancers after organ transplantation," *The New England Journal of Medicine*, vol. 348, no. 17, pp. 1681–1691, 2003.

[30] P. O'Donovan, C. M. Perrett, and X. Zhang, "Azathioprine and UVA light generate mutagenic oxidative DNA damage," *Science*, vol. 309, no. 5742, pp. 1871–1874, 2005.

[31] J. Pedersen-Bjergaard, S. Olesen Larsen, J. Struck et al., "Risk of therapy-related leukaemia and preleukaemia after Hodgkin's disease. Relation to age, cumulative dose of alkylating agents, and time from chemotherapy," *The Lancet*, vol. 330, no. 8550, pp. 83–88, 1987.

[32] V. Bîrluțiu, E. C. Rezi, R. M. Bîrluțiu, and I. S. Zaharie, "A rare association of chronic lymphocytic leukemia with c-ANCA-positive Wegener's granulomatosis: A case report," *World Journal of Surgical Oncology*, vol. 14, no. 1, article no. 145, 2016.

[33] D. Jayne, N. Rasmussen, K. Andrassy et al., "A randomized trial of maintenance therapy for vasculitis associated with anti-neutrophil cytoplasmic autoantibodies," *The New England Journal of Medicine*, vol. 349, no. 1, pp. 36–44, 2003.

[34] K. Aasarod, B. M. Iversen, J. Hammerstrom, L. Bostad, L. Vatten, and S. Jorstad, "Wegener's granulomatosis: clinical course in 108 patients with renal involvement," *Nephrology Dialysis Transplantation*, vol. 15, no. 5, pp. 611–618, 2000.

[35] C. Newlands, R. Currie, A. Memon, S. Whitaker, and T. Woolford, "Non-melanoma skin cancer: United Kingdom National Multidisciplinary Guidelines," *The Journal of Laryngology & Otology*, vol. 130, no. S2, pp. S125–S132, 2016.

21

Apolipoprotein C-I Levels Are Associated with the Urinary Protein/Urinary Creatinine Ratio in Pediatric Idiopathic Steroid-Sensitive Nephrotic Syndrome: A Case Control Study

Jun Odaka, Takahiro Kanai, Takane Ito, Takashi Saito, Jun Aoyagi, Hiroyuki Betsui, and Takanori Yamagata

Department of Pediatrics, Jichi Medical University, 3311-1 Yakushiji, Shimotsuke, Tochigi 329-0498, Japan

Correspondence should be addressed to Jun Odaka; mrjo@jichi.ac.jp

Academic Editor: Jochen Reiser

Humoral factors may cause idiopathic steroid-sensitive nephrotic syndrome (ISSNS). In the present study, we analyzed serum proteins using mass spectrometry (MS) to identify proteins associated with the pathophysiology of pediatric ISSNS. We collected serial serum samples from 33 children during each ISSNS phase; Phase A1 is the acute phase prior to steroid treatment (STx), Phase A2 represents the remission period with STx, and Phase A3 represents the remission period after completion of STx. Children with normal urinalyses (Group B) and children with a nephrotic syndrome other than ISSNS (Group C) served as controls. No significant differences in urinary protein/urinary creatinine (UP/UCr) ratios were observed between the children with phase A1 ISSNS and Group C. We used surface-enhanced laser desorption/ionization time of flight MS for sample analysis. Four ion peaks with a mass-to-charge ratio (m/z) of 6,444, 6,626, 8,695, and 8,915 were significantly elevated during ISSNS Phase A1 compared to Phase A2, Phase A3, and Group C. The intensity of an m/z of 6,626 significantly correlated with the UP/UCr ratio and an m/z of 6,626 was identified as apolipoprotein C-I (Apo C-I). Apo C-I levels correlate with the UP/UCr ratio in pediatric ISSNS. Our findings provide new insights into the pathophysiology of ISSNS.

1. Introduction

Idiopathic steroid-sensitive nephrotic syndrome (ISSNS) is one of the most common chronic renal diseases in children and is caused by increased permeability of the glomerular filtration barrier [1]. A number of studies have suggested that the permeability factors underlying glomerular filtration barrier dysfunction are associated with the pathophysiology of ISSNS [2–5], but these factors have not yet been identified. Conventional serum proteomic analysis has the limitations of interference and charge suppression from high-abundance proteins, in addition to the hindrances caused by the extremely wide dynamic range (>10 orders of magnitude) of serum protein concentrations. Furthermore, the 22 most common protein species comprise approximately 99% of the total serum protein [6].

Surface-enhanced laser desorption/ionization time of flight mass spectrometry (SELDI-TOF MS) can overcome these problems. Using this technique, we have associated apolipoprotein A-II (Apo A-II) levels in serum with the status of ISSNS [7]; Apo A-II was found to induce type 2 helper T-cells (Th2) [7], which are predominantly found in the nephrotic phase in ISSNS [8]. In the present study, we tried to identify another protein associated with the status of ISSNS using SELDI-TOF MS.

2. Methods

This study was performed in accordance with the principles of the Declaration of Helsinki and was approved by the Ethics Committee of Jichi Medical University (A08-13, A14-055). Informed consent was obtained from all patients and/or their parents.

2.1. Patients and Controls. The study investigated 33 patients with ISSNS that were admitted to our department between

March 2004 and November 2009. The study cohort consisted of three groups of children, those in Phase A1–A3 ISSNS and two age- and sex-matched control groups (Groups B and Group C) [7]. The characteristics of the groups are described in Table 1. The common inclusion criteria for the Phase A group were the presence of ISSNS, a selectivity index < 0.1 as determined by the immunoglobulin (Ig)G/transferrin clearance ratio, no infections for 1 week before the study began, and a 6-month absence of immunosuppressant therapy before the study began. Thirty-three patients were in the nephrotic phase of ISSNS before steroid therapy (STx) initiation (Phase A1), 33 patients were in the remission phase of ISSNS during STx (Phase A2), and 12 patients were in the remission phase of ISSNS after completing STx (Phase A3). The reason for fewer patients in Phase A3 is that 21 of 33 patients were STx-dependent.

Group B consisted of 15 healthy children with normal urinalyses, and Group C consisted of eight children with a nephrotic syndrome other than ISSNS (i.e., $n = 1$ with Alport syndrome, lupus nephritis, purpura nephritis, hemolytic uremic syndrome, IgA nephritis, or non-IgA mesangial proliferative glomerulonephritis; $n = 2$ with membranoproliferative glomerulonephritis type I).

No significant differences in the protein/urinary creatinine (UP/UCr) ratios ($P = 0.26$), the serum albumin (sAlb) level ($P = 0.95$), and the serum total cholesterol (T. chol.) level ($P = 0.16$) were found between Phase A1 and Group C. The sAlb level was significantly reduced in Phase A1 compared with Phase A3 ($P < 0.05$) or Group B ($P < 0.05$). The T. chol. level ($P < 0.05$) was significantly increased in Phase A1 compared with Phase A3 ($P < 0.05$). Student's t-test was applied to compare the differences between Phase A1 and each group. Anticholesterol agents had not yet been administered to any of the study participants.

2.2. Surface-Enhanced Laser Desorption/Ionization Time of Flight Mass Spectrometry.

SELDI-TOF MS was performed according to the manufacturer's instructions with some previously described modifications [7].

2.3. Purification and Identification of ISSNS-Associated Peptides.

Human serum samples (100 μL) were diluted with 50 mM Tris buffer (pH 9.0) and loaded onto an anion-exchange column (Q Sepharose Fast Flow; GE Healthcare, Little Chalfont, UK). The samples were fractionated by applying buffer with declining pH values and the purification was confirmed using the Q10 ProteinChip® (Bio-Rad Laboratories, Inc., Hercules, CA). The desired fraction was diluted with 50 mM acetate buffer (pH 4.0) and loaded onto a cation-exchange column (CM Sepharose Fast Flow; GE Healthcare). The sample was fractionated by applying buffer with increasing sodium concentrations and the purification was confirmed using the NP20 ProteinChip (Bio-Rad Laboratories, Inc.). The desired fraction was separated by reverse-phase high-performance liquid chromatography (HPLC) (2 × 100 mm columns, TSK-GEL Super ODS; TOSOH, Tokyo, Japan) and the purification progress was confirmed using the NP20 ProteinChip (Bio-Rad Laboratories, Inc.). The desired fraction was purified using HPLC columns (2 × 150 mm)

(TSK-GEL Amide-80; TOSOH, Tokyo, Japan), and the purification progress was monitored and it was confirmed using the NP20 ProteinChip (Bio-Rad Laboratories, Inc.). After a series of steps, we electrophoresed the desired fractions on Tris-tricine sodium dodecyl sulfate-polyacrylamide gels (polyacrylamide gel 16.2% T, 6% C) to evaluate the purity. Tandem mass spectrometry was used to analyze the purified fractions using a Nanoflow-LC ESI in positive mode (Q-TOF Ultima API®; Waters Corporation, Milford, MA, USA). Database searches were performed using Mascot® (Matrix Science Ltd., London, UK).

2.4. Serum Apolipoprotein C-I Measurements.

Serum samples were collected from 11 patients in the Phase A1 subgroup and seven individuals in Group C to determine the serum Apo C-I levels. These two groups were matched for age and sex (Table 2). The two groups did not differ significantly with respect to their UP/UCr, serum albumin, and total cholesterol levels ($P = 0.99$, $P = 0.21$, and $P = 0.33$, resp.).

An enzyme-linked immunosorbent assay (ELISA) was performed to determine the Apo C-I levels in the serum samples from the two groups, using the Human Apolipoprotein C-I ELISA Kit (Assaypro LLC, MO, USA) according to the manufacturer's instructions. This assay employs a quantitative sandwich enzyme immunoassay technique. The standards and each sample were diluted to 100-fold concentration with diluent concentrate (EIA Diluent Concentrate; Assaypro LLC), and 50 μL of each of the standards and samples was added to individual wells and the plate was incubated at room temperature for 2 h. After washing the plate with the wash buffer (Wash Buffer Concentrate; Assaypro LLC), 50 μL of the biotinylated antibody (Biotinylated Apo C-I Antibody; Assaypro LLC) was added to each well, and the plate was incubated at room temperature for 2 h. After washing the plate with the wash buffer, 50 μL of the streptavidin-peroxidase conjugate (Streptavidin-Peroxidase Conjugate, Assaypro LLC) was added to each well, and the plate was incubated at room temperature for 30 min. After washing the plate with the wash buffer, 50 μL of a peroxidase enzyme substrate (Chromogen Substrate, Assaypro LLC) was added to each well, and the plate was incubated at room temperature for 30 min. After adding 50 μL of stop solution (Stop Solution, Assaypro LLC) to each well, the absorbances were read by a microplate reader (Benchmark Plus Microplate Reader; Bio-Rad Laboratories, Inc.) at a wavelength of 450 nm.

2.5. Statistical Analyses.

The data were analyzed using a two-tailed Kruskal-Wallis H test, followed by a two-tailed Mann–Whitney U test with Bonferroni correction to detect the peaks specific to the Phase A1 subgroup. We also analyzed the data to determine correlations between the intensities of each peak and the UP/UCr ratios using a two-tailed Spearman rank test.

Student's t-test was used to compare the differences in serum Apo C-I levels between the Phase A1 subgroup and Group C. $P < 0.05$ was considered significant.

TABLE 1: Characteristics of the study groups [7].

Group	Criteria	N	M : F	Median age (range), years	Mean UP/UCr (g/gCr)	Mean serum albumin (g/dL)	Mean T. chol. (mg/dL)	Mean serum Cr (mg/dL)	Mean eGFR (ml/min/1.73 m^2)	Mean disease duration, months	Mean systolic blood pressure (mmHg)
Phase A1	Nephrotic phase in ISSNS before STx initiation	33	21:12	7 (1–15)	8.3 ± 7.5	2.5 ± 1.1	319 ± 145	0.36 ± 0.14	136 ± 21	17 ± 35	110 ± 12
Phase A2	Remission phase in ISSNS during STx	33	21:12	7 (1–15)		2.8 ± 0.9	328 ± 113	0.38 ± 0.14	126 ± 19		110 ± 10
Phase A3	Remission phase in ISSNS after completing STx	12	8:4	6.5 (2–13)		4.0 ± 0.4	155 ± 20	0.34 ± 0.15	150 ± 25		103 ± 11
Group B	Normal urinalysis	15	7:8	5 (1–13)		4.6 ± 0.2	176 ± 3	0.32 ± 0.13	138 ± 22		97 ± 11
Group C	Nephrotic phase in nephrotic syndrome other than ISSNS before STx initiation	8	3:5	10 (4–14)	5.2 ± 3.2	2.6 ± 0.5	211 ± 59	0.73 ± 0.65	111 ± 46	17 ± 45	119 ± 22

M: male; F: female; UP/UCr: urinary protein/urinary creatinine; T. chol.: total cholesterol; Cr: creatinine; eGFR: estimated glomerular filtration rate; ISSNS: idiopathic steroid-sensitive nephrotic syndrome; STx: steroid treatment.

TABLE 2: Characteristics of groups analyzed for serum apolipoprotein C-I.

Group	Criteria	N	M : F	Median age (range), years	Average UP/UCr
Phase A1	Nephrotic phase in ISSNS before STx initiation	11	7 : 4	7 (1–13)	10.7
Group C	Nephrotic phase in nephrotic syndrome other than ISSNS before STx initiation	7	4 : 3	10 (4–15)	10.6

M: male; F: female; UP/UCr: urinary protein/urinary creatinine; ISSNS: idiopathic steroid-sensitive nephrotic syndrome; STx: steroid treatment.

3. Results

3.1. Detection of Peaks Associated with the Nephrotic Phase of ISSNS. Representative protein mass spectra for each ISSNS phase and Groups B and C are presented in Figure 1. To compensate for variations in the concentrations of the loaded samples, the peak intensities were normalized using a normal ion current and analyzed in Biomarker Wizard software (Bio-Rad Laboratories, Inc.). The data are presented as arbitrary units. The spectra of 101 samples exhibited 207 peaks with mass-to-charge ratios (m/z) between 2,000 and 10,000 using the following parameters for all spectra: first pass, 5.0; signal-to-noise ratio, 5.0 valley depth; minimum peak threshold, 5.0 valley depth; and minimum peak threshold 20.0%. Four peaks specific for Phase A1 were detected with an m/z of 6,444, 6,626, 8,695, and 8,915 (Figure 2). The intensities of these peaks were significantly greater for the Phase A1 subgroup than Phases A2 and A3 or Group C. No significant differences were observed between the patients in the Phase A3 subgroup and Group B with respect to the intensities of the peaks with an m/z of 6,626 or 8,915. The intensities of the peaks with an m/z of 6,444 and 8,695 were greater for the patients in the Phase A3 subgroup than those in Group B.

3.2. Correlations between Peak Intensities and UP/UCr Ratio. Significant correlations were found between the intensities of the peaks with an m/z of 6,626, 8,695, or 8,915 and the UP/UCr ratios (Figure 3). The peak at m/z 6,626 was the only peptide ion with a P value < 0.01 between the Phase A1 subgroup and Phase A3 or Group C. Therefore, we tried to identify the original protein with an m/z of 6,626.

3.3. Mascot Identification of the Peak with m/z 6,626. We identified the protein with an m/z of 6,626, the intensity of which correlated significantly with the UP/UCr ratio. We purified this protein from several mixed samples (Figure 4) and, by searching the Mascot database, were able to identify it as an Apo C-I fragment that has a score of 407. A score > 41 indicated identity or extensive homology ($P < 0.05$).

3.4. Serum Apo C-I Analysis. The mean serum Apo C-I levels were significantly higher in the Phase A1 subgroup than in Group C ($87 \pm 18\,\mu g/mL$ *versus* $64 \pm 21\,\mu g/mL$, $P < 0.05$). The mean serum Apo C-I levels in the Phase A1 subgroup were higher than the plasma reference value of 40–$70\,\mu g/mL$ and were within the normal range in Group C.

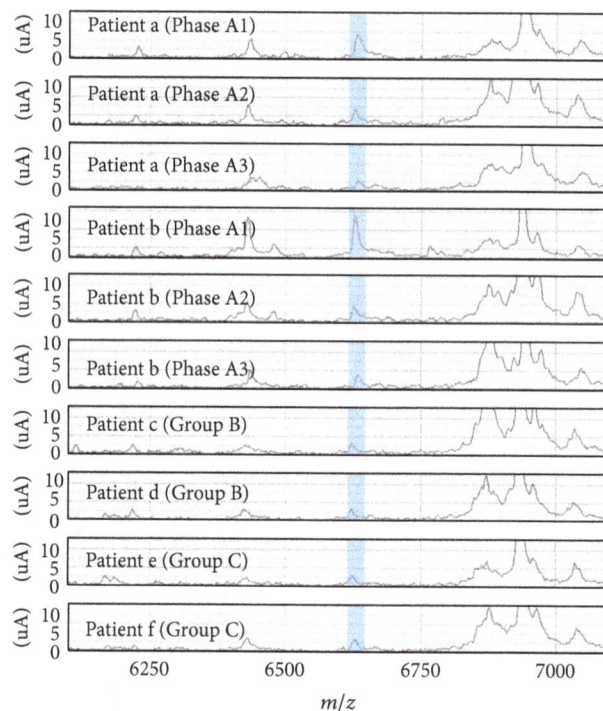

FIGURE 1: Representative spectra of six patients for the mass-to-charge ratio (m/z) of 6,626 (Q10, pH 5.0). The gray zone represents peaks at m/z 6,626. The upper six lanes show the serial change from Phase A1 to Phase A3 in patients a and b. The lower four lanes show the spectra of four patients from the control groups.

4. Discussion

In the present study, we identified Apo C-I as a protein that is specifically elevated during Phase A1 of pediatric ISSNS, and its intensity correlated significantly with the UP/UCr ratio. In addition, the serum Apo C-I levels in Phase A1, which were determined by ELISA, were significantly higher than those found in Group C. Therefore, we conclude that this elevation is not secondary to the hyperlipidemia that is associated with nephrotic syndrome. To the best of our knowledge, these data are the first to suggest an association between Apo C-I levels and ISSNS status.

We suggest that Apo C-I may be associated with the pathophysiology of ISSNS.

One mechanism underlying this potential association is an increase in the serum Apo C-I levels reflecting the activation of macrophages during the nephrotic phase of pediatric

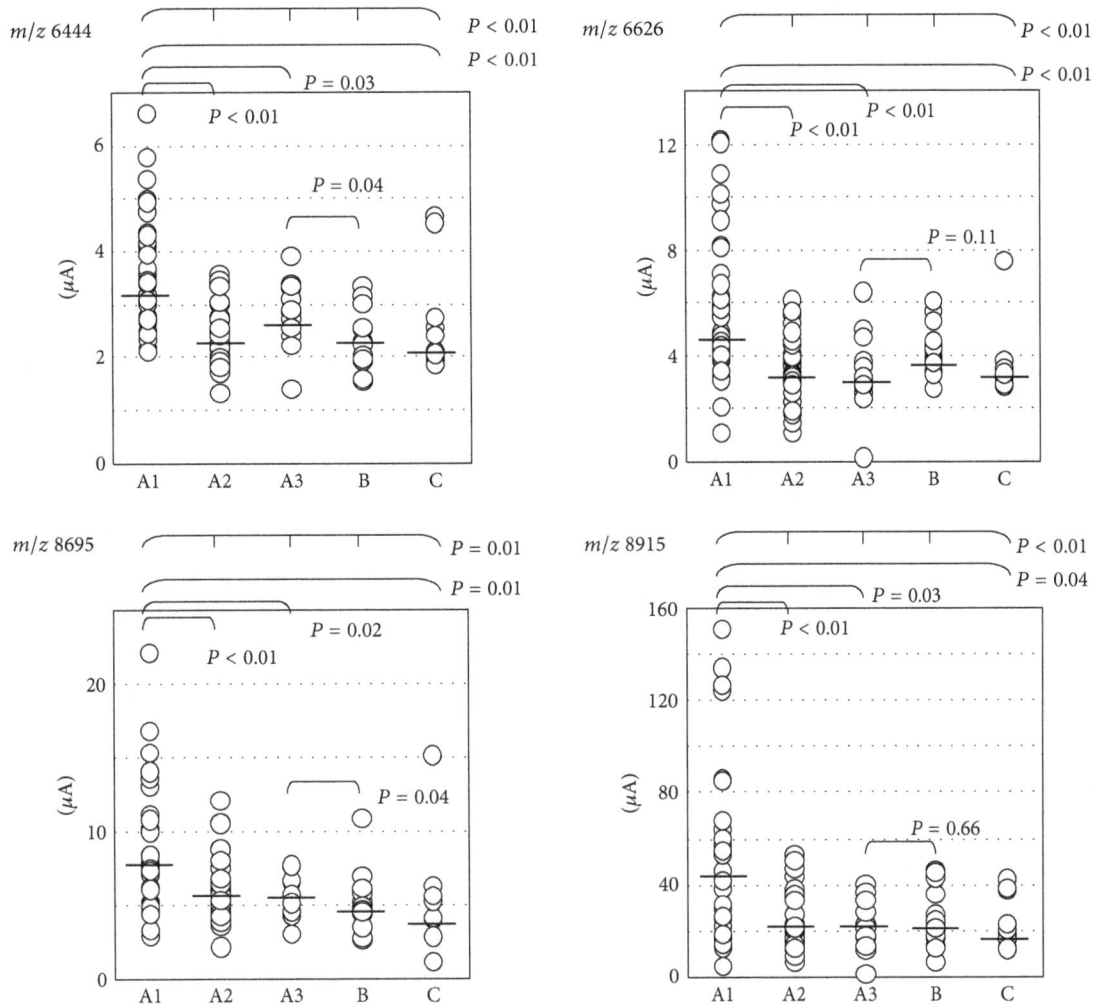

FIGURE 2: Intensity of each mass-to-charge ratio (m/z) level. Horizontal bars show each median value. The intensity of each m/z increased during Phase A1 [7].

ISSNS. Apo C-I is the smallest apolipoprotein (6.6 kDa) identified to date and comprises 57 amino acids [9, 10]. *Apo C-I* mRNA is upregulated when monocytes differentiate into macrophages [11]. Shalaby et al. [12] reported that levels of interleukin-18, which is largely regarded as a product of macrophages [13], are significantly higher during the active stage of pediatric ISSNS compared to remission and controls. In previous studies, we found significantly increased levels of serum macrophage inflammatory protein-1β (MIP-1β) during the nephrotic phase of pediatric ISSNS before STx and during the remission phase during STx compared to the remission phase after completing STx [14]. These results suggest that macrophages are activated during the nephrotic phase of ISSNS, which may increase the production of MIP-1β. On the other hand, Chen et al. [15] reported a decrease in the expression of CD14, a monocyte marker, on the surface of peripheral monocytes from pediatric ISSNS patients during active relapses. However, patients who had already completed STx were included in their study, so the findings did not precisely reflect the phenomena associated with the pathophysiology of pediatric ISSNS. Schlecker et al. [16]

demonstrated that intratumoral injections of MIP-1β increase the number of tumor-infiltrating regulatory T-cells (Tregs), suggesting that MIP-1β recruits high numbers of Tregs, which may play a role in the pathogenesis of pediatric ISSNS [17]. Accordingly, macrophage activation during the nephrotic phase of ISSNS may increase MIP-1β production and induce remission through the recruitment of Tregs. Furthermore, the increase in serum Apo C-I levels during the nephrotic phase of pediatric ISSNS may reflect macrophage activation rather than hypoalbuminemia.

Another potential mechanism is Apo C-I interacting with Th2 cell responses. Patients with pediatric ISSNS have a high incidence of atopic diseases [18], and atopy is characterized by Th2-dominant immune mechanisms [19], suggesting that Th2 plays an important role in the pathogenesis of ISSNS in children [8]. Nagelkerken et al. [10] demonstrated that mice transgenic for the expression of human Apo C-I in the liver and skin spontaneously develop symptoms associated with atopic dermatitis. One of the possible pathogenic mechanisms was enhanced Th2 activity facilitating a loss of skin integrity. Similarly, Apo C-I overexpression may cause

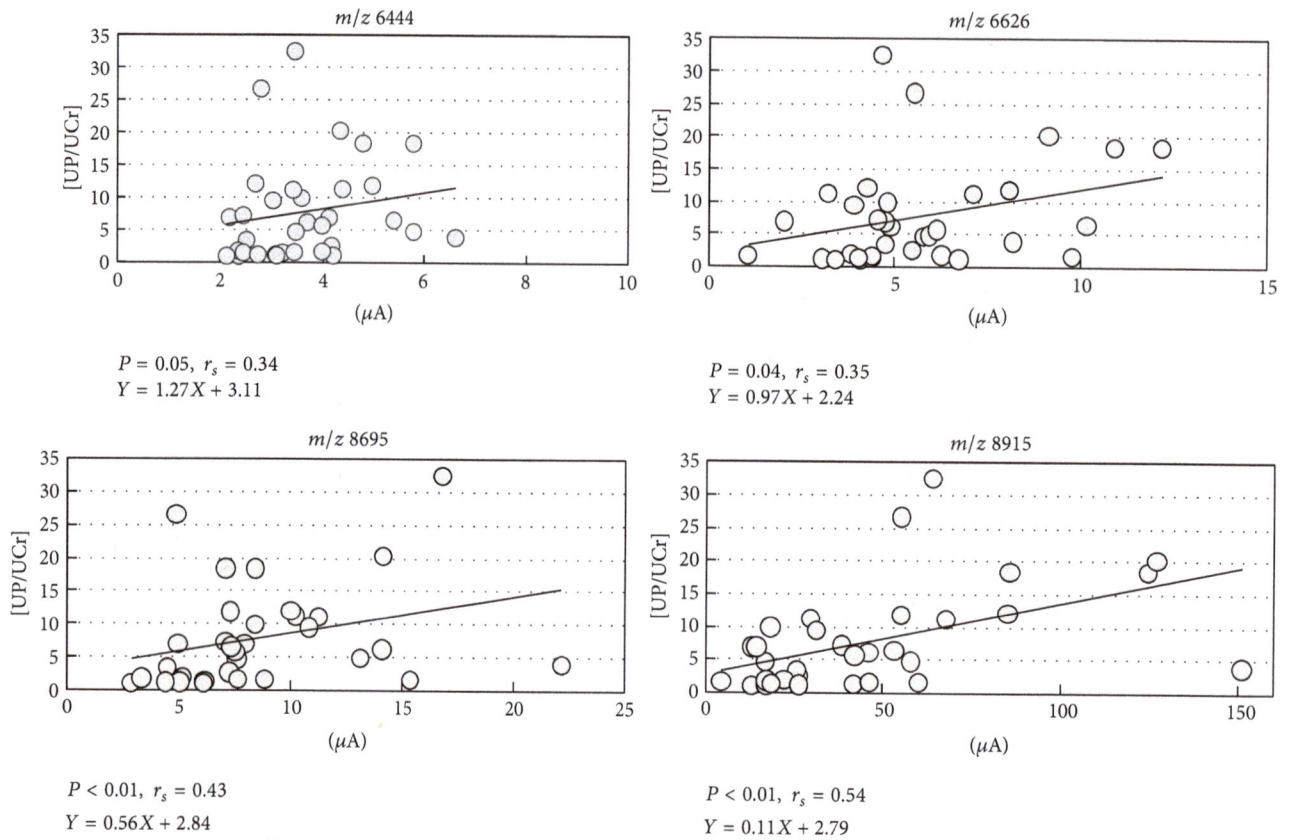

FIGURE 3: Correlations between the intensities of each mass-to-charge ratio (m/z) and each urinary protein/urinary creatinine (UP/UCr) ratio. Significant correlations were found between the intensities of the peaks at m/z ratios 6,626, 8,695, and 8,915 and their UP/UCr ratio [7].

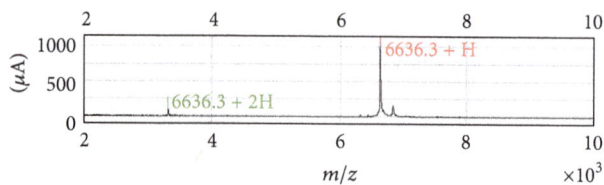

FIGURE 4: Peaks of mass-to-charge ratio (m/z) 6,626 after purification. The lower peak is the dication of m/z 6,626.

functional or structural abnormalities in podocytes, and these abnormalities could induce the development of Th2-dominant immune mechanisms, which may be associated with the pediatric ISSNS phases. In our previous study, we identified m/z of 8,695 as an Apo A-II fragment [7]. Apo A-II inhibits interferon-γ production in human CD4 T-cells [20] and could lead to Th2-dominant immune mechanisms. Apo C-I may work in cooperation with Apo A-II.

A third mechanism is CD80 expression in podocytes being influenced by Apo C-I. Mice given lipopolysaccharide (LPS) expressed CD80 in their podocytes, which leads to podocyte foot process effacement and proteinuria [21]. These findings suggest that innate immunity to LPS may be involved in the pathogenesis of minimal-change nephrotic syndrome (MCNS). Berbé et al. [22] demonstrated that Apo C-I binds to LPS, which enhances the LPS-binding inflammatory response. Thus, Apo C-I might facilitate the expression of CD80 in podocytes and may be involved in the pathogenesis of MCNS in children.

5. Conclusions

We detected elevated Apo C-I levels during the nephrotic phase of pediatric ISSNS, and the Apo C-I levels were associated with the UP/UCr ratio. Since the sample size of Group C in this study is small, whether the elevation in Apo C-I was a secondary response to the hyperlipidemia associated with nephrotic syndrome or not is open to discussion. Nevertheless, these findings are an interesting starting point for further investigations into the pathophysiology of ISSNS.

Disclosure

The authors obtained permission from the copyright holder to reproduce Figures 2 and 3 and Table 1 that had previously been published [7].

References

[1] P. Pais and E. D. Avner, "Nephrotic syndrome," in *Nelson Textbook of Pediatrics*, R. M. Kliegman, B. F. Stanton, J. W. St Geme III, and N. F. Schor, Eds., pp. 2521–2528, Elsevier, Philadelphia, Pa, USA, 2015.

[2] K. Maruyama, S. Tomizawa, N. Shimabukuro, T. Fukuda, T. Johshita, and T. Kuroume, "Effect of supernatants derived from T lymphocyte culture in minimal change nephrotic syndrome on rat kidney capillaries," *Nephron*, vol. 51, no. 1, pp. 73–76, 1989.

[3] A. A. Ali, E. Wilson, J. F. Moorhead et al., "Minimal-change glomerular nephritis: normal kidneys in an abnormal environment?" *Transplantation*, vol. 58, no. 7, pp. 849–852, 1994.

[4] R. J. Glassock, "Circulating permeability factors in the nephrotic syndrome: a fresh look at an old problem," *Journal of the American Society of Nephrology*, vol. 14, no. 2, pp. 541–543, 2003.

[5] P. E. C. Brenchley, "Vascular permeability factors in steroid-sensitive nephrotic syndrome and focal segmental glomerulosclerosis," *Nephrology Dialysis Transplantation*, vol. 18, supplement 6, pp. vi21–vi25, 2003.

[6] N. L. Anderson and N. G. Anderson, "The human plasma proteome: history, character, and diagnostic prospects," *Molecular & Cellular Proteomics*, vol. 1, no. 11, pp. 845–867, 2002.

[7] T. Kanai, T. Yamagata, T. Ito et al., "Apolipoprotein AII levels are associated with the UP/UCr levels in idiopathic steroid-sensitive nephrotic syndrome," *Clinical and Experimental Nephrology*, vol. 19, no. 1, pp. 107–113, 2015.

[8] T. Kanai, H. Shiraishi, T. Yamagata et al., "Th2 cells predominate in idiopathic steroid-sensitive nephrotic syndrome," *Clinical and Experimental Nephrology*, vol. 14, no. 6, pp. 578–583, 2010.

[9] M. C. Jong, K. Willems Van Dijk, V. E. H. Dahlmans et al., "Reversal of hyperlipidaemia in apolipoprotein C1 transgenic mice by adenovirus-mediated gene delivery of the low-density-lipoprotein receptor, but not by the very-low-density-lipoprotein receptor," *Biochemical Journal*, vol. 338, no. 2, pp. 281–287, 1999.

[10] L. Nagelkerken, P. Verzaal, T. Lagerweij et al., "Development of atopic dermatitis in mice transgenic for human apolipoprotein C1," *Journal of Investigative Dermatology*, vol. 128, no. 5, pp. 1165–1172, 2008.

[11] M. Westerterp, M. Van Eck, W. de Haan et al., "Apolipoprotein CI aggravates atherosclerosis development in ApoE-knockout mice despite mediating cholesterol efflux from macrophages," *Atherosclerosis*, vol. 195, no. 1, pp. e9–e16, 2007.

[12] S. A. Shalaby, H. M. Al-Edressi, S. A. El-Tarhouny, M. F. El-Bab, and M. A. Zolaly, "Type 1/type 2 cytokine serum levels and role of interleukin-18 in children with steroid-sensitive nephrotic syndrome," *Arab Journal of Nephrology and Transplantation*, vol. 6, no. 2, pp. 83–88, 2013.

[13] E. I. Franke, B. A. Vanderbrink, K. L. Hile et al., "Renal IL-18 production is macrophage independent during obstructive injury," *PLoS ONE*, vol. 7, no. 10, Article ID e47417, 2012.

[14] T. Kanai, T. Yamagata, and M. Y. Momoi, "Macrophage inflammatory protein-1β and interleukin-8 associated with idiopathic steroid-sensitive nephrotic syndrome," *Pediatrics International*, vol. 51, no. 4, pp. 443–447, 2009.

[15] S. P. Chen, W. Cheung, C. K. Heng, S. C. Jordan, and H.-K. Yap, "Childhood nephrotic syndrome in relapse is associated with down-regulation of monocyte CD14 expression and lipopolysaccharide-induced tumour necrosis factor-α production," *Clinical and Experimental Immunology*, vol. 134, no. 1, pp. 111–119, 2003.

[16] E. Schlecker, A. Stojanovic, C. Eisen et al., "Tumor-infiltrating monocytic myeloid-derived suppressor cells mediate CCR5-dependent recruitment of regulatory T cells favoring tumor growth," *The Journal of Immunology*, vol. 189, no. 12, pp. 5602–5611, 2012.

[17] C. Araya, L. Diaz, C. Wasserfall et al., "T regulatory cell function in idiopathic minimal lesion nephrotic syndrome," *Pediatric Nephrology*, vol. 24, no. 9, pp. 1691–1698, 2009.

[18] C.-Y. Lin, B.-H. Lee, C.-C. Lin, and W.-P. Chen, "A study of the relationship between childhood nephrotic syndrome and allergic diseases," *Chest*, vol. 97, no. 6, pp. 1408–1411, 1990.

[19] J. M. Hopkin, "The rise of asthma and atopy," *QJM*, vol. 91, no. 3, pp. 169–170, 1998.

[20] J. Yamashita, C. Iwamura, T. Sasaki et al., "Apolipoprotein A-II suppressed concanavalin a-induced hepatitis via the inhibition of CD4 T cell function," *The Journal of Immunology*, vol. 186, no. 6, pp. 3410–3420, 2011.

[21] E. H. Garin, L. N. Diaz, W. Mu et al., "Urinary CD80 excretion increases in idiopathic minimal-change disease," *Journal of the American Society of Nephrology*, vol. 20, no. 2, pp. 260–266, 2009.

[22] J. F. P. Berbé, C. P. Coomans, M. Westerterp, J. A. Romijn, L. M. Havekes, and P. C. N. Rensen, "Apolipoprotein CI enhances the biological response to LPS via the CD14/TLR4 pathway by LPS-binding elements in both its N- and C-terminal helix," *Journal of Lipid Research*, vol. 51, no. 7, pp. 1943–1952, 2010.

22

Overview of Pregnancy in Renal Transplant Patients

Silvi Shah[1] and Prasoon Verma[2]

[1]Department of Nephrology and Hypertension, University of Cincinnati, Cincinnati, OH, USA
[2]Division of Neonatal/Perinatal Medicine, Brown University, Providence, RI, USA

Correspondence should be addressed to Silvi Shah; shah2sv@ucmail.uc.edu

Academic Editor: Franca Anglani

Kidney transplantation offers best hope to women with end-stage renal disease who wish to become pregnant. Pregnancy in a kidney transplant recipient continues to remain challenging due to side effects of immunosuppressive medication, risk of deterioration of allograft function, risk of adverse maternal complications of preeclampsia and hypertension, and risk of adverse fetal outcomes of premature birth, low birth weight, and small for gestational age infants. The factors associated with poor pregnancy outcomes include presence of hypertension, serum creatinine greater than 1.4 mg/dL, and proteinuria. The recommended maintenance immunosuppression in pregnant women is calcineurin inhibitors (tacrolimus/cyclosporine), azathioprine, and low dose prednisone; and it is considered safe. Sirolimus and mycophenolate mofetil should be stopped 6 weeks prior to conception. The optimal time to conception continues to remain an area of contention. It is important that counseling for childbearing should start as early as prior to getting a kidney transplant and should be done at every clinic visit after transplant. Breast-feeding is not contraindicated and should not be discouraged. This review will help the physicians in medical optimization and counseling of renal transplant recipients of childbearing age.

1. Introduction

The first successful pregnancy in kidney transplant recipient occurred in 1958 to 23-year-old Edith Helm who received a kidney from her identical twin sister in 1956 and she delivered a healthy full-term boy of 3300 grams by cesarean section. Her twin sister, Wanda Foster, also gave birth four times successfully after donating the kidney [1]. Since then, there have been many successful pregnancies that have been reported in kidney transplant recipients offering hope to women who have always wished to conceive.

Current knowledge of outcomes of pregnancy in kidney transplant is limited from case reports, single-center studies, and four voluntary registries including National Transplantation Pregnancy Registry (NTPR) in the United States established in 1991 which is the only active registry, National Transplant Pregnancy Registry in the United Kingdom initiated in 1997, European Dialysis and Transplant Association Registry, and the Australian and New Zealand Dialysis and Transplant Registry. Small patient numbers and unavoidable reporting bias limit all these registries [2–5]. We have to keep in mind that most of our current knowledge that guides

the management of pregnancy in renal transplant recipients comes from these retrospective studies.

2. Sexual Function

Women with chronic kidney disease (CKD) have abnormal hypothalamus-pituitary-ovarian axis that leads to menstrual cycle irregularity, anovulation, decreased libido, and impaired fertility. There is an earlier onset of menopause in women with CKD on an average by 4.5 years as compared to general population [6, 7]. Among women on hemodialysis, 73% have menstrual disorders and amenorrhea present in half of them [8]. Women with end-stage renal disease (ESRD), especially with amenorrhea, have high serum prolactin due to impaired renal clearance, increased luteinizing hormone (LH) and follicular stimulating hormone (FSH), and reduced estradiol and progesterone concentration. The persistently elevated gonadotropins due to loss of negative feedback on hypothalamic and pituitary centers and absence of LH surge lead to anovulation [6, 8, 9]. Pregnancy is therefore rare in women on dialysis with very low incidence of conception ranging from 0.9 to 7%. Even after conceiving successfully, the incidence of viable fetal outcome remains low at 20 to 40% [10].

However, the temporary change to hypogonadotropic hypogonadism takes place as soon as 2-3 weeks with return of circulating sex steroids to normal range within 6 months after successful renal transplantation [11]. Due to rapid restoration of hypothalamic-pituitary-gonadal axis, it becomes imperative that contraception should be started immediately after transplant in women with childbearing potential [12].

3. Effect of Pregnancy on Allograft Function

A normal pregnancy leads to hyperfiltration, intrarenal vasodilation, and increase in effective plasma flow with no concomitant increase in intraglomerular pressure. There is an increase in the glomerular filtration rate by about 50% with decrease in the serum concentration of creatinine and urea [13]. Renal allograft is able to adapt to physiological changes of pregnancy with an increase in creatinine clearance of approximately 30% in the first trimester which is sustained with a small decrease in the second trimester and returns to prepregnancy level during the third trimester [14]. Davison reported that the increase in 24-hour creatinine clearance in healthy women was comparable to allograft recipients at 10 weeks of gestation (38% versus 34%). Allograft recipients also have a higher 24-hour protein excretion as compared to healthy women which increases throughout pregnancy, becomes threefold higher by third trimester regularly exceeding 500 mg (versus 200 mg in healthy women), and returns to prepregnancy levels at 3 months postpartum [15]. Proteinuria in pregnancy should never be attributed to normal pregnancy related changes and common comorbidities like urinary tract infection and preeclampsia should be ruled out.

4. Risk of Maternal Complications

4.1. Hypertension and Preeclampsia. Hypertension is common in kidney transplant recipients with a reported incidence of 52% to 69%. The incidence of preeclampsia in renal transplant recipients ranges between 24% and 38% with a 6-fold higher risk compared to incidence of 4-5% in general population [4, 16–18]. It is difficult to distinguish preeclampsia from hypertension in renal transplant recipients because of the frequent increase in blood pressure after 20 weeks in previously normotensive women and hyperfiltration related worsening of preexisting proteinuria. Hyperuricemia becomes a less reliable marker for diagnosing preeclampsia since renal transplant recipients are usually on calcineurin inhibitors which also increase uric acid levels [19]. In addition, sudden worsening of hypertension and marked increase in the proteinuria are also noted in acute rejection, which further makes the diagnosis of preeclampsia challenging. Hypertension during pregnancy increases the risk of preterm delivery, intrauterine growth retardation, and the risk of graft loss [18].

Antihypertensives should be initiated if the blood pressure is consistently higher than 140/90 mmHg. Alpha-methyldopa and hydralazine are the traditional agents that have been used safely for controlling blood pressure during pregnancy. Other antihypertensives that are safe to be used in pregnancy include beta-blockers and calcium channel blockers. Angiotensinogen converting enzyme inhibitors are contraindicated due to their association with pulmonary hypoplasia and oligohydramnios in fetus. Low dose aspirin reduces the risk of preeclampsia in high-risk population and should be given to all renal transplant recipients [20].

4.2. Allograft Function. Pregnancy in the absence of risk factors does not increase the rate of graft loss. The graft failure rate did not differ in pregnant women as compared to nonpregnant allograft recipients at follow-up of 10 years (19% versus 21%) [14]. Risk factors associated with graft loss include history of drug treated hypertension, prepregnancy creatinine ≥ 1.4 mg/dL, and proteinuria. It was demonstrated in the NTPR registry that, out of 133 female renal transplant recipients, 20 who lost graft within 5 years had higher serum creatinine before pregnancy (1.6 mg/dL versus 1.1 mg/dL), higher serum creatinine after pregnancy (2.2 mg/dL versus 1.3 mg/dL), and higher incidence of rejection during or within 3 months after pregnancy (45% versus 4.6%). The risk of allograft loss at 5 years was 3.3-fold higher if prepregnancy creatinine was >1.3 mg/dL and 7.4-fold higher if prepregnancy creatinine was >1.6 mg/dL [4]. Keitel et al. reported that prepregnancy creatinine was >1.5 mg/dL in all six women who suffered graft loss within 2 years postpartum [21]. Sibanda et al. showed that there was no evidence of increased renal allograft loss after pregnancy in matched case control study but the 2-year postpregnancy graft survival was lower in allograft recipients with hypertension as compared to those without (100% versus 87%) [18]. The presence of nephrotic range proteinuria increases the risk of spontaneous abortion, intrauterine growth retardation, and prematurity in pregnant women and therefore it is recommended that proteinuria should be ≤500 mg before pregnancy in renal transplant recipients [22].

4.3. Risk of Rejection and Its Treatment. Pregnancy is a state of immunological tolerance associated with immunodepressant activity of lymphocytes which creates tolerance to fetus and may benefit the renal allograft; however, there is a possibility that the antigenic stimulus provided by the fetus may trigger graft rejection as well. In addition, acute rejection may be higher in the postpartum period due to return to normal immunosurveillance status [23]. The rate of allograft rejection is not increased during pregnancy or 3 months postpartum and varies between 1 and 14.5%, which is comparable to nonpregnant transplant recipients [4, 22]. Risk factors that increase the risk of rejection include high serum creatinine, rejection before pregnancy, and changing levels of immunosuppressive drugs but not the different immunosuppression regime [24]. The diagnosis of rejection is difficult, since rejection is frequently associated with a small rise in creatinine and could be confounded due to hyperfiltration related decrease in creatinine during pregnancy. It is safe to do ultrasound guided allograft biopsy during pregnancy to diagnose rejection [25]. High dose steroids have been successful in treating allograft rejection during pregnancy and remain first-line treatment. Data on the use of other agents like antithymocyte globulin and rituximab for treatment of rejection in pregnancy are limited and there are no specific recommendations [26].

4.4. Infections. Pregnant renal transplant recipients have a higher risk of infections, especially bacterial urinary tract infections (UTI) and acute pyelonephritis, due to use of immunosuppressive medications. UTI is present in up to 40% of women due to reflux, mild hydronephrosis after transplant, and pregnancy related dilation of renal collecting ducts and ureters. Screening for UTI should be performed with dipstick at every visit and with urine cultures at 4-week intervals. Asymptomatic bacteria should be treated with antibiotics for 2 weeks and then prophylaxis should be continued throughout pregnancy. Antibiotics used to treat UTI include nitrofurantoin and cephalexin [22]. Primary cytomegalovirus (CMV) infection results in 40–50% transmission to fetus with 5–18% of them being symptomatic at birth; however, secondary infection has a lower risk of affecting fetus (~2%). The diagnosis of fetal CMV is done by culture of the amniotic fluid. Congenital CMV is associated with hearing loss, learning problems, microcephaly, mental retardation, and perinatal death. The treatment of mother with ganciclovir or CMV hyperimmunoglobulin to prevent fetal CMV disease has not been demonstrated [27]. Herpes simplex infection in mother is associated with increased risk of abortion and can be transmitted from mother to the child during birth. Treatment is with acyclovir and caesarean section is preferred since it attenuates the risk of neonatal herpes. Infants born to mothers who carry hepatitis B antigen should be given hepatitis B immunoglobulin and hepatitis B vaccine to prevent neonatal infection, which offers protection for more than 90% of infants. Vertical transmission with hepatitis C remains low at <7%.

4.5. Other Obstetrical Complications. The risk of cesarean section in renal transplant recipients is higher than the general populations with a reported incidence of 43–64% [4, 16, 17]. Bramham et al. reported that the likelihood of cesarean section in renal transplant recipients in UK transplant registry was 5-fold higher and was twice as common as compared to general population (64% versus 24%), with majority being for fetal distress and 3% being performed merely due to the presence of renal allograft [17]. The incidence of gestational diabetes mellitus is not increased in pregnant women with renal transplants and ranges between 3% and 8% [16, 17].

5. Risk of Fetal Complications

The rate of live births in allograft recipients is comparable to general population and ranges from 71 to 79% [4, 18]. The incidence of preterm delivery has been reported to be as high as 40 to 60% versus 5 to 15% in general population and occurs mostly due to maternal or fetal compromise rather than spontaneous preterm labor [4]. High serum creatinine ≥1.7 mg/dL and presence of maternal hypertension predispose to preterm delivery [18]. In addition, they have high incidence of preterm birth (52 to 53%), low birth weight (42 to 46%), and IUGR (30 to 50%) [4, 23, 28]. Renal allograft

recipients have a 13-fold higher risk of preterm deliveries, 12-fold higher risk of low birth weight babies, and 5-fold high risk of small for gestation babies as compared to general population as reported in a study by Bramham et al. [17]. The mean gestational age for newborn is 35.6 weeks with mean birth weight of 2420 grams [16]. The miscarriage rate ranges from 11 to 26% (versus 8 to 9% in general population) but there is no higher risk of perinatal mortality in the absence of risk factors of hypertension, proteinuria, and impaired allograft dysfunction [4, 17, 18].

6. Predictors of Pregnancy Outcomes

Risk factors described in association with poor pregnancy outcomes are hypertension, elevated prepregnancy creatinine ≥1.4 mg/dL, proteinuria, and history of ≥2 renal transplants. There was about 6-fold higher likelihood of poor fetal outcome (still birth, miscarriage, neonatal death, birth < 32 weeks, and congenital anomalies) in women with high prepregnancy creatinine and high diastolic pressure during second and third trimesters as reported in a study by Bramham et al. [17]. The presence of nephrotic range proteinuria increases the risk of spontaneous abortion, intrauterine growth retardation, and prematurity in pregnant women [22]. Therefore, prepregnancy creatinine ≤1.4 mg/dL, absence of hypertension, and minimal proteinuria <500 mg before pregnancy are associated with successful pregnancy outcomes. In addition, young age at pregnancy and young age at transplantation are associated with a higher likelihood of successful outcomes of live births. The duration of dialysis or history of living donation is not a predictor of successful pregnancy [14].

7. Optimal Time to Conception

The optimal time to conception after renal transplant continues to remain an area of contention. The ideal time of conception in women with renal transplant is between 1 and 2 years according to guidelines by American Society of Transplantation. European best practice guidelines recommend delaying pregnancy for a period of 2 years after transplantation [22, 29]. However, it is safe to conceive even after 6 months of getting a kidney transplant provided that the graft function is stable and that women are not on teratogenic medications. There is a higher likelihood of viable fetal outcome when conception is within 2 years of getting a transplant [16]. In addition, by that time, the viral prophylaxis has been completed and the immunosuppressive medication is at its nadir. Waiting longer may also result in impaired renal function postpartum which may fail to recover with already declining renal function due to chronic allograft nephropathy. However, a recent study reported that there is an increased risk of allograft failure to pregnancies in both first posttransplant year (HR: 1.25; 95% CI: 1.04, 1.50) and second posttransplant year (HR: 1.26; 95% CI: 1.06, 1.50), while pregnancy in the third posttransplant year was not associated with an increased risk of death censored graft loss [30].

8. Immunosuppression

Management of immunosuppression in pregnant renal transplant recipients is important due to the concern for teratogenic risk and potential adverse effects. All the immunosuppressive drugs cross the maternal-fetal circulation and have been detected in variable degrees in fetal circulation [31]. The Food and Drug Administration (FDA) categorizes drugs for pregnancy safety as follows: A (no human risk), B (animal studies showing risk but no evidence of human risk), C (human risk not ruled out), D (evidence of human risk), and X (absolutely contraindicated). The majority of the drugs fall into category C, where risk and benefits have to be weighed. The commonly used immunosuppressive drugs used in renal transplant recipients and their pregnancy information are summarized in Table 1 [32].

8.1. Calcineurin Inhibitors. Calcineurin inhibitors including tacrolimus and cyclosporine are considered safe during pregnancy. Calcineurin inhibitors cross the placenta and enter the fetal circulation; the blood levels detected in the fetus are about half that of the mother [33]. The prevalence of major congenital structural malformation in women on calcineurin inhibitors is approximately 4 to 5% and is comparable to the reported incidence in general population of 3 to 4% [4, 34]. Cyclosporine has been shown to increase the production of thromboxane and endothelin increasing vascular bed resistance, which is implicated in the pathogenesis of preeclampsia. It also increases the risk of low birth weight babies, IUGR, and small for gestational age babies. Animal studies have shown that in utero exposure to calcineurin inhibitors causes hypoplastic peripheral lymphatic organs, immature T cells, and nonfunctional T cell reactivity [35]. In human neonates, cyclosporine may cause immature T cell and low number of B cells which may possibly lead to development of autoimmunity [36]. Developmental delays were found in 16% of children with mean age of 4.4 years who received cyclosporine in utero [37]. However, data on pediatric neurocognitive follow-up are limited and the long-term consequence of in utero exposure to calcineurin inhibitors remains limited [38, 39]. There is a 20–25% dose elevation of calcineurin inhibitors of prepregnancy levels required during gestation due to increase in both the volume of distribution and metabolic activity of cytochrome P450 3A pathway. Cyclosporine trough levels decrease by an average of 23% in the first trimester, 39% in the second trimester, and 29% in the third trimester [40]. We recommend more frequent monitoring of the whole blood trough level during pregnancy with biweekly levels in first and second trimesters, weekly levels in third trimester, and repeating levels within a week postpartum.

8.2. Azathioprine. Azathioprine is a prodrug that is metabolized rapidly to 6-mercaptopurine and is safe to be used as immunosuppression in pregnancy, even though it has been listed a class D drug by FDA. 6-Mercaptopurine passes into the fetal circulation but fetal liver lacks the enzyme inosinate pyrophosphorylase required for the conversion to active metabolite thioinosinic acid and therefore the fetus

TABLE 1: Common immunosuppressive drugs use in transplantation.

	FDA pregnancy category
Induction	
Basiliximab	B
Alemtuzumab	C
Antithymocyte globulin	C
Methylprednisolone	C
Maintenance	
Azathioprine	D
Cyclosporine	C
Tacrolimus	C
Mycophenolate mofetil	D
Sirolimus, rapamycin	C
Prednisone	B
Belatacept	C
Leflunomide	X
Treatment of rejection	
Antithymocyte globulin	C
Basiliximab	B

is protected from its adverse effect [41]. Azathioprine is teratogenic in rats in high doses of 6 mg/kg of body weight but no anomalies have been described in doses ≤2 mg/kg in the offspring. It is also associated with dose related myelosuppression in fetus but neonatal leukopenia is usually rare, if maternal white cell count is greater than 7500/mm^3 [42].

8.3. Corticosteroids. Commonly used steroids in renal transplant recipients include prednisone (category B) and methylprednisolone (category C) [16, 22, 32]. The placental metabolism of corticosteroids is efficient with 90% of the maternal dose being metabolized in placenta before it reaches fetus; and maternal to cord blood ratio is approximately 10 : 1 [43]. Sporadic cases of fetal adrenal immunosuppression, thymic hypoplasia, and cleft palate have been reported usually at doses more than 20 g/day [44]. In addition, steroids increase the risk of premature rupture of membranes and maternal hypertension during pregnancy. Treatment of allograft rejection with steroids if warranted during pregnancy is not contraindicated.

8.4. Mycophenolate Mofetil. Mycophenolate mofetil is a category D drug and is associated with increased risk of spontaneous abortion and congenital malformation. Limb and facial anomalies are the most common congenital malformations and include microtia, hypoplastic nails, shortened fifth finger, cleft lip and palate, congenital diaphragmatic hernia, and congenital heart defects [45]. Mycophenolate mofetil is contraindicated in pregnancy and should be stopped 6 weeks prior to conception. It remains unclear as to what to do in the setting of unplanned pregnancy; however, decision should be based on each individual patient after appropriate counseling has been provided. The risk of malformations is not increased in pregnancies fathered by transplant recipients taking mycophenolate [46]. The incidence of congenital anomalies is 23% and miscarriage rate is 49% in babies born to women on mycophenolate as reported in NTPR [4]. Risk evaluation and mitigation strategy (REMS) should be done in all women with childbearing potential and must be on contraception while taking mycophenolate.

8.5. Sirolimus. Sirolimus is a category C drug. In animal studies, it has been associated with increased fetal mortality, decreased fetal weights, and delayed ossification of skeletal structure, but no teratogenicity was noted [26]. Data is limited with human exposure but sirolimus is contraindicated in pregnancy and should be stopped 6 weeks prior to conception [22, 47].

9. Labor and Delivery

Vaginal delivery is the preferred route of delivery and cesarean section is indicated only for obstetric indications. The renal allograft, which is located in the false pelvis, is not obstructive to the delivery of the fetus. Spontaneous labor can be allowed up to 38 to 40 weeks if there are no obstetrical complications. Stress dose steroids should be given to women during labor who are maintained on steroids for immunosuppression [25]. Pregnancy in renal transplant recipient is high risk and should be managed by a multidisciplinary team of high-risk obstetrician, neonatologist, and transplant nephrologist [22]. We recommend a close follow-up with transplant nephrologist every 2 weeks during the prenatal care.

10. Contraception

An unplanned pregnancy after transplantation may expose both mother and fetus to risk of adverse outcomes and puts them at higher risk for induced abortion. More than 90% of the pregnancies were unplanned after transplantation as reported in British transplantation clinic. Among the women who received a transplant, only 48.7% were advised to use contraception and 72.1% were actually using the contraceptive method [12]. It is therefore recommended that women in childbearing age should receive contraceptive counseling as part of their routine care, which should start before transplantation and effective contraceptive method should be started immediately after transplantation. Women who have not been immunized to rubella should receive the vaccination before transplantation, since live viral vaccines are contraindicated after transplantation. Data on the ideal contraceptive method in renal transplant recipients remain limited. Barrier method is not an optimal form of contraception due to potential for contraception failure. Intrauterine devices may increase the chances of infection and in addition lead to contraceptive failure due to reduced anti-inflammatory properties and decreased effectiveness in association with immunosuppressive drugs [48]. The American Society of Transplantation Consensus Conference has suggested the use of low dose estrogen/progesterone or progestin only oral contraceptives in renal transplant recipients if hypertension is well controlled [29]. Center for Disease Control recommends use of either hormonal methods or intrauterine device in uncomplicated solid organ transplant recipients. However, in complicated solid organ transplant patients with acute or chronic allograft failure, combined estrogen/progesterone methods pose unacceptable health risks [49]. Surgical contraception like tubal ligation should be advised in women who have completed their families. Physicians must discuss risk and benefit of each contraceptive method with renal transplant recipients and take into account their desire and lifestyle to determine the most effective contraception.

11. Breast-Feeding

Transplant recipients taking prednisone, azathioprine, cyclosporine, and tacrolimus should not be discouraged from breast-feeding [50]. It is well established now that the infants who are breast-fed by mothers on prednisone, azathioprine, and cyclosporine/tacrolimus have a lesser exposure via breast milk than in utero and they do not have adverse effects. The estimated absorption of tacrolimus from breast milk is equivalent to 0.23% of the weight-adjusted maternal dose, which is negligible; and breast-feeding does not slow the decline of tacrolimus levels in infant from higher levels at birth [51]. Infants breast-fed by women on cyclosporine receive less than 300 mcg per day of cyclosporine and absorb undetectable amounts [52]. Exposure of breast milk to corticosteroids is at most 0.1% of total maternal dose and maternal dose of prednisone up to 20 mg/day does not cause adverse effects in infants [53]. Similarly, the amount of azathioprine in breast milk and infant serum is negligible; and breast-feeding is considered safe [54]. Clinical information on breast-feeding is inadequate for mycophenolic acid, sirolimus, everolimus, and belatacept; and breast-feeding should be avoided.

12. Conclusion

Renal transplant restores fertility and pregnancy requires careful planning. There should be an expansion of effort by primary care physicians and nephrologists to include the discussion of menstrual and reproductive issues in women with renal transplant. Women of childbearing age wishing to consider pregnancy should receive complete information and counseling from the transplant team. The following summarizes the criteria for renal transplant recipients contemplating pregnancy [29, 32]:

At least 6 months after transplantation

Stable allograft function and creatinine < 1.4 mg/dL

No recent episodes of acute rejection

Blood pressure ≤ 140/90 mmHg

No or minimal proteinuria ≤ 500 mg/24 hours

Prednisone ≤ 15 mg/day

Azathioprine ≤ 2 mg/kg/day

Stopping mycophenolate mofetil and sirolimus 6 weeks prior to conception

Prepregnancy counseling with the potential risks will enable pregnancy planning and help parents make an informed decision. A multidisciplinary approach by the transplant nephrologist and maternal-fetal medicine is essential throughout pregnancy and can result in good outcomes for mother and infant. Due to lack of prospective data, further research is needed in this field which will help us expand our current knowledge.

References

[1] J. E. Murray, D. E. Reid, J. H. Harrison, and J. P. Merrill, "Successful pregnancies after human renal transplantation," *The New England Journal of Medicine*, vol. 269, pp. 341–343, 1963.

[2] J. M. Davison and C. W. G. Redman, "Pregnancy post-transplant: the establishment of a UK registry," *British Journal of Obstetrics and Gynaecology*, vol. 104, no. 10, pp. 1106–1107, 1997.

[3] G. Rizzoni, J. H. H. Ehrich, M. Broyer et al., "Successful pregnancies in women on renal replacement therapy: report from the EDTA Registry," *Nephrology Dialysis Transplantation*, vol. 7, no. 4, pp. 279–287, 1992.

[4] L. A. Coscia, S. Constantinescu, M. J. Moritz et al., "Report from the National Transplantation Pregnancy Registry (NTPR): outcomes of pregnancy after transplantation," *Clinical Transplants*, pp. 65–85, 2010.

[5] V. Levidiotis, S. Chang, and S. McDonald, "Pregnancy and maternal outcomes among kidney transplant recipients," *Journal of the American Society of Nephrology*, vol. 20, no. 11, pp. 2433–2440, 2009.

[6] J. L. Holley, R. J. Schmidt, F. H. Bender, F. Dumler, and M. Schiff, "Gynecologic and reproductive issues in women on dialysis," *American Journal of Kidney Diseases*, vol. 29, no. 5, pp. 685–690, 1997.

[7] J. R. Weisinger and E. Bellorin-Font, "Outcomes associated with hypogonadism in women with chronic kidney disease," *Advances in Chronic Kidney Disease*, vol. 11, no. 4, pp. 361–370, 2004.

[8] J. Matuszkiewicz-Rowińska, K. Skórzewska, S. Radowicki et al., "Endometrial morphology and pituitary-gonadal axis dysfunction in women of reproductive age undergoing chronic haemodialysis—a multicentre study," *Nephrology Dialysis Transplantation*, vol. 19, no. 8, pp. 2074–2077, 2004.

[9] J. Matuszkiewicz-Rowińska, K. Skórzewska, S. Radowicki et al., "Menstrual disturbances and alternations in hypophyseal gonadal axis in end-stage premenopausal women undergoing hemodialysis: a multi-center study," *Polskie Archiwum Medycyny Wewnetrznej*, vol. 109, no. 6, pp. 609–615, 2003.

[10] I. Giatras, D. P. Levy, F. D. Malone, J. A. Carlson, and P. Jungers, "Pregnancy during dialysis: case report and management guidelines," *Nephrology Dialysis Transplantation*, vol. 13, no. 12, pp. 3266–3272, 1998.

[11] M.-T. Saha, H. H. T. Saha, L. K. Niskanen, K. T. Salmela, and A. I. Pasternack, "Time course of serum prolactin and sex hormones following successful renal transplantation," *Nephron*, vol. 92, no. 3, pp. 735–737, 2002.

[12] C. A. F. Guazzelli, M. R. Torloni, T. F. Sanches, M. Barbieri, and J. O. M. A. Pestana, "Contraceptive counseling and use among 197 female kidney transplant recipients," *Transplantation*, vol. 86, no. 5, pp. 669–672, 2008.

[13] J. M. Davison and W. Dunlop, "Renal hemodynamics and tubular function in normal human pregnancy," *Kidney International*, vol. 18, no. 2, pp. 152–161, 1980.

[14] H. W. Kim, H. J. Seok, T. H. Kim, D.-J. Han, W. S. Yang, and S.-K. Park, "The experience of pregnancy after renal transplantation: pregnancies even within postoperative 1 year may be tolerable," *Transplantation*, vol. 85, no. 10, pp. 1412–1419, 2008.

[15] J. M. Davison, "The effect of pregnancy on kidney function in renal allograft recipients," *Kidney International*, vol. 27, no. 1, pp. 74–79, 1985.

[16] N. A. Deshpande, N. T. James, L. M. Kucirka et al., "Pregnancy outcomes in kidney transplant recipients: a systematic review and meta-analysis," *American Journal of Transplantation*, vol. 11, no. 11, pp. 2388–2404, 2011.

[17] K. Bramham, C. Nelson-Piercy, H. Gao et al., "Pregnancy in renal transplant recipients: a UK national cohort study," *Clinical Journal of the American Society of Nephrology*, vol. 8, no. 2, pp. 290–298, 2013.

[18] N. Sibanda, J. D. Briggs, J. M. Davison, R. J. Johnson, and C. J. Rudge, "Pregnancy after organ transplantation: a report from the U.K. Transplant Pregnancy Registry," *Transplantation*, vol. 83, no. 10, pp. 1301–1307, 2007.

[19] J. M. Morales, G. Hernandez Poblete, A. Andres, C. Prieto, E. Hernandez, and J. L. Rodicio, "Uric acid handling, pregnancy and cyclosporin in renal transplant women," *Nephron*, vol. 56, no. 1, pp. 97–98, 1990.

[20] L. Duley, D. J. Henderson-Smart, S. Meher, and J. F. King, "Antiplatelet agents for preventing pre-eclampsia and its complications," *The Cochrane Database of Systematic Reviews*, no. 2, Article ID CD004659, 2007.

[21] E. Keitel, R. M. Bruno, M. Duarte et al., "Pregnancy outcome after renal transplantation," *Transplantation Proceedings*, vol. 36, no. 4, pp. 870–871, 2004.

[22] "European best practice guidelines for renal transplantation. Section IV: long-term management of the transplant recipient. IV.10. Pregnancy in renal transplant recipients," *EBPG Expert Group on Renal Transplantation*, vol. 17, supplement 4, pp. 50–55, 2002.

[23] P. Stratta, C. Canavese, F. Giacchino, P. Mesiano, M. Quaglia, and M. Rossetti, "Pregnancy in kidney transplantation: satisfactory outcomes and harsh realities," *Journal of Nephrology*, vol. 16, no. 6, pp. 792–806, 2003.

[24] V. T. Armenti, C. H. McGrory, J. R. Cater, J. S. Radomski, and M. J. Moritz, "Pregnancy outcomes in female renal transplant recipients," *Transplantation Proceedings*, vol. 30, no. 5, pp. 1732–1734, 1998.

[25] J. M. Davidson and M. D. Lindheimer, *Maternal-Fetal Medicine: Principles and Practice*, Saunders, Philadelphia, Pa, USA, 2004.

[26] V. T. Armenti, M. J. Moritz, E. H. Cardonick, and J. M. Davison, "Immunosuppression in pregnancy: choices for infant and maternal health," *Drugs*, vol. 62, no. 16, pp. 2361–2375, 2002.

[27] R. S. Gibbs, R. L. Sweet, and P. Duff, *Maternal Fetal Medicine Principles and Practice*, Saunders, 2004.

[28] M. del Mar Colon and J. U. Hibbard, "Obstetric considerations in the management of pregnancy in kidney transplant recipients," *Advances in Chronic Kidney Disease*, vol. 14, no. 2, pp. 168–177, 2007.

[29] D. B. McKay, M. A. Josephson, V. T. Armenti et al., "Reproduction and transplantation: report on the AST consensus conference on reproductive issues and transplantation," *American Journal of Transplantation*, vol. 5, no. 7, pp. 1592–1599, 2005.

[30] C. Rose, J. Gill, N. Zalunardo, O. Johnston, A. Mehrotra, and J. S. Gill, "Timing of pregnancy after kidney transplantation and risk of allograft failure," *American Journal of Transplantation*, vol. 16, no. 8, pp. 2360–2367, 2016.

[31] C. D. Chambers, S. R. Braddock, G. G. Briggs A et al., "Postmarketing surveillance for human teratogenicity: a model approach," *Teratology*, vol. 64, no. 5, pp. 252–261, 2001.

[32] L. A. Coscia, S. Constantinescu, J. M. Davison, M. J. Moritz, and V. T. Armenti, "Immunosuppressive drugs and fetal outcome," *Best Practice & Research: Clinical Obstetrics & Gynaecology*, vol. 28, no. 8, pp. 1174–1187, 2014.

[33] R. Venkataramanan, B. Koneru, C.-C. P. Wang, G. J. Burckart, S. N. Caritis, and T. E. Starzl, "Cyclosporine and its metabolites in mother and baby," *Transplantation*, vol. 46, no. 3, pp. 468–469, 1988.

[34] R. H. Finnell, "Teratology: general considerations and principles," *The Journal of Allergy and Clinical Immunology*, vol. 103, no. 2, pp. S337–S342, 1999.

[35] K. Heeg, S. Bendigs, and H. Wagner, "Cyclosporine A prevents the generation of single positive (Lyt2$^+$ L3T4$^-$, Lyt2$^-$ L3T4$^+$) mature T cells, but not single positive (Lyt2$^+$ T3$^-$) immature thymocytes, in newborn mice," *Scandinavian Journal of Immunology*, vol. 30, no. 6, pp. 703–710, 1989.

[36] F. P. Schena, G. G. Stallone, A. Schena et al., "Pregnancy in renal transplantation: immunologic evaluation of neonates from mothers with transplanted kidney," *Transplant Immunology*, vol. 9, no. 2-4, pp. 161–164, 2001.

[37] C. W. Stanley, R. Gottlieb, R. Zager et al., "Developmental well-being in offspring of women receiving cyclosporine post-renal transplant," *Transplantation Proceedings*, vol. 31, no. 1-2, pp. 241–242, 1999.

[38] M. Avramut, A. Zeevi, and C. L. Achim, "The immunosuppressant drug FK506 is a potent trophic agent for human fetal neurons," *Developmental Brain Research*, vol. 132, no. 2, pp. 151–157, 2001.

[39] R. G. Victor, G. D. Thomas, E. Marban, and B. O'Rourke, "Presynaptic modulation of cortical synaptic activity by calcineurin," *Proceedings of the National Academy of Sciences of the United States of America*, vol. 92, no. 14, pp. 6269–6273, 1995.

[40] H. Kim, J. C. Jeong, J. Yang et al., "The optimal therapy of calcineurin inhibitors for pregnancy in kidney transplantation," *Clinical Transplantation*, vol. 29, no. 2, pp. 142–148, 2015.

[41] S. Saarikoski and M. Seppälä, "Immunosuppression during pregnancy: transmission of azathioprine and its metabolites from the mother to the fetus," *American Journal of Obstetrics and Gynecology*, vol. 115, no. 8, pp. 1100–1106, 1973.

[42] J. M. Davison, H. Dellagrammatikas, and J. M. Parkin, "Maternal azathioprine therapy and depressed haemopoiesis in the babies of renal allograft patients," *British Journal of Obstetrics and Gynaecology*, vol. 92, no. 3, pp. 233–239, 1985.

[43] I. Z. Beitins, F. Bayard, I. G. Ances, A. Kowarski, and C. J. Migeon, "The transplacental passage of prednisone and prednisolone in pregnancy near term," *The Journal of Pediatrics*, vol. 81, no. 5, pp. 936–945, 1972.

[44] S. Chhabria, "Aicardi's syndrome: are corticosteroids teratogens?" *Archives of Neurology*, vol. 38, article 70, 1981.

[45] N. M. Sifontis, L. A. Coscia, S. Constantinescu, A. F. Lavelanet, M. J. Moritz, and V. T. Armenti, "Pregnancy outcomes in solid organ transplant recipients with exposure to mycophenolate mofetil or sirolimus," *Transplantation*, vol. 82, no. 12, pp. 1698–1702, 2006.

[46] A. Jones, M. J. Clary, E. McDermott et al., "Outcomes of pregnancies fathered by solid-organ transplant recipients exposed to mycophenolic acid products," *Progress in Transplantation*, vol. 23, no. 2, pp. 153–157, 2013.

[47] D. B. McKay and M. A. Josephson, "Pregnancy after kidney transplantation," *Clinical Journal of the American Society of Nephrology*, vol. 3, supplement 2, pp. S117–S125, 2008.

[48] J. Zerner, K. L. Doil, J. Drewry, and D. A. Leeber, "Intrauterine contraceptive device failures in renal transplant patients," *The Journal of Reproductive Medicine*, vol. 26, no. 2, pp. 99–102, 1981.

[49] K. M. Curtis, T. C. Jatlaoui, N. K. Tepper et al., "U.S. selected practice recommendations for contraceptive use, 2016," *MMWR. Recommendations and Reports: Morbidity and Mortality Weekly Report*, vol. 65, no. 4, pp. 1–66, 2016.

[50] S. Constantinescu, A. Pai, L. A. Coscia, J. M. Davison, M. J. Moritz, and V. T. Armenti, "Breast-feeding after transplantation," *Best Practice & Research: Clinical Obstetrics & Gynaecology*, vol. 28, no. 8, pp. 1163–1173, 2014.

[51] K. Bramham, G. Chusney, J. Lee, L. Lightstone, and C. Nelson-Piercy, "Breastfeeding and tacrolimus: serial monitoring in breast-fed and bottle-fed infants," *Clinical Journal of the American Society of Nephrology*, vol. 8, no. 4, pp. 563–567, 2013.

[52] G. Nyberg, U. Haljamäe, C. Frisenette-Fich, M. Wennergren, and I. Kjellmer, "Breast-feeding during treatment with cyclosporine," *Transplantation*, vol. 65, no. 2, pp. 253–255, 1998.

[53] P. A. Greenberger, Y. K. Odeh, M. C. Frederiksen, and A. J. Atkinson Jr., "Pharmacokinetics of prednisolone transfer to breast milk," *Clinical Pharmacology and Therapeutics*, vol. 53, no. 3, pp. 324–328, 1993.

[54] L. A. Christensen, J. F. Dahlerup, M. J. Nielsen, J. F. Fallingborg, and K. Schmiegelow, "Azathioprine treatment during lactation," *Alimentary Pharmacology & Therapeutics*, vol. 28, no. 10, pp. 1209–1213, 2008.

23

Serial Galactose-Deficient IgA1 Levels in Children with IgA Nephropathy and Healthy Controls

John T. Sanders,[1] **M. Colleen Hastings,**[2,3] **Zina Moldoveanu,**[4] **Jan Novak,**[4] **Bruce A. Julian,**[4] **Zoran Bursac,**[2] **and Robert J. Wyatt**[2,3]

[1]*Sanford Children's Hospital, Sioux Falls, SD 57117, USA*
[2]*University of Tennessee Health Sciences Center, Memphis, TN 38013, USA*
[3]*Children's Foundation Research Institute, Memphis, TN 38013, USA*
[4]*University of Alabama at Birmingham, Birmingham, AL 35294, USA*

Correspondence should be addressed to Robert J. Wyatt; rwyatt@uthsc.edu

Academic Editor: Laszlo Rosivall

Galactose-deficient IgA1 (Gd-IgA1) is a key pathogenic factor for IgA nephropathy (IgAN) and a potential biomarker for the disease. This study examined serial serum Gd-IgA1 levels over 1 year in 13 children with IgAN and 40 healthy children, to determine whether or not serum Gd-IgA1 levels changed over time. Subjects were younger than 18 years of age. Follow-up measurements were scheduled 6 and/or 12 months later. Analysis of variance and regression models for repeated measures were used to estimate group and time effects. Serum Gd-IgA1 level was higher in initial samples for IgAN patients compared to those of healthy children ($P < 0.0001$). Serum Gd-IgA1 levels did not change over time for healthy controls but increased for IgAN patients ($P = 0.001$). Serum Gd-IgA1 level was elevated for 9 children with IgAN at study entry and remained elevated. Two of the 4 IgAN patients with initially normal Gd-IgA1 levels had a subsequent elevated level. The persistent elevation of the serum Gd-IgA1 level in children with IgAN enhances its utility as a potential diagnostic test for IgAN.

1. Introduction

IgA nephropathy (IgAN) is the most common type of chronic glomerulonephritis worldwide [1]. However, the true incidence of IgAN is difficult to determine because a renal biopsy is required for diagnosis. Diagnosis of IgAN may not be made in the milder cases or may be delayed until clinical manifestations are severe enough to necessitate this invasive procedure [2]. Development of a reliable serologic test for diagnosis of IgAN would be a major advance for early detection and treatment of this condition.

The pathogenesis of IgAN is related to aberrantly glycosylated IgA1 wherein some *O*-linked glycans in the hinge region contain terminal *N*-acetylgalactosamine (GalNAc) rather than a GalNAc-galactose structure [3]. The galactose-deficient IgA1 (Gd-IgA1) is recognized by anti-Gd-IgA1 autoantibodies [4]. This process results in formation of circulating immune complexes and then some complexes deposit in the glomerular mesangium, subsequently activating mesangial cells to proliferate and overproduce extracellular-matrix proteins and cytokines, thus inciting injury of the glomerulus [5–7].

In 2007, we found that serum levels of Gd-IgA1 were elevated in 75% of adult and pediatric patients with IgAN, suggesting that this measurement may be a useful diagnostic test for the condition [8, 9]. Subsequently, serum Gd-IgA1 level has been proposed as biomarker for IgAN [2, 10–12]. Serial levels of Gd-IgA1 have not previously been examined to determine if these levels remain stable over time in patients with IgA nephropathy or healthy controls. The only published data are for serial levels after kidney transplantation of adults with IgAN that showed that immunosuppressants, particularly corticosteroids, lowered serum Gd-IgA1 levels [11]. In addition, serum levels of Gd-IgA1 are significantly lower in children and adolescents as compared to adults [9] and African Americans have slightly lower levels than Caucasians [13]. The purpose of this study was to examine serial serum Gd-IgA1 levels over a period of 1 year in children with IgAN and healthy pediatric controls, to determine the effect of time on serum Gd-IgA1 level.

2. Materials and Methods

2.1. Ethical Considerations. The University of Tennessee Health Science Center Institutional Review Board approved the study protocol, "Non-Invasive Diagnosis of IgA Nephropathy" (IRB number 08-08771-XP). Informed written consent was obtained from each subject's legal guardian(s) and signed assent was obtained from all children 8 years of age or older.

2.2. Study Population. Children over 4 and less than 18 years of age were eligible for recruitment from the outpatient pediatric nephrology clinics and the Pediatric Clinical Research Unit at Le Bonheur Children's Hospital. Healthy controls were screened for renal disease by questionnaire at study entry and by urinalysis. Potential control subjects were excluded if more than trace blood or protein was detected on urine dipstick. The following demographic characteristics were obtained: date of birth, gender, and self-reported race/ethnicity. Subjects were excluded if they were a first-degree relative of previously entered patients or controls. Seventy-seven healthy controls were initially enrolled, but only 40 of them returned for follow-up visits.

The diagnosis of IgAN required renal biopsy showing IgA as the dominant or codominant immunoglobulin in a typical mesangial distribution in the absence of clinical and laboratory evidence for other systemic disease. No subject with IgAN was treated with a corticosteroid or nonsteroidal immunosuppressant during the study and no subject was studied during an episode of macroscopic hematuria. Children with IgA vasculitis (Henoch Schonlein purpura) were excluded.

2.3. Sample Handling. Blood and urine were obtained at study entry and at approximately 6 and 12 months later. The serum fractions of whole-blood specimens were frozen at −70°C and sent overnight in batches to the Department of Microbiology at the University of Alabama at Birmingham for determination of serum levels of Gd-IgA1 and total IgA. Samples were labelled by a unique code and the samples were analyzed in a blinded manner.

2.4. Serum Total IgA and Gd-IgA1 Levels. Serum levels of total IgA and Gd-IgA1 were determined by ELISA [8]. Serum total IgA was determined using IgA-calibrated human sera (Binding Site, Birmingham, UK) and the serum Gd-IgA1 was standardized to a polymeric Gd-IgA1 myeloma protein [8]. One unit/mL of Gd-IgA1 was equivalent to 1.0 μg/ml of the Gd-IgA1 (Ale) standard. Total serum IgA levels are reported in μg/ml.

2.5. Statistical Analysis. Depending on the underlying distribution, continuous variables are reported as a mean ± standard deviation or median (range) and categorical variables are reported as percentages. One-way analysis of variance

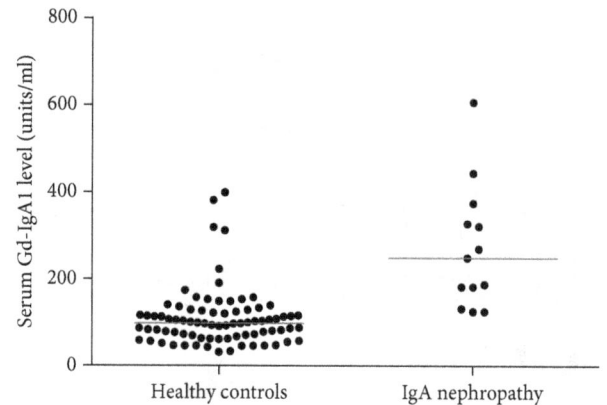

FIGURE 1: Serum Gd-IgA1 level at study baseline visit is shown for each study group. The red bars indicate median serum levels. Levels were significantly higher for the IgA nephropathy group as compared to the healthy-control group ($P < 0.0001$).

(ANOVA) was used to compare mean serum levels of Gd-IgA1, total IgA, and percent Gd-IgA1/total IgA at baseline in patients with IgAN and healthy controls. To test the correlation and association between the outcome measures and age at baseline, we fit a simple linear regression model. Finally, we applied a repeated measure regression model with group, visit, and their interaction term using unstructured covariance structure, to test the group and visit marginal means and account for correlation in the data. This model made use of all available data points, regardless of the number of completed visits. Both ANOVA and regression methods incorporated Bonferroni adjustments for multiple comparisons between groups and visit time points. The 90th percentile for healthy controls was the cutoff point for elevated level of Gd-IgA1 as levels in patients were not normally distributed.

All statistical analyses were performed with SAS/STATv14.1 (SAS Institute Inc., Cary, NC, USA) and GraphPad Prism 6.0 (Graphpad Inc., San Diego, CA, USA). Statistical associations were considered significant at the alpha level of 0.05.

3. Results

Table 1 shows the demographic characteristics of both groups. The age of subjects in the healthy-control group versus the IgAN group did not significantly differ. African-American children comprised about two-thirds of the healthy controls, but only about one-third of the children with IgAN.

Data from the initial visit showed that children with IgAN had significantly elevated serum Gd-IgA1 levels compared to the healthy-control group ($P < 0.0001$) (Figure 1). The group of children with IgAN also had significantly higher serum total IgA levels as compared to the healthy-control group ($P = 0.025$) (Figure S1, supplemental appendix, in Supplementary Material, available online at https://doi.org/10.1155/2017/8210641). The percentage of Gd-IgA1 of total IgA was also higher in patients with IgAN than healthy controls ($P < 0.0001$) (Figure S2, supplemental appendix). Serum Gd-IgA1

TABLE 1: Demographic characteristics for subject groups.

Group	Number	Males	Caucasians	Age at study entry median (range) years
Healthy controls	77	48 (62%)	32 (41%)	11.7 (6.8–17.6)
Patients with IgAN	13	6 (46%)	9 (69%)	14.3 (8.6–17.2)

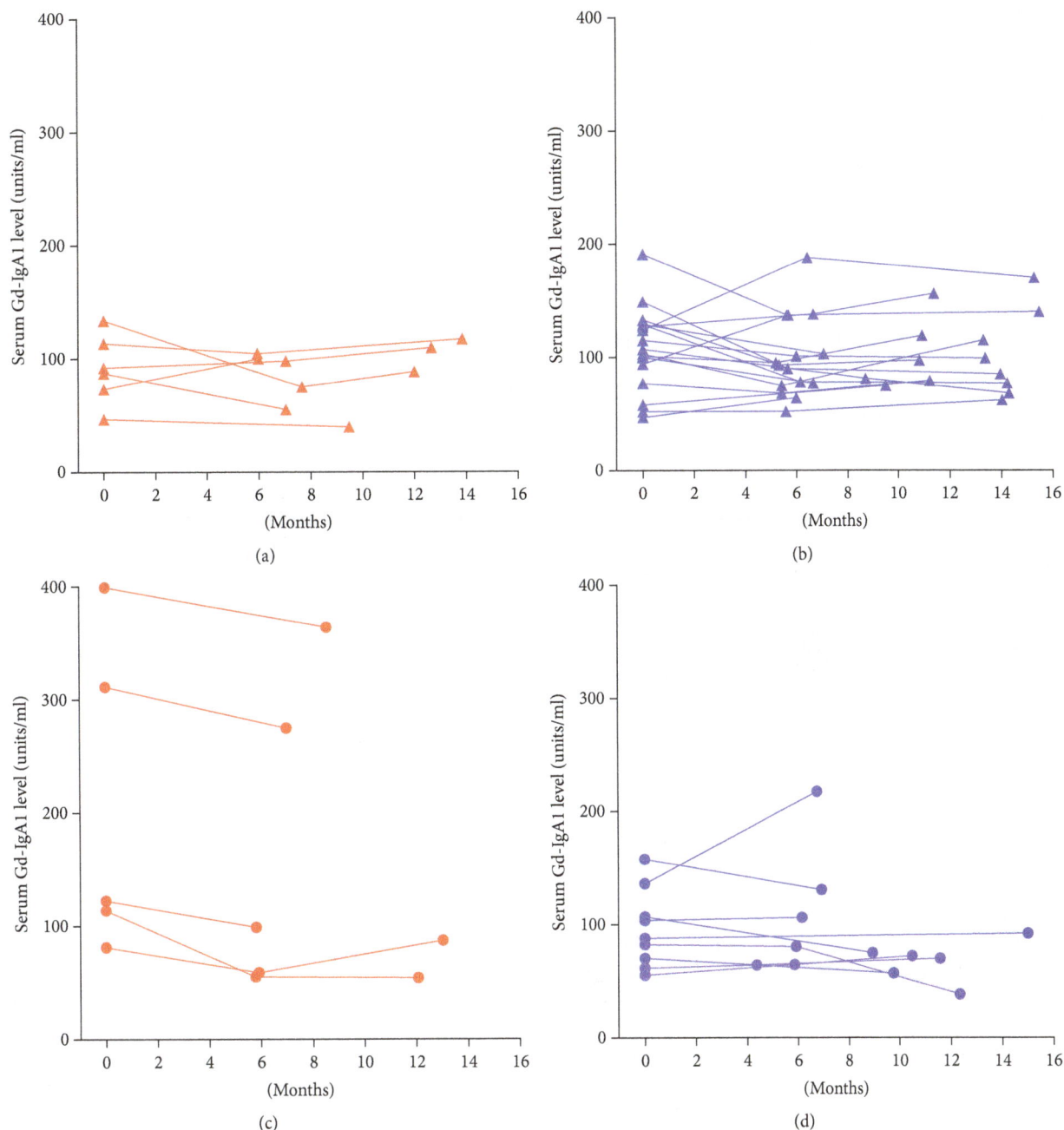

FIGURE 2: Spaghetti plots of serial serum Gd-IgA1 levels for healthy-control group are shown in Panel (a)—Caucasian males, Panel (b)—African-American males, Panel (c)—Caucasian females, and Panel (d)—African-American females.

level did not have a significant association with age at study baseline for healthy controls of both races ($P = 0.36$).

Serum Gd-IgA1 levels over the course of the study were plotted for each ethnicity-gender combination (Figure 2). The levels for each subject in these four groups appeared to be stable over the course of the study. Serum Gd-IgA1 level in the initial sample was above the 90th percentile for 9 of 13 (69%) subjects with IgAN (Figure 3). All 9 subjects with an elevated initial level had elevated levels in subsequent samples. Two of the 4 IgAN patients with an initially normal

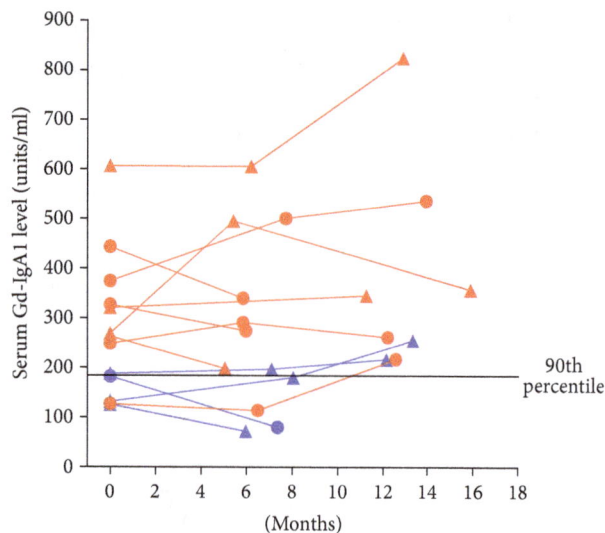

FIGURE 3: Spaghetti plots of serial Gd-IgA1 serum levels in pediatric patients with IgAN. Red symbols and lines represent Caucasian patients, while blue lines and symbols represent African Americans. Circles represent females and triangles represent males.

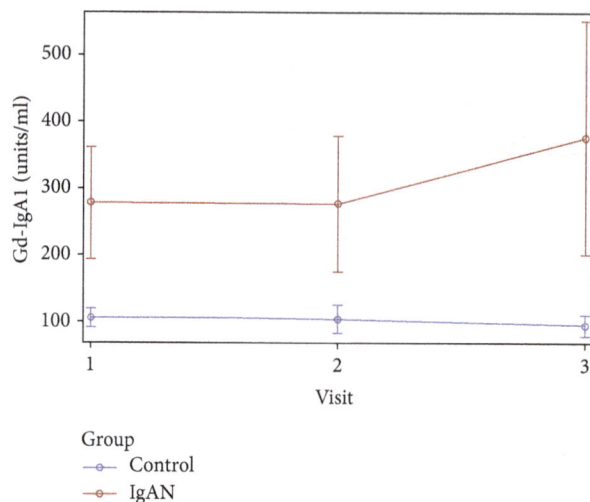

FIGURE 4: Mean and 95% confidence interval of serum Gd-IgA1 levels for each of the two study groups across three data collection points. The red line and circles represent IgAN patients and the blue line and circles represent healthy controls.

serum Gd-IgA1 level had an elevated level at 1-year of follow-up.

Figure 4 shows that, for the healthy-control group, the mean serum Gd-IgA1 levels did not significantly change over time ($P = 0.13$). For the children with IgAN, there was no significant difference between baseline and the 6-month follow-up measurement ($P = 0.99$); however, Gd-IgA1 levels at the 12-month follow-up were significantly higher than at the first 2 time points ($P = 0.001$ and $P = 0.046$, resp.).

4. Discussion

Our group previously demonstrated significantly elevated serum Gd-IgA1 levels in 22 pediatric patients with IgAN compared to 16 pediatric-control subjects [9]. No data from that previous study were included in the present study. This study further establishes that serum Gd-IgA1 levels are significantly elevated in pediatric patients with IgAN compared to levels in healthy-control pediatric subjects.

Serum IgA levels are known to increase during childhood and total serum IgA levels in young children are very low [14]. One study showed serum IgA levels in children to approach adult levels by the age of 6 to 7 years [14], although, in another study, adult levels for serum IgA were not achieved until the age of 16 years [15]. None of our healthy controls was younger than 6 years. If serum Gd-IgA1 levels parallel the total IgA levels for younger children, one must be careful in interpreting whether the Gd-IgA1 level is normal or elevated for children under age of 6 years.

Few studies have evaluated variation in serum total IgA levels using serial sampling. Veys et al. [16] showed that serum IgA levels fluctuate as much as 20% in samples collected 2 weeks apart, but changes over a month were not significant. Serum Gd-IgA1 levels showed little variation over 1 year for

pediatric healthy-control subjects. However, almost half of the control subjects entered in the study did not return for serial measurements. Although the number of remaining healthy controls was more than 3 times higher than the number of IgAN patients in the study, it is possible that the noncomplying subjects differed somehow from the ones that continued in the study, introducing a source of bias for the results of our study.

Our study showed an increase in mean serum Gd-IgA1 levels at the 1-year visit in children with IgAN. This finding may be explained, in part, by the 4 IgAN patients with an initially normal serum Gd-IgA1 level. Two of those subjects returned for a 6-month but not for a 12-month blood draw, while for the other 2 the level increased at the final blood draw. Thus, the significant increase in Gd-IgA1 level might not be found in study with a larger sample size of subjects having levels for all 3 time points.

Although there appeared to be more variation in children with IgAN, those with an initially elevated level maintained an elevated level over the course of 1 year. Sustained elevations of serum Gd-IgA1 levels over time for most children with IgAN contributes to the utility of this biomarker as a potential diagnostic test.

Acknowledgments

Dr. Sanders was supported by a National Kidney Foundation/Strides for IgA Nephropathy fellowship grant. Other support was provided by grants from the National Institutes of Health (DK082753 and DK07824) and the General Clinical Research Center of the University of Tennessee Health Science Center (M01 RR00211) and by a generous gift to the University of Tennessee Pediatric Nephrology Research Support Fund from Anna and Donald Waite. The authors regret to report that, during this study, Dr. Grant Somes died unexpectedly on March 18, 2010. He provided significant early input on the statistical analysis of the data. Andrew Bush, Emeritus Professor of Preventive Medicine, served on Dr. Sanders project committee for his M.S. degree in epidemiology and provided important input with regards to design of the study. They also appreciate the work of Sherry Walker, BSN, and Olivia Hancox, LPN, in the recruitment and retention of study subjects, collection of blood samples, and management of clinical data.

References

[1] G. D'Amico G, "The commonest glomerulonephritis in the world: IgA nephropathy," *Quarterly Journal of Medicine*, vol. 64, no. 245, pp. 709–727, 1987.

[2] R. J. Wyatt and B. A. Julian, "Medical progress: IgA nephropathy," *The New England Journal of Medicine*, vol. 368, no. 25, pp. 2402–2414, 2013.

[3] M. Tomana, K. Matousovic, B. A. Julian, J. Radl, K. Konecny, and J. Mestecky, "Galactose-deficient IgA1 in sera of IgA nephropathy patients is present in complexes with IgG," *Kidney International*, vol. 52, no. 2, pp. 509–516, 1997.

[4] H. Suzuki, R. Fan, Z. Zhang et al., "Aberrantly glycosylated IgA1 in IgA nephropathy patients is recognized by IgG antibodies with restricted heterogeneity," *The Journal of Clinical Investigation*, vol. 119, no. 6, pp. 1668–1677, 2009.

[5] K. Ebefors, P. Liu, E. Lassén et al., "Mesangial cells from patients with IgA nephropathy have increased susceptibility to galactose-deficient IgA1," *BMC Nephrology*, vol. 17, no. 1, article no. 251, 2016.

[6] G. Seki, M. Tanaka, T. Someya, M. Nagata, and T. Fujita, "Aberrantly glycosylated IgA1 as a factor in the pathogenesis of IgA nephropathy," *Clinical and Developmental Immunology*, vol. 2011, Article ID 470803, 2011.

[7] H. Suzuki, K. Kiryluk, J. Novak et al., "The pathophysiology of IgA nephropathy," *Journal of the American Society of Nephrology*, vol. 22, no. 10, pp. 1795–1803, 2011.

[8] Z. Moldoveanu, R. J. Wyatt, J. Y. Lee et al., "Patients with IgA nephropathy have increased serum galactose-deficient IgA1 levels," *Kidney International*, vol. 71, no. 11, pp. 1148–1154, 2007.

[9] K. K. Lau, R. J. Wyatt, Z. Moldoveanu et al., "Serum levels of galactose-deficient IgA in children with IgA nephropathy and Henoch-Schönlein purpura," *Pediatric Nephrology*, vol. 22, no. 12, pp. 2067–2072, 2007.

[10] Q. Sun, Z. Zhang, H. Zhang, and X. Liu, "Aberrant IgA1 glycosylation in IgA nephropathy: A systematic review," *PLoS ONE*, vol. 11, no. 11, Article ID e0166700, 2016.

[11] M. J. Kim, S. Schaub, K. Molyneux, M. T. Koller, S. Stampf, and J. Barratt, "Effect of immunosuppressive drugs on the changes of serum galactose-deficient IgA1 in patients with IgA nephropathy," *PLoS ONE*, vol. 11, no. 12, Article ID e0166830, 2016.

[12] R. Coppo, "Biomarkers and targeted new therapies for IgA nephropathy," *Pediatric Nephrology*, vol. 32, no. 5, pp. 725–731, 2017.

[13] M. C. Hastings, Z. Moldoveanu, B. A. Julian et al., "Galactose-deficient IgA1 in African Americans with IgA nephropathy: serum levels and heritability," *Clinical Journal of the American Society of Nephrology*, vol. 5, no. 11, pp. 2069–2074, 2010.

[14] R. H. Buckley, S. C. Dees, and W. M. O'Fallon, "Serum immunoglobulins. I. Levels in normal children and in uncomplicated childhood allergy," *Pediatrics*, vol. 41, no. 3, pp. 600–611, 1968.

[15] E. R. Stiehm and H. H. Fudenberg, "Serum levels of immune globulins in health and disease: a survey," *Pediatrics*, vol. 37, no. 5, pp. 715–727, 1966.

[16] E. M. Veys, R. J. Wieme, J. Van Egmond, P. Gabriel, and J. Van Der Jeught, "Short term variation of human immunoglobulin levels with an estimation of the day to day physiological variability," *Clinica Chimica Acta*, vol. 75, no. 2, pp. 275–285, 1977.

24

Denosumab for Male Hemodialysis Patients with Low Bone Mineral Density: A Case-Control Study

Hiroya Takami,[1,2] Kazunori Washio,[1] and Hiromichi Gotoh[3]

[1]*Saiyu Kawaguchi Clinic, Kawaguchi, Japan*
[2]*Saitama Honoka Clinic, Saitama, Japan*
[3]*Saiyu Souka Clinic, Souka, Japan*

Correspondence should be addressed to Hiroya Takami; daruma5454daruma@yahoo.co.jp

Academic Editor: Laszlo Rosivall

Denosumab increases bone mineral density (BMD) in patients not receiving hemodialysis therapy. However, limited data are available in the literature concerning the use of denosumab in hemodialysis patients. We treated male hemodialysis patients with low radius BMD with denosumab therapy for 1 year and evaluated its effect on radius BMD. Seventeen patients were treated with denosumab 60 mg every 6 months, and 20 patients were not treated with denosumab (control group). At seven days, the mean corrected calcium level decreased from 9.2 ± 0.5 mg to 8.5 ± 0.5 mg ($P < 0.01$), and mean serum phosphorus decreased from 5.0 ± 1.3 mg/dl to 4.2 ± 0.9 mg/dl ($P < 0.01$). At 1 month, the corrected calcium and serum phosphorus levels were 9.2 ± 0.9 mg/dl and 4.0 ± 1.1 mg/dl, respectively. At 1 year, BMD increased by $2.6\% \pm 4.4\%$ in the denosumab group and decreased by $4.5\% \pm 7.7\%$ in the control group ($P < 0.001$). In our observational study, denosumab therapy represents an effective treatment for male dialysis patients with low BMD.

1. Introduction

Low bone mass is a worldwide public health concern that results in increased risk of fractures.

Bone fractures are relatively common among hemodialysis patients and pose a significant health burden [1–3]. Some studies suggested that bone mineral density (BMD) was lower in patients with chronic kidney disease who had fractures [4, 5].

Denosumab is a monoclonal antibody against the receptor activator of nuclear factor-$\kappa\beta$ ligand (RANKL), a cytokine that is essential for the formation, function, and survival of osteoclasts [6]. By binding RANKL, denosumab prevents the interaction of RANKL with RANK on osteoclasts and reversibly inhibits osteoclast-mediated bone resorption. Many effective antiosteoporotic drugs are available, but, generally, they are contraindicated in patients with chronic kidney disease because of their progressive accumulation.

Although denosumab increased BMD in women without renal failure [7], effects in hemodialysis male patients are not well known.

Unlike other antiosteoporotic drugs, denosumab is not contraindicated in advanced chronic kidney disease, as its pharmacokinetics does not differ from that in patients with normal kidney function [8, 9]. Use of bisphosphonates in advanced chronic kidney disease requires considerable caution, and adequate clinical investigations were not reported [10]. A case report [11] and noncontrolled studies [12–14] indicated that denosumab could be efficacious in hemodialysis patients.

For 1 year, we used denosumab to treat male hemodialysis patients with low BMD at Saiyuu Kawaguchi Clinic and evaluated its effects on the BMD at the distal third of the radius in comparison with those in a control group.

As a hemodialysis patient treated with denosumab was reported to have developed severe hypocalcemia [15, 16], we carefully evaluated serum calcium levels.

2. Materials and Methods

This was an observational retrospective case-control study. At Saiyuu Kawaguchi Clinic in Japan, approximately 160 male patients underwent maintenance hemodialysis. Each patient was continuously taken care of by one of the two physicians. Each patient was randomly assigned to one of the two physicians at the first visit to the clinic. One physician administered treatment with denosumab, and the other physician did not use denosumab. Male patients with low BMD (<70% of the young adult mean) at Saiyuu Kawaguchi Clinic were eligible for inclusion.

Patients were excluded if they had conditions that influence bone metabolism or if they had taken bisphosphonates, parathyroid hormone (PTH), corticosteroids, or selective estrogen-receptor modulators. Patients were also excluded if they had active peptic ulcer, abnormal hepatic function, malignant disease, a history of severe brain stroke, or a history of parathyroidectomy.

BMD at the distal third of the radius was measured by using dual-energy X-ray absorptiometry on a DTX-200 densitometer before treatment and after 1 year. Dialysates with a calcium content of 2.5 mEq/l were used.

Biochemical parameters including phosphorus (P), calcium (Ca), whole PTH, total alkaline phosphatase (ALP), and albumin were measured by using standard laboratory techniques. Serum calcium values were corrected for serum albumin concentration by using the following formula: corrected calcium (mg/dl) = total calcium (mg/dl) + 4 − albumin (g/dl).

A combination of calcium-based phosphate binder, sevelamer, lanthanum carbonate hydrate, calcitriol, alfacalcidol, maxacalcitol, and cinacalcet was titrated according to the serum calcium, phosphate, or PTH levels.

Most of the laboratory tests were performed once a month and blood samples were withdrawn at the start of the second dialysis session of each week.

ALP level was measured as bone turnover marker [17].

Data were expressed as mean ± standard deviation (SD). Data comparisons between two groups were performed by t-test. Data for whole PTH were expressed as median and interquartile range. Data comparison for whole PTH levels was performed by using the Wilcoxon signed-rank test. P values of <0.05 were considered significant.

3. Results

Seventeen patients (mean age: 72.8 years) were treated with denosumab 60 mg every 6 months. Their original disease was diabetes mellitus in nine patients, hypertensive nephropathy in three patients, glomerulonephritis in three patients, and rapid progressive glomerulonephritis in one patient and it was unknown in one patient. One patient had a fragility fracture at baseline in the denosumab group. Twenty patients (mean age: 71.2 years) were not treated with denosumab (control group). Their original disease was diabetes mellitus in eleven patients, hypertensive nephropathy in two patients, and glomerulonephritis in five patients and it was unknown

TABLE 1: Baseline characteristics of the patients.

	Denosumab	Control	P value
n	17	20	
Age (years)	72.8 ± 9.5	71.2 ± 11.0	NS
Body mass index (kg/m²)	21.6 ± 2.3	20.8 ± 2.3	NS
HD duration (years)	7.1 ± 4.9	6.4 ± 5.3	NS
BMD (% of young mean)	56.7 ± 7.2	54.7 ± 11.0	NS

Continuous values are given as mean ± SD. The body mass index is the weight in kilograms divided by the square of the height in meters. BMD: bone mineral density; NS: not significant.

TABLE 2: Baseline parameters of the patients.

	Denosumab	Control	P value
Corrected Ca (mg/dl)	9.2 ± 0.5	9.0 ± 0.5	NS
Phosphate (mg/dl)	5.0 ± 1.3	4.8 ± 1.2	NS
W-PTH (pg/ml)	164 (58.5–228)	157 (108–231)	NS
ALP (U/l)	276 ± 129	270 ± 69	NS

W-PTH: whole PTH. Median and interquartile range are shown for whole PTH. The reference range for ALP level is from 115 to 359 U/l.

in two patients. Three patients in the control group had a fragility fracture at baseline.

None of the patients was excluded from the analysis. The baseline characteristics or parameters in both groups were not significantly different (Tables 1 and 2).

The administration of denosumab was clinically well tolerated. In the denosumab group, at 7 days, the mean serum albumin-corrected calcium (Ca [alb]) decreased from 9.2 ± 0.5 mg/dl to 8.5 ± 1.1 mg/dl (P < 0.01), and the mean serum P decreased from 5.0 ± 1.3 mg/dl to 4.2 ± 0.9 mg/dl (P < 0.01). At one month, serum albumin-corrected calcium (Ca [alb]) was 9.2 ± 0.9 mg/dl and mean serum P was 4.0 ± 1.1 mg/dl (Table 3). Five patients who showed hypocalcemia (<8.0 mg/dl at 1 week), without clinical symptom, recovered soon after increased doses of vitamin D receptor activators and/or calcium-based phosphate binder.

Tables 4(a) and 4(b) show mean medication doses and number of treated patients by each medication during the treatment course. Alfacalcidol appears to have been used more in the denosumab group, and maxacalcitol was used more in the control group.

ALP level decreased in the denosumab group at 1 year (Table 5) and showed decreased bone turnover.

At 1 year, BMD at the distal third of the radius increased by 2.6 ± 4.4% in the denosumab group and decreased by 4.5 ± 7.7% in the control group (P < 0.001) (Table 6).

4. Discussion

The present study demonstrated that male hemodialysis patients with low BMD who received subcutaneous administration of 60 mg of denosumab every 6 months had significantly increased BMD at the distal third of the radius at 12 months, in comparison with a control group.

TABLE 3: Serum albumin-corrected calcium, P, and whole-PTH levels during the denosumab treatment course.

	Baseline*	1 week**	1 month	P value * versus **
Corrected Ca (mg/dl)	9.2 ± 0.5	8.5 ± 1.1	9.2 ± 0.9	$P < 0.01$
Phosphate (mg/dl)	5.0 ± 1.3	4.2 ± 0.9	4.0 ± 1.1	$P < 0.01$
W-PTH (pg/dl)	164 (58.5 to 228)	224 (96 to 355.5)	161 (82.5 to 234)	NS

W-PTH: whole PTH. Median and interquartile range are shown for whole PTH.

TABLE 4

(a) Mean medication dose in the treatment course of the denosumab group

	Baseline	3 months	6 months	12 months
CaCo$_3$ (g/day)	1.47 (15)	1.65 (16)	1.18 (15)	1.32 (15)
Alfacalcidol (μg/day)	0.31 (11)	0.43 (11)	0.34 (10)	0.34 (11)
Calcitriol (μg/day)	0.01 (1)	0.03 (1)	0.03 (1)	0 (0)
Maxacalcitol (μg/week)	5.0 (2)	4.41 (2)	2.94 (2)	4.71 (3)
Cinacalcet (mg/day)	2.94 (8)	2.94 (10)	2.94 (8)	4.41 (9)

The number in the parentheses denotes the number of patients treated with each medication among the 17 patients.

(b) Mean medication dose in the treatment course in the control group

	Baseline	3 months	6 months	12 months
CaCo$_3$ (g/day)	1.50 (14)	1.73 (15)	1.10 (15)	1.6 (15)
Alfacalcidol (μg/day)	0.03 (2)	0.01 (1)	0.01 (1)	0.01 (1)
Calcitriol (μg/day)	0 (0)	0 (0)	0 (0)	0 (0)
Maxacalcitol (μg/week)	10.0 (7)	8.75 (7)	10.0 (6)	10.0 (14)
Cinacalcet (mg/day)	6.75 (16)	11.25 (17)	7.50 (17)	11.25 (17)

The number in the parentheses denotes the number of patients treated with each medication among the 20 patients.

TABLE 5: Parameters of the patients at 12 months.

	Denosumab group	Control group	P value
Corrected Ca (mg/dl)	9.1 ± 0.6	9.1 ± 0.4	NS
Phosphate (mg/dl)	5.1 ± 1.4	4.6 ± 0.9	NS
W-PTH (pg/ml)	128 (72 to 191)	140 (76 to 215)	NS
ALP (U/l)	185 ± 59	249 ± 65	$P < 0.01$

The reference range for ALP is from 115 to 359 U/l. Median and interquartile range are shown for whole PTH.

TABLE 6: BMD at the distal third of radius.

	Baseline (% of YAM)	1 year (% of YAM)	% change
Denosumab	56.7 ± 7.2	58 ± 7.9	2.6 ± 4.4%
Control	54.7 ± 11	52.3 ± 10.1	−4.5 ± 7.7%
P value			<0.001

BMD: bone mineral density; YAM: young adult mean.

Although the patient selection was not randomized, selection was not intentional, because denosumab was used as treatment only by one of the primary physicians. The primary physician was assigned randomly during the initial visit of each patient at the clinic.

BMD measurement alone is known to show no correlation with fracture risk in this population. However, as BMD is a major factor reflecting bone strength [18], it seems logical that low BMD alone would increase the risk of fractures, and monitoring BMD is therefore a sensible means of measuring therapeutic effects.

Denosumab therapy prevents the interaction of RANKL with RANK, its receptor, on osteoclasts and their precursors, thereby blocking the formation, function, and survival of osteoclasts. By contrast, bisphosphonates chemically bind to calcium hydroxyapatite in bone; they reduce bone resorption by blocking the function and survival but not the formation of osteoclasts.

Although successful studies concerning the use of denosumab in hemodialysis patients were reported, those studies did not have a control group [12–14]. Denosumab led to significant increase in lumbar spine BMD and femoral neck BMD but not radius BMD in eleven hemodialysis patients in one year [12]. We cannot explain why radius BMD increased in our study and did not significantly increase in the previous study. We speculate that if they compared the treated group with a control group, they may find a significant difference. The BMD increased in both the femoral neck (mean increase:

23.7% ± 4.0%) and lumbar spine (17.1% ± 2.6%) after 6 months in the hemodialysis patients with severe secondary hyperparathyroidism [13].

A meta-analysis of studies that reported on BMD and fractures in chronic kidney disease showed that BMD was significantly lower in the subjects with fractures than in those without fractures [5]. This study was too small to show the effect of therapy on the incidence of fracture.

The common adverse effect of denosumab is hypocalcemia. Two case reports warned against the use of denosumab because of severe hypocalcemia [15, 16]. In another case, hypocalcemia was also observed but was overcome with adjustment of the concomitant treatment [11]. Although we also observed hypocalcemia, we adjusted hypocalcemia by increasing calcium-based phosphate binder and/or vitamin D receptor activators. What is this mechanism? Secondary hyperparathyroidism is a hallmark of chronic renal failure. It results in accelerated bone resorption and bone formation. Calcium is supplied by bone resorption and utilized by bone formation. Denosumab reduces mainly bone resorption. This imbalance may cause hypocalcemia.

During the treatment course, four kinds of medications that increase Ca levels were used (Tables 4(a) and 4(b)). Those are calcium carbonate, alfacalcidol, calcitriol, and maxacalcitol. Cinacalcet reduced calcium levels. It appears that alfacalcidol was used more in the denosumab group, and maxacalcitol was used more in the control group. Which group was treated by stronger medications to increase Ca levels? A comparison was not possible, because no formula exists to convert the effects of each medication.

Our study has limitations. It is too small to evaluate the safety of denosumab and did not have a randomized control group. A large-scale, randomized controlled study is necessary to confirm the efficacy of the treatment. Bone biopsy with quantitative histomorphometric analysis is the gold standard for the diagnosis of renal osteodystrophy. Nonetheless, bone biopsy is an invasive procedure that is not routinely performed. We did not measure bone specific ALP, osteocalcin, TRACP-5b, and intact N-terminal propeptide of type I procollagen levels, which would have been informative for bone metabolism. We did not measure bone mineral density at the lumbar spine, total hip, or femoral neck.

In summary, in this observational study, denosumab administered at 6-month intervals over a period of 12 months increased bone mineral density at the distal third of the radius in male hemodialysis patients with low BMD. This result supports the continued investigation for the use of denosumab in the treatment for male hemodialysis patients with bone loss.

References

[1] F. Tentori, K. McCullough, R. D. Kilpatrick et al., "High rates of death and hospitalization follow bone fracture among hemodialysis patients," Kidney International, vol. 85, no. 1, pp. 166–173, 2014.

[2] A. M. Alem, D. J. Sherrard, D. L. Gillen et al., "Increased risk of hip fracture among patients with end-stage renal disease," Kidney International, vol. 58, no. 1, pp. 396–399, 2000.

[3] M. Wakasugi, J. J. Kazama, M. Taniguchi et al., "Increased risk of hip fracture among Japanese hemodialysis patients," Journal of Bone and Mineral Metabolism, vol. 31, no. 3, pp. 315–321, 2013.

[4] S. Iimori, Y. Mori, W. Akita et al., "Diagnostic usefulness of bone mineral density and biochemical markers of bone turnover in predicting fracture in CKD stage 5D patients—a single-center cohort study," Nephrology Dialysis Transplantation, vol. 27, no. 1, pp. 345–351, 2012.

[5] S. A. Jamal, J. A. Hayden, and J. Beyene, "Low bone mineral density and fractures in long-term hemodialysis patients: a meta-analysis," The American Journal of Kidney Diseases, vol. 49, no. 5, pp. 674–681, 2007.

[6] D. L. Lacey, E. Timms, H.-L. Tan et al., "Osteoprotegerin ligand is a cytokine that regulates osteoclast differentiation and activation," Cell, vol. 93, no. 2, pp. 165–176, 1998.

[7] S. R. Cummings, J. S. Martin, M. R. McClung et al., "Denosumab for prevention of fractures in postmenopausal women with osteoporosis," New England Journal of Medicine, vol. 361, no. 8, pp. 756–765, 2009.

[8] S. A. Jamal, Ö. Ljunggren, C. Stehman-Breen et al., "Effects of denosumab on fracture and bone mineral density by level of kidney function," Journal of Bone and Mineral Research, vol. 26, no. 8, pp. 1829–1835, 2011.

[9] G. A. Block, H. G. Bone, L. Fang, E. Lee, and D. Padhi, "A single-dose study of denosumab in patients with various degrees of renal impairment," Journal of Bone and Mineral Research, vol. 27, no. 7, pp. 1471–1479, 2012.

[10] W. C. Liu, J. F. Yen, C. L. Lang, M. T. Yan, and K. C. Lu, "Bisphophonates in CKD patients with low bone mineral density," The Scientific World Journal, vol. 2013, Article ID 837573, 11 pages, 2013.

[11] S. Dusilová Sulková, J. Horáček, R. Šafránek, P. Gorun, O. Viklický, and V. Palička, "Denosumab associated with bone density increase and clinical improvement in a long-term hemodialysis patient. Case report and review of the literature," Acta Medica, vol. 57, no. 1, pp. 30–33, 2014.

[12] R. Hiramatsu, Y. Ubara, N. Sawa et al., "Denosumab for low bone mass in hemodialysis patients: a noncontrolled trial," American Journal of Kidney Diseases, vol. 66, no. 1, pp. 175–177, 2015.

[13] C.-L. Chen, N.-C. Chen, C.-Y. Hsu et al., "An open-label, prospective pilot clinical study of denosumab for severe hyperparathyroidism in patients with low bone mass undergoing dialysis," Journal of Clinical Endocrinology & Metabolism, vol. 99, no. 7, pp. 2426–2432, 2014.

[14] F. Festuccia, M. T. Jafari, A. Moioli et al., "Safety and efficacy of denosumab in osteoporotic hemodialysed patients," Journal of Nephrology, vol. 30, no. 2, pp. 271–279, 2017.

[15] B. B. Mccormick, J. Davis, and K. D. Burns, "Severe hypocalcemia following denosumab injection in a hemodialysis patient," The American Journal of Kidney Diseases, vol. 60, no. 4, pp. 626–628, 2012.

[16] M. Agarwal, E. Csongradi, and A. C. Koch, "Severe symptomatic hypocalcemia after denosumab administration in an end-stage renal disease patient on peritoneal dialysis with controlled secondary hyperparathyroidism," British Journal of Medicine and Medical Research, vol. 3, no. 4, pp. 1398–1406, 2013.

25

Population Based Trends in the Incidence of Hospital Admission for the Diagnosis of Hepatorenal Syndrome: 1998–2011

Manish Suneja,[1] **Fan Tang,**[2] **Joseph E. Cavanaugh,**[2]
Linnea A. Polgreen,[3] **and Philip M. Polgreen**[1]

[1]*Department of Internal Medicine, University of Iowa Hospitals and Clinics, Iowa City, IA 52242, USA*
[2]*Department of Biostatistics, University of Iowa, Iowa City, IA 52242, USA*
[3]*Department of Pharmacy Practice and Science, University of Iowa, Iowa City, IA 52242, USA*

Correspondence should be addressed to Manish Suneja; manish-suneja@uiowa.edu

Academic Editor: Suresh C. Tiwari

Background and Objectives. Hepatorenal syndrome carries a high risk of mortality. Understanding the incidence and mortality trends in hepatorenal syndrome will help inform future studies regarding the safety and efficacy of potential therapeutic interventions. *Design and Methods.* We conducted a retrospective cohort study using the Nationwide Inpatient Sample. We identified hospitalizations from January 1998–June 2011 with a primary diagnosis of hepatorenal syndrome. To characterize the incidence trends in monthly hepatorenal syndrome hospitalizations, we fit a piecewise linear model with a change point at January 2008. We examined hospital and patient characteristics before and after the change point. *Results.* Hospital admissions with a diagnosis of hepatorenal syndrome increased markedly between September of 2007 and March of 2008. Comparing patients who were admitted with a diagnosis of hepatorenal syndrome prior to 2008 with those after 2008, we found that length of stay increased while the mortality of patients admitted for hepatorenal syndrome decreased. *Conclusion.* The revision of the diagnostic criteria for hepatorenal syndrome may have contributed to the increase in the incidence of admissions for hepatorenal syndrome. However, the changes in the principles of hepatorenal syndrome management may have also contributed to the increase in incidence and lower mortality.

1. Introduction

Hepatorenal syndrome (HRS) is a distinct form of functional kidney injury seen in end-stage liver disease. HRS is characterized by intense renal vasoconstriction in the setting of systemic and splanchnic arterial vasodilatation. The association between liver disease and renal failure had been known for more than a hundred years, but the first consensus definition of HRS was developed in 1994 by the International Ascites Club (IAC) with a new revised criterion introduced in 2006-07 [1]. HRS has a reported incidence of 10% among hospitalized patients with cirrhosis and ascites and is associated with a high mortality [1]. HRS is classified into 2 types: type-1 HRS is characterized by a rapid and often precipitous decline in renal function with a median survival of about 2 weeks, whereas with type-2 HRS, kidney failure occurs over a longer period of time, with a median

survival of 6 months [2–5]. To date, reports on the incidence and mortality associated with HRS have mostly been based on single-center experiences, which may not reflect the nationwide incidence and burden of HRS-related hospital admissions.

A recent systematic review of HRS patients suggested an epidemiologic improvement in short-term mortality between 2005 and 2010 when compared to the 27 years between 1977 and 2004 [6]. Understanding the nationwide incidence and mortality trends in HRS will help hospitals plan for the resources needed to care for these patients and inform future studies regarding the safety and efficacy of potential interventions for the management of HRS.

The objective of this study was to determine how the rate of hospital admissions for HRS has changed over the past decade in the United States. To our knowledge, this is the first study that has examined the national incidence and mortality trends for hospital admissions with a diagnosis of HRS.

2. Methods

2.1. Data Source. We conducted a retrospective cohort study using the Nationwide Inpatient Sample (NIS). The NIS is the largest all-payer database of national discharges in the US. The database is maintained as part of the Healthcare Cost and Utilization Project by the Agency for Healthcare Research and Quality (AHRQ) and contains data from a 20% stratified sample of nonfederal acute care hospitals. To adjust for yearly changes in the sampling design, we applied the weights provided by AHRQ. All analyses were performed using R, version 2.15.1 (R Foundation for Statistical Computing).

We first identified all hospitalizations over the period from January 1998 through June 2011 during which a primary diagnosis of HRS was recorded. For HRS case ascertainment, we used the *International Classification of Diseases, 9th Revision, Clinical Modification (ICD-9-CM)* code 572.4. We then aggregated all cases by month to produce a national sample of cases of HRS over time. Cases were assigned to a calendar month on the basis of the date that the patient was admitted to the hospital. In a similar fashion, we compiled a sample of AKI- (acute kidney injury) cirrhosis cases. We identified all hospitalizations over the same time period during which a primary diagnosis of AKI was received and a secondary diagnosis of cirrhosis was also recorded, or a primary diagnosis of cirrhosis was received and a secondary diagnosis of AKI was then recorded. For AKI-cirrhosis case ascertainment, we used ICD-9-CM codes 574.5, 584.6, 584.7, 584.8, and 584.9 for AKI and 571.5, 571.2, and 571.6 for cirrhosis.

2.2. Statistical Analysis. We fit a piecewise (or segmented) linear regression model. A piecewise linear model is comprised of a series of linear models connected at "change points," where shifts in the slope may occur. In our case, we determined a single change point for the HRS series by visual inspection. We detrended the series and conducted residual diagnostics to investigate whether there was any autocorrelation pattern in the residuals, as failure to account for such autocorrelation may lead to incorrect inferential conclusions. Temporal correlation in the residuals was examined by the autocorrelation function (ACF) and the partial autocorrelation function (PACF).

To examine if changes occurred in demographics and characteristics before and after the change point, the sample was divided into two groups based on the identified change point (based on the HRS series). For binary outcomes (e.g., gender, mortality) and categorical outcomes (e.g., race, hospital bed size), comparisons of proportions were conducted using the Pearson chi-square test. For continuous outcomes (e.g., length of stay and age), comparisons of means were conducted using Wilcoxon rank sum test.

3. Results

The overall time series plot of HRS incidence from 1998 to 2011 is shown in Figure 1. Based on a visual inspection of

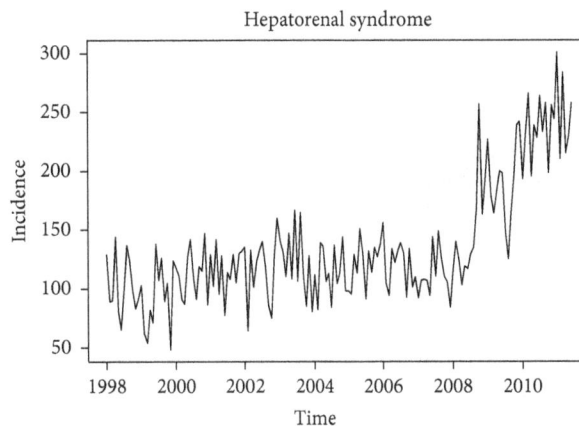

FIGURE 1: Monthly hospitalizations of patients diagnosed with hepatorenal syndrome in the United States (Nationwide Inpatient Sample, 1998–2011).

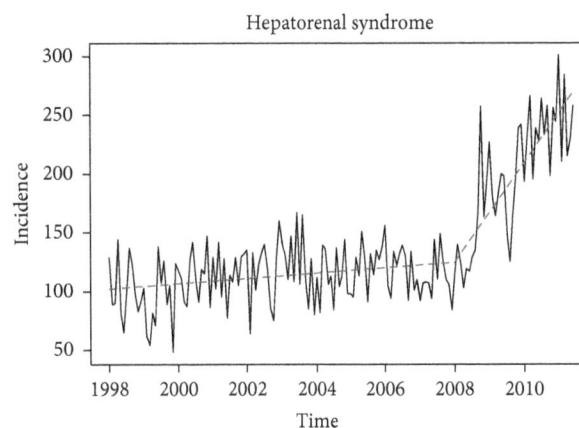

FIGURE 2: Fitted segmented linear regression model for hepatorenal syndrome incidence series based on monthly hospitalizations.

the plot, we chose January of 2008 to be the change point for our piecewise linear regression model. Upon inspection of the ACF and PACF for the residuals from the fitted model (Figure 2), we found no evidence of temporal correlation in the detrended HRS series, which implies that a segmented linear regression model based on independent errors is sufficient to characterize HRS incidence (data not shown).

Table 1 summarizes the model results for the HRS series. The yearly slope coefficient for the period before the change point (January of 2008) is positive and significant (P value = 0.0030) but small (slope estimate = 2.26; 95% CI: (0.81, 3.71)). In January of 2008, a substantial increase in the yearly slope is evident (change in slope estimate = 40.1; 95% CI: (33.84, 46.34); and P value < 0.0001).

Table 2 summarizes the means and proportions in the demographics and characteristics of HRS hospitalizations before and after January 2008. Specifically, mean age decreased after January 2008, and patients had a longer mean length of stay (P value < 0.0001). In addition, a significant decrease in the mortality rate was found with HRS patients after January 2008 (P value < 0.0001), and a higher proportion

TABLE 1: Results of the fitted segmented linear regression model, characterizing the change in the yearly slope after 2008.

Diagnosis	Parameter	Estimate	Std. error	t-value	P value
HRS	Slope before change point	2.26	0.74	3.02	0.0030
	Change of slope	40.09	3.19	12.56	<0.0001[*]

[*]Note that because the change point was identified based on visual inspection, this P value must be interpreted liberally, since it is based on a post hoc test.

TABLE 2: Demographics and characteristics of patients diagnosed with HRS during hospitalization.

	Before the change point	After the change point	P value
Age, mean (SD), years	59.26 (13.99)	58.00 (12.22)	0.0048
Length of stay, mean (SD), days	7.74 (9.19)	8.91 (11.37)	<0.0001
Race, n (%)			0.1480
White	1594 (71.38)	1163 (72.64)	
Black	245 (10.97)	155 (9.68)	
Hispanic	275 (12.32)	180 (11.24)	
Asian or Pacific Islander	45 (2.02)	28 (1.75)	
Native American	21 (0.94)	26 (1.62)	
Other	53 (2.37)	49 (3.06)	
Mortality, n (%)			<0.0001
Alive	1615 (53.89)	1246 (67.98)	
Died	1382 (46.11)	587 (32.02)	
Gender, n (%)			0.6347
Male	1911 (63.59)	1180 (64.27)	
Female	1094 (36.41)	656 (35.73)	
Hospital teaching status, n (%)			<0.0001
Nonteaching	1677 (56.24)	878 (48.35)	
Teaching	1305 (43.76)	938 (51.65)	
Hospital bed size			<0.0001
Small	446 (14.96)	207 (11.40)	
Medium	856 (28.71)	438 (24.12)	
Large	1680 (56.34)	1171 (64.48)	
Procedures, n (%)			<0.0001
Dialysis	391 (13.01)	405 (22.06)	
Primary payer, n (%)			0.7733
Medicare	1198 (39.92)	706 (38.54)	
Medicaid	526 (17.53)	339 (18.50)	
Private insurance	917 (30.56)	557 (30.40)	
Self-pay	221 (7.36)	134 (7.31)	
No charge	20 (0.67)	17 (0.93)	
Other	119 (3.97)	79 (4.31)	

of patients received dialysis (P value < 0.0001). Finally, more patients were admitted to teaching and large hospitals after January 2008 (P value < 0.0001).

Table 3 summarizes the means and proportions in the demographics and characteristics of AKI-cirrhosis hospitalizations before and after January 2008 (i.e., based on the change point for the HRS series). Specifically, average age increased after January 2008 and patients had a shorter mean length of stay (P value < 0.0001). In addition, a significant decrease in the mortality rate was found with AKI-cirrhosis patients after January 2008 (P value < 0.0001). In contrast to the HRS cohort, patients had a lower probability of receiving dialysis after the change point (P value < 0.0001).

4. Discussion

Our results show that hospital admissions with a diagnosis of HRS increased markedly after January 2008. In addition, when we compared patients who were admitted with a diagnosis of HRS prior to January 2008 with those after January 2008, we found that length of stay increased over time. However, during the same period of time, the mortality of patients admitted for HRS decreased. Finally, the incidence of HRS patients treated with dialysis increased over this period of time.

Interestingly, multiple randomized controlled trials demonstrating the short-term efficacy of medical management of

TABLE 3: Demographics and characteristics of patients diagnosed with AKI-cirrhosis during hospitalization.

	Before the change point	After the change point	P value
Age, mean (SD), years	58.83 (13.03)	60.00 (12.47)	<0.0001
Length of stay, mean (SD), days	11.02 (12.91)	9.30 (11.36)	<0.0001
Race, n (%)			0.0335
White	13564 (65.14)	9555 (65.57)	
Black	2507 (12.04)	1685 (11.56)	
Hispanic	3634 (17.45)	2489 (17.08)	
Asian or Pacific Islander	419 (2.01)	272 (1.87)	
Native American	185 (0.89)	138 (0.95)	
Other	513 (2.46)	433 (2.97)	
Mortality, n (%)			<0.0001
Alive	19115 (70.98)	14047 (84.43)	
Died	7816 (29.02)	2590 (15.57)	
Gender, n (%)			0.8224
Male	17256 (64.00)	10679 (64.11)	
Female	9706 (36.00)	5979 (35.89)	
Hospital teaching status, n (%)			0.2657
Nonteaching	11117 (41.50)	6732 (40.95)	
Teaching	15673 (58.50)	9706 (59.05)	
Hospital bed size			<0.0001
Small	2349 (8.77)	1324 (8.05)	
Medium	6552 (24.46)	3538 (21.52)	
Large	17889 (66.77)	11576 (70.42)	
Procedures, n (%)			<0.0001
Dialysis	4017 (14.90)	1922 (11.54)	
Primary payer, n (%)			<0.0001
Medicare	11104 (41.31)	7158 (43.09)	
Medicaid	5394 (20.07)	3418 (20.58)	
Private insurance	7513 (27.95)	4230 (25.47)	
Self-pay	1702 (6.33)	1050 (6.32)	
No charge	198 (0.74)	133 (0.80)	
Other	967 (3.60)	622 (3.74)	

HRS were published in 2007-2008 [7–11]. Thus, it is possible that the publication of these studies was associated with a change in the management of HRS and perhaps improved outcomes. New recommendations included changing the choice of volume expander from saline to albumin. Albumin improves circulatory function in cirrhosis by expanding central blood volume and increasing cardiac output [12]. Some recent studies have shown that the administration of albumin to cirrhotic patients with SBP causes arterial vasoconstriction and blood pressure increase, probably attributable to the ability of albumin to bind to vasodilators [13]. A large body of evidence, based on observational studies and randomized controlled trials, has accumulated in the last decade showing that some of the new therapies represent a milestone in the management of HRS [14]. The demonstration that type-1 HRS can be improved by vasoconstrictors or norepinephrine alone or in conjunction with intravascular volume expansion with albumin and that reversal of type-1 HRS may be associated with improved survival represents a major change in our understanding of the syndrome. It is therefore conceivable

that an improvement of renal function in patients with HRS treated with vasoconstrictors and albumin could be due to the additive effects that the compounds have on cardiac function and peripheral arterial circulation. Finally the use of high dose albumin in cases of HRS might have a favorable effect on effective circulating volume and thus improving clinical outcomes.

The change in the admissions for HRS and changes in outcomes could have been due to changes in practice management. Alternatively, the change we observed could also be in part due to the change in definition of HRS or inclusion criteria for HRS [4], which also occurred during the same period of time. The change in definition of HRS expanded the syndrome to include elements that were considered non-inclusive in the older criteria; for example, an active infection is no longer an exclusion criterion. Finally, the increase in the incidence of HRS and a decrease in mortality in the HRS series could be due to a change in coding. However, we also analyzed the mortality rates of patients diagnosed with both AKI and cirrhosis (AKI-cirrhosis series). We found that the mortality rate for this series also decreased. Thus, it appears that outcomes have improved irrespective of the diagnostic codes after the change point.

Regardless of the cause of the increase in admissions for HRS, we anticipate a corresponding increase in healthcare resources used to treat this condition. If the treatment for HRS is truly more effective, it follows that it will be used more frequently, potentially leading to a dramatic increase in hospital charges related to the care for HRS. In addition to the number of admissions, we also noted that the length of stay associated with HRS admissions has increased during our study period and length of stay is one of the major drivers of healthcare costs [15]. Accurate estimates of the cost of HRS need to take into account readmissions and other posthospitalization events. Unfortunately, we cannot explore these issues using the NIS database. However, future HRS research should focus on readmissions and other outcome measures.

Our study has several limitations including the retrospective nature of the data. First, the NIS (similar to other administrative and hospital databases) is subject to coding errors and variability in coding illnesses. Also, NIS data does not allow for detailed individual chart reviews. Second, NIS data do not include medication records; thus we cannot investigate changes regarding specific therapeutics (e.g., national prevalence of albumin use). Third, as mentioned previously, we cannot follow patients following discharge. This is an important limitation to note because it limits our ability to determine if patients with HRS received liver transplants during subsequent hospitalizations during our study period. Furthermore, although the admissions for HRS increased, we are not able to determine how frequently readmissions occur nor can we attribute the increased volume of admissions to one-time versus multiple admissions. Finally lack of availability of specific therapies (e.g., terlipressin) in United States makes our findings less generalizable in countries where these therapies are available.

Despite the limitations of the study, we were able to explore the incidence and rate of hospitalizations for the diagnosis of HRS on a population level across the United States, and our results will help inform future studies both regarding resource use and longer-term studies of the efficacy of new approaches to HRS treatments. Our results also highlight the need for future studies to estimate the attributable cost of HRS.

5. Conclusions

The national trend in management of HRS shows that it continues to be a significant source of morbidity and mortality in patients with end-stage liver disease in the United States. The revision and broadening of the diagnostic criteria may have partially contributed to the increase in the incidence of admissions for HRS. Although we are unable to conclusively comment on the decrease in the overall mortality of HRS since 2008, we speculate that the widespread changes in the principles of management, including the use of volume expansion and vasopressors, may have played a part. The HRS patient cohort deserves further prospective examination in the near future.

Acknowledgments

Linnea A. Polgreen has received funding from the National Heart Lung and Blood Institute at the National Institutes of Health (Grant no. K25 HL 122305).

References

[1] G. C. de Carvalho, C. de Andrade Regis, J. R. Kalil et al., "Causes of renal failure in patients with decompensated cirrhosis and its impact in hospital mortality," *Annals of Hepatology*, vol. 11, no. 1, pp. 90–95, 2012.

[2] V. Arroyo, P. Ginès, A. L. Gerbes et al., "Definition and diagnostic criteria of refractory ascites and hepatorenal syndrome in cirrhosis," *Hepatology*, vol. 23, no. 1, pp. 164–176, 1996.

[3] R. Bataler, P. Sort, P. Gines, and V. Arroyo, "Hepatorenal syndrome: definition, pathophysiology, clinical features and management," *Kidney International, Supplement*, vol. 53, no. 66, pp. S47–S53, 1998.

[4] F. Salerno, A. Gerbes, P. Ginès, F. Wong, and V. Arroyo, "Diagnosis, prevention and treatment of hepatorenal syndrome in cirrhosis," *Gut*, vol. 56, no. 9, pp. 1310–1318, 2007.

[5] P. Ginès, M. Guevara, V. Arroyo, and J. Rodés, "Hepatorenal syndrome," *The Lancet*, vol. 362, no. 9398, pp. 1819–1827, 2003.

[6] G. Fede, G. D'Amico, V. Arvaniti et al., "Renal failure and cirrhosis: a systematic review of mortality and prognosis," *Journal of Hepatology*, vol. 56, no. 4, pp. 810–818, 2012.

[7] C. Alessandria, A. Ottobrelli, W. Debernardi-Venon et al., "Noradrenalin vs terlipressin in patients with hepatorenal syndrome: a prospective, randomized, unblinded, pilot study," *Journal of Hepatology*, vol. 47, no. 4, pp. 499–505, 2007.

[8] P. Sharma, A. Kumar, B. C. Shrama, and S. K. Sarin, "An open label, pilot, randomized controlled trial of noradrenaline versus terlipressin in the treatment of type 1 hepatorenal syndrome and predictors of response," *The American Journal of Gastroenterology*, vol. 103, no. 7, pp. 1689–1697, 2008.

[9] S. Neri, D. Pulvirenti, M. Malaguarnera et al., "Terlipressin and albumin in patients with cirrhosis and type I hepatorenal syndrome," *Digestive Diseases and Sciences*, vol. 53, no. 3, pp. 830–835, 2008.

[10] A. J. Sanyal, T. Boyer, G. Garcia-Tsao et al., "A randomized, prospective, double-blind, placebo-controlled trial of terlipressin for type 1 hepatorenal syndrome," *Gastroenterology*, vol. 134, no. 5, pp. 1360–1368, 2008.

[11] M. Martín-Llahí, M.-N. Pépin, M. Guevara et al., "Terlipressin and albumin vs albumin in patients with cirrhosis and hepatorenal syndrome: a randomized study," *Gastroenterology*, vol. 134, no. 5, pp. 1352–1359, 2008.

[12] K. Brinch, S. Møller, F. Bendtsen, U. Becker, and J. H. Henriksen, "Plasma volume expansion by albumin in cirrhosis. Relation to blood volume distribution, arterial compliance and severity of disease," *Journal of Hepatology*, vol. 39, no. 1, pp. 24–31, 2003.

[13] J. Fernández, M. Navasa, J. C. Garcia-Pagan et al., "Effect of intravenous albumin on systemic and hepatic hemodynamics and vasoactive neurohormonal systems in patients with cirrhosis and spontaneous bacterial peritonitis," *Journal of Hepatology*, vol. 41, no. 3, pp. 384–390, 2004.

[14] F. Fabrizi, A. Aghemo, and P. Messa, "Hepatorenal syndrome and novel advances in its management," *Kidney and Blood Pressure Research*, vol. 37, no. 6, pp. 588–601, 2013.

[15] E. Polverejan, J. C. Gardiner, C. J. Bradley, M. Holmes-Rovner, and D. Rovner, "Estimating mean hospital cost as a function of length of stay and patient characteristics," *Health Economics*, vol. 12, no. 11, pp. 935–947, 2003.

26

The Factors Affecting Survival in Geriatric Hemodialysis Patients

Murat Tuğcu ⓘ,[1] Umut Kasapoğlu,[2] Gülizar Şahin,[3] and Süheyla Apaydın[4]

[1]Department of Nephrology, Marmara University Pendik Training and Research Hospital, Istanbul, Turkey
[2]Department of Nephrology, Ağrı Public Hospital, Ağrı, Turkey
[3]Department of Nephrology, Sultan Abdulhamid Han Training and Research Hospital, Istanbul, Turkey
[4]Department of Nephrology, Bakirkoy Sadi Konuk Training and Research Hospital, Istanbul, Turkey

Correspondence should be addressed to Murat Tuğcu; drmrttgc@hotmail.com

Academic Editor: Suresh C. Tiwari

Introduction. The number of geriatric patients is increasing in hemodialysis population over the years and mortality is higher in this group of patients. This study evaluated the factors affecting geriatric hemodialysis patient survival. *Materials and Methods.* This retrospective cohort study enrolled patients discharged from our nephrology clinic from 2009 to 2014. Data collected included demographics, Eastern Cooperative Oncology Group-Performance Status, vascular access type, and metabolic parameters. Comorbidity was quantified using the modified Liu comorbidity index. The outcome measure was mortality. *Results.* The study enrolled 99 elderly dialysis patients (42.4% women (n = 42); mean age 75 ± 7 years). The mean follow-up duration was 19.7 ± 11 months. The mortality rate over the four years was 47.5% (n = 46). The modified Liu comorbidity index score, patient age, and Eastern Cooperative Oncology Group-Performance Status were significantly related to mortality in univariate and multivariate analyses. *Conclusion.* The present study revealed that comorbidities and low performance status at the onset of dialysis had shortened the survival time in the geriatric hemodialysis patient group.

1. Introduction

The elderly dialysis population has grown with the increase in the number of elderly people in many countries [1]. However, treatment decisions are difficult because the older dialysis population has a high burden of chronic health conditions and their limited life expectancy [2]. Several comorbidity index scoring systems have also been used to evaluate the prognosis of these patients objectively [3–6]. And, also, performance status generally reflects comorbidity burden and has prognostic significance, especially chronic diseases such as chronic kidney disease.

In fact, no established guidelines exist to inform the practice of hemodialysis in the elderly population. And also hemodialysis practice in elderly patients was different and tended to follow region-specific practices. This study is one of the few studies in this field in Turkey and evaluated the relationship between the Eastern Cooperative Oncology Group-Performance Status (ECOG-PS) and modified Liu comorbidity index (mLCI) score in survival in a geriatric hemodialysis population. We hypothesized that there would be negative correlations between comorbid diseases and performance status and survival outcome.

2. Materials and Methods

Geriatric dialysis patients (age > 65 years) who were started on hemodialysis between January 1, 2011, and December 31, 2014, at our nephrology clinic were analyzed retrospectively. Maintenance hemodialysis was defined as undergoing dialysis for more than 90 days and patients who died or switched from hemodialysis to peritoneal dialysis or transplanted were excluded. The hemodialysis is performed at the different private dialysis centers three times per week. The patients were followed from the first reported hemodialysis date to the date of death or December 31, 2014.

TABLE 1: Liu Comorbidity Index, 11 comorbid conditions, and weighing score.

Comorbid Conditions	Weighing Score
Diabetic Mellitus	1
Coronary Artery Disease	3
Congestive Heart Disease	1
Cerebrovascular Disease	2
Peripheral Vascular Disease	2
Other Cardiac	2
Dysrhythmia	2
Chronic Obstructive Pulmonary Disease	2
Gastrointestinal Bleeding	2
Liver Disease	2
Cancer	2

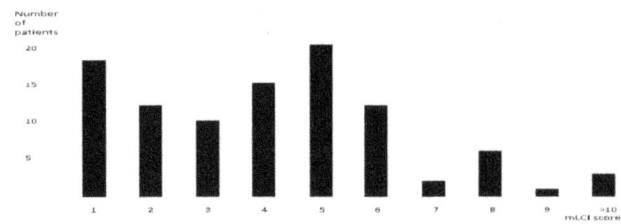

FIGURE 1: Distribution of mLCI score according to number of patients.

Patient demographic data, comorbidities, and date of death information were obtained from the National Dialysis Management System and computerized hospital records. Baseline metabolic parameters were taken at the 3rd month after starting of hemodialysis. Patient general health status before initiating dialysis was graded according to the ECOG-PS, ranging from 0 to 5, with 0 indicating that the patient is active and capable of normal everyday activity and 5 indicating that he or she is dead [7].

We calculated the mLCI (we allowed claims-based diagnosis capture to commence immediately upon initiating dialysis for a 90-day period). Briefly, this index assigns the following weights for 11 conditions: 1 point for atherosclerotic heart disease and diabetes; 2 points for cerebrovascular accident/transient ischemic attack, peripheral vascular disease, dysrhythmia, other cardiac diseases, chronic obstructive pulmonary disease, gastrointestinal bleeding, liver disease, and cancer; and 3 points for congestive heart failure (Table 1).

The data were analyzed using the Statistical Package for the Social Sciences for Windows 20.0 (SPSS, Chicago, IL, USA). Study subjects were censored if they were alive until December 31, 2014. The primary outcome (event) was death from any cause. Numeric data were presented as mean ± standard deviation. Either the Student's t-test or the Mann–Whitney U test was used for comparing the two groups. In univariate and multivariate analyses, mortality was the dependent variable and other variables were independent variables. We used the method of subtracting the mean to remove the multicollinearity produced by interaction of variables. Significance was set at $P < 0.05$.

3. Results

This study enrolled 99 elderly dialysis patients with a mean age of 75 ± 7 years; 42.4% were women (n = 42). The mean duration of follow-up was 19.7 ± 11 months. During the four-year study period, 47 (47.5%) patients died. Although most patients (68.7%) had chronic renal failure before initiating dialysis, a temporary hemodialysis catheter was the main vascular access (87.9%). Baseline metabolic parameters, primary renal disease, vascular access type, and gender did not differ significantly between survivors and nonsurvivors (Table 2).

Chronic comorbidities were very common in the nonsurvivors; the mean mLCI was 3, 7±2,3, and also the mean age (77.4±7.80 years) and ECOG-PS (2.8±1) were higher in this group. In the univariate and multivariate model, age, ECOG-PS, and mLCI score were significantly associated with mortality (Table 3).

The mLCI score distribution is shown in Figure 1. Patients with low mLCI score had a significantly better survival rate than those with a high mLCI score ($p = 0.027$). Older age group were significantly associated with mortality ($p = 0.047$).

4. Discussion

Approximately one-third of elderly patients with end-stage renal disease (ESRD) have four or more chronic health conditions and most are not candidates for kidney transplantation [2]. When geriatric patients need dialysis, treatment decisions based on the patient's underlying condition and probable outcome are difficult [8, 9].

Mortality in elderly patients is closely correlated with many comorbidities independent of age [10, 11]. Therefore, multiple scoring systems have been developed and more than 80 randomized trials have been published to help physicians assess whether a dialysis patient could benefit from therapy and have their lifespan prolonged [12–15].

Liu et al. developed an improved comorbidity index for dialysis patients, the Liu comorbidity index (LCI) [16], which covers comorbid conditions, but not age, which is already a strong predictor of mortality. Recently, Rigler et al. modified the Liu comorbidity index because of the 270-day survival requirement for patient selection. Consequently, they could include sicker patients more prone to early mortality and reduce sample size loss without survivor bias. They found that the mLCI was as effective as the original [17].

Because mortality may be high in the first few months after initiating dialysis therapy, especially for elderly patients [1], we used mLCI for scoring our patients comorbidities and found that patients with higher mLCI scores had a shorter life expectancy ($p = 0.009$). Similar to our results, Khan et al. also found that patients in the highest LCI score group had the highest mortality risk and lowest survival rate [18].

Multiple comorbidities limit physical functioning; performance status is a vital instrument because it significantly influences morbidity and mortality [19]. Clinicians worldwide consider the ECOG-PS when planning new treatments

TABLE 2: Univariate analysis of clinical and metabolic parameters (at the 3rd month after starting hemodialysis). Significance was set at P < 0.05.

Variables	SURVIVORS N: 52	NON-SURVIVORS N: 47	P
Age	73±6	77.4±7.80	0,012
Gender, Women (%)	39	47	0,545
mLCI score	2,5±2,2	3,7±2,3	0,009
ECOG-PS	2.3±0.8	2.8±1	0,023
Temporary Vascular Access (%)	87	89	0,722
Ischemic / Atherosclerotic (Primary Kidney Diseases)	8	11	0,255
Interstitial Nephritis (Acute / Chronic) (Primary Kidney Diseases)	4	3	0,476
Diabetic mellitus (Primary Kidney Diseases)	16	12	0,149
Unknown Etiology (Primary Kidney Diseases)	10	17	0,24
Other (Primary Kidney Diseases)	8	8	0,65
Serum Creatinine (mg/dl)	7±3	6.1±2.4	0,11
Serum Albumin (gr/dl)	2.7±0.5	2.6±0.6	0,232
Venous Bicarbonate (mmol/L)	16.6±6	17.3±5.2	0,72
Hemoglobin (g/dl)	8.7±1.3	9.2±1.3	0,74
C-Reactive Protein (mg/dl)	5.1±5.7	6±7	0,77
Ferritin (ng/ml)	400±336	836±1855	0,10
Proteinuria (g/day)	3.2±3	2.6±2.5	0,36
Cardiac Ejection Fraction (%)	51	49	0,85

TABLE 3: Multivariate analysis of clinical and metabolic parameters. All variables in Table 2 were included in multivariate analysis, but only statistically significant results are presented in Table 3. Significance was set at $P < 0.05$.

Dependent Variable	Multivariate Analysis		
	Odds ratio	%95 CI	P value
Age	5,520	1,8-18,1	0,021
mLCI score	4,944	1,6-12,2	0,029
ECOG-PS	3,986	2,09-5,15	0,049

for elderly patients [20]. We found that the ECOG-PS was related to mortality. Similar to our results, in a Japanese study, ECOG-PS was a prognostic factor in a multivariate analysis of hemodialysis patients aged ≥ 80 years [9]. However, we could not find a significant linear correlation between the mLCI score and ECOG-PS. However, the addition of functional status/fragility can help develop comorbidity scoring systems [21].

Age is a strong independent predictor in all existing scoring systems and we also found that older age was related to higher mortality. Another recent study found that dialysis may not benefit the survival of patients over 75 years old who have multiple comorbidities [22]. Nevertheless, older age should not be an obstacle to dialysis treatment because

patients with a low mLCI may have an acceptable mean life expectancy.

This study has several important limitations. The number of subjects was small and we did not classify the severity of each comorbid condition. However, we recorded the ECOG-PS and it may indirectly quantify the severity of all comorbidities. And, also, the study was retrospective and the patients included were from a single institution.

5. Conclusion

Treatment of ESRD in geriatric population is complex and there is a lot of questions on how to best manage these patients. Our study evaluated the life expectancy of geriatric hemodialysis patients using mLCI score, age, and ECOG-PS. Our findings may help suggesting the prognosis of geriatric patients after starting dialysis and mortality is high in geriatric hemodialysis patients who have many comorbidities (i.e., higher mLCI scores), especially those with poor daily living status (i.e., higher ECOG-PS) and our findings contribute to international clinical experience.

References

[1] A. J. Collins, R. N. Foley, and B. Chavers, "United States Renal Data System 2011 Annual Data Report: atlas of chronic kidney disease & end-stage renal disease in the United States," *American Journal of Kidney Diseases*, vol. 59, no. 1, supplement 1, p. A7, 2012.

[2] J. W. Chae, C. S. Song, H. Kim, K. B. Lee, B. S. Seo, and etal., "Prediction of mortality in patients undergoing maintenance hemodialysis by Charlson Comorbidity Index using ICD," *Nephron Clinical Practice*, vol. 117, no. 4, pp. c379–c384, 2011.

[3] N. V. Athienites, D. C. Miskulin, G. Fernandez et al., "Comorbidity assessment in hemodialysis and peritoneal dialysis using the index of coexistent disease," *Seminars in Dialysis*, vol. 13, no. 5, pp. 320–326, 2000.

[4] M. Kurella, K. E. Covinsky, A. J. Collins, and G. M. Chertow, "Octogenarians and nonagenarians starting dialysis in the United States," *Annals of Internal Medicine*, vol. 146, no. 3, pp. 177–183, 2007.

[5] R. Werb, "Palliative Care in the Treatment of End-Stage Renal Failure," *Primary Care—Clinics in Office Practice*, vol. 38, no. 2, pp. 299–309, 2011.

[6] M. E. Charlson, P. Pompei, K. L. Ales, and C. R. MacKenzie, "A new method of classifying prognostic comorbidity in longitudinal studies: development and validation," *Journal of Chronic Diseases*, vol. 40, no. 5, pp. 373–383, 1987.

[7] M. M. Oken, R. H. Creech, and D. C. Tormey, "Toxicity and response criteria of the Eastern Cooperative Oncology Group," *American Journal of Clinical Oncology*, vol. 5, no. 6, pp. 649–655, 1982.

[8] F. E. M. Murtagh, J. E. Marsh, P. Donohoe, N. J. Ekbal, N. S. Sheerin, and F. E. Harris, "Dialysis or not? A comparative survival study of patients over 75 years with chronic kidney disease stage 5," *Nephrology Dialysis Transplantation* , vol. 22, no. 7, pp. 1955–1962, 2007.

[9] A. Burns, "Conservative management of end-stage renal failure: masterly inactivity or benign neglect? See Smith et al., pp. c40-c46.," *Nephron Clinical Practice*, vol. 95, no. 2, pp. c37–39, 2003.

[10] D. Joly, D. Anglicheau, C. Alberti et al., "Octogenarians reaching end-stage renal disease: cohort study of decision-making and clinical outcomes," *Journal of the American Society of Nephrology*, vol. 14, no. 4, pp. 1012–1021, 2003.

[11] D. L. Lamping, N. Constantinovici, P. Roderick et al., "Clinical outcomes, quality of life, and costs in the North Thames dialysis study of elderly people on dialysis: a prospective cohort study," *The Lancet*, vol. 356, no. 9241, pp. 1543–1550, 2000.

[12] J. G. Van Manen, J. C. Korevaar, F. W. Dekker, E. W. Boeschoten, P. M. M. Bossuyt, and R. T. Krediet, "How to adjust for comorbidity in survival studies in ESRD patients: A comparison of different indices," *American Journal of Kidney Diseases*, vol. 40, no. 1, pp. 82–89, 2002.

[13] L. Fried, J. Bernardini, and B. Piraino, "Charlson comorbidity index as a predictor of outcomes in incident peritoneal dialysis patients," *American Journal of Kidney Diseases*, vol. 37, no. 2, pp. 337–342, 2001.

[14] B. Di Iorio, N. Cillo, M. Cirillo, and N. Gaspare De Santo, "Charlson Comorbidity Index is a predictor of outcomes in incident hemodialysis patients and correlates with phase angle and hospitalization," *The International Journal of Artificial Organs*, vol. 27, no. 4, pp. 330–336, 2004.

[15] D. C. Miskulin, A. A. Martin, R. Brown et al., "Predicting 1 year mortality in an outpatient haemodialysis population: A comparison of comorbidity instruments," *Nephrology Dialysis Transplantation* , vol. 19, no. 2, pp. 413–420, 2004.

[16] J. Liu, Z. Huang, D. T. Gilbertson, R. N. Foley, and A. J. Collins, "An improved comorbidity index for outcome analyses among dialysis patients," *Kidney International*, vol. 77, no. 2, pp. 141–151, 2010.

[17] S. K. Rigler, J. B. Wetmore, J. D. Mahnken, L. Dong, E. F. Ellerbeck, and T. I. Shireman, "Impact of a modified data capture period on Liu comorbidity index scores in Medicare enrollees initiating chronic dialysis," *BMC Nephrology*, vol. 14, no. 1, article no. 51, 2013.

[18] W.-C. Kan, J.-J. Wang, S.-Y. Wang et al., "The New Comorbidity Index for Predicting Survival in Elderly Dialysis Patients: A Long-Term Population-Based Study," *PLoS ONE*, vol. 8, no. 8, Article ID e68748, 2013.

[19] E. L. Knight, N. Ofsthun, M. Teng, J. M. Lazarus, and G. C. Curhan, "The association between mental health, physical function, and hemodialysis mortality," *Kidney International*, vol. 63, no. 5, pp. 1843–1851, 2003.

[20] S. Hatakeyama, H. Murasawa, I. Hamano et al., "Prognosis of elderly Japanese patients aged ≥80 Years undergoing hemodialysis," *The Scientific World Journal*, vol. 2013, Article ID 693514, 7 pages, 2013.

[21] M. Thamer, J. S. Kaufman, Y. Zhang, Q. Zhang, D. J. Cotter, and H. Bang, "Predicting early death among elderly dialysis patients: Development and validation of a risk score to assist shared decision making for dialysis initiation," *American Journal of Kidney Diseases*, vol. 66, no. 6, pp. 1024–1032, 2015.

[22] S. M. Chandna, M. Da Silva-Gane, C. Marshall, P. Warwicker, R. N. Greenwood, and K. Farrington, "Survival of elderly patients with stage 5 CKD: Comparison of conservative management and renal replacement therapy," *Nephrology Dialysis Transplantation* , vol. 26, no. 5, pp. 1608–1614, 2011.

27

Vascular Calcification in Chronic Kidney Disease: The Role of Inflammation

Kerstin Benz,[1] **Karl-Friedrich Hilgers,**[2] **Christoph Daniel ⓘ,**[1] **and Kerstin Amann ⓘ**[1]

[1]*Department of Nephropathology, Friedrich-Alexander University (FAU) Erlangen-Nürnberg, Germany*
[2]*Department of Nephrology and Hypertension, Friedrich-Alexander University (FAU) Erlangen-Nürnberg, Germany*

Correspondence should be addressed to Kerstin Amann; kerstin.amann@uk-erlangen.de

Academic Editor: Nicolas Verheyen

Cardiovascular complications are extremely frequent in patients with chronic kidney disease (CKD) and death from cardiac causes is the most common cause of death in this particular population. Cardiovascular disease is approximately 3 times more frequent in patients with CKD than in other known cardiovascular risk groups and cardiovascular mortality is approximately 10-fold more frequent in patients on dialysis compared to the age- and sex-matched segments of the nonrenal population. Among other structural and functional factors advanced calcification of atherosclerotic plaques as well as of the arterial and venous media has been described as potentially relevant for this high cardiovascular morbidity and mortality. One potential explanation for this exceedingly high vascular calcification in animal models as well as in patients with CKD increased systemic and most importantly local (micro)inflammation that has been shown to favor the development of calcifying particles by multiple ways. Of note, local vascular upregulation of proinflammatory and proosteogenic molecules is already present at early stages of CKD and may thus be operative for vascular calcification. In addition, increased expression of costimulatory molecules and mast cells has also been documented in patients with CKD pointing to a more inflammatory and potentially less stable phenotype of coronary atherosclerotic plaques in CKD.

1. Introduction

Patients with chronic kidney disease (CKD) and chronic renal failure (CRF) develop early on in the course of the disease structural and functional alterations of the heart and the vascular tree that represent a major clinical problem in these patients. In addition, cardiovascular diseases are a major contributor to the high incidence of cardiovascular complications and particularly death from cardiovascular causes in this population [1, 2]. Apart from left ventricular hypertrophy (LVH) which is present very early in the course of the renal disease even in normotensive CKD patients structural alterations of the myocardium as well as the intra- and extracardiac arteries and veins are hallmarks of this disease. With respect to the myocardium reduced myocardial capillary supply, interstitial fibrosis and thickening of the intramyocardial arteries can be seen [3–5]. These intramyocardial structural alterations increase the susceptibility of the hypertrophied heart of CKD patients towards ischemic damage and

favor the development of arrhythmias, myocardial infarction, and sudden cardiac death [6]. The pathogenesis of these myocardial alterations is certainly multifactorial, but only partly understood. Among the mechanisms that have been described for LVH and the associated myocardial alterations are the so-called classical or traditional risk factors like hypertension, hyperlipidemia, and diabetes but also CKD-specific changes such as anemia, hypervolemia, increased sympathetic activity, hyperphosphatemia, oxidative stress, and altered expression of the fibroblast growth factor 23 (FGF-32) [7, 8]. As a consequence clinical strategies to prevent or ameliorate LVH and associated structural alterations in CKD comprise prevention of anemia by normalization of the hemoglobin value (Hb), prevention of hypervolemia, and strict blood pressure control particularly with ACE-inhibitors. In experimental models of chronic renal failure blockade of the renin-angiotensin system (RAS), the endothelin (ET) system, pharmacological and mechanical

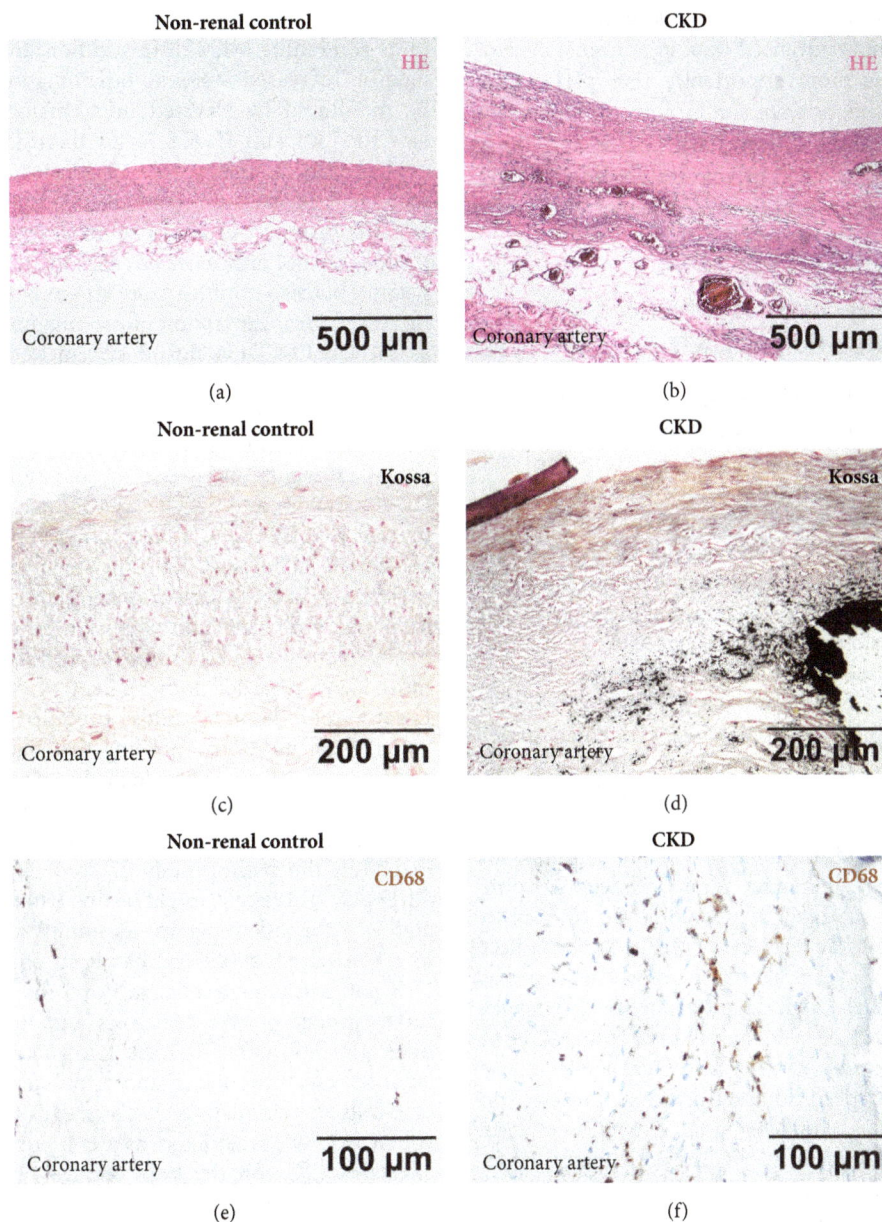

FIGURE 1: (a-f) Representative vascular findings in nonrenal control patients (a, c, e) and patients with chronic kidney disease (CKD). (a, b) Marked thickening of coronary arteries in CKD patients (b) compared to nonrenal controls (a). HE-stain. (c, d) Marked calcification of the arterial intima and media and atherosclerotic coronary plaques in CKD patients (d) compared to nonrenal controls (d). Von Kossa stain. (e, f) Increased number of CD68 positive macrophages in the vascular wall of CKD patients (f) compared to nonrenal controls (e). Immunohistochemistry.

inhibition of the sympathetic nervous system, and blockade of the FGF23-axis [9–13] were also shown to be successful.

In addition to the cardiac alterations specific structural changes of the extracardiac arteries and veins are present which consist of vessel thickening (Figures 1(a) and 1(b)) but more importantly of marked calcification of the arterial intima and media as well as of venous walls and atherosclerotic coronary plaques giving rise to complications such as coronary artery thrombosis and myocardial infarction [14–18]. Based on their clinical experience the group of Lindner and coworkers in 1974 [19] were the first to show that

atherosclerosis in CKD patients is different from that of nonrenal patients. They particularly showed that the lesions were more advanced and the course of atherosclerosis in these patients was more aggressive. Consequently, they speculated that this may contribute to the exceedingly high cardiovascular morbidity and mortality in these patients. The functional consequences of increase vascular and plaques calcification are manifold: it leads to increased stiffness of the vessel which in the case of the arterial tree increases the cardiac afterload and impairs coronary artery perfusion [20–22]. In an autoptic study Schwarz and coworkers [23, 24] were able to confirm that indeed the coronary atherosclerotic lesions in CKD patients were more advanced than in nonrenal control patients and perhaps more importantly that particularly the calcified plaque lesions were significantly more present in CKD patients (Figures 1(c) and 1(d)). This and other findings prompted in vitro and in vivo studies investigating the underlying pathogenesis of increased plaque and vessel calcification in CKD.

2. Potential Pathogenesis of Advanced Vascular Calcification in CKD

Although the exact pathogenesis of increased vascular calcification in CKD is not fully understood there are some very plausible hypotheses and candidates: from the very beginning disturbances in the phosphorus (P) and calcium (Ca) metabolism [25, 26], altered expression of many factors, which are involved or regulate the mineral metabolism [27, 28], and perhaps most importantly chronic microinflammation which is present in CKD patients early on in the disease and comes along with increased CRP levels [29, 30] have been discussed as important pathogenetic factors. Particularly, early on a major pathogenetic role of P and Ca has emerged from clinical [31, 32] and experimental studies [33, 34] where a strong correlation between serum values of both P and Ca and perhaps more importantly the Ca-P product (CaxP) and cardiovascular events could be shown [35]. On the other hand, experimental manipulation with high and low phosphate diet in an animal model of chronic renal failure, i.e., the subtotally nephrectomized rat (SNX), could clearly document the deleterious cardiovascular effect of high phosphate [34]. It has also been shown in vitro that increased P and Ca levels can induce osteoblast-like changes in vascular smooth muscle cells (VSMC) via stimulation of Na-dependent P-cotransporters [36, 37]. This is reflected by de novo expression of specific marker proteins of osteogenic differentiation like cbfa-1 und osteocalcin which coincide with a change in phenotype of VSMC from a contractile to a secretory calcifying cell. In patients with CKD the expression of calcification-inhibiting proteins like Fetuin-A, MGP, beta-Glucosidase, and osteoprotegerin is reduced which may also contribute to a procalcific milieu [38, 39]. Very recently, serum calciprotein particles and circulating nanostructures, such as extracellular vesicles, have been identified as important players in the mechanism of calcification in CKD mainly by promoting cell osteochondrogenic differentiation and inflammation [40]. Vice versa, a role for inhibition of mineral crystal formation by Gla-rich protein which in vitro could prevent calciprotein particles induced calcification was postulated.

3. Role of Systemic and Local Inflammation in Vascular Calcification

The above-mentioned recent study by Viegas and coworkers [40] more emphasizes a potential role of inflammation for vascular calcification in CKD. Systemic and local effects of inflammation on vascular alterations in CKD but also in other

segments of the general population are being discussed for quite some time [41, 42]. In addition, to the many excellent data on increased systemic inflammation in CKD that can be monitored by elevated inflammatory biomarkers such as CRP [30] and IL-6 [43–45] there is also experimental evidence for a major role of local inflammation in the pathogenesis of advanced atherosclerosis in renal failure [24]. In CKD patients our group could show that coronary artery plaques are not only more advanced than in nonrenal control patients but also exhibit a more inflammatory phenotype with increased local expression of proinflammatory systems such as the CD40-CD154 ligand system and also macrophages (Figures 1(e) and 1(f)) which has been associated with increased risk of atherosclerotic events [46]. In addition, we could recently show [47] that local upregulation of proinflammatory and proosteogenic molecules such as CRP, CD40, CD154, and SATB2 as well as galectin-3 is already present at early stages of CKD in various vessels (Figure 2), i.e., the A. mammaria int., the V. saphena magna, and the aorta taken at the occasion of cardiac surgery [47]. Of note, local microinflammation was even seen in the absence of major disturbances of the CaxP product and could thus be most likely regarded independent of changes in P or Ca. Local microinflammation also preceded the development of vascular calcification, a finding that may point to an early and important pathophysiological role of (pro)inflammatory changes. In addition, we recently investigated a potential role for dendritic cells (DCs) and particularly mast cells (MCs) in the pathogenesis of coronary atherosclerosis in CKD [48]. These cells might be important since a role of DCs and MCs for inflammation, immunity, and T-cell-activation in atherosclerosis [49–55] has been shown. Consequently, DCs and MCs may represent novel therapeutic targets [56] for treatment of atherosclerosis and its complications. Of note, patients with CKD are known to show clinical and laboratory features of immunosuppression with low numbers of T-cells and circulating DCs as well as impaired T-cell activation [57–59], most likely as a consequence of suppressive effects of CKD on the bone marrow and cell maturation. Using immunohistochemistry, Hueso et al. [60] investigated aortic lesions of CKD and control patients, i.e., adaptive as well as pathological intimal thickening of the aorta and fibroatheromas and found a significantly higher percentage of DCs in CKD patients compared to non-CKD controls. In contrast, in coronary arteries we found a lower number of DCs in CKD compared to nonrenal control patients. DCs were predominantly located in the shoulder, boundary, and basis subregions of plaques in good correlation with the Stary classification of atherosclerotic lesions. In addition, in the shoulder and cap region DCs positivity correlated with T-cells and macrophages potentially indicating a proinflammatory role of DCs that might be important in terms of plaque instability. It is also speculated that DCs activation by nicotine, stress, hypoxia, or CRP may stimulate the local immune response [61]. This might be of interest in view of our previous finding of an increased in situ expression of CRP in atherosclerotic plaques of CKD patients compared to controls [46]. With respect to the effect of CKD on MC number and distribution we found a tendency for more

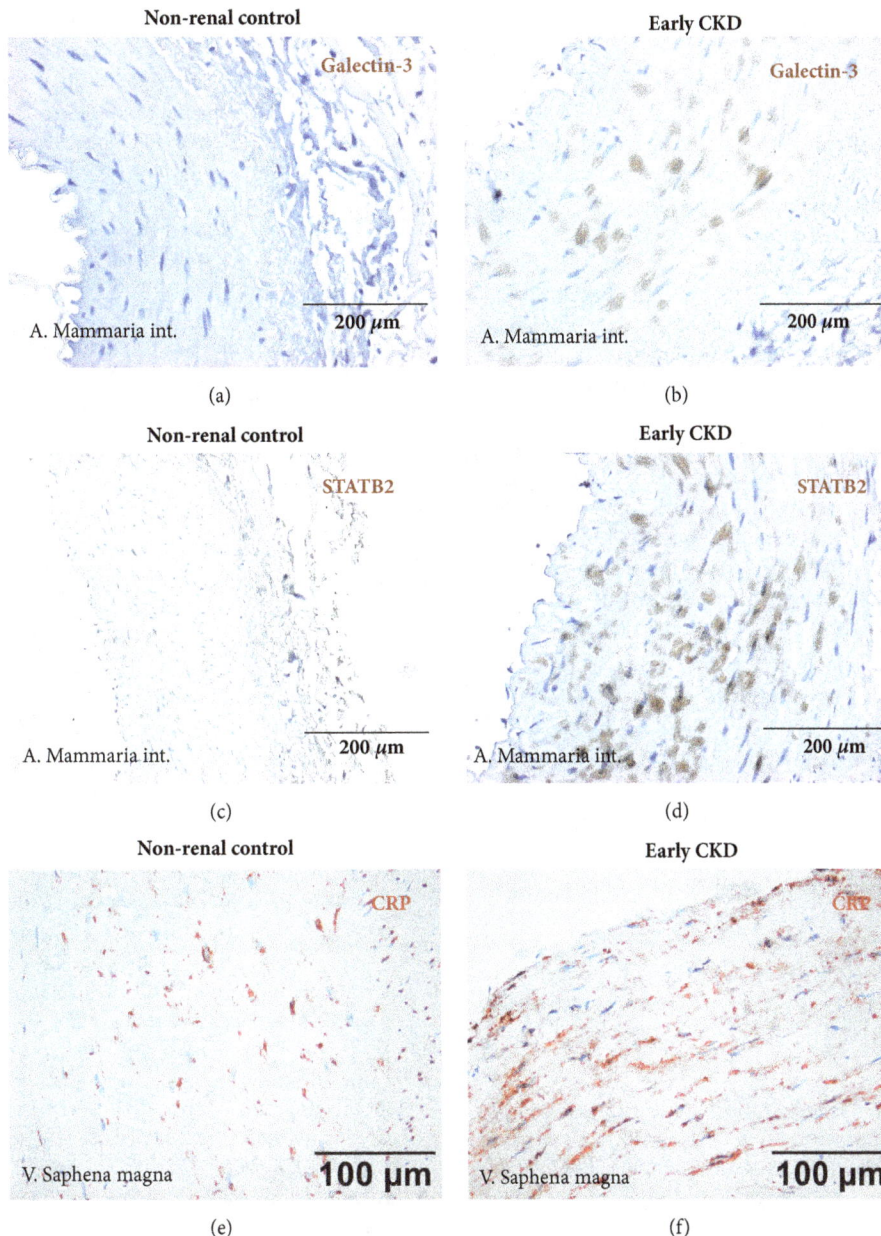

FIGURE 2: (a-f) Representative vascular changes in nonrenal control patients (a, c, e) and patients with early chronic kidney disease (CKD). (a, b) Increased expression of galectin-3 in arteria mammaria int. in early CKD patients (b) compared to nonrenal controls (a). Immunohistochemistry. (c, d) Marked increase in STAB2 expression in arteria mammaria int. in early CKD patients (d) compared to nonrenal controls (d). Immunohistochemistry. (e, f) Increased staining for C-reactive protein (CRP) in vena saphena magna in early CKD patients (f) compared to nonrenal controls (e). Immunohistochemistry.

MCs in vessels from end-stage CKD patients particularly in calcified ones. This finding potentially points to a specific role of MCs compared to DCs under the condition of renal failure and particularly in vessel calcification. Detailed correlation analysis of MCs with inflammatory cells such as T-cells and macrophages inside plaques subregions revealed a positive association with T-cells in end-stage CKD specimens and a significant correlation between the MC score within the plaque and the serum C-reactive protein (CRP) levels, again suggesting a potential link of MCs to local intraplaque T-cell and macrophage activation and also to systemic inflammation.

4. Summary and Conclusion

Advanced stages of atherosclerotic plaques particularly with plaque and vessel calcification are specific features in patients with CKD that might contribute to the high cardiovascular morbidity and mortality in these patients. Our findings of a more inflammatory phenotype of coronary atherosclerotic plaques and particularly of a potential role of MCs for advanced atherosclerosis in CKD might be particularly important in view of recent experimental findings in the animal model of the ApoE knockout mouse [62] where pharmacological MC chymase inhibition using the protease inhibitor RO5066852 was shown to reduce atherosclerotic plaque progression and to improve plaque stability. If this novel experimental finding could be successfully translated into the human situation pharmacological MC inhibition might possibly evolve as a new therapeutic target in the treatment of atherosclerosis particularly in the advanced condition of chronic renal failure. In order to find adequate and effective treatment strategies it is tremendously important to gain further insight into the exact mechanisms of calcification under the conditions of CKD [63, 64]. It is most likely that in the near future we aim at specific treatment options for hyperphosphatemia, chronic microinflammation, and increased FGF-23 levels and may be also MC chymase inhibition in patients with CKD that might help to lower the exceedingly high cardiovascular risk in this particular population group.

Acknowledgments

The authors acknowledge support by Deutsche Porschungsgemeinschaft and Friedrich-Alexander-Universität Erlangen-Nürnberg (FAU) within the funding programme Open Access Publishing.

References

[1] K. Amann, C. Wanner, and E. Ritz, "Cross-talk between the kidney and the cardiovascular system," *Journal of the American Society of Nephrology*, vol. 17, no. 8, pp. 2112–2119, 2006.

[2] C. Wanner, K. Amann, and T. Shoji, "The heart and vascular system in dialysis," *The Lancet*, vol. 388, no. 10041, pp. 276–284, 2016.

[3] K. Amann and E. Ritz, "Microvascular disease—the Cinderella of uraemic heart disease," *Nephrology Dialysis Transplantation*, vol. 15, no. 10, pp. 1493–1503, 2000.

[4] K. Amann, "Cardiovascular changes in chronic renal failure—pathogenesis and therapy," *Clinical Nephrology*, vol. 58, 1, pp. S62–S72, 2002.

[5] K. Amann and E. Ritz, "The heart in renal failure: morphological changes of the myocardiom - new insights," *Journal of Clinical and Basic Cardiology*, vol. 4, pp. 109–113, 2001.

[6] R. Dikow, L. P. Kihm, M. Zeier et al., "Increased infarct size in uremic rats: Reduced ischemia tolerance?" *Journal of the American Society of Nephrology*, vol. 15, no. 6, pp. 1530–1536, 2004.

[7] J. Himmelfarb, P. Stenvinkel, T. A. Ikizler, and R. M. Hakim, "The elephant in uremia: oxidant stress as a unifying concept of cardiovascular disease in uremia," *Kidney International*, vol. 62, no. 5, pp. 1524–1538, 2002.

[8] C. Faul, A. P. Amaral, B. Oskouei et al., "FGF23 induces left ventricular hypertrophy," *The Journal of Clinical Investigation*, vol. 121, no. 11, pp. 4393–4408, 2011.

[9] K. Amann, P. Gassmann, M. Buzello et al., "Effects of ACE inhibition and bradykinin antagonism on cardiovascular changes in uremic rats," *Kidney International*, vol. 58, no. 1, pp. 153–161, 2000.

[10] K. Amann, J. Hofstetter, V. Câmpean et al., "Nonhypotensive dose of β-adrenergic blocker ameliorates capillary deficits in the hearts of rats with moderate renal failure," *Virchows Archiv*, vol. 449, no. 2, pp. 207–214, 2006.

[11] K. Amann, K. Münter, S. Wessels et al., "Endothelin a receptor blockade prevents capillary/myocyte mismatch in the heart of uremic animals," *Journal of the American Society of Nephrology*, vol. 11, no. 9, pp. 1702–1711, 2000.

[12] K. Amann, K. Tyralla, M.-L. Gross et al., "Cardiomyocyte loss in experimental renal failure: Prevention by ramipril," *Kidney International*, vol. 63, no. 5, pp. 1708–1713, 2003.

[13] G. S. Di Marco, S. Reuter, D. Kentrup et al., "Treatment of established left ventricular hypertrophy with fibroblast growth factor receptor blockade in an animal model of CKD," *Nephrology Dialysis Transplantation*, vol. 29, no. 11, pp. 2028–2035, 2014.

[14] V. Campean, D. Neureiter, I. Varga et al., "Atherosclerosis and vascular calcification in chronic renal failure," *Kidney and Blood Pressure Research*, vol. 28, no. 5-6, pp. 280–289, 2006.

[15] K. Amann, "Media calcification and intima calcification are distinct entities in chronic kidney disease," *Clinical Journal of the American Society of Nephrology*, vol. 3, no. 6, pp. 1599–1605, 2008.

[16] W. G. Goodman, "Vascular calcification in end-stage renal disease," *Journal of Nephrology*, vol. 15, no. 6, pp. S82–S85, 2002.

[17] W. G. Goodman, J. Goldin, B. D. Kuizon et al., "Coronary-artery calcification in young adults with end-stage renal disease who are undergoing dialysis," *The New England Journal of Medicine*, vol. 342, no. 20, pp. 1478–1483, 2000.

[18] M.-L. Gross, H.-P. Meyer, H. Ziebart et al., "Calcification of coronary intima and media: Immunohistochemistry, backscatter imaging, and x-ray analysis in renal and nonrenal patients," *Clinical Journal of the American Society of Nephrology*, vol. 2, no. 1, pp. 121–134, 2007.

[19] A. Lindner, B. Charra, D. J. Sherrard, and B. H. Scribner, "Accelerated atherosclerosis in prolonged maintenance hemodialysis," *The New England Journal of Medicine*, vol. 290, no. 13, pp. 697–701, 1974.

[20] G. M. London, A. P. Guérin, S. J. Marchais, F. Métivier, B. Pannier, and H. Adda, "Arterial media calcification in end-stage renal disease: Impact on all-cause and cardiovascular mortality," *Nephrology Dialysis Transplantation*, vol. 18, no. 9, pp. 1731–1740, 2003.

[21] G. M. London, S. J. Marchais, and A. P. Guerin, "Arterial stiffness and function in end-stage renal disease," *Advances in Chronic Kidney Disease*, vol. 11, no. 2, pp. 202–209, 2004.

[22] K. Amann and E. Ritz, "Cardiovascular abnormalities in ageing and in uraemia - Only analogy or shared pathomechanisms?" *Nephrology Dialysis Transplantation*, vol. 13, no. 7, pp. 6–11, 1998.

[23] U. Schwarz, M. Buzello, E. Ritz et al., "Morphology of coronary atherosclerotic lesions in patients with end-stage renal failure," *Nephrology Dialysis Transplantation*, vol. 15, no. 2, pp. 218–223, 2000.

[24] S. B. Schwedler, K. Amann, K. Wernicke et al., "Native C-reactive protein increases whereas modified C-reactive protein

reduces atherosclerosis in apolipoprotein E-knockout mice," *Circulation*, vol. 112, no. 7, pp. 1016–1023, 2005.

[25] W. G. Goodman, "Importance of hyperphosphataemia in the cardio-renal axis," *Nephrology Dialysis Transplantation*, vol. 19, no. 1, pp. i4–i8, 2004.

[26] K. Amann, M.-L. Gross, G. M. London, and E. Ritz, "Hyperphosphataemia - A silent killer of patients with renal failure?" *Nephrology Dialysis Transplantation*, vol. 14, no. 9, pp. 2085–2087, 1999.

[27] M. Ketteler, C. Wanner, T. Metzger et al., "Deficiencies of calcium-regulatory proteins in dialysis patients: A novel concept of cardiovascular calcification in uremia," *Kidney International Supplements*, vol. 63, no. 84, pp. S84–S87, 2003.

[28] C. Schäfer, A. Heiss, A. Schwarz et al., "The serum protein α_2-Heremans-Schmid glycoprotein/fetuin-A is a systemically acting inhibitor of ectopic calcification," *The Journal of Clinical Investigation*, vol. 112, no. 3, pp. 357–366, 2003.

[29] E. Ishimura, S. Okuno, K. Kitatani et al., "C-reactive protein is a significant predictor of vascular calcification of both aorta and hand arteries," *Seminars in Nephrology*, vol. 24, no. 5, pp. 408–412, 2004.

[30] J. Zimmermann, S. Herrlinger, A. Pruy, T. Metzger, and C. Wanner, "Inflammation enhances cardiovascular risk and mortality in hemodialysis patients," *Kidney International*, vol. 55, no. 2, pp. 648–658, 1999.

[31] G. A. Block, "Prevalence and clinical consequences of elevated Ca x P product in hemodialysis patients," *Clinical Nephrology*, vol. 54, no. 4, pp. 318–324, 2000.

[32] G. A. Block, T. E. Hulbert-Shearon, N. W. Levin, and F. K. Port, "Association of serum phosphorus and calcium x phosphate product with mortality risk in chronic hemodialysis patients: a national study," *American Journal of Kidney Diseases*, vol. 31, no. 4, pp. 607–617, 1998.

[33] K. Amann, E. Ritz, G. Wiest, G. Klaus, and G. Mall, "A role of parathyroid hormone for the activation of cardiac fibroblasts in uremia," *Journal of the American Society of Nephrology*, vol. 4, no. 10, pp. 1814–1819, 1994.

[34] K. Amann, J. Törnig, B. Kugel et al., "Hyperphosphatemia aggravates cardiac fibrosis and microvascular disease in experimental uremia," *Kidney International*, vol. 63, no. 4, pp. 1296–1301, 2003.

[35] S. M. Moe, "Current issues in the management of secondary hyperparathyroidism and bone disease," *Peritoneal Dialysis International*, vol. 21, no. 3, pp. S241–S246, 2001.

[36] C. M. Giachelli, "Vascular calcification: in vitro evidence for the role of inorganic phosphate," *Journal of the American Society of Nephrology*, vol. 14, 4, no. 9, pp. S300–S304, 2003.

[37] N. X. Chen, K. D. O'Neill, D. Duan, and S. M. Moe, "Phosphorus and uremic serum up-regulate osteopontin expression in vascular smooth muscle cells," *Kidney International*, vol. 62, no. 5, pp. 1724–1731, 2002.

[38] S. M. Moe, D. Duan, B. P. Doehle, K. D. O'Neill, and N. X. Chen, "Uremia induces the osteoblast differentiation factor Cbfa1 in human blood vessels," *Kidney International*, vol. 63, no. 3, pp. 1003–1011, 2003.

[39] S. M. Moe, K. D. O'Neill, D. Duan et al., "Medial artery calcification in ESRD patients is associated with deposition of bone matrix proteins," *Kidney International*, vol. 61, no. 2, pp. 638–647, 2002.

[40] C. S. Viegas, L. Santos, A. L. Macedo et al., "Chronic Kidney Disease Circulating Calciprotein Particles and Extracellular Vesicles Promote Vascular Calcification: A Role for GRP (Gla-Rich Protein)," *Arteriosclerosis, Thrombosis, and Vascular Biology*, vol. 38, no. 3, pp. 575–587, 2018.

[41] A. Mehta, J. Patel, M. Al Rifai et al., "Inflammation and coronary artery calcification in South Asians: The Mediators of Atherosclerosis in South Asians Living in America (MASALA) study," *Atherosclerosis*, vol. 270, pp. 49–56, 2018.

[42] Y. S. Hamirani, S. Pandey, J. J. Rivera et al., "Markers of inflammation and coronary artery calcification: A systematic review," *Atherosclerosis*, vol. 201, no. 1, pp. 1–7, 2008.

[43] R. Pecoits-Filho, B. Lindholm, and P. Stenvinkel, "The malnutrition, inflammation, and atherosclerosis (MIA) syndrome—the heart of the matter," *Nephrology Dialysis Transplantation*, vol. 17, 11, pp. 28–31, 2002.

[44] J. P. Kooman, M. J. Dekker, L. A. Usvyat et al., "Inflammation and premature aging in advanced chronic kidney disease," *American Journal of Physiology-Renal Physiology*, vol. 313, no. 4, pp. F938–F950, 2017.

[45] L. Dai, E. Golembiewska, B. Lindholm, and P. Stenvinkel, "End-Stage Renal Disease, Inflammation and Cardiovascular Outcomes," *Contributions to Nephrology*, vol. 191, pp. 32–43, 2017.

[46] V. Campean, D. Neureiter, B. Nonnast-Daniel, C. Garlichs, M.-L. Gross, and K. Amann, "CD40-CD154 expression in calcified and non-calcified coronary lesions of patients with chronic renal failure," *Atherosclerosis*, vol. 190, no. 1, pp. 156–166, 2007.

[47] K. Benz, I. Varga, D. Neureiter et al., "Vascular inflammation and media calcification are already present in early stages of chronic kidney disease," *Cardiovascular Pathology*, vol. 27, pp. 57–67, 2017.

[48] D. L. Wachter, D. Neureiter, V. Campean, K. Hilgers et al., "In-situ analysis of mast cells and dendritic cells in coronary atherosclerosis in chronic kidney disease (CKD)," *Histology and Histopathology*, 2018.

[49] J. Swedenborg, M. I. Mäyränpää, and P. T. Kovanen, "Mast cells: Important players in the orchestrated pathogenesis of abdominal aortic aneurysms," *Arteriosclerosis, Thrombosis, and Vascular Biology*, vol. 31, no. 4, pp. 734–740, 2011.

[50] Y. V. Bobryshev, R. S. A. Lord, S. Rainer, O. S. Jamal, and V. F. Munro, "Vascular dendritic cells and atherosclerosis," *Pathology - Research and Practice*, vol. 192, no. 5, pp. 462–467, 1996.

[51] Y. V. Bobryshev and R. S. A. Lord, "Langhans cells of human arterial intima: Uniform by stellate appearance but different by nature," *Tissue & Cell*, vol. 28, no. 2, pp. 177–194, 1996.

[52] Y. V. Bobryshev and R. S. A. Lord, "Detection of vascular dendritic cells accumulating calcified deposits in their cytoplasm," *Tissue & Cell*, vol. 30, no. 3, pp. 383–388, 1998.

[53] Y. V. Bobryshev and R. S. A. Lord, "Mapping of vascular dendritic cells in atherosclerotic arteries suggests their involvement in local immune-inflammatory reaction," *Cardiovascular Research*, vol. 37, no. 3, pp. 799–810, 1998.

[54] Y. V. Bobryshev, "Dendritic cells and their role in atherogenesis," *Laboratory Investigation*, vol. 90, no. 7, pp. 970–984, 2010.

[55] K. E. Paulson, S.-N. Zhu, M. Chen, S. Nurmohamed, J. Jongstra-Bilen, and M. I. Cybulsky, "Resident intimal dendritic cells accumulate lipid and contribute to the initiation of atherosclerosis," *Circulation Research*, vol. 106, no. 2, pp. 383–390, 2010.

[56] I. Bot and E. A. L. Biessen, "Mast cells in atherosclerosis," *Thrombosis and Haemostasis*, vol. 106, no. 5, pp. 820–826, 2011.

[57] T. Eleftheriadis, G. Antoniadi, V. Liakopoulos, C. Kartsios, and I. Stefanidis, "Disturbances of acquired immunity in hemodialysis patients," *Seminars in Dialysis*, vol. 20, no. 5, pp. 440–451, 2007.

[58] M. Girndt, M. Sester, U. Sester, H. Kaul, and H. Köhler, "Molecular aspects of T- and B-cell function in uremia," *Kidney International Supplements*, vol. 59, no. 78, pp. S206–S211, 2001.

[59] W. H. Lim, S. Kireta, E. Leedham, G. R. Russ, and P. T. Coates, "Uremia impairs monocyte and monocyte-derived dendritic cell function in hemodialysis patients," *Kidney International*, vol. 72, no. 9, pp. 1138–1148, 2007.

[60] M. Hueso, J. Torras, M. Carrera, A. Vidal, E. Navarro, and J. Grinyó, "Chronic Kidney Disease is associated with an increase of Intimal Dendritic cells in a comparative autopsy study," *Journal of Inflammation*, vol. 12, p. 26, 2015.

[61] E. A. Van Vré, H. Bult, V. Y. Hoymans, V. F. I. Van Tendeloo, C. J. Vrints, and J. M. Bosmans, "Human C-reactive protein activates monocyte-derived dendritic cells and induces dendritic cell-mediated T-cell activation," *Arteriosclerosis, Thrombosis, and Vascular Biology*, vol. 28, no. 3, pp. 511–518, 2008.

[62] I. Bot, M. Bot, S. H. Van Heiningen et al., "Mast cell chymase inhibition reduces atherosclerotic plaque progression and improves plaque stability in ApoE-/- mice," *Cardiovascular Research*, vol. 89, no. 1, pp. 244–252, 2011.

[63] Y. V. Bobryshev, "Targeting vascular calcification: Up-date," *Current Pharmaceutical Design*, vol. 20, no. 37, pp. 5799-5800, 2014.

[64] B. F. Sena, J. L. Figueiredo, and E. Aikawa, "Cathepsin S As an Inhibitor of Cardiovascular Inflammation and Calcification in Chronic Kidney Disease," *Frontiers in Cardiovascular Medicine*, vol. 4, p. 88, 2018.

28

Complex Monitoring of Biochemical and Radionuclide Parameters in Patients with Metastatic Renal Cell Carcinoma during Immunotherapy

M. S. Sayapina,[1] **S. G. Averinova,**[1] **T. V. Zacharova,**[1] **A. V. Kashkadaeva,**[1] **S. V. Shiryaev,**[1] **M. V. Poluectova,**[2] **and O. A. Vorob'eva**[2]

[1]*N.N. Blokhin Russian Cancer Research Center, Ministry of Health of Russia, 23 Kashirskoe Shosse, Moscow 115478, Russia*
[2]*A. Tsyb Medical Radiological Research Centre, Branch of the National Medical Research Radiological Centre of The Ministry of Health of The Russian Federation, 10 Zhukov St., Obninsk, Kaluga 249036, Russia*

Correspondence should be addressed to M. S. Sayapina; maria.sayapina@mail.ru

Academic Editor: Jochen Reiser

Study Objective. To study the effectiveness of complex monitoring of the kidney function, based on biochemical and radionuclide methods in patients with metastatic renal cell carcinoma (mRCC). *Materials and Methods.* 41 mRCC patients after nephrectomy received nivolumab ($n = 23$) and interferon-α ($n = 18$) from 2015 to 2017. At baseline and 2 months after, all patients underwent blood chemistry, urinalysis, Rehberg test, and ELISA to determine serum levels of IL-17A, TGF-β, and erythropoietin. The monitoring of the renal function and urodynamics by complex renal scintigraphy (CRS) was used for all patients using a dual-detector gamma camera and simultaneous data recording in 2 projections. The interpretation of CRS data used the original SENS CRS technology. *Study Results.* Statistically significant correlations were established between IL-17A, TGF-β, and D (excretion rate of 99mTc-technephore from the parenchyma) and Rnfsc (a stable sign of nephrosclerosis), respectively. A significant correlation was established between the parameters of the complex functional monitoring with the prognosis for the risk of renal failure (RF) and efficacy of immunotherapy in mRCC. *Conclusions.* All mRCC patients after nephrectomy were recommended to undergo biochemical monitoring with inclusion of TGF-β and IL-17A, as well as radionuclide monitoring (CRS) to determine the RF risk at an early stage.

1. Introduction

Literature describe cases of proteinuria and irreversible renal failure during immunotherapy and targeted therapy in patients with mRCC, resulting in a dose reduction and/or drug withdrawal, which can affect the objective response [1–4]. All patients with mRCC after nephrectomy should be assigned to a high risk group for developing chronic kidney disease (CKD).

Until recently, clearance of endogenous creatinine was the most widely used method for determining GFR in clinical practice. However, in moderate to severe renal insufficiency, GFR values calculated from the endogenous creatinine clearance are significantly overestimated, since creatinine is secreted by the proximal tubule in the settings of renal failure and uremia [5, 6].

In order to estimate GFR, formulas such as MDRD (Modification of Diet in Renal Disease), Cockcroft-Gault, CKD-EPI (Chronic Kidney Disease Epidemiology Collaboration), and MCQ (Mayo Clinic Quadratic) are widely put into practice. Currently, there is evidence allowing suggesting that the screening diagnosis of CKD should be based on only a simultaneous estimation of GFR and albuminuria/proteinuria, which allows estimation of the prognosis and risk of cardiovascular events [7].

The KDIGO (Kidney Disease: Improving Global Outcomes) classification, as is the case with RIFLE (risk, injury, failure, loss, and end-stage kidney disease) and AKIN (acute kidney injury network), based on serum creatinine levels and the volume of diuresis, allow timely diagnosing acute kidney damage and have a prognostic value, but do not allow to take into account causes of kidney damage and, therefore, do not always help determine preventive and treatment tactics [8, 9]. In this regard, the search for the most accurate biomarkers that would allow for early diagnosis of CKD and establishing the cause of its development is of current concern. At the moment, a number of biomarkers associated with nephrotoxicity are known, but FDA (Food and Drug Administration) and EMEA (European Medicines Agency) have approved only KIM-1 (kidney injury molecule-1), albumin, total protein, β2-microglobulin, cystatin C, clusterin, and TFF3 (trefoil factor 3) for routine use in practice [10, 11].

The rate of progression of chronic renal failure (CRF) is noted to be proportional to the rate of the renal parenchyma sclerosis, a fundamental component of the CRF pathogenesis [6]. Transforming growth factor-β (TGF-β) plays the most prominent role in this process. The signaling pathways of this growth factor (Smad, p38, Erk1/2, PI3K, JNK, etc.) can cause glomerulosclerosis and tubulointerstitial fibrosis via multiple pathological processes [12]. An increase in TGF-β activity stimulates the cell proliferation and accumulation of extracellular matrix (ECM) components, such as collagen types I, III, and IV, laminin, and cellular and plasma forms of fibronectin, which contributes to the development of glomerulosclerosis [12].

Hemodynamic effects of glomerular hypertrophy caused by the loss of the renal mass are closely related to the mechanisms of persisting kidney inflammation and fibrosis via interaction of angiotensin II, TGF-β, and other growth factors. In addition to hemodynamic effects, primarily a systemic vasoconstrictor action also transmitted to the glomerular capillaries. So angiotensin II has so-called inherent nonhemodynamic effects, including the ability to induce endothelial dysfunction, as well as to enhance local renal expression of TGF-β. A nonhemodynamic component of the angiotensin II effect plays the main role in aggravation of proteinuria, which is why the drugs that block its formation (ACE inhibitors) or interaction with type 1 receptors (angiotensin II receptor blockers) have prominent antiproteinuric properties [6].

Of interest is investigation of IL-17 concentrations in the serum, having strong proinflammatory properties and inducing severe autoimmune pathology, including nephritis [13, 14].

In recent years, glomerulotropic radiopharmaceuticals labeled with radioisotopes are widely used as marker substances allowing determining GFR [15]. The diagnostic value of renal purification from nephrotropic substances (^{99m}Tc-MAG$_3$, ^{123}I-hippuran, and ^{99m}Tc-DTPA) closely correlates with inulin clearance [16–18]. However, GFR studies using radioactive isotopes are used only if specialized radiological laboratories are available [19, 20]. In this regard, the Laboratory for Radioisotope Diagnosis of Russian N.N. Blokhin Cancer Research Center, a federal state-funded scientific institution, has developed the systemic examination of nephrourological status based on complex renoscintigraphy

(SENS-CRS) and has been using it in pediatric and adult clinical practice for more than 15 years [19, 21–23]. SENS-CRS is a high technology implemented in the development of an automated workplace (AWP) for a radionephrologist (Project Manager A.P. Alekhin) (Figure 1).

SENS-CRS is designed for a rapid assessment of the functional reserves of the urinary system and the risk of renal failure. The CRS method provides not only the monitoring of the concentration levels in the parenchyma, but also early detection of relative stagnation in the parenchyma, its edema, urine stasis in the departments of the pyelocaliceal system (PCS), and lower urinary tract, that is, at all functional structural levels. Biochemical parameters of the kidney function, such as serum creatinine and urea, reflect quite gross morphologic alterations in the renal parenchyma and become diagnostically significant when 50 to 70% of active nephron mass (ANM) have already become dysfunctional [19].

When planning this study, it was assumed that complex monitoring of the renal function based on biochemical and RN methods will allow diagnosis of the risk factors for RF at an early stage, differentiate the structural kidney damage from the functional one, determine their relationship with immunotherapy toxicity and efficacy in patients with mRCC, and timely prescribe concomitant therapy.

2. Materials and Methods

This study included 41 mRCC patients after nephrectomy within the period from 2015 to 2017. 18 patients were treated with interferon (IFN-α) and 23 patients were treated with nivolumab (as part of the BMS expanded access program). Of 18 patients treated with IFN-α, 16 patients (88.8%) received it as the first line therapy. The median age was 56 years. Before (within a week) and during the treatment (every 2 months), all patients underwent blood chemistry, urinalysis, and Rehberg test.

The serum levels of proteins studied were determined according to the standard procedure prior to the treatment (within a week) and 2 months after. The serum was obtained after blood centrifugation at 3000 rpm, 4°C for 10 min using RS-6 model centrifuge ("Technocom", Russia). 300–400 μL of serum were dispensed in 2 plastic tubes and stored at −80°C until the analysis. ELISA tests for IL-17 (eBioscience, USA), TGF-β1 (eBioscience, USA), and EPO (erythropoietin) (Biomerica, USA) were performed using standard kits for direct immunoassay according to manufacturer's instructions.

Complex renoscintigraphy (CRS) was carried out on a dual-detector gamma camera (E-com, Siemens) with simultaneous recording in 2 projections, which allowed studying the entire renal clearance system, starting with the heart blood flow and ending with the bladder. Diagnostic simulation of renal clearance from nephrotropic substances begins with intravenous administration of ^{99m}Tc-technephore. ^{99m}Tc-technephore, a Russian product from the group of bisphosphonates, has hemodynamics of a glomerulotropic product, concentrating mainly in the nephrons via filtration, with partial involvement of secretion. The

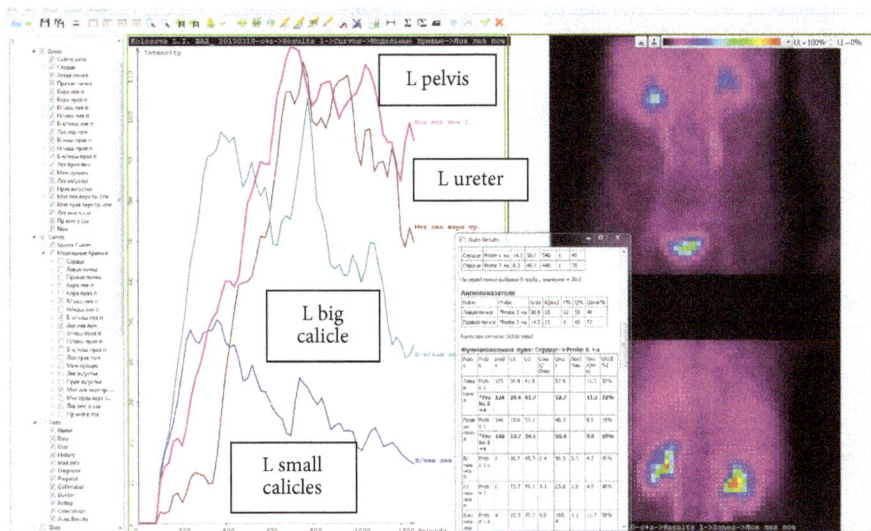

FIGURE 1: An automated workstation implementing the SENS-CRS technology on a personal computer by processing CRS DICOM (Digital Imaging and Communications in Medicine) files generated by a modern dual-detector gamma camera. In the upper band a set of tool icons is used in the workstation in the analysis of data of functional radionuclide studies of the kidneys. In the left part there is a set of zones of interest (an interphase in Russian language), selected on scintigraphic images of the kidneys and urinary tract according to the SENS-CRS technology. The curves obtained from the automated workstation represent the dynamics of the concentration of urine labeled with a nephrotropic radiopharmaceutical agent (99mTc-MAG3) in the structures of the left (L) kidney: the group of small upper calices, the big upper calices, the pelvis, and the ureter (delay of labeled urine in the middle third). Scintigrams on the right: top, image of the urinary system in the front projection; bottom, in the back projection. At the top there is a color scale (the red color corresponds to the maximum score on scintigrams). In a separate window (in the center): results of a quantitative estimation on original algorithms of function parameters of urinary system are shown.

visualization quality (even with a weak kidney function) of ^{99m}Tc-technephore is comparable to that of tubulotropic ^{99m}Tc-MAG$_3$ (mercaptoacetyltriglycine) and ^{123}I-hippuran, significantly outperforming conventional glomerulotropic ^{99m}Tc-DTPA (diethylenetriaminepentaacetic acid) [21]. The data registered in 2 projections is processed based on 2-phase registration: the first step is a 21-minute (1 min, angiophase) basic test with administration of the labeled substance; the second phase is delayed (after a 25-minute break) 21-minute examination (sometimes a 7-minute test) without administration of RP, but with administration of small amounts of water (200–300 ml) and/or an antispasmodic (less frequently diuretic). The bladder emptying by the patient before the baseline test and examination is a mandatory functional test. Complex renoscintigraphy allowed achieving the lowest radiation doses for patients and staff. When CRS is performed, adults are administered intravenously 74 MBq of ^{99m}Tc-technephore (an effective equivalent dose of 0.6 mSv), less frequently ^{99m}Tc-technephore; children are given a radiopharmaceutical based on their age and body weight. When kidneys and bones are investigated on the same day, adults are given 370 to 555 MBq of ^{99m}Tc-technephore (an effective equivalent dose of 3.0–4.5 mSv). The interpretation of CRS data used a concentration-rate model of urinary excretion and the original SENS CRS technology developed in the laboratory of radioisotope diagnostics, Russian N.N. Blokhin Cancer Research Center. The level of concentration of both glomerulo- and tubulotropic radiopharmaceuticals in the

parenchyma is proved to be a well reproducible measure of the kidney concentration function [21, 24]. The statistical analysis of the results was performed using software Statistica 13.0 with the Spearman nonparametric method (R_{Sp} is a correlation coefficient; the result was considered insignificant at $p \geq 0.05$).

3. Study Results and Discussion

This study included 41 mRCC patients after nephrectomy within the period from 2015 to 2017; 18 patients were treated with IFN-α and 23 patients were treated with nivolumab. Of 18 patients treated with IFN-α, 16 patients (88.8%) received it as the first line therapy. Twelve (12) patients (52%) and 11 patients (48%) in the nivolumab group received nivolumab as their second line and third or further line therapy. Thus, given the large number of previous lines of therapy, the nivolumab group had a higher risk of developing tubulointerstitial nephritis (TIN). Thus, the incidence of stage-3 CKD at the time of treatment was 35% in the nivolumab group and 17% in the IFN-α group.

Inflammation of the renal tubulointerstitium is always clinically characterized by impairment of the renal concentration function and often renal filtration function. Renal glomeruli can be abnormal, but abnormalities have a secondary nature [7]. As a result, the amount of the radiopharmaceutical concentrates reduced during a radionuclide study, which determines the fundamental premise of the

TABLE 1: Relationship between CKD and FSS gradation: a radionuclide estimate for the total renal function.

CKD stage	Renal function characteristic	GFR level (mL/min/1.73 m^2)	FSS characteristic	FSS index gradation
1	High and optimal	>90	*Status 1* high level slightly decreased (stable or conditionally stable compensation)	1a
2	Slightly decreased	60–89		1b
3a	Slightly decreased	45–59	*Status 2* moderately decreased (conditionally stable compensation, transitionally unsustainable level of compensation)	2a
3b	Significantly decreased	30–44		2b
4	Severely decreased	15–29	*Status 3* moderately to severely decreased (unstable compensation or decompensation)	3a 3b
5	End-stage renal failure	<15	Decompensation	4

complex renography (CR), the "concentration function" as a total result of all processes in the renal parenchyma [25]. In SENS-CRS, an algorithm was developed that determines the level of compensation and the risk of destabilization of the total renal function in gradations of FSS (Functional Systems Scores), the total prognostic index of the urinary system functional state, and stability. The relationship between different degrees of clinical parameter gradations—CKD according to KDOQI (Kidney Disease Outcomes Quality Initiative) and KDIGO—and RN parameter—total prognostic index (FSS) according to CRS findings with nephrotropic radiopharmaceuticals (^{99m}Tc-technephore, ^{99m}Tc-DTPA, ^{99m}Tc-technemag, ^{99m}Tc-MAG3)—are presented in Table 1.

The grades of the FSS index are the same for the above radiopharmaceuticals (the differences between these drugs are taken into account within the SENS-CRS algorithm). A single concentration-rate approach to the study of kidney function and urodynamics of the urinary tract with different nephrotropic radiopharmaceuticals is described in detail in the publication [21, 26].

The rate of irreversible deterioration of the kidney function in most variants of TIN is much slower than that in other chronic progressive nephropathies. In our study, only 1 patient (2.4%) developed acute renal failure (ARF) after 2 injections of nivolumab. It should be noted that this was the only patient who initially had the lowest RN estimate for the total urinary system function, FSS = 3b (significantly reduced). The cause elimination is crucial in the management of patients with TIN. In this particular case, the patient probably developed tubular necrosis as early as during previous therapy with everolimus (for 2 years); however, at the time of the initiation of nivolumab treatment, GFR, calculated by the MDRD formula, was 41 ml/min. Due to the development of acute renal failure, nivolumab treatment was discontinued. The patient was switched to dialysis.

The presence of confounding factors that can increase the severity of renal disease should be taken into account: chronic heart failure; type 2 diabetes; impaired uric acid metabolism. Elderly patients can have a combination of several forms of renal disease ("multimorbidity"), such as analgesic, urate, and diabetic nephropathy, as well as ischemic renal disease (IRD)

TABLE 2: The relationship between biochemical and radionuclide parameters in the monitoring of the urinary system function.

$N = 97$	Plasma creatinine level (112.3 ± 24.4 mcmol/L)	Plasma urea level (7.3±2.4 mmol/L)
RK, compensation level	$R_{Sp} = +0.3$, $p < 0.01$	Trend → $R_{Sp} = +0.2$ ($p > 0.05$)
FSS, a total prognostic index for the urinary system	$R_{Sp} = +0.3$, $p < 0.005$	$p > 0.05$
G_{ren}, a measured level of ^{99m}Tc-technephore in the renal parenchyma	$R_{Sp} = -0.3$, $p < 0.001$	$R_{Sp} = -0.3$, $p < 0.01$
A [s], an arterial index of renal parenchyma	$p > 0.05$	$p > 0.05$
IF_{ost}, a speed index of the ureteral orifice (during examination)	$R_{Sp} = -0.3$, $p < 0.01$	$p > 0.05$

and chronic pyelonephritis [6]. In our study, hypertension was observed in 15 patients (36.5%), type 2 diabetes in 4 patients (9.7%), urinary infection in 4 patients (9.7%), urolithiasis in 2 patients (4.8%), and obesity in 2 patients (4.8%).

3.1. Analysis of Biochemical and Radionuclide Parameters during Immunotherapy.

The analysis of blood chemistry parameters (creatinine, urea), daily Rehberg test, total protein in the urine, and total and partial RN parameters established their relationship, which confirmed the diagnostic value of both methods—biochemical and CRS (Table 2). We analyzed 97 clinical cases (during the monitoring) constituting the group of patients after nephrectomy during therapy with IFN-α and nivolumab.

There was also a statistically significant relationship between the total GFR based on the 24-hour Rehberg test and RN parameters, D, % (RP excretion rate from the parenchyma at the "cortex-medulla" level) and GB_{20} (a 20-minute level of

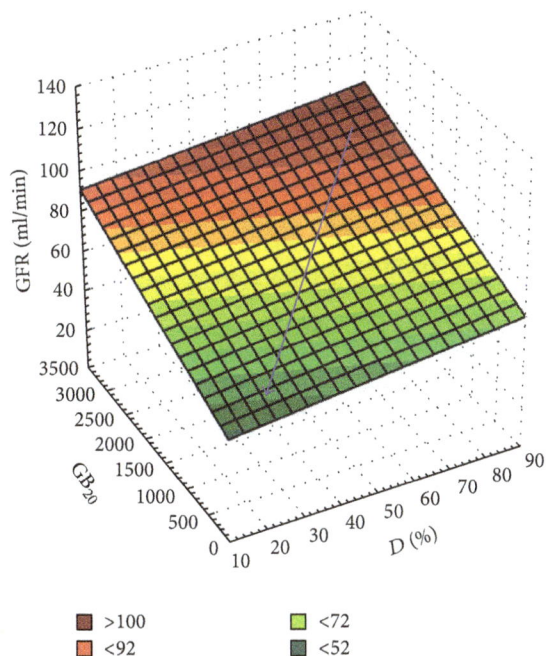

■ >100   □ <72
■ <92   ■ <52

FIGURE 2: A linearly smoothed 3D-surface showing the relationship between GFR in the Rehberg test and RN parameters, D and GB_{20}. The blue arrow shows the development of CTIN (chronic tubulointerstitial nephritis) and an increase in the risk of RF, followed by a decrease in the urine excretion rate in the renal parenchyma (D), the level of concentration of labeled urine that entered in the bladder within 20 minutes of the basic CSR test (GB_{20}), and GFR estimated by the Rehberg method (R_{Sp} = +0.4, $p < 0.01$).

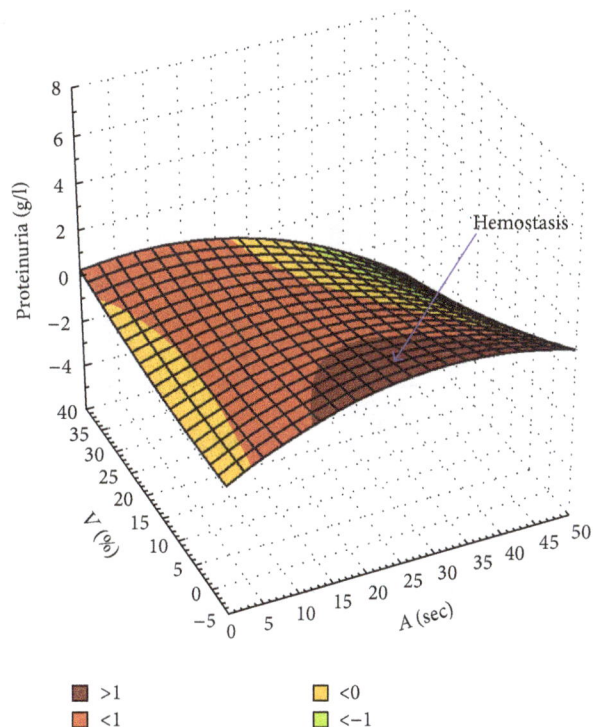

■ >1   □ <0
■ <1   □ <−1

FIGURE 3: The 3D surface (spline-smoothing) showing a relationship between proteinuria and hemodynamic parameters of kidney parenchyma, A [s] and V [%]. The blue arrow points to an area corresponding to pronounced hemostasis (parameters A-V) observed with an increase in proteinuria with the development of CTIN and a possible urinary tract infection (UTI).

RP concentration in the urinary bladder in the basic CRS test) (Figure 2).

An increase in proteinuria up to the nephrotic level is determined primarily by the loss of the selectivity of the glomerular basement membrane and progressive podocyte dysfunction. This disorder is also accompanied by inappropriate activation of the renin-angiotensin-aldosterone system, typical of many variants of nephrotic syndrome and resulting in sodium retention and osmotically bound water aggravating the edema in addition to the developed resistance of respective nephron segments to natriuretic peptides [7]. Hypercoagulability typical for nephrotic syndrome is determined primarily by the activation of serum and endothelial hemostasis, which results in an increased risk of venous thrombosis and thromboembolism. This phenomenon is reflected during CRS, demonstrating the relationship between proteinuria and hemodynamic parameters of the renal parenchyma, A [s] (a perfusion rate of renal blood labeled with RP, an arterial index of renal parenchyma) and V [%] (a clearance rate of RP-labeled blood via the renal venous system, a venous index of renal parenchyma) (Figure 3).

With regard to the search of diagnostic markers of early stages of renal dysfunction, we analyzed transforming growth factor-β (TGF-β) as a factor of renal parenchyma sclerosis and IL-17 having strong proinflammatory properties and inducing severe autoimmune pathology, including nephritis,

in the serum of 40 patients with mRCC prior to immunotherapy (IFN and nivolumab) and 2 months after. Against the backdrop of immunotherapy with the inclusion of INF-α and nivolumab, there was a significant increase in IL-17A from 0 ± 4.29 (median ± SD) to 0.166 ± 1.714 pg/ml ($p <$ 0.0005) and a trend toward TGF-β growth from 11.3 ± 12.4 to 13 ± 10.1 ng/ml ($p = 0.1$) (Figure 4). The study was able to compare TGF-β and IL-17 values with RN parameters, Rnfss, a stable sign of nephrosclerosis (presumably sclerosis of interlobar renal arteries), and D, an excretion rate of ^{99m}Tc-technephore from the parenchyma (at the "cortex-medulla" level), respectively (Table 3).

Thus, an increase in TGF-β concentrations correlates with Rnfsc during CRS, which confirms the diagnostic value of Rnfsc as a visual radionuclide sign of "nephrosclerosis", whose assessment was carried out according to the grading specified in Table 4. Moreover, in the nivolumab group, nephrosclerosis was much more pronounced than in the IFN-α group, which may be due to a larger number of previous lines of targeted therapy.

At the same time, an increased IL-17 level both prior to immunotherapy and 2 months after corresponded to a decrease in the RP excretion rate from the parenchyma (D) due to increasing interstitial edema, confirming the importance of cytokine IL-17 in the pathogenesis of autoimmune nephritis.

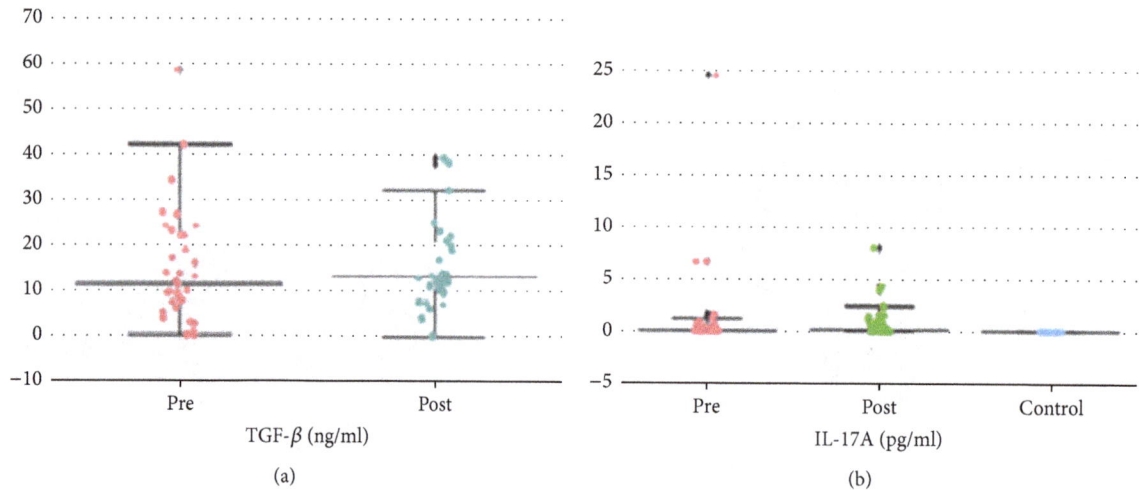

FIGURE 4: (a) TGF-β content in the serum of 40 mRCC patients before the initiation of immunotherapy with the inclusion of INF-α and nivolumab and after 2 months. (b) IL-17A content in the serum of 40 mRCC patients before the initiation of immunotherapy with the inclusion of INF-α and nivolumab and after 2 months (in comparison with the parameters of the control group, $n = 10$).

TABLE 3: Relationship between ELISA findings and RN parameters.

$N = 40$ (before the treatment initiation)	TGF-β		IL-17	
	Before therapy	In 2 months	Before therapy	In 2 months
D, %, an excretion rate of ^{99m}Tc-technephore from the parenchyma (at the "cortex-medulla" level)	Trend → $R_{Sp} = -0.3$ ($p = 0.08$)	Trend → $R_{Sp} = -0.3$ ($p = 0.06$)	$R_{Sp} = -0.3$, $p < 0.05$	$R_{Sp} = -0.5$, $p < 0.005$
Rnfsc, a visual sign of nephrosclerosis (sclerosis of interlobar renal arteries)	$R_{Sp} = +0.5$, $p < 0.005$	$p > 0.05$	$p > 0.05$	$R_{Sp} = -0.3$, $p < 0.05$ (polyuria?)

It should be noted that these biochemical and RN markers not only allow establishing impairment of the renal function at an early stage, but also differentiating the cause of this disease, nephrosclerosis or an autoimmune condition, which is extremely important in determining the treatment strategy for CKD.

Also, in the IFN-α group, endogenous erythropoietin levels were evaluated by ELISA in 15 mRCC patients after nephrectomy prior to the treatment. The findings had a significant correlation with creatinine levels before the treatment ($R_{Sp} = -0.6$, $p < 0.05$). Thus, reduced erythropoietin levels correlated with increased creatinine concentrations, which is consistent with the pathophysiological basis of the renal function (Figure 5).

In the SENS-CRS technology, radionuclide (CRS with 99mTc-technefor or 99mTc-MAG3, rarely with 99mTc-DTPA) images of the kidneys in the gray scale are obtained using a 64 × 64 matrix, chosen to minimize the dose of the radiopharmaceutical administered and the patient's radiation load.

3.2. The Prognostic Value of Laboratory Diagnostic and Biochemical Parameters. At the first stage, we evaluated the effect of RN and biochemical parameters on the RF risk estimated based on an increase in creatinine and urea levels during

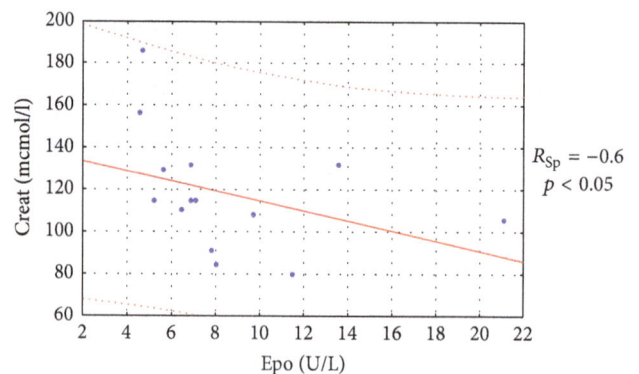

FIGURE 5: Correlation between erythropoietin (Epo) and creatinine (Creat) in the serum of mRCC patients prior to the treatment with IFN-α ($n = 15$).

immunotherapy with IFN-α and nivolumab. The data of the nonparametric correlation analysis for parameters potentially significant for the prognosis of RN risks are presented in Table 5.

Statistically significant correlations are established between an increase in creatinine levels and IL-17, FSS, G_{eff}, and Rnfss (Figure 6) and an increase in urea and protein levels in the urine, IL-17, D, T_{ev}, and T_{pelv} (Figure 7). Thus,

TABLE 4: The rating scale of an RN visual sign of "nephrosclerosis" in points.

Rnfsc, a visual sign of nephrosclerosis	Points	Typical scintigrams	
		Left kidney Basic test (left), examination (right)	*Right kidney* Basic test (left), examination (right)
None (?)	0		
Contradictory picture of initial changes	0.5		
Unsure sign of "nephrosclerosis"	1		
Picture of irreversible "nephrosclerosis"	2		

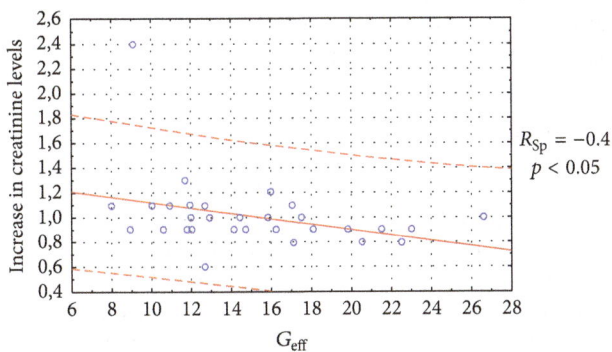

$R_{Sp} = -0.4$
$p < 0.05$

FIGURE 6: Correlation between a 1.2-fold increase in creatinine levels (± 0.4) during immunotherapy and G_{eff} prior to the treatment initiation.

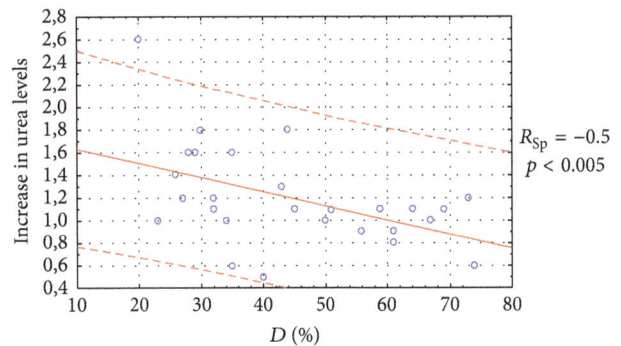

$R_{Sp} = -0.5$
$p < 0.005$

FIGURE 7: Correlation between a 1.6-fold increase in urea levels (± 0.6) during immunotherapy and D, % prior to the treatment initiation.

the initial IL-17 value in the serum can be an early predictor for RF development in CKD during immunotherapy, whereas serum creatinine and urea levels gave no statistically significant results in terms of the RF prognosis.

TABLE 5: An effect of biochemical and radionuclide parameters on the prognosis for RF risk during immunotherapy.

Before initiation of immunotherapy	A 1.2-fold increase in plasma creatinine level (± 0.4)	A 1.6-fold increase in plasma urea level (± 0.6)
Parameters of laboratory blood and urine tests (n = 40)		
Plasma creatinine level	$p > 0.05$	$p > 0.05$
Plasma urea level	$p > 0.05$	$p > 0.05$
Protein in urine	Trend → $R_{Sp} = +0.3$ ($p = 0.06$)	$R_{Sp} = +0.5$, $p < 0.05$
Plasma TGF-β_1	Trend → $R_{Sp} = +0.3$ ($p = 0.08$)	Trend → $R_{Sp} = +0.3$ ($p = 0.08$)
Plasma IL-17	$R_{Sp} = +0.4$, $p < 0.05$	$R_{Sp} = +0.4$, $p < 0.05$
Parameters of complex renoscintigraphy with ^{99m}Tc-technephore (n = 31)		
FSS, a total prognostic index for the urinary system	$R_{Sp} = +0.4$, $p < 0.05$	$p > 0.05$
G_{eff}, an effective index of the renal concentration function	$R_{Sp} = -0.4$, $p < 0.05$	$p > 0.05$
D, %, an excretion rate of ^{99m}Tc-technephore from parenchyma	$p > 0.05$	$R_{Sp} = -0.5$, $p < 0.005$
T_{ev} [min], the time of start of excretion of the labeled urine from the pyelocaliceal system	$R_{Sp} = +0.4$, $p < 0.05$	$R_{Sp} = +0.5$, $p < 0.01$
T_{ev} [min], the time of start of excretion of the labeled urine from the renal pelvis	Trend → $R_{Sp} = +0.3$ ($p = 0.06$)	$R_{Sp} = +0.5$, $p < 0.005$
Rnfsc, a visual sign of nephrosclerosis	$R_{Sp} = +0.4$, $p < 0.05$	$p > 0.05$

TABLE 6: An effect of biochemical and RN parameters on the immunotherapy effectiveness.

Before initiation of immunotherapy (n = 40)	Treatment effect
Parameters of laboratory blood and urine tests	
Plasma creatinine level	
Plasma urea level	
Protein in urine	$p > 0.05$
TGF-β_1	
IL-17	
Parameters of complex renoscintigraphy with ^{99m}Tc-technephore	
FSS, total prognostic index of the urinary system	$R_{Sp} = -0.4$, $p < 0.05$
G_{eff}, an effective index of the renal concentration function	$R_{Sp} = +0.3$, $p < 0.05$
T_{ev} [min], the time of start of excretion of the labeled urine from the pyelocaliceal system	$R_{Sp} = -0.4$, $p < 0.05$
T_{ev} [min], the time of start of excretion of the labeled urine from the renal pelvis	$R_{Sp} = -0.3$, $p < 0.05$

Also, a correlation was observed between the RN sign of nephrosclerosis (Rnfss) and an increase in creatinine levels. Thus, despite the lack of a statistically significant correlation between serum TGF-β_1 and an increase in creatinine levels, but given the correlation between TGF-β_1 and Rnfss ($p < 0.005$), TGF-β_1 can be considered as a relative risk factor for RF development during immunotherapy in patients with mRCC who underwent nephrectomy.

At the next stage, we evaluated the effect of RN and biochemical parameters on the effectiveness of immunotherapy estimated according to the RECIST criteria (Table 6).

As it turned out, the CRS findings have prognostic significance in relation to not only the RF risk, but also the efficacy of immunotherapy in patients with mRCC after nephrectomy. It should be noted that most of correlations were obtained due to statistically significant relationships in the IFN-α group. Thus, patients with mRCC with better kidney function parameters have a better prognosis regarding the efficacy of immunotherapy.

4. Conclusion

Thus, immunotherapy has no pronounced nephrotoxicity. All mRCC patients after nephrectomy were recommended, prior to the treatment initiation, to undergo biochemical monitoring with inclusion of TGF-β_1 and IL-17, as well as radionuclide monitoring (SENS-CRS) to determine the RF risk at an early stage and to establish prognosis for the underlying disease and timely adjust the treatment in order to improve their response to immunotherapy.

References

[1] G. Khan, A. Golshayan, P. Elson et al., "Sunitinib and sorafenib in metastatic renal cel," *Annals of Oncology*, vol. 21, pp. 1618–1622, 2010.

[2] D. Takahashi, K. Nagahama, Y. Tsuura, H. Tanaka, and T. Tamura, "Sunitinib-induced nephrotic syndrome and irreversible renal dysfunction," *Clinical and Experimental Nephrology*, vol. 16, no. 2, pp. 310–315, 2012.

[3] P. Selby, J. Kofin, J. Raymond, I. Judson, and T. M. Wain, "Nephrotic syndrome during treatment with interferon," *British Medical Journal*, vol. 290, no. 6476, p. 1180, 1985.

[4] H. Ha, H. Park, R. Jang et al., "Increased risk of everolimus-associated acute kidney injury in cancer patients with impaired kidney function," *BMC Cancer*, vol. 14, no. 1, article 906, 2014.

[5] A. S. Levey, R. Atkins, J. Coresh et al., "Chronic kidney disease as a global public health problem: approaches and initiatives—a position statement from Kidney Disease Improving Global Outcomes," *Kidney International*, vol. 72, no. 3, pp. 247–259, 2007.

[6] E. M. Shilov, *The Textbook of Nephrology*, GEOTAR-Media Publishing, 2010 (Russian).

[7] National Kidney Foundation, "K/DOQI clinical practice guidelines for chronic kidney disease: evaluation, classification, and stratification," *American Journal of Kidney Diseases*, vol. 39, no. 2, supplement 1, pp. S1–S266, 2002.

[8] R. Bellomo, C. Ronco, J. A. Kellum, R. L. Mehta, and P. Palevsky, "Acute renal failure—definition, outcome measures, animal models, fluid therapy and information technology needs: the Second International Consensus Conference of the Acute Dialysis Quality Initiative (ADQI) Group," *Critical Care*, vol. 8, no. 4, pp. R204–R212, 2004.

[9] R. L. Mehta, J. A. Kellum, S. V. Shah et al., "Acute Kidney Injury Network: report of an initiative to improve outcomes in acute kidney injury," *Critical Care*, vol. 11, no. 2, article R31, 2007.

[10] N. V. Lyubimova, Z. K. Kumykova, and N. E. Kushlinsky, "Biochemical indices in the diagnosis of nephrotoxicity of antitumor chemotherapy in children," *Questions of Oncology*, vol. 4, pp. 448–453, 1997 (Russian).

[11] F. Dieterle, F. Sistare, F. Goodsaid et al., "Renal biomarker qualification submission: a dialog between the FDA-EMEA and Predictive Safety Testing Consortium," *Nature Biotechnology*, vol. 28, no. 5, pp. 455–462, 2010.

[12] I. Loeffler and G. Wolf, "Transforming growth factor-β and the progression of renal disease," *Nephrology Dialysis Transplantation*, vol. 29, supplement 1, pp. i37–i45, 2014.

[13] K. Peliçari, M. Postal, N. Sinicato et al., "Serum interleukin-17 levels are associated with nephritis in childhood-onset systemic lupus erythematosus," *Clinics*, vol. 70, no. 5, pp. 313–317, 2015.

[14] J. C. Waite and D. Skokos, "Th17 response and inflammatory autoimmune diseases," *International Journal of Inflammation*, vol. 2012, Article ID 819467, 10 pages, 2012.

[15] E. Durand and A. Prigent, "The basics of renal imaging and functional studies," *The Quarterly Journal of Nuclear Medicine*, vol. 46, pp. 249–267, 2002.

[16] F. P. Esteves, R. K. Halkar, M. M. Issa, S. Grant, and A. Taylor, "Comparison of camera-based 99mTc-MAG3 and 24-hour creatinine clearances for evaluation of kidney function," *American Journal of Roentgenology*, vol. 187, no. 3, pp. W316–W319, 2006.

[17] A. Prigent, "Monitoring renal function and limitations of renal function tests," *Seminars in Nuclear Medicine*, vol. 38, no. 1, pp. 32–46, 2008.

[18] G. F. Gates, "Filtration fraction and its implications for radionuclide renography using diethylenetriaminepentaacetic acid and mercaptoacetyltriglycine," *Clinical Nuclear Medicine*, vol. 29, no. 4, pp. 231–237, 2004.

[19] M. I. Davydov and B. I. Dolgushin, *Radionuclide Studies of Kidney Function and Urodynamics in Oncology*, Practical Medicine, Moscow, Russia, 2007 (Russian).

[20] W. He and A. J. Fischman, "Nuclear imaging in the genitourinary tract: recent advances and future directions," *Radiologic Clinics of North America*, vol. 46, no. 1, pp. 25–43, 2008.

[21] A. V. Kashkadayeva, S. G. Averinova, A. P. Alekhin et al., "The method of diagnosis of the risk factors for renal failure based on "concentration-rate" approach to the analysis of the complex renoscintigraphy data," *Russian Electronic Journal of Radiology*, vol. 3, pp. 47–62, 2013.

[22] A. V. Kashkadayev, S. G. Averinova, G. D. Dmitrieva et al., "Method of radionuclide diagnosis of urinary system function," The Patent of the Russian Federation No. 2001113119 (priority of May 2001).

[23] A. V. Kashkadayeva, A. P. Alekhin, S. G. Averinova, G. D. Dmitrieva, and T. V. Zakharova, "Iterative optimization procedure for visually-quantitative analysis of functional delays in the renal purification system based on complex renoscintigraphy on a 2-detector gamma camera," *Collection of Scientific Works of MEPhI Camera*, vol. 1, pp. 7-8, 2013 (Russian).

[24] M. Rutland, L. Que, and I. M. Hassan, "'FUR'—one size suits all," *European Journal of Nuclear Medicine and Molecular Imaging*, vol. 27, no. 11, pp. 1708–1713, 2000.

[25] A. C. Guiton and J. E. Hall, *The Textbook of Medical Physiology*, Elsevier, New York, NY, USA, 2006.

[26] S. G. Averinova, A. V. Kashkadaeva, S. V. Shiryaev, A. M. Nechipai, and G. D. Dmitrieva, "Nephrourological monitoring technology based on functional radionuclide tests: Functions of an automated workplace," *Biomedical Engineering Online*, vol. 33, no. 3, pp. 115–127, 1999.

29

Dialysis Provision and Implications of Health Economics on Peritoneal Dialysis Utilization: A Review from a Malaysian Perspective

Mohd Rizal Abdul Manaf,[1] Naren Kumar Surendra,[1] Abdul Halim Abdul Gafor,[2] Lai Seong Hooi,[3] and Sunita Bavanandan[4]

[1]*Department of Community Health, Faculty of Medicine, Pusat Perubatan Universiti Kebangsaan Malaysia, Jalan Yaacob Latif, Bandar Tun Razak, 56000 Cheras, Kuala Lumpur, Malaysia*
[2]*Nephrology Unit, Faculty of Medicine, Pusat Perubatan Universiti Kebangsaan Malaysia, Jalan Yaacob Latif, Bandar Tun Razak, 56000 Cheras, Kuala Lumpur, Malaysia*
[3]*Hospital Sultanah Aminah, Jalan Persiaran Abu Bakar Sultan, 80100 Johor Bahru, Johor, Malaysia*
[4]*Hospital Kuala Lumpur, Jalan Pahang, 50586 Kuala Lumpur, Malaysia*

Correspondence should be addressed to Naren Kumar Surendra; naren.cruise@gmail.com

Academic Editor: Franca Anglani

End-stage renal disease (ESRD) is managed by either lifesaving hemodialysis (HD) and peritoneal dialysis (PD) or a kidney transplant. In Malaysia, the prevalence of dialysis-treated ESRD patients has shown an exponential growth from 504 per million population (pmp) in 2005 to 1155 pmp in 2014. There were 1046 pmp patients on HD and 109 pmp patients on PD in 2014. Kidney transplants are limited due to lack of donors. Malaysia adopts public-private financing model for dialysis. Majority of HD patients were treated in the private sector but almost all PD patients were treated in government facilities. Inequality in access to dialysis is visible within geographical regions where majority of HD centres are scattered around developed areas. The expenditure on dialysis has been escalating in recent years but economic evaluations of dialysis modalities are scarce. Evidence shows that health policies and reimbursement strategies influence dialysis provision. Increased uptake of PD can produce significant economic benefits and improve patients' access to dialysis. As a result, some countries implemented a PD-First or Favored Policy to expand PD use. Thus, a current comparative costs analysis of dialysis is strongly recommended to assist decision-makers to establish a more equitable and economically sustainable dialysis provision in the future.

1. Introduction

Malaysia is a federation of 13 states and 2 territories in a parliamentary democracy, with the Prime Minister the head of government and a constitutional monarch elected by the Conference of Rulers. Malaysians make up 0.4% of the world's total population at 31 million with gross domestic product (GDP) at US$272 billion in 2015 [1]. Life expectancy for newborn baby boy and girl was 72.6 years and 77.2 years, respectively [2]. Malaysia has a dual-tiered system of healthcare services consisting of a government-led public sector and a coexisting private sector creating a dichotomous yet synergistic public-private model [3]. The total health expenditure in 2013 was 4.53% of GDP (US$ 14, 205.7 million) [4].

Both developing and developed nations may have an ageing population with modifiable lifestyle risk factors causing chronic diseases particularly chronic kidney disease (CKD) [5]. CKD is characterized by progressive, irreversible kidney function deterioration culminating in end-stage renal disease (ESRD), which requires treatment by renal replacement therapy (RRT), either hemodialysis (HD) or peritoneal dialysis (PD) when kidney transplantation is limited or contraindicated. HD is usually performed at hospital or separate dialysis unit three times per week or sometimes at home. PD is administered at home and several PD modalities are available. The most common is continuous ambulatory PD (CAPD). Total ESRD patients were 3,200,000 but only 2,519,000 were being treated in 2013 with approximately 7% annual growth rate [6].

CKD is a global health threat with socioeconomic and public health consequences. Estimates on the Global Burden of Disease (GBD) indicated that kidney diseases were responsible for 2,993,000 years of life lost (YLL) and 38,104,000 disability adjusted life years (DALYs) lost globally [7]. In Malaysia, kidney disease ranked 8th from ten causes of death with 365.7 (YLL) per 100,000 population which accounted for 2.3% of total premature deaths [8]. Persons with CKD and ESRD have poor health related quality of life as compared to the general population [9–11]. Kidney transplantation is the best RRT option. However, the new kidney transplants' rate in Malaysia is very low at 3 per million population (pmp) due to organ shortage [12].

In addition, the healthcare costs and economic burden of CKD are huge [13]. The expenditure for the management of patients with ESRD in developed countries accounted for 2-3% of total healthcare expenditure, while ESRD patients represent only 0.02–0.03% of the total population [14]. PD is known as the most cost-effective dialysis modality in most developed countries and some developing countries [15, 16]. However, PD is underutilized around the world [17]. This article aims to review the dialysis provision, issues, and implications of health economics on PD utilization from a Malaysian perspective.

2. Methodology

A review of dialysis provision, issues, and implications of health economics on PD utilization was conducted from a Malaysian perspective. The 22nd Malaysian Dialysis and Transplant Registry report and other published articles through limited literature search on key resources including PubMed, Medline, and a focused Internet search were used in this review.

3. Results

3.1. Dialysis Provision in Malaysia. Malaysian Dialysis and Transplant Registry (MDTR) collects information on patients with ESRD on RRT in Malaysia. Hence, most of the data on dialysis provision are from the registry's annual report. The latest report published is the 22nd MDTR 2014 report [12]. The acceptance rate of dialysis patients had increased since 2004 with 203 pmp new HD cases and 31 pmp new PD cases in 2014. A total of 31,497 HD patients and 3,270 PD patients were dialyzing in 2014 giving a prevalence rate of 1046 pmp and 109 pmp, respectively. The dialysis treatment rate exceeded 100 pmp for all states in Malaysia except Sabah with the lowest rates in Kelantan and Sabah. In terms of gender, the treatment gap between men and women accepted for dialysis had remained constant over the years with male 55% and female 45%. Meanwhile, 58% of new dialysis patients were 55 years or older at the onset of dialysis and 61% of new

patients had diabetes mellitus as the primary renal disease [12].

An influx of dialysis patients had resulted in an increase of dialysis centres especially in the private sector [18]. The number of dialysis centres for the whole of Malaysia increased from 205 in 2000 to 758 in 2014, mainly contributed by private dialysis centres which had almost tripled from 6 pmp in 2005 to 14 pmp in 2014. Nongovernmental organization (NGO) centres had only increased from 4 pmp in 2005 to 5 pmp in 2014. Meanwhile, the rate was stagnant in the public sector, 5 pmp in 2005 and 2014 [12]. Private dialysis centres are mainly distributed in economically developed west coast states of Peninsular Malaysia. The government operates most of the dialysis centres in less developed states. Majority of HD patients were in the private sector (54%) but almost all PD patients were treated in government facilities (97%) [12].

3.2. Survival of Dialysis Patients in Malaysia. There were 4,015 dialysis deaths reported in 2014. Modality specific death rate over the last 10 years ranged from 12 to 13% for HD and 16 to 18% for PD. The annual death rate among HD patients remained relatively unchanged while the annual death rate of PD patients began to increase in mid-2000s and appeared to have improved over the last 3 years [12].

The apparent survival difference between PD and HD patients in Malaysia began to widen after the first year. The overall unadjusted 5-year and 10-year patient survival for all dialysis was 54% and 30%, respectively. At 10 years the unadjusted patient survival on HD was 31% compared with 27% for those on PD. There were various factors associated with better patient survival including younger age and absence of diabetes. It is important to highlight that the persistent difference in annual death rate between the two modalities was partly associated with negative selection of patients for PD. After adjustments patients on PD have a 4.8% lower mortality risk compared to those on HD [12].

3.3. Dialysis Funding in Malaysia. Malaysia has a mixed healthcare financing system. Public healthcare services are funded through general taxation, with annual health budgets allocated by Ministry of Finance (MOF) to the MOH. Within the private sector, individuals can purchase health insurance on voluntary basis, with variable premiums charged based on their health status and the level of coverage or covered by negotiated packages with Managed Care Organizations (MCOs) and private insurance companies [19]. Civil servants and their dependents would be reimbursed by the government. Social Security Organization (SOCSO), a government-run social insurance body that receives mandatory contributions from private-sector employees earning below US$950 per month and the state-run Islamic social welfare organizations reimburse eligible patients for certain treatments and dialysis, was included as a rehabilitation therapy [18].

The government is the main source of funding for dialysis therapy for new and existing patients from 2004 to 2014. Out of pocket payment or self-funding for dialysis was about 26 to 30% and funding from NGOs remained at 11–15% over the years [12].

3.4. Issues Related to Dialysis Provision in Malaysia. The increasing prevalence of ESRD patients in Malaysia is of concern. Some options that have been proposed to tackle this issue include early medical intervention to slow the progression of CKD in high-risk patients, promotion of kidney transplantation, and use of the most cost-effective dialysis therapy that can be offered to a patient without compromising outcome [10, 20–22]. In Malaysia, renal failure prevention initiatives are carried out nationwide including patient screening at primary care settings, prevention of renal failure workshops targeting primary care doctors and allied healthcare staff, development of clinical practice guidelines (CPG) on CKD management and nephrology services operational policy [23], and national public awareness for World Kidney Day. Despite all these efforts, the ESRD population is increasing at an alarming rate. As kidney transplants are limited due to lack of donors, the choice of RRT lies between HD and PD.

Analysis of the expenditure of dialysis provision in Malaysia has been limited to a few studies. Total spending on dialysis in 2005 was US\$ 100 million accounted for 1.72% of the total health expenditure [18]. A recent forecast data shows that the estimated cost incurred to treat 51,269 patients with dialysis in the year 2020 is US\$ 384.5 million [24]. This burden will have implications for healthcare financing in the future.

Although PD is associated with lower costs than HD, it is underutilized around the world including Malaysia. Only 9% of ESRD patients are on PD and 97% of them are treated in MOH [12]. An economic evaluation study of centre HD and CAPD among MOH hospitals in Malaysia published in 2005 found that CAPD was marginally more cost-effective than HD (US\$ 8325 versus US\$ 8853 life year saved) [25]. PD also offer a number of medical advantages over HD including better preservation of residual renal function and less requirement for Erythropoiesis Stimulating Agents (ESAs) [26, 27]. Many nephrologists believe that home dialysis including PD is better for the patients as opposed to their current practice [28, 29].

Although dialysis treatment rates reached a level comparable to rates in developed countries [18], there is an inequitable distribution. Economically developed west coast states of Peninsular Malaysia have higher rates compared to east coast states, Sabah and Sarawak. Federal territory of Kuala Lumpur has the hugest dialysis rate at 1741 pmp and Federal Territory of Labuan and state of Sabah has the lowest dialysis rate at 486 pmp [12]. Registries capture information on patients who are on RRT, not all those who develop ESRD. Recently published article show that there is a gap between incidence of ESRD and use of RRT which was estimated through the prevalence of diabetes and hypertension [30, 31]. In Malaysia, overall prevalence of hypertension and diabetes (known and undiagnosed) among adults of 18 years and above was 30.3% and 17.5%, respectively [32]. In a population-based study by Hooi et al., it was reported that the prevalence of CKD stage 5 in Malaysia was 0.36% in people above 18 years old [33]. However, only 0.17% of people above 18 years old were on RRT at the same year; that is, about half of the CKD stage 5 were on RRT. Although some patients might not be suitable for dialysis or do not need it yet (dialysis is started at

about GFR 5–7 ml/min, CKD stage 5 is GFR < 15 ml/min) or die before dialysis is started, a gap is observed between CKD stage 5 and RRT provision in Malaysia.

3.5. Factors Influencing Selection of Dialysis Modalities. Medical and nonmedical factors including social conditions, geographic considerations, economic/reimbursement, and patient choice dictate the selection of PD or HD, with patient choice being an important factor [34]. In Malaysia, the selection of patients for long-term hemodialysis in MOH is under the purview of a selection committee according to selection criteria including waiting time and priority group (failed graft following kidney transplant at MOH hospitals, children, change of modality) [23]. The criteria for selection of patients for long-term PD include patient choice with absence of contraindications to PD. There are factors to consider including vision, manual dexterity and availability of assistant, home environment, and lack of vascular access [23].

Although many factors affect the selection of one dialysis modality, absolute medical contraindications for the use of either modality are few [23, 35]. Differences in outcome between modalities or patient preference do not justify these variations [36]. Economic factors including financial and reimbursement strategy have been recognized as the main nonmedical factors in dialysis modality selection in countries around the world [34, 37, 38].

3.6. Implications of Health Economics on Peritoneal Dialysis Utilization. Economic evaluation is an analytical tool for decision making because it involves both cost and benefit which are being evaluated against each other [39]. A cost-effectiveness analysis includes life years gained, a cost utility analysis includes quality adjusted life years (QALY), and a cost benefit analysis includes monetary units as primary outcome, respectively [39]. Relevant perspectives to be considered include provider, payer, or society because in one situation items may be considered as costs but in other cases not [39]. For a proper evaluation, activity based costing (primary data) is the most appropriate cost approach to be carried out which could be resource intensive [40]. Costs are generally described in four categories: direct medical costs, direct nonmedical costs, indirect costs, and intangible costs [39]. Direct medical costs of dialysis include staff salaries, costs of dialyzers and extracorporeal circuits in HD, costs of solutions and disposables in PD, costs associated with radiology, laboratory, medications, capital costs of HD machines, and PD cyclers, costs of hospitalizations, and costs of outpatient consultations from other specialties. Direct nonmedical costs include building costs, facility utilities, and other overhead costs. Intangible costs are the costs associated with pain, suffering, and impairment in quality of life as well as the value of extending life. Intangible costs are often omitted from economic evaluations [39].

Some argue that economic evaluation such as cost-effectiveness or cost utility is only suitable to compare new against existing treatment. However, since economic factors influence dialysis provision, many countries conduct economic evaluation of HD and PD (both are established therapies). Economic evaluation studies are vital for health policy decisions. For example, in Thailand, the "PD-First" Policy has been promoted in 2008 as a model of initial treatment for ESRD patients under the Universal Coverage scheme [41] after the benefit of PD over HD has been shown in terms of medical expenses and cost-effectiveness [42]. Similarly, the government of Hong Kong developed the PD-First Policy based on its basis of cost-effectiveness [43]. Meanwhile, some other countries including Canada, China, Guatemala, India, Mexico, Spain, Taiwan, and the United States adopt a PD-Favored Policy. Cost-effectiveness plays a significant role on their policy decision [44]. Hong Kong has the highest proportion of PD in the world (72%) in 2013 [45]. HD remains an integral part of dialysis to cater for patients' preference, PD contraindicated patients, and transfer of PD to HD due to complications. In Malaysia, there is no clear PD-Favored Policy although PD is found to be marginally more cost-effective than HD. However, the acceptance and prevalence rate of PD treatment have increased twofold between 2004 and 2014 [12].

There are suggestions to revise the reimbursement structure in a way to provide incentives for home-based dialysis including PD and home HD to improve sustainability and patient outcome [34]. In the Canadian province of Ontario, the dialysis reimbursement system was changed from fee-for-service system with higher rates for in-centre HD to a modality-independent weekly capitation fee in 1998. PD use increased in Ontario while in the rest of Canada there were declines in PD use [46]. In Japan, reimbursement for dialysis was determined on a fee-for-service basis until 1999. Reimbursement for HD has been reduced based on recommendation by the Council on Economic and Fiscal Policy [47]. In Taiwan, there were four policies proposed by the Ministry of Health and Welfare relating to modality selection to increase the incidence of patients receiving PD as initial RRT [48]. In the US, the near 25-year-old fee-for-service payment method for dialysis was replaced by new prospective payment system (PPS). The new PPS places most costs for dialysis care, including injected medications within a bundle of services where the dialysis facility and the nephrologist both have financial incentives to promote PD [49]. There was an increased PD use in the 2-year period after the implementation of PPS [50].

The most frequently cited motivations for PD-First or PD-Favored Policies were to increase patient access to care, control costs through lower infrastructure and capital investments, empower patients, and optimize treatment provision [44]. This is particularly important in Malaysia as 97% of PD patients are being treated at public settings and there is geographical imbalance of dialysis access. PD is managed by salaried public-sector nurses and nephrologists and it is believed that more profits are obtained from private centre HD [51]. Recently, a budget impact analysis of HD versus PD was developed to estimate dialysis associated costs from Malaysian government perspective [52]. It was reported that increasing the use of PD for eligible patients could improve patients' access to dialysis in rural areas of Malaysia as the current funding model favors the setting up of HD centres in urban areas. Only government and NGOs are willing to open HD centres in less developed areas. Reliance on HD

extensively in the current economic condition will further aggravate the healthcare budget [52].

Decision-analytical modeling in economic evaluation has been widely used to examine overall cost over time. Modeling may have low validity due to data simulations, but it remains an essential aspect of economic evaluation [53]. Several decision-analytical models are used including decision tree and Markov model, discrete event simulation, and mathematical modeling [52]. Studies conducted in UK [54], Austria [55], and Australia [56] using Markov modeling found that increasing the allocation of PD patients using simulated data versus current practice had resulted in significant cost savings from a payer perspective. Similar findings were reported in Malaysia through the budget impact analysis of PD versus HD [52].

4. Discussion

CKD is an important cause of death and disability but it remains asymptomatic till late stage when intervention cannot stop the progression of the disease [57]. Hence, detection and prevention of CKD at early stage are a necessity. Measures used to improve detection include training of nephrologists, urologists, and allied healthcare staff as well as continuous improvements in various allied services including radiology services, laboratory tests, and renal pathology [58]. CPG of management of CKD in adults was developed to assist in prevention and reduction in risk of CKD, screening and early detection of CKD, treatment of early CKD to prevent its progression to ESRD, and reduction in risk of cardiovascular disease [59]. Since diabetes and hypertension are two major risk factors to CKD in Malaysia, CPG of these diseases were also developed with strong emphasis on CKD detection via screening of proteinuria, microalbuminuria, and serum creatinine level to determine GFR. Numerous initiatives have been undertaken by the government to promote lifelong wellness and healthy lifestyle among the community. The Malaysia Health Promotion Board (MySihat) was established by MOH in 2006 where the main objective is to set and develop the health promotion agenda across different sectors and settings particularly with the active participation of the NGOs.

However, the increasing incidence and prevalence of ESRD seem inevitable. Kidney transplantation is significantly associated with improved survival and quality of life, as well as substantial cost savings, compared with dialysis [21]. Malaysia has one of the lowest organ donation rates in the world [60] making dialysis the only viable option for majority of ESRD patients. Some patients, however, are managed by palliative care when dialysis support is not feasible or being withdrawn and the operational policy was established in 2010 [61]. Palliative care is an important aspect of medical service offered by some major hospitals in this country to minimize suffering by early identification, assessment, and prompt intervention of physical, psychosocial, and spiritual problems related to ESRD.

Dialysis is a costly treatment with substantial impact on healthcare budget especially when HD, a costlier treatment than PD, dominates dialysis provision. Malaysia's dialysis financing system (public-private partnership) is in alignment with WHO recommendation of health system and financing for RRT [21]. This review suggests that some countries tend to widen their PD utilization amid positive economic implications and improved dialysis access. Nevertheless, increasing PD utilization require strong coordinated effort. Liu et al. in their overview of the impact of PD-First or PD-Favored Policies around the world indicated that barriers to policy implementation are generally associated with government policy, economics, provider or healthcare professional education, modality-related factors, and patient-related factors [44]. Education and training for healthcare professionals including nephrologists, doctors, nurses, and other dialysis staff as well as patients' successful PD catheter placement and technique survival are crucial for its expansion [34, 62–65]. Collaboration between various departments such as the Ministry of Health, National Kidney Foundation (NKF), and other NGOs is vital to ensure expansion of the PD program. For example, in Thailand, improved survival rates and technique were observed after three-year PD-First Policy implementation. There was support from the National Health Security Office, the Nephrology Society of Thailand, the Dialysis Nurse Association, the Kidney Foundation of Thailand, and other NGOs [41]. Resource availability and reimbursement or incentives are important for these initiatives [34].

Reliance on an economic evaluation research conducted many years ago could be a concern. The cost of treatments has changed tremendously. Cost of HD is driven mainly by fixed costs of facility space and staff while cost of PD is determined mainly by variable costs such as solutions and disposables. There have been large reductions in the price of erythropoietin (EPO) albeit PD patients have a lower requirement for ESAs [12, 26, 27]. Salaries of dialysis staff have increased accompanied by rising costs of land, building, and utilities. There are also variations in costs of dialysis machines, dialyzers, medications, and dialysis consumables. Since most HD is conducted at hospital or clinic while PD is performed at home, the costs of both treatments could change significantly. The recent budget impact analysis of HD versus PD reported several limitations including reliance on previously conducted economic evaluation of dialysis and costs of hospitalizations being not included [52]. Hence, a current comprehensive global cost evaluation of PD and HD (either from provider or societal perspective) is vital for any potential changes in policy and reimbursement strategies.

5. Conclusion

In conclusion, increasing ESRD prevalence in Malaysia is imposing a heavy financial burden on the healthcare budget especially when kidney transplants are limited. This paper addresses the dialysis provision in Malaysia, issues and implications of health economics on PD utilization. The literature show that PD is more cost-effective than HD but PD is underutilized in many countries including Malaysia. Some countries adopt "PD-First Policy" or "PD Favored Policy" from economic perspectives ensuring patients' quality of care, outcomes and widening PD utilization. Finding sustainable health polices and reimbursement strategies is essential to

contain spending on ESRD treatment and improve patients' disparities in access to dialysis through economic evaluation studies.

Abbreviations

CAPD: Continuous Ambulatory Peritoneal Dialysis
CKD: Chronic kidney disease
CPG: Clinical practice guidelines
DALYs: Disability adjusted life years
EPO: Erythropoietin
ESA: Erythropoiesis Stimulating Agent
ESRD: End-stage renal disease
GDB: Global Burden of Disease
GDP: Gross domestic product
HD: Hemodialysis
MCO: Managed Care Organization
MDTR: Malaysian Dialysis and Transplant Registry
MOF: Ministry of Finance
MOH: Ministry of Health
NGO: Nongovernmental organization
PD: Peritoneal dialysis
PMP: Per million population
PPS: Prospective payment system
QALY: Quality adjusted life years
RRT: Renal replacement therapies
SOCSO: Social Security Organization
YLL: Years of life lost
WHO: World Health Organization.

Ethical Approval

Ethics approval was obtained from Pusat Perubatan Universiti Kebangsaan Malaysia (JEP-2016-360) and Medical Research Ethics Committee (NMRR-16-1341-30856).

Disclosure

Submitted manuscript is a review article. This review was conducted as part of the study "Cost Utility Analysis of End Stage Renal Disease Treatment in Ministry of Health Dialysis Centres, Malaysia: Hemodialysis versus Continuous Ambulatory Peritoneal Dialysis." This Ph.D. project is currently in the data collection stage. This review article received no specific grant from any funding agency in the public, commercial, or not-for-profit sectors.

Acknowledgments

The authors acknowledge the National Renal Registry for access to the data used as a reference in this review paper.

References

[1] Economic Planning Unit, "The Malaysian Economy in Figures," *Prime Minister's Department*, 2017.

[2] Department of Statistics Malaysia, "Population and Demography: Abridged Life Tables, Malaysia," 2013–2016, https://www.dosm.gov.my/v1/index.php?r=column/cthemeByCat&cat=116&bul_id=TkpmM05EK3NBV0JRU1pmOUJnS3RCQT09&menu_id=L0pheU43NWJwRWVSZklWdzQ4TlhUUT09.

[3] World Health Organization, "Malaysian Health System review," 2013.

[4] Ministry of Health Malaysia, "Health Expenditure Report 1997-2013," Planning Division, 2015.

[5] O. E. Ayodele and C. O. Alebiosu, "Burden of chronic kidney disease: an international perspective," Advances in Chronic Kidney Disease, vol. 17, no. 3, pp. 215–224, 2010.

[6] Fresinius Medical Care, "Magazine 2013 Perspectives," http://www.equitystory.com/download/companies/fmc/Annual%20Reports/DE0005785802-JA-2013-EQ-E-00.pdf.

[7] World Health Organization, "Global Burden of Disease.: Regional Estimates for 2000–2015, DALY Estimates," http://www.who.int/healthinfo/global_burden_disease/estimates/en/index2.html.

[8] Institute of Health Metrics and Evaluation, "Global Burden of Disease Study 2015," http://ghdx.healthdata.org/gbd-results-tool.

[9] S. Bele, T. N. Bodhare, N. Mudgalkar, A. Saraf, and S. Valsangkar, "Health-related quality of life and existential concerns among patients with end-stage renal disease," Indian Journal of Palliative Care, vol. 18, no. 2, pp. 103–108, 2012.

[10] W. G. Couser, G. Remuzzi, S. Mendis, and M. Tonelli, "The contribution of chronic kidney disease to the global burden of major noncommunicable diseases," Kidney International, vol. 80, no. 12, pp. 1258–1270, 2011.

[11] B. G. Jaar, A. Chang, and L. Plantinga, "Can we improve quality of life of patients on dialysis?" Clinical Journal of the American Society of Nephrology, vol. 8, no. 1, pp. 1–4, 2013.

[12] The National Renal Registry, 22nd Report of the Malaysian Dialysis and Transplant Registry, 2015.

[13] A. Ojo, "Addressing the global burden of chronic kidney disease through clinical and translational research," Transactions of the American Clinical and Climatological Association, vol. 125, pp. 6–229, 2014.

[14] A. S. Levey, R. Atkins, J. Coresh et al., "Chronic kidney disease as a global public health problem: approaches and initiatives—a position statement from Kidney Disease Improving Global Outcomes," Kidney International, vol. 72, no. 3, pp. 247–259, 2007.

[15] F. X. Liu, T. P. Quock, and J. Burkart, "Economic evaluations of peritoneal dialysis and hemodialysis: 2004–2012," F1000Research, vol. 2, no. 273, pp. 1–13, 2013.

[16] A. N. Karopadi, G. Mason, E. Rettore, and C. Ronco, "Cost of peritoneal dialysis and haemodialysis across the world," Nephrology Dialysis Transplantation, vol. 28, no. 10, pp. 2553–2569, 2013.

[17] E. Grapsa, "Is the underutilization of peritoneal dialysis in relation to hemodialysis, as renal replacement therapy, justifiable worldwide? yes or no," Hippokratia, vol. 15, no. 1, pp. 13–15, 2011.

[18] T.-O. Lim, A. Goh, Y.-N. Lim, Z. M. M. Zaher, and A. B. Suleiman, "How public and private reforms dramatically improved access to dialysis therapy in Malaysia," Health Affairs, vol. 29, no. 12, pp. 2214–2222, 2010.

[19] H. T. Chua and J. C. H. Cheah, "Financing universal coverage in Malaysia: A case study," BMC Public Health, vol. 12, no. 1, article no. S7, 2012.

[20] J. B. Wetmore and A. J. Collins, "Global challenges posed by the growth of end-stage renal disease," Renal Replacement Therapy, vol. 2, no. 1, pp. 1–7, 2016.

[21] S. L. White, S. J. Chadban, S. Jan, J. R. Chapman, and A. Cass, "How can we achieve global equity in provision of renal replacement therapy?" Bulletin of the World Health Organization, vol. 86, no. 3, pp. 229–237, 2008.

[22] C. Tan, C. Chan, C. Ho, K. S. Wong, E. J. Lee, and K. T. Woo, "Health economics of renal replacement therapy: Perspectives from Singapore," Kidney International, vol. 67, no. 94, pp. S19–S22, 2015.

[23] Medical Development Division, "Ministry of Health Malaysia, Nephrology services operational policy, 2010".

[24] M. A. Bujang, T. H. Adnan, N. H. Hashim et al., "Forecasting the Incidence and Prevalence of Patients with End-Stage Renal Disease in Malaysia up to the Year 2040," International Journal of Nephrology, vol. 2017, Article ID 2735296, 2017.

[25] L. S. Hooi, T. O. Lim, A. Goh et al., "Economic evaluation of centre haemodialysis and continuous ambulatory peritoneal dialysis in Ministry of Health hospitals, Malaysia," Nephrology, vol. 10, no. 1, pp. 25–32, 2005.

[26] N. Lameire and W. van Biesen, "Epidemiology of peritoneal dialysis: a story of believers and nonbelievers," Nature Reviews Nephrology, vol. 6, no. 2, pp. 75–83, 2010.

[27] P. Dalal, H. Sangha, and K. Chaudhary, "In peritoneal dialysis, is there sufficient evidence to make 'PD first' therapy?" International Journal of Nephrology, vol. 2011, Article ID 239515, 5 pages, 2011.

[28] M. Novak, F. Bender, and B. Piraino, "Why is peritoneal dialysis underutilized in the United States?" Dialysis & Transplantation, vol. 37, no. 3, p. 1, 2008.

[29] R. J. Fluck, D. Fouque, and R. S. Lockridge Jr., "Nephrologists' perspectives on dialysis treatment: Results of an international survey," BMC Nephrology, vol. 15, no. 1, article no. 16, 2014.

[30] S. Anand, A. Bitton, and T. Gaziano, "The Gap between Estimated Incidence of End-Stage Renal Disease and Use of Therapy," PLoS ONE, vol. 8, no. 8, Article ID e72860, 2013.

[31] T. Liyanage, T. Ninomiya, V. Jha et al., "Worldwide access to treatment for end-stage kidney disease: a systematic review," The Lancet, vol. 385, no. 9981, pp. 1975–1982, 2015.

[32] Institute for Public Health, "National Health and Morbidity Survey 2015 Vol. II: Non-Communicable Diseases, Risk Factors and Other Health Problems," Ministry of Health Malaysia, 2015.

[33] L. S. Hooi, L. M. Ong, G. Ahmad et al., "A population-based study measuring the prevalence of chronic kidney disease among adults in West Malaysia," Kidney International, vol. 84, no. 5, pp. 1034–1040, 2013.

[34] P. M. Just, F. T. De Charro, E. A. Tschosik, L. L. Noe, S. K. Bhattacharyya, and M. C. Riella, "Reimbursement and economic factors influencing dialysis modality choice around the world," Nephrology Dialysis Transplantation, vol. 23, no. 7, pp. 2365–2373, 2008.

[35] National Kidney Foundation, "A-Z Health Guide," https://www.kidney.org/atoz.

[36] M. J. Oliver, R. R. Quinn, E. P. Richardson, A. J. Kiss, D. L. Lamping, and B. J. Manns, "Home care assistance and the utilization of peritoneal dialysis," Kidney International, vol. 71, no. 7, pp. 673–678, 2007.

[37] N. Lameire, P. Peeters, R. Vanholder, and W. Van Biesen, "Peritoneal dialysis in Europe: An analysis of its rise and fall," Blood Purification, vol. 24, no. 1, pp. 107–114, 2006.

[38] J.-P. Wauters and D. Uehlinger, "Non-medical factors influencing peritoneal dialysis utilization: The Swiss experience," *Nephrology Dialysis Transplantation* , vol. 19, no. 6, pp. 1363–1367, 2004.

[39] M. F. Drummond, M. J. Sculpher, G. W. Torrance, B. J. OBrien, and G. L. Stoddart, *Methods for the Economic Evaluation of Health Care Programmes*, Oxford University Press, 3rd edition, 2005.

[40] J. B. Oostenbrink, M. A. Koopmanschap, and F. F. H. Rutten, "Standardisation of costs: The Dutch Manual for Costing in Economic Evaluations," *PharmacoEconomics*, vol. 20, no. 7, pp. 443–454, 2002.

[41] P. Dhanakijcharoen, D. Sirivongs, S. Aruyapitipan, P. Chuengsaman, and A. Lumpaopong, "The 'PD First' policy in Thailand: three-years experiences (2008–2011)," *Journal of the Medical Association of Thailand*, vol. 94, supplement 4, pp. S153–S161, 2011.

[42] Y. Teerawattananon, M. Mugford, and V. Tangcharoensathien, "Economic evaluation of palliative management versus peritoneal dialysis and hemodialysis for end-stage renal disease: Evidence for coverage decisions in Thailand," *Value in Health*, vol. 10, no. 1, pp. 61–72, 2007.

[43] A. S.-M. Choy and P. K.-T. Li, "Sustainability of the Peritoneal Dialysis-First Policy in Hong Kong," *Blood Purification*, vol. 40, no. 4, pp. 320–325, 2015.

[44] F. X. Liu, X. Gao, G. Inglese, P. Chuengsaman, R. Pecoits-Filho, and A. Yu, "A global overview of the impact of peritoneal dialysis first or favored policies: an opinion," *Peritoneal Dialysis International*, 2014.

[45] United States Renal Data System (USRD), "Chapter 13: Mortality," https://www.usrds.org/2015/view/v2_13.aspx.

[46] D. C. Mendelssohn, N. Langlois, and P. G. Blake, "Peritoneal dialysis in Ontario: A natural experiment in physician reimbursement methodology," *Peritoneal Dialysis International*, vol. 24, no. 6, pp. 531–537, 2004.

[47] H. Naito, "The Japanese health-care system and reimbursement for dialysis," *Peritoneal Dialysis International*, vol. 26, no. 2, pp. 155–161, 2006.

[48] Y.-C. Lin, Y.-C. Lin, C.-C. Kao, H.-H. Chen, C.-C. Hsu, and M.-S. Wu, "Health policies on dialysis modality selection: A nationwide population cohort study," *BMJ Open*, vol. 7, no. 1, Article ID e013007, 2017.

[49] T. A. Golper, "The possible impact of the us prospective payment system ("bundle") on the growth of peritoneal dialysis," *Peritoneal Dialysis International*, vol. 33, no. 6, pp. 596–599, 2013.

[50] Q. Zhang, M. Thamer, O. Kshirsagar, and Y. Zhang, "Impact of the End Stage Renal Disease Prospective Payment System on the Use of Peritoneal Dialysis," *Kidney International Reports*, vol. 2, no. 3, pp. 350–358, 2017.

[51] Z. Morad, D. G. Lee, Y. N. Lim, and P. C. Tan, "Peritoneal dialysis in Malaysia," *Peritoneal Dialysis International*, vol. 25, no. 5, pp. 426–431, 2005.

[52] S. Bavanandan, G. Ahmad, A.-H. Teo, L. Chen, and F. X. Liu, "Budget Impact Analysis of Peritoneal Dialysis versus Conventional In-Center Hemodialysis in Malaysia," *Value in Health Regional Issues*, vol. 9, pp. 8–14, 2016.

[53] X. Sun, "Markov modelling in healthcare economic evaluations," *Chinese Journal of Evidence-Based Medicine*, vol. 7, no. 10, pp. 750–756, 2007.

[54] C. Treharne, F. X. Liu, M. Arici, L. Crowe, and U. Farooqui, "Peritoneal dialysis and in-centre haemodialysis: A cost-utility analysis from a UK payer perspective," *Applied Health Economics and Health Policy*, vol. 12, no. 4, pp. 409–420, 2014.

[55] M. Haller, G. Gutjahr, R. Kramar, F. Harnoncourt, and R. Oberbauer, "Cost-effectiveness analysis of renal replacement therapy in Austria," *Nephrology Dialysis Transplantation* , vol. 26, no. 9, pp. 2988–2995, 2011.

[56] K. Howard, G. Salkeld, S. White et al., "The cost-effectiveness of increasing kidney transplantation and home-based dialysis," *Nephrology*, vol. 14, no. 1, pp. 123–132, 2009.

[57] Y. Almualm and H. Zaman Huri, "Chronic kidney disease screening methods and its implication for Malaysia: an in depth review," *Global Journal of Health Science*, vol. 7, no. 4, pp. 96–109, 2015.

[58] L. S. Hooi, H. S. Wong, and Z. Morad, "Prevention of renal failure: the Malaysian experience," *Kidney International Supplements*, vol. 67, no. 94, pp. S70–S74, 2005.

[59] Medical Development Division, "Ministry of Health Malaysia, Management of Chronic Kidney Disease in Adults," 2011.

[60] International Registry for organ donation and transplantation, "Final numbers 2014. 2015," http://www.irodat.org/img/database/pdf/NEWSLETTER2015_December2.pdf.

[61] Medical Development Division, "Ministry of Health Malaysia, Palliative Care Services Operational Policy," 2010.

[62] L. P. Wong, K. T. Yamamoto, V. Reddy et al., "Patient education and care for peritoneal dialysis catheter placement: A quality improvement study," *Peritoneal Dialysis International*, vol. 34, no. 1, pp. 12–23, 2014.

[63] P. G. Blake, R. R. Quinn, and M. J. Oliver, "Peritoneal dialysis and the process of modality selection," *Peritoneal Dialysis International*, vol. 33, no. 3, pp. 233–241, 2013.

[64] K. Chaudhary, H. Sangha, and R. Khanna, "Peritoneal dialysis first: rationale," *Clinical Journal of the American Society of Nephrology*, vol. 6, no. 2, pp. 447–456, 2011.

[65] A. Figueiredo, B.-L. Goh, S. Jenkins et al., "Clinical practice guidelines for peritoneal access," *Peritoneal Dialysis International*, vol. 30, no. 4, pp. 424–429, 2010.

30

Effects of Therapy on Urine Neutrophil Gelatinase-Associated Lipocalin in Nondiabetic Glomerular Diseases with Proteinuria

Amnuay Sirisopha,[1] Somlak Vanavanan,[2] Anchalee Chittamma,[2] Bunyong Phakdeekitcharoen,[1] Ammarin Thakkinstian,[3] Amornpan Lertrit,[1] Nuankanya Sathirapongsasuti,[4] and Chagriya Kitiyakara[1]

[1]Department of Medicine, Faculty of Medicine Ramathibodi Hospital, Mahidol University, Bangkok 10400, Thailand
[2]Department of Pathology, Faculty of Medicine Ramathibodi Hospital, Mahidol University, Bangkok 10400, Thailand
[3]Section for Clinical Epidemiology and Biostatistics, Faculty of Medicine Ramathibodi Hospital, Mahidol University, Bangkok 10400, Thailand
[4]Graduate Program in Translational Medicine, Research Center, Faculty of Medicine Ramathibodi Hospital, Mahidol University, Bangkok 10400, Thailand

Correspondence should be addressed to Chagriya Kitiyakara; kitiyakc@yahoo.com

Academic Editor: Kazunari Kaneko

Urine neutrophil gelatinase-associated lipocalin (NGAL) is widely used as a biomarker for acute kidney injury. Cross-sectional studies have shown that NGAL may be elevated in glomerular diseases, but there is limited information on the value of NGAL in predicting treatment response or on the changes of NGAL levels after therapy. We prospectively evaluated the effects of therapy on NGAL in nondiabetic glomerular diseases. Urine NGAL was collected at biopsy and follow-up at 12 months. At baseline, NGAL in glomerular disease patients ($n = 43$) correlated with proteinuria, but not with glomerular filtration rate (GFR). After therapy with renin-angiotensin blockers and/or immune modulating agents, change of NGAL correlated with change of proteinuria, but not with change of GFR. NGAL at baseline was not different between patients in complete remission (CR) at follow-up compared to those not in remission (NR). Compared to baseline, NGAL at follow-up decreased in CR ($n = 10$), but not in NR. Change of NGAL was greater in CR than NR. In conclusion, the change of urine NGAL correlated with the change of proteinuria. Baseline NGAL was not a predictor of complete remission. Future studies will be necessary to determine the role of NGAL as a predictor of long term outcome in proteinuric glomerular diseases.

1. Background

Glomerular disease consists of a group of disorders that together constitutes one of the leading causes of end-stage renal disease (ESRD) worldwide [1]. Once established, proteinuric glomerular disease causes activation of pathogenic processes leading to chronic tubular injury, fibrosis with subsequent nephron loss, and progressive decline in renal function [2]. Proteinuria is an important direct mediator of tubular epithelial cell injury and is a strong predictor of renal disease progression [3]. Reducing proteinuria with immune modulating therapy or renin-angiotensin system blockers has been shown to improve outcome in diverse types of glomerular diseases. However, response to therapy is variable and progressive nephron loss could still occur at dissimilar rates. A noninvasive biomarker that could predict response to treatment or prognosis would be useful in the management of glomerular diseases.

Neutrophil gelatinase-associated lipocalin (NGAL) is a small 25-kDa protein of the lipocalin family. After acute kidney injury, intrarenal NGAL is markedly upregulated [4] and NGAL is excreted in the urine in parallel with the severity of tubular injury. Urine NGAL is now widely used as a biomarker for acute kidney injury (AKI). Recently, urine

NGAL has also been shown to be elevated in patients with chronic kidney diseases (CKD) of different etiologies. Cross-sectional studies found that urine NGAL was higher in patients with glomerulonephritis [5], diabetic nephropathy [6], and adult polycystic kidney disease [7] compared with healthy controls. Prospective studies suggest that urine NGAL, measured once at baseline, may be a useful predictor for loss of renal function in CKD patients with low level protein excretion [8] or the general population [9]. While several investigators have proposed that NGAL might be a useful biomarker in CKD subjects without significant proteinuria, there is still limited information on the prognostic role of NGAL in proteinuric glomerular diseases. Preliminary studies have shown that baseline NGAL levels may correlate with adverse prognosis in adults with membranous nephropathy and in nephrotic children [5, 10]. However, there are few prospective data on the value of NGAL for predicting therapeutic response in common glomerular diseases. Moreover, previous studies have evaluated NGAL only once at baseline and the relationship between changes of urine NGAL over time in response to treatment has not been fully studied. This information is important if NGAL is to be considered as a biomarker to monitor disease progression. In this study, we will test the hypothesis that NGAL levels can predict medium term response to therapy and that treatment of glomerular diseases will decrease urine NGAL and assess the relationship between changes in urine NGAL excretion with changes of clinical parameters in proteinuric patients with common biopsy-proven, nondiabetic glomerular diseases.

2. Materials and Methods

2.1. Patients and Baseline Data. This single center, prospective cohort study enrolled adult patients with glomerular diseases referred to the nephrology outpatient clinic of Ramathibodi Hospital during 2013 to 2015. All procedures performed in studies involving human participants were in accordance the 1964 Helsinki Declaration and its later amendments and approved by the Ethics Committee of the Ramathibodi Hospital. Written informed consent was obtained.

Inclusion criteria were biopsy-proven glomerulonephritis and the presence of proteinuria (urine protein creatinine ratio > 0.50 g/g creatinine) and a stable renal function. Patients with kidney transplant, diabetic nephropathy, active infections, or other severe intercurrent illnesses were excluded from the study. The patients' history and clinical examination data were carefully recorded. Patients were given standard treatment including renin-angiotensin system blockade (ACEi-angiotensin converting enzyme inhibitors or ARB-angiotensin receptor blockers) and/or immunosuppressive agents (corticosteroids or other immune modulating drugs or both) according to standard guidelines [11].

Urine samples were also collected from healthy volunteers and from patients with acute kidney injury (AKI). Healthy controls were recruited from volunteers with no chronic illnesses including hypertension or kidney diseases after detailed history taking, physical examination, and routine blood tests including urinalysis and serum creatinine. AKI controls were recruited from hospitalized patients without glomerular

diseases who developed acute kidney injury due to nephrotoxic or ischemic insults (defined by KDIGO guideline 2012) [12].

2.2. Pathologic Studies. Kidney biopsies were fixed in histological fixative (Glyo-Fixx, Thermo scientific, USA) and paraffin embedded, and sections ($2\,\mu m$) were processed for light microscopy (hematoxylin and eosin, periodic acid-Schiff, Masson's trichrome, and silver staining), immunofluorescence, and electronmicroscopy and evaluated by a nephropathologist blinded to the laboratory and NGAL data. Glomerular diseases were classified according standard criteria [11]. *Tubular injury* was present if there were apical blebs, attenuation of brush border epithelium, sloughed epithelium, or evidence of tubular regeneration. The severity of interstitial fibrosis and tubular atrophy (IFTA) was assessed semiquantitatively as a proportion relative to the total section area as follows: none, <5%; mild, 5–25%; moderate, 26–50%; and severe, >50%.

2.3. Laboratory Measurements and Definitions. Baseline blood and second void urine samples were collected on the day of the biopsy and follow-up samples were collected 12 months later.

Common biochemical parameters were measured in a laboratory in compliance with ISO 15189. Creatinine was measured by enzymatic method. Urine samples were centrifuged at 3000 rpm for 10 minutes at $4^{\circ}C$ and the supernatant was sent for analysis for NGAL using a chemiluminescent microparticle immunoassay (CMIA) kit (The ARCHITECT Urine NGAL assay). Coefficient of variation at the low (20.2 ng/mL), medium (196.7 ng/mL), and high (1174.4 ng/mL) urine NGAL levels was 4.4%, 3.0%, and 2.2% for intra-assay variation, respectively, while that for the interassay was 2.1%, 1.7%, and 1.4%, respectively. Using the same aliquot, urine protein was measured by modified pyrogallol red-molybdate method and urine creatinine by enzymatic method on the Dimension ExL analyzer (Siemens Healthcare Diagnostics, Newark, DE, USA).

Glomerular filtration rate (GFR in mL/min/1.73 m^2) was calculated by using the CKD-EPI equation [13]. Urine protein was reported as urine protein creatinine ratio (UPCR in mg/mgCr).

Nephrotic range proteinuria was defined as UPCR more than 2000 mg/mg [11]. *Low GFR* was defined as GFR < 60 [14]. *Complete remission* was defined as UPCR < 0.3 at the follow-up period [11]. Subjects not in complete remission *(not in remission)* were further subclassified *as partial remission*, defined as 50% or greater reductions in proteinuria, or *resistant disease*, defined as less than 50% reduction in proteinuria or greater than 30 mL/min/1.73 m^2 decrease in GFR at follow-up.

2.4. Statistical Analysis. Data are presented as mean ± standard deviation, median (range), or percentage (frequency), as appropriate. Change in parameters was calculated by subtracting follow-up values from baseline such that positive values represent an increase. These within-individual changes

TABLE 1: Baseline characteristics according to remission status at follow-up.

Baseline characteristics	All patients ($N = 43$)	By response to treatment		p value
		Complete remission ($N = 10$)	Not in remission ($N = 33$)	
Male, n (%)	15 (34.9%)	5 (55.6%)	10 (29.4%)	0.143
Age, years	45 ± 17	42 ± 17	47 ± 17	0.409
BMI, kg/m^2	25.5 ± 3.9	26.7 ± 3.2	25 ± 4.1	0.19
Systolic BP, mmHg	135 ± 21	133 ± 12	137 ± 23	0.52
Diastolic BP, mmHg	79 ± 11	82 ± 7	79 ± 12	0.26
ACEI and/or ARB use	38 (88.3%)	8 (80%)	30 (90.9%)	0.52
Corticosteroids $\pm$ immunosuppressive agents (%)	25 (58%)	9 (90%)	16 (48.5%)	0.035*
Albumin, g/dL	3.14 (0.59–3.88)	1.86 (0.78–3.88)	3.21 (0.59–3.88)	0.035*
Cholesterol, mg/dL	250 (143–669)	338 (150–594)	240 (143–669)	0.060
Serum creatinine, mg/dL	1.21 (0.43–4.17)	1.21 (0.54–1.42)	1.21 (0.43–4.17)	0.141
Baseline GFR, mL/min/1.73 m^2	66.2 (12.3–143.4)	77 (54–137)	59 (12–143)	0.09
Proteinuria, g/g creatinine	2.17 (0.09–9.23)	3.06 (0.11–9.23)	2.15 (0.09–9.15)	0.55

Data shown as mean $\pm$ SD or median (min–max). *$p < 0.05$ considered significant.
ACEI, angiotensin converting enzyme inhibitor; ARB, angiotensin receptor blockade; BMI, body mass index; BP, blood pressure; GFR, glomerular filtration rates.

were compared by Wilcoxon test, and changes between groups were compared using independent t-test if data were normally distributed; otherwise Mann-Whitney U test or Kruskal-Wallis test was applied. Chi-square test was applied to compare distributions for categorical variables. In addition, Spearman's rank correlation was used to assess the correlations between urine NGAL and other variables. A mixed-effect logistic regression was used to assess correlation between GFR group and other variables. All analyses were performed using STATA version 14. All results were considered significant if p was <0.05.

3. Results

3.1. Patient Characteristics. A total of 43 patients of glomerular disease were enrolled (IgA nephropathy ($n = 10$), lupus nephritis class III/IV ($n = 9$), focal segmental glomerulosclerosis ($n = 7$), minimal change disease ($n = 8$), membranous nephropathy ($n = 5$), and others ($n = 4$)). The main baseline characteristics of the study cohort are summarized in Table 1. Mean age of patients was 45 ± 17 years and 34.9% were male. Thirty-eight patients (88.3%) received ACEI or ARB therapy. Twenty-five (58%) patients received immune modulating agents; 7 (16.3%) received only corticosteroids and 18 (41.9%) received a combinations of corticosteroids and immunosuppressive agents.

3.2. Proteinuria, GFR, and NGAL at Baseline and Follow-Up. Overall, protein excretion tended to decrease from baseline ($t = 1$) to follow-up ($t = 2$) (UPCR$_1$, 2.17 (0.09–9.23) versus UPCR$_2$, 0.67 (0.06–16.96) g/g, $p = 0.12$). GFR did not change significantly (GFR$_1$, 66 (12–143) versus GFR$_2$, 71 (12–140) mL/min/1.73 m^2, $p = 0.76$) and neither did NGAL (NGAL$_1$, 26.1 (2.3–213.0) versus NGAL$_2$, 20.8 (0.5–359.7) ng/mL, $p = 0.96$).

Median NGAL in glomerular disease patients at baseline was about 6-fold higher than healthy subjects (NGAL$_1$ GN: 26.1 (2.3–213.0) versus healthy, 4.4 (3.1–10.6), $n = 10$, $p < 0.001$), and about 12-fold lower than AKI controls (NGAL$_1$ GN: 26.1 (2.3–213.0) versus AKI, 302.6 (85.9–4808), $n = 19$, $p < 0.001$).

3.3. Relationship between Urine NGAL with Proteinuria and GFR at Baseline. Overall, baseline NGAL$_1$ (Figure 1(a)) correlated significantly with baseline UPCR$_1$ ($r_s = 0.346$, $p = 0.023$). Twenty-four patients (55.8%) had nephrotic range proteinuria. As expected, nephrotic subjects had higher degrees of proteinuria (UPCR$_1$: *nephrotic*, 3.57 (2.14–9.23) versus *subnephrotic*, 1.02, (0.54–1.95, $p < 0.001$)), but GFR was not different (GFR$_1$: *nephrotic*, 59 (25–143) versus *subnephrotic*, 71 (12–143), $p = 0.56$). NGAL was higher in nephritic subjects (NGAL$_1$: *nephrotic*, 39.2 (5.0–213.0) versus *subnephrotic*, 23.5 (2.3–70.4), $p < 0.042$).

Overall, baseline NGAL did not correlate with baseline GFR (Figure 1(b)). Nineteen patients (44.1%) had *Low GFR* (GFR < 60) with median GFR$_1$ of 46.3 (12–57). Baseline GFR in those with preserved GFR ($\geq$60) was 81 (61–143). Baseline proteinuria (UPCR$_1$; *low GFR*, 2.18 (0.54–8.40) *versus preserved GFR*, 2.22 (0.54–9.23), $p = 0.56$) and baseline NGAL (NGAL$_1$: *Low GFR*, 37.9 (2.3–213.1) versus *preserved GFR*, 25.8 (2.4–120.3), $p = 0.63$) were similar between the two GFR groups.

3.4. Relationship between Change of Urine NGAL and Change of Proteinuria or GFR. From baseline to follow-up, the change of proteinuria (ΔUPCR$_{2-1}$) was −1.38 (−9.03–14.1) g/g Cr, change of GFR (ΔGFR$_{2-1}$) was −0.5 (−39.2–71.7) mL/min/1.73 m^2, and change of NGAL (ΔNGAL$_{2-1}$) was −0.300 (−211.4–289.3) ng/mL. ΔNGAL$_{2-1}$ significantly correlated

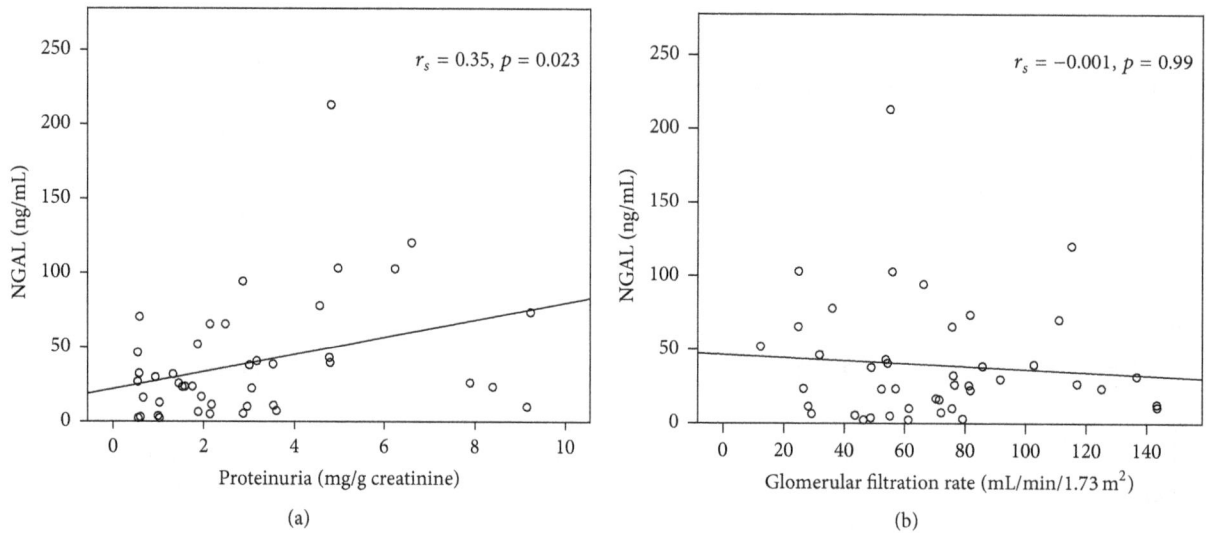

FIGURE 1: Relationship between NGAL and other laboratory parameters at baseline. (a) Proteinuria at baseline and (b) glomerular filtration rate at baseline ($n = 43$).

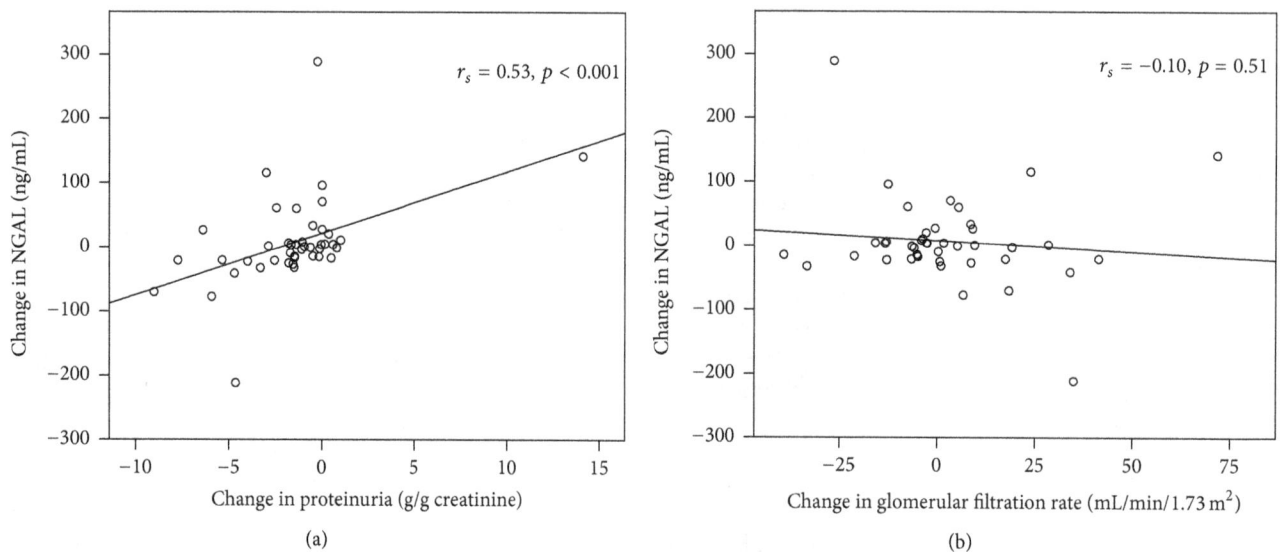

FIGURE 2: Relationship between change in NGAL and change in other laboratory parameters. (a) Change in proteinuria and (b) change in glomerular filtration rate ($n = 43$) from baseline to follow-up.

with $\Delta UPCR_{2-1}$ ($r_s = 0.530$, $p < 0.001$), but not with ΔGFR_{2-1} (Figure 2).

3.5. Relationship between Urine NGAL and Renal Histopathology.
To explore the relationship between acute tubular injury and NGAL levels, we divided patients into *tubular injury* ($n = 32$) and *no injury* ($n = 11$) groups according renal histology findings. GFR_1 at baseline and GFR_2 at follow-up were higher in *tubular injury*, but there were no differences in proteinuria. There was considerable overlap in baseline NGAL such that there was no statistical difference between the 2 groups. ($NGAL_1$: *no injury*, 26.8 (2.4–73.4) versus *tubular injury*, 26.1 (2.3–213.1) ng/mL, $p = 0.92$). No differences were observed in ΔGFR_{2-1}, $\Delta UPCR_{2-1}$, and $\Delta NGAL_{2-1}$ between the 2 groups. It is worth noting that only patients with features of tubular

injury ($n = 5$) had baseline NGAL above 85 ng/mL (the lowest level in nonglomerular AKI controls). All five patients had nephrotic syndrome and 4 of these patients had serum albumin less than 2.5 g/dL.

To explore relationship between NGAL and chronic tubulointerstitial changes, subjects were divided into 2 groups according to the severity of interstitial fibrosis and tubular atrophy (IFTA): *none to mild* ($n = 36$) and *moderate to severe* ($n = 7$). GFR at baseline and at follow-up were lower in *moderate to severe* IFTA, but there were no differences in proteinuria (*data not shown*). NGAL tended to be higher in *moderate to severe* IFTA at baseline ($NGAL_1$: *none to mild*, 24.6 (2.3–213.0) versus *moderate to severe*, 46.4 (5.4–103.2) ng/mL, $p = 0.19$) but were similar at follow-up ($NGAL_2$: *none to mild*, 18.4 (0.5–359.7) versus *moderate to severe*, 25.6 (9.1–80.9) ng/mL,

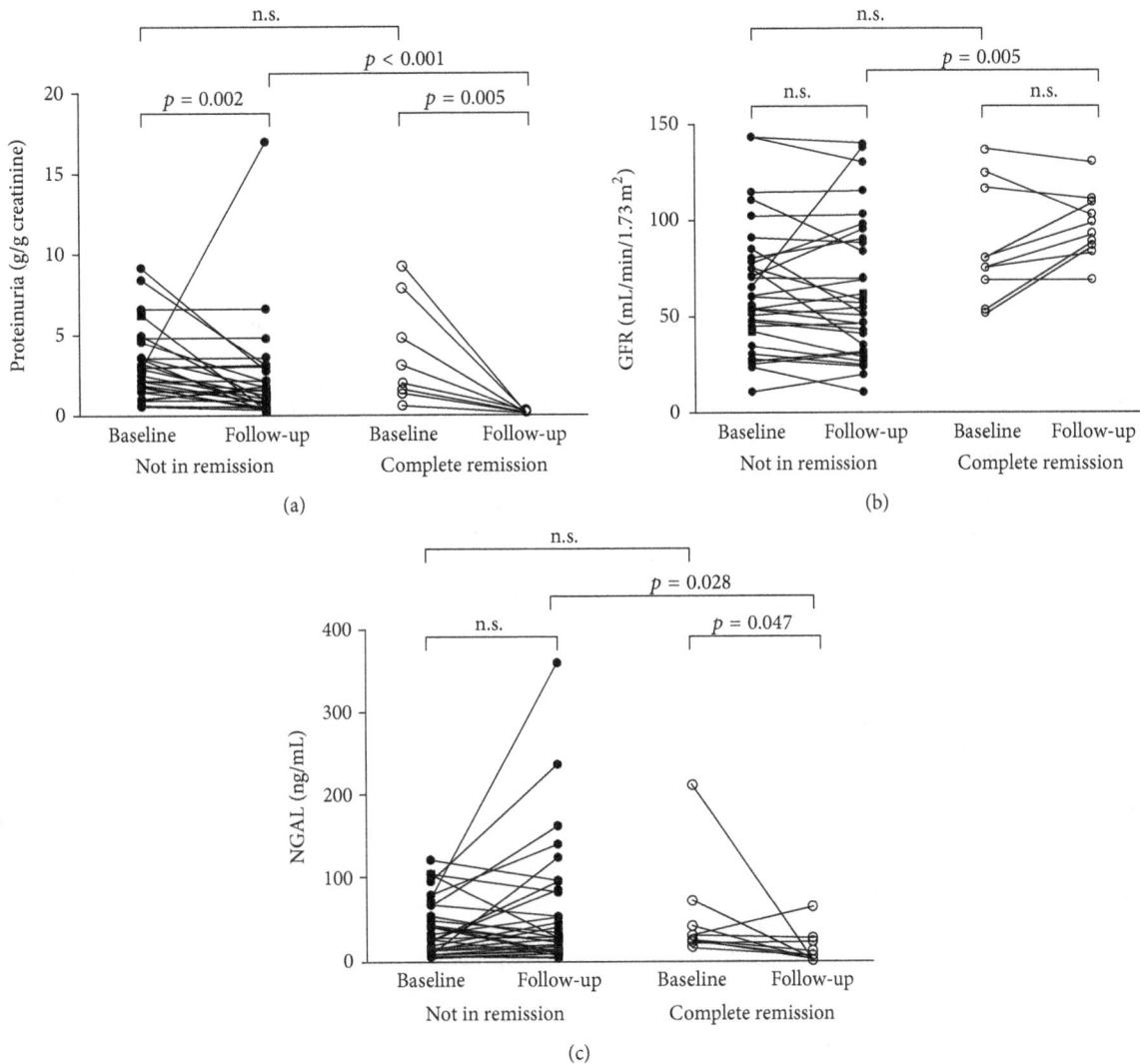

FIGURE 3: Laboratory parameters according to remission status at follow-up. (a) Proteinuria, (b) glomerular filtration rate, and (c) NGAL at baseline and follow-up. Complete remission ($n = 10$); not in remission ($n = 33$).

$p = 0.63$). Reduction in NGAL was greater in *moderate to severe* IFTA (ΔNGAL$_{2-1}$: *none to mild*, -2.8 (-211.4– 289.3) versus *moderate to severe*, -15.0 (-77.3–3.7) ng/mL, $p = 0.046$). No differences were observed in ΔGFR$_{2-1}$ or ΔUPCR$_{2-1}$ between the 2 groups.

3.6. NGAL in Patients with or without Complete Remission. At follow-up, 10 patients (23.2%) were *incomplete remission* (CR) (Table 1). CR was more likely in those who received immune modulating drugs compared to those not in remission (NR). In CR patients, the pathologies were lupus nephritis ($n = 2$), minimal change disease ($n = 5$), IgA nephropathy ($n = 1$), and focal segmental glomerulosclerosis ($n = 2$). Four patients were treated with prednisolone, four had prednisolone and immunosuppressive agents (azathioprine, cyclophosphamide, or mycophenolate mofetil), and 2 had ACEi or ARB without immune modulating agents. All patients received ACEi or ARB except one patient with minimal change disease who had prednisolone alone.

Baseline protein (UPCR$_1$) was not significantly different between patients who were in CR compared to NR (Figure 3(a)). UPCR decreased significantly at follow-up in both groups (CR: UPCR$_1$, 2.51 (0.54–9.23) versus UPCR$_2$, 0.15 (0.06–0.26), $p = 0.005$, and NR: UPCR$_1$, 2.18 (0.54–9.15), versus UPCR$_2$, 1.22 (0.23–16.96), $p = 0.002$). As expected, protein levels at follow-up (UPCR$_2$) were lower in CR group compared to NR ($p < 0.001$). Change of proteinuria was greater in those with CR (ΔUPCR$_{2-1}$: CR, -2.28 (-9.03– -0.48), versus NR, -1.05 (-6.40–14.10), $p = 0.031$).

There was no difference in baseline GFR$_1$ (Figure 3(b)) between CR versus NR ($p = 0.28$). In NR group, GFR did not change at follow-up (NR: GFR$_1$, 57 (12–143), versus GFR$_2$, 56 (12–140), $p = 0.48$). In CR group, GFR tended to increase (CR: GFR$_1$, 79 (54–137), versus GFR$_2$, 97 (71–131), $p = 0.11$). Change in GFR tended to be greater in CR, but this was not significant (ΔGFR$_{2-1}$: CR, +13 (-21–35), versus NR -3 (-39– 72), $p = 0.11$). GFR$_2$ at follow-up was higher in CR compared to NR ($p = 0.005$).

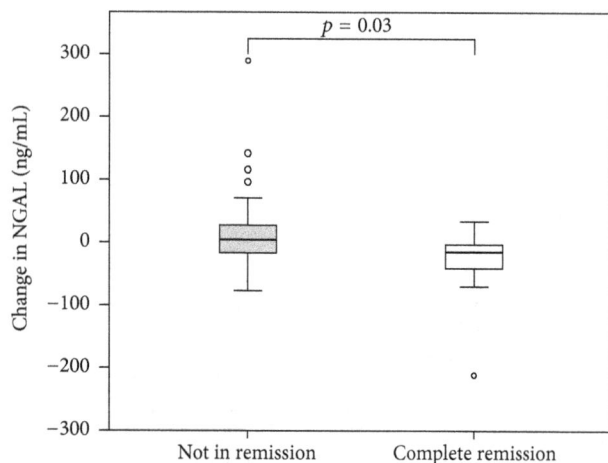

FIGURE 4: Change in NGAL (ng/mL) levels according to remission status at follow-up. Change in urine NGAL levels from baseline to follow-up between complete remission ($n = 10$) versus not in remission ($n = 33$).

Median NGAL at baseline (Figure 3(c)) were similar between patients with or without remission ($p = 0.286$). Compared to baseline values, NGAL decreased in CR subjects (CR: $NGAL_1$, 29.3 (16.7–213.2), versus $NGAL_2$, 7.4 (1.6–66.1) ng/mL, $p = 0.047$), but not in patients without remission (NR: $NGAL_1$, 23.5 (2.3–120.3), versus $NGAL_2$, 25.2 (0.5–359.7) ng/mL, $p = 0.31$). At follow-up, $NGAL_2$ was lower in CR compared to NR ($p = 0.028$). Of note, the follow-up level of $NGAL_2$ in CR was comparable to those of healthy subjects ($p = 0.393$). The reduction in NGAL was greater in CR compared to NR ($\Delta NGAL_{2\text{-}1}$: CR, −15.150 (−211.4–33.7), versus NR, 3.9 (−77.3–289.3) ng/mL, $p = 0.033$) (Figure 4).

A simple logistic regression showed that baseline urine NGAL was not a predictor of the remission status (*data not shown*). For all analyses, using log transformed NGAL or adjusting NGAL with urine creatinine concentrations (NGAL/Cr) produced similar results to NGAL alone (*data not shown*).

3.7. Partial Remission and Resistant Disease. Not in remission subjects (see Supplementary Table 1 in Supplementary Material available online at http://dx.doi.org/10.1155/2016/4904502) were further subclassified into *partial remission* ($n = 17$) and *resistant disease* ($n = 16$). Compared to *resistant disease* (resistant), *partial remission* (PR) had similar proteinuria at baseline, but lower proteinuria and greater reduction in proteinuria at follow-up ($UPCR_2$: PR, 0.80 (0.31–13.04), versus resistant, 1.62 (0.34–16.96) g/g, $p = 0.023$; $\Delta UPCR_{2\text{-}1}$, −2.12 (−6.44––0.93), versus 0.01 (−1.78–14.1) g/g, $p < 0.001$). GFR and NGAL at baseline or follow-up and $\Delta NGAL_{2\text{-}1}$ or $\Delta GFR_{2\text{-}1}$ were similar.

When PR subjects were compared to CR, there were no differences in proteinuria at baseline, but CR patients had lower proteinuria level and greater reduction in proteinuria at follow-up ($UPCR_2$: CR, 00.15 (0.06–0.26), versus PR, 0.80 (0.31–3.04) g/g creatinine, $p < 0.001$; $\Delta UPCR_{2\text{-}1}$, CR −2.28 (−9.03––0.48), versus PR, −2.12 (−6.44––0.93) g/g

creatinine, $p < 0.001$). GFR at baseline and at follow-up or change in GFR were similar. Although baseline and follow-up NGAL levels were not different, the reduction in NGAL was greater in CR than PR ($\Delta NGAL_{2\text{-}1}$: CR, −15.2 (−211.3–33.7), versus PR, 2.2 (−77.2–116.1) ng/mL, $p = 0.046$).

4. Discussion

Although urine NGAL has long been studied for its usefulness in acute kidney injury, few studies have evaluated the changes of urine NGAL over time in CKD. This study examined prospectively the effects of therapy on urine NGAL levels and the relationship of the change of NGAL with other clinical parameters in common glomerular diseases. The novel aspects of this study are that baseline NGAL level was not predictive of response to therapy and that there was a strong relationship between proteinuria and NGAL at baseline and at follow-up. Patients who were in complete remission with normal protein excretion had reduced NGAL at follow-up with levels comparable to healthy subjects, whereas NGAL levels in patients who were not in remission remained elevated. Changes in NGAL excretion correlated with changes in proteinuria, but not with changes in GFR.

In contrast to serum creatinine, which measures renal excretory function, NGAL is specifically induced in the damaged tubule and then released into the urine [15]. Only low levels of NGAL are detectable in the urine of healthy subjects [4]. Acute kidney injury leads to rapid NGAL mRNA upregulation in kidney tubules followed by marked increase in urine NGAL protein excretion [16]. More recently, urine NGAL has been shown to be elevated in patients with chronic tubulointerstitial disease [17, 18] and urine NGAL may be predictive of long term decline in renal function in nonproteinuric CKD, but limited data are available in glomerular diseases. Ding et al. found increases in urinary but not serum NGAL in patients with advanced IgA nephropathy levels consistent with local renal generation as the major source of urinary NGAL [19]. Hammad et al. found levels of urinary NGAL were higher in systemic lupus erythematosus patients with nephritis than those without nephritis [20]. Bolignano et al. showed that patients with membranous nephropathy had increased urine NGAL compared to controls [5]. Consistent with this, we found the levels of NGAL in glomerular diseases to be elevated by about 6-fold in glomerular diseases compared to normal subjects.

Proteinuria is an important direct mediator of tubular epithelial cell injury and is a strong predictor of renal disease progression [3]. Reducing proteinuria with immune modulating therapy or renin-angiotensin system blockers is the cornerstone of therapy for glomerular diseases [14]. Cross-sectional studies have shown that urinary NGAL increased in parallel with degree of proteinuria in glomerular diseases [5, 18, 19], but few studies have examined the changes of NGAL after treatment. In streptozotocin-diabetic mice, angiotensin receptor blockade which decreased proteinuria also lowered NGAL excretion [21]. Kuwabara et al. showed a reduction of NGAL in 4 nephrotic syndrome patients after treatment of proteinuria with immunosuppressive therapy [21]. In this study, we treated patients with biopsy-proven glomerular diseases according to standard guidelines [11] and found that the change in proteinuria strongly correlated with the change in NGAL excretion. Moreover, NGAL levels in patients with complete remission decreased to levels similar to healthy subjects. Our prospective data is consistent with a cross-sectional study in children with steroid-sensitive nephrotic syndrome in which subjects with active disease had higher NGAL than children in remission [18].

Several mechanisms may account for the strong correlation between proteinuria and urinary NGAL levels [22]. Passive loss of circulating NGAL through the damaged glomeruli could contribute to the increase in urinary NGAL level. Increased filtered albumin and other proteins could also overload the megalin-cubilin dependent reabsorption of NGAL in the proximal tubule leading to increased urinary NGAL excretion [21]. Excessive reabsorption of protein could result in direct tubular toxicity and increased synthesis of cytokines and complement activation leading to inflammatory cell infiltration, tubulointerstitial fibrosis, and subsequent nephron loss [2, 3]. Augmented production of NGAL may be a defensive compensatory response to prevent tubular cell apoptosis induced by proteinuria [23]. Increased NGAL production by damaged distal tubules might contribute to NGAL excretion in glomerular diseases [19]. Previous investigators found that NGAL excretion increased with the severity of chronic tubulointerstitial changes [19, 24]. A similar trend was observed in our study and would probably reach statistical significance if more patients with moderate to severe tubulointerstitial changes were included.

Acute tubular necrosis due to ischemia or nephrotoxins leads to a marked increase in NGAL excretion [4]. In nephrotic syndrome, low oncotic pressure can result in reduced renal perfusion and reversible acute tubular injury [25]. The levels of NGAL in patients with glomerular diseases were on average 10–100 times lower than levels in non-glomerular disease AKI controls. Despite clear differences in GFR, there were no overall differences in baseline NGAL levels between glomerular disease patients with histological features of tubular injury and those without, although a few patients with tubular injury had high NGAL levels in the same range as AKI controls. Correlations of urine NGAL and GFR have been observed in previous cross-sectional studies in CKD [5, 8, 26]. Lower numbers of patients with advanced disease and higher mean GFR in our subjects as well as the interfering effects of proteinuria could also account for the lack of relationship between NGAL and GFR. Taken together, this suggests that a combination of mechanisms likely contributes to the elevated NGAL excretion in glomerular disease [21]. Excess filtration of systemic NGAL and mal-processing in the proximal tubules appear to be dominant mechanisms given the strong correlations of NGAL with proteinuria although coexisting tubular injury might account for the very high levels of NGAL in some patients. GFR and chronic tubulointerstitial change appear to have less dominant roles.

Complete remission is a good predictor of long term prognosis in many types of glomerular diseases including lupus nephritis [27] and focal segmental glomerulosclerosis [28]. In our study, the baseline levels of NGAL in subjects with complete remission at follow-up were similar to those not in remission and the baseline NGAL level did not correlate with GFR at follow-up (*data not shown*). Thus NGAL level at baseline was not predictive of response to therapy but rather NGAL decreased with the resolution of proteinuria. Our results suggest that NGAL is not a useful biomarker for predicting therapeutic response in nondiabetic glomerular disease and raise cautions on the benefit of NGAL for predicting long term outcome in proteinuric CKD. Data showing predictive value of NGAL on outcome in GN is limited. A previous study found that high baseline NGAL was predictive of decline of renal function in membranous glomerular diseases [5]. In contrast to our subjects, many of these patients had low GFR at baseline and most subjects still had persistent proteinuria at follow-up. Residual proteinuria after therapy has been shown to be a strong predictor of adverse outcome in CKD [14]. In our study, patients with partial remission or resistant disease had no reduction of NGAL at follow-up. Future studies will be necessary to determine if the persistent elevation or progressive increase of NGAL during the course of therapy can serve as a useful prognostic marker of disease prognosis independent of residual proteinuria.

This study had several limitations which may have influenced the results. We included various types of glomerular diseases with varying severity of proteinuria and GFR. Patients were not given standardized regimen but were treated by individual physicians according to broad guidelines recommended by KDIGO. These factors may have influenced the numbers of patients achieving remission or the ability of baseline NGAL to predict outcome. However, this unselected group of patients is quite representative of patients with nondiabetic glomerular diseases in our nephrology practice and the results serve further to emphasize the importance of proteinuria on NGAL excretion, although we cannot determine the exact mechanism of this relationship. The follow-up period was quite short so we cannot fully evaluate the predictive value of baseline or posttreatment NGAL levels on long term outcome. This study is small in size so detailed disease specific differences cannot be evaluated.

5. Conclusions

In glomerular diseases, the prevailing level of proteinuria at baseline and at follow-up is a strong determinant of NGAL, whereas tubulointerstitial disease severity and GFR have lesser roles. Patients who achieve complete remission have greater reduction of urine NGAL with follow-up levels being similar to normal subjects. In contrast to the proposed benefit of NGAL in predicting long term outcome in nonproteinuric CKD, baseline NGAL levels may not be a useful biomarker to predict medium-term therapeutic response in proteinuric glomerular diseases with relatively preserved tubulointerstitium. Larger studies with longer follow-up involving patients with a broader spectrum of disease severity will be essential to determine if baseline or posttherapy levels of urine NGAL can provide additional prediction of long term outcome in proteinuric CKD beyond that of residual proteinuria.

Acknowledgments

The authors would like to thank all Nephrology Staff at Ramathibodi Hospital for inclusion of their patients. This study is supported by grants from Faculty of Medicine, Ramathibodi Hospital, and the National Science and Technology Development Agency (NSTDA), Thailand.

References

[1] V. Jha, G. Garcia-Garcia, K. Iseki et al., "Chronic kidney disease: global dimension and perspectives," *The Lancet*, vol. 382, no. 9888, pp. 260–272, 2013.

[2] K. S. Hodgkins and H. W. Schnaper, "Tubulointerstitial injury and the progression of chronic kidney disease," *Pediatric Nephrology*, vol. 27, no. 6, pp. 901–909, 2012.

[3] P. Cravedi and G. Remuzzi, "Pathophysiology of proteinuria and its value as an outcome measure in chronic kidney disease," *British Journal of Clinical Pharmacology*, vol. 76, no. 4, pp. 516–523, 2013.

[4] P. Devarajan, "Neutrophil gelatinase-associated lipocalin: a promising biomarker for human acute kidney injury," *Biomarkers in Medicine*, vol. 4, no. 2, pp. 265–280, 2010.

[5] D. Bolignano, G. Coppolino, A. Lacquaniti, G. Nicocia, and M. Buemi, "Pathological and prognostic value of urinary neutrophil gelatinase-associated lipocalin in macroproteinuric patients with worsening renal function," *Kidney and Blood Pressure Research*, vol. 31, no. 4, pp. 274–279, 2008.

[6] K.-S. Woo, J.-L. Choi, B.-R. Kim, J.-E. Kim, W.-S. An, and J.-Y. Han, "Urinary neutrophil gelatinase-associated lipocalin levels in comparison with glomerular filtration rate for evaluation of renal function in patients with diabetic chronic kidney disease," *Diabetes and Metabolism Journal*, vol. 36, no. 4, pp. 307–313, 2012.

[7] D. Bolignano, G. Coppolino, S. Campo et al., "Neutrophil gelatinase-associated lipocalin in patients with autosomal-dominant polycystic kidney disease," *American Journal of Nephrology*, vol. 27, no. 4, pp. 373–378, 2007.

[8] E. R. Smith, D. Lee, M. M. Cai et al., "Urinary neutrophil gelatinase-associated lipocalin may aid prediction of renal decline in patients with non-proteinuric Stages 3 and 4 chronic kidney disease (CKD)," *Nephrology Dialysis Transplantation*, vol. 28, no. 6, pp. 1569–1579, 2013.

[9] N. A. Bhavsar, A. Köttgen, J. Coresh, and B. C. Astor, "Neutrophil gelatinase-associated lipocalin (NGAL) and kidney injury molecule 1 (KIM-1) as predictors of incident CKD stage 3: the atherosclerosis risk in communities (ARIC) study," *American Journal of Kidney Diseases*, vol. 60, no. 2, pp. 233–240, 2012.

[10] M. R. Bennett, N. Piyaphanee, K. Czech, M. Mitsnefes, and P. Devarajan, "NGAL distinguishes steroid sensitivity in idiopathic nephrotic syndrome," *Pediatric Nephrology*, vol. 27, no. 5, pp. 807–812, 2012.

[11] Kidney Disease: Improving Global Outcomes (KDIGO) Glomerulonephritis Work Group, "KDIGO 2012 clinical practice guideline for glomerulonephritis," *Kidney International Supplements*, vol. 2, pp. 139–274, 2012.

[12] A. Khwaja, "KDIGO clinical practice guidelines for acute kidney injury," *Nephron—Clinical Practice*, vol. 120, no. 4, pp. c179–c184, 2012.

[13] A. S. Levey, L. A. Stevens, C. H. Schmid et al., "A new equation to estimate glomerular filtration rate," *Annals of Internal Medicine*, vol. 150, no. 9, pp. 604–612, 2009.

[14] Kidney Disease: Improving Global Outcomes (KDIGO) CKD Work Group, "KDIGO 2012 clinical practice guideline for the evaluation and management of chronic kidney disease," *Kidney International Supplements*, vol. 3, pp. 1–150, 2013.

[15] E. Singer, L. Markó, N. Paragas et al., "Neutrophil gelatinase-associated lipocalin: pathophysiology and clinical applications," *Acta Physiologica*, vol. 207, no. 4, pp. 663–672, 2013.

[16] J. Mishra, M. A. Qing, A. Prada et al., "Identification of neutrophil gelatinase-associated lipocalin as a novel early urinary biomarker for ischemic renal injury," *Journal of the American Society of Nephrology*, vol. 14, no. 10, pp. 2534–2543, 2003.

[17] Y. Wu, L. Yang, T. Su, C. Wang, G. Liu, and X.-M. Li, "Pathological significance of a panel of urinary biomarkers in patients with drug-induced tubulointerstitial nephritis," *Clinical Journal of the American Society of Nephrology*, vol. 5, no. 11, pp. 1954–1959, 2010.

[18] M. Nishida, H. Kawakatsu, Y. Okumura, and K. Hamaoka, "Serum and urinary neutrophil gelatinase-associated lipocalin levels in children with chronic renal diseases," *Pediatrics International*, vol. 52, no. 4, pp. 563–568, 2010.

[19] H. Ding, Y. He, K. Li et al., "Urinary neutrophil gelatinase-associated lipocalin (NGAL) is an early biomarker for renal tubulointerstitial injury in IgA nephropathy," *Clinical Immunology*, vol. 123, no. 2, pp. 227–234, 2007.

[20] A. Hammad, Y. Mosaad, S. Elhanbly et al., "Urinary neutrophil gelatinase-associated lipocalin as a marker of severe lupus nephritis in children," *Lupus*, vol. 22, no. 5, pp. 486–491, 2013.

[21] T. Kuwabara, K. Mori, M. Mukoyama et al., "Urinary neutrophil gelatinase-associated lipocalin levels reflect damage to glomeruli, proximal tubules, and distal nephrons," *Kidney International*, vol. 75, no. 3, pp. 285–294, 2009.

[22] D. Bolignano, V. Donato, G. Coppolino et al., "Neutrophil Gelatinase-Associated Lipocalin (NGAL) as a marker of kidney damage," *American Journal of Kidney Diseases*, vol. 52, no. 3, pp. 595–605, 2008.

[23] J. A. Gwira, F. Wei, S. Ishibe, J. M. Ueland, J. Barasch, and L. G. Cantley, "Expression of neutrophil gelatinase-associated lipocalin regulates epithelial morphogenesis in vitro," *The Journal of Biological Chemistry*, vol. 280, no. 9, pp. 7875–7882, 2005.

[24] T. L. Nickolas, C. S. Forster, M. E. Sise et al., "NGAL (Lcn2) monomer is associated with tubulointerstitial damage in chronic kidney disease," *Kidney International*, vol. 82, no. 6, pp. 718–722, 2012.

[25] M. B. Tavares, M. D. C. C. D. Almeida, R. T. C. Martins, A. C. G. P. De Sousa, R. Martinelli, and W. L. C. Dos-Santos, "Acute tubular necrosis and renal failure in patients with glomerular disease," *Renal Failure*, vol. 34, no. 10, pp. 1252–1257, 2012.

[26] D. Bolignano, A. Lacquaniti, G. Coppolino et al., "Neutrophil gelatinase-associated lipocalin (NGAL) and progression of chronic kidney disease," *Clinical Journal of the American Society of Nephrology*, vol. 4, no. 2, pp. 337–344, 2009.

[27] Y. E. Chen, S. M. Korbet, R. S. Katz, M. M. Schwartz, E. J. Lewis, and Collaborative Study Group, "Value of a complete or partial remission in severe lupus nephritis," *Clinical Journal of the American Society of Nephrology*, vol. 3, no. 1, pp. 46–53, 2008.

31

The Urinary Phosphate to Serum Fibroblast Growth Factor 23 Ratio, Deemed the Nephron Index, Is a Useful Clinical Index for Early Stage Chronic Kidney Disease in Patients with Type 2 Diabetes: An Observational Pilot Study

Hodaka Yamada ⓘ,[1] **Makoto Kuro-o** ⓘ,[2] **Shunsuke Funazaki** ⓘ,[1] **San-e Ishikawa**,[3] **Masafumi Kakei**,[1] and **Kazuo Hara**[1]

[1]*Department of Medicine, Division of Endocrinology and Metabolism, Jichi Medical University Saitama Medical Center, 1-847 Amanuma-cho, Omiya-ku, Saitama 330-8503, Japan*
[2]*Center for Molecular Medicine, Jichi Medical University, 3311-1 Yakushiji Shimotsuke, Tochigi 329-0498, Japan*
[3]*Division of Endocrinology and Metabolism, International University of Health and Welfare Hospital, 537-3 Iguchi, Nasushiobara, Tochigi 329-2763, Japan*

Correspondence should be addressed to Hodaka Yamada; hyamada0510@jichi.ac.jp

Academic Editor: Anil K. Agarwal

Renal function decline is associated with progressive type 2 diabetes mellitus, which causes mineral and bone disorders. In the present study, we defined the ratio of urinary phosphate excretion (mg/day) to serum fibroblast growth factor 23 as the nephron index. We examined changes in the nephron index in type 2 diabetes patients with early stage chronic kidney disease (stages 1–3), enrolling 15 patients and retrospectively analysing the follow-up data. After follow-up at 5.4 years, we observed no significant changes in the estimated glomerular filtration rate; the nephron index, however, was significantly reduced between the baseline and the follow-up. We propose that the nephron index may be potentially useful as a biomarker for monitoring the decline of renal function in the early stages of diabetic chronic kidney disease patients.

1. Introduction

Several biomarkers relevant to bone and mineral metabolism in chronic kidney disease (CKD)—for which type 2 diabetes mellitus (T2DM) is an important risk—are associated with cardiovascular complications. Among them, serum levels of fibroblast growth factor 23 (FGF23) have been identified, from as early as stage 2 CKD, as one of the earliest biomarkers that start increasing, and correlate with cardiac hypertrophy, heart failure, and all-cause mortality [1, 2].

Following phosphate intake, the bone secretes the peptide hormone FGF23, which acts on the kidney to induce urinary phosphate excretion, thereby maintaining the phosphate balance. However, for several hours after oral phosphate administration, T2DM patients reportedly showed higher serum phosphate and lower serum FGF23 levels than non-diabetes patients, even when there was no difference in their renal function [3]. The measurement of serum FGF23 levels alone—as suggested by these results—may not be sufficient for the early detection of renal dysfunction in CKD patients with differing pathogeneses.

FGF23 exerts phosphaturic activity through its ability to suppress phosphate resorption in the renal proximal tubule. FGF23 is thus thought to correlate with phosphate excretion per nephron. Namely,

$$phosphate\ excretion\ per\ nephron$$
$$= \frac{urinary\ phosphate\ excretion}{nephron\ number} \propto FGF23 \tag{1}$$

$$\therefore nephron\ number \propto \frac{urinary\ phosphate\ excretion}{FGF23} \tag{2}$$

$$\equiv nephron index$$

We hypothesise the ratio of urinary phosphate excretion (mg/day) to serum FGF23 to serve as an index correlating with the nephron number, which we define as the nephron index [4, 5].

In a recent cross-sectional study, we reported the nephron index to be decreased in T2DM patients with stages 1–3 CKD and associated with macrovascular complications [6]. In the present pilot study, during longitudinal follow-up, we examined changes in the nephron index in T2DM patients.

2. Material and Methods

We enrolled 18 patients with T2DM who had been admitted twice to Jichi Medical University Saitama Medical Center for diabetes control between October 2006 and January 2017 depending on the 2-week diabetes education program. The 24-hour urine collections were performed 10 days after the hospitalization. All the patients had an estimated glomerular filtration rate (eGFR) greater than 45 mL/min/1.73 m^2. Because 3 patients had incomplete urine collection records, we did not consider them for this study, and finally we analysed the present data for 15 patients (CKD categories, number of patients: G1, 4; G2, 8; G3a, 3; A1, 11; and A2, 4). Daily phosphate intake had been managed between 600 and 700 mg/day by a nutritionist. We used fasting blood samples to measure 24 h urinary phosphate excretion (mg/day) and other mineral and metabolic parameters. We collected the clinical parameters based on medical records and laboratory data. Intact FGF23 had been measured using an enzyme-linked immunosorbent assay (ELISA) (Kainos, Tokyo, Japan) in our previous study [6]. We compared the parameters from baseline (the first admission) with those after follow-up (the second admission). Other variables had been measured at a central laboratory section of the Jichi Medical University Saitama Medical Center. Renal function was determined with calculation of eGFR using the modification of diet in renal disease equation revised for the Japanese population by the Japanese Society of Nephrology as follows: eGFR (mL/min/1.73 m^2) = 194 × serum creatinine (mg/dL)$^{-1.094}$ × age$^{-0.287}$ × 0.739 (if female). Baseline and follow-up eGFR was calculated by blood test for each hospitalization. We compared the data relating to the two dates using a paired t test. Data are expressed as the mean ± standard deviation or median with interquartile range. We considered a p value < 0.05 to be statistically significant. We performed all analyses using EZR (Saitama Medical Center, Jichi Medical University), a graphical user interface for R (the R Foundation for Statistical Computing, ver. 2.13.0) and a modified version of the R Commander (ver. 1.6-3), with additional frequently used biostatistical functions [7].

This study was approved by the Ethics Committee at Jichi Medical University Saitama Medical Center (No. S17-007) and performed in compliance with the Declaration of Helsinki.

3. Results

The average age and follow-up period were 64 ± 8 and 5.4 ± 2.9 years, respectively (Table 1). We observed no significant

TABLE 1: Baseline characteristics of patients.

Variables and parameters	Baseline
Age (years)	64 ± 8
Sex, male (%)	4 (27)
BMI (kg/m^2)	26.5 ± 3.3
Duration of diabetes (years)	11 ± 6.2
Diabetic retinopathy, n (%)	9 (60)
Dyslipidemia, n (%)	14 (93)
Hypertension, n (%)	10 (67)
HbA1c (%)	10.3 ± 2.2
HbA1c (mmol/L)	89 ± 24.5
BUN (mg/dL)	14 ± 3.1
Cr (mg/dL)	0.59 [0.50–0.74]
eGFR (mL/min/1.73 m^2)	83 ± 24
Serum magnesium (mg/dL)	1.9 [1.75–2.00]
Serum phosphate (mg/dL)	3.5 ± 0.60
Creatinine clearance (mL/min)	77 ± 23
Urinary albumin excretion (mg/day)	11 (7.9–34)
Urinary phosphate excretion (mg/day)	511 ± 176

Data are expressed as means ± standard deviation (SD), and skewed variables are described as medians with an interquartile range. BMI, body mass index; HbA1c, glycated haemoglobin; BUN, blood urea nitrogen; Cr, creatinine; eGFR, estimated glomerular filtration rate.

changes in the eGFR at the baseline and at the follow-up (83 ± 24 mL/min/1.73 m^2 and 75 ± 25 mL/min/1.73 m^2, p = 0.082). However, we found a significant reduction in the nephron index from 13.7 ± 6.5 to 9.1 ± 4.6 (p = 0.001) and a significant elevation in the serum FGF23 from 43.3 ± 18.2 to 55.0 ± 20.8 ng/mL (p = 0.022). We did not find any change in fractional excretion of phosphate (FEP) (%) after the follow-up (21 ± 12% and 19 ± 9.0%, p = 0.211) (Figure 1) and in serum phosphate and calcium levels (data not shown). In addition, there was no significant change in the measured GFR (Ccr: creatinine clearance) between the baseline and the follow-up period (77.0 ± 22.9 mL/min and 73.8 ± 22.8 mL/min, p = 0.1999). The eGFR decline slope was −1.11 ± 2.64 mL/min/1.73 m^2/year. During the follow-up, there were no cardiovascular events.

4. Discussion

In this retrospective observational study, we detected the decline in renal function during the ~5-year follow-up period using the nephron index, but not the eGFR. We propose that the nephron index may potentially be useful as a biomarker for monitoring the decline of renal function in the early stages of diabetic CKD patients.

Because the hormone FGF23 increases phosphate excretion per nephron, it is thought to correlate with FEP, which is defined as the ratio of phosphate clearance (= $(Up \times V)/Pp$) to creatinine clearance (= $(Ucr \times V)/Pcr$).

$$FEP = \frac{(Up \times V)/Pp}{(Ucr \times V)/Pcr} = \frac{Up \times V}{Ccr \times Pp} \quad (3)$$

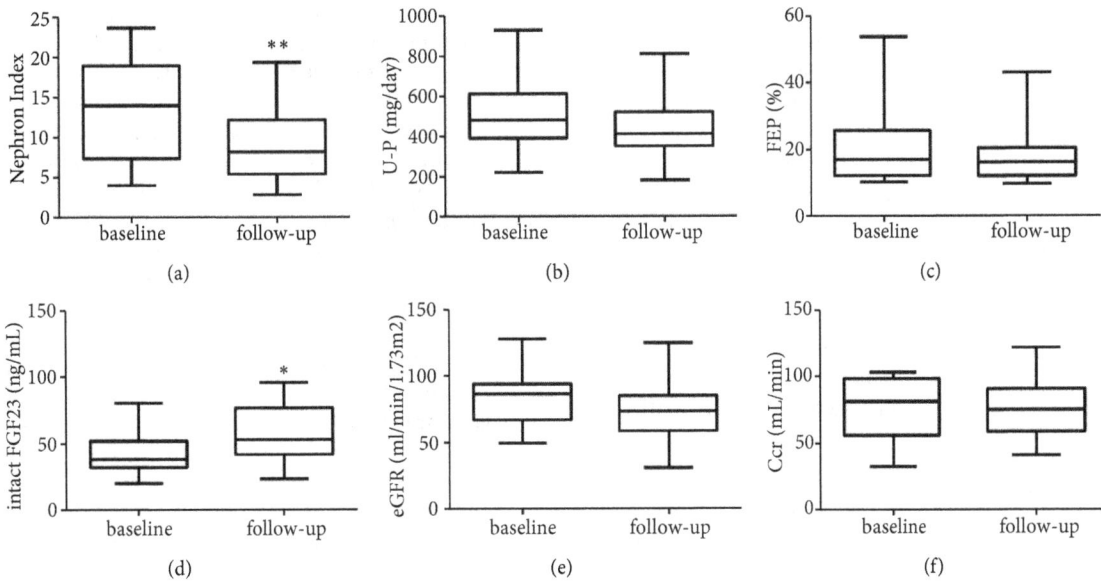

FIGURE 1: Comparisons of nephron index (a), daily (24 h) urinary phosphate excretion (U-P) (b), fractional excretion of phosphate (FEP) (c), serum intact FGF23 (d), estimated glomerular filtration rate (eGFR) (e), and creatinine clearance (Ccr) (f) between baseline and time after follow-up in the patients with type 2 diabetes. $*p < 0.05$ vs. baseline, $**p < 0.01$ vs. baseline.

where Up is urinary phosphate concentration, V is urine volume (24 h), Pp is serum phosphate concentration, Ucr is urinary creatinine concentration, Pcr is serum creatinine concentration, and Ccr is creatinine clearance.

Higher serum FGF23 levels are, in fact, associated with higher FEP. However, in early to moderate CKD, some patients have a lower FEP than others with the same serum FGF23 level, suggesting the variability among individuals in renal sensitivity to FGF23. Those considered resistant to FGF23 because they exhibit low FEP relative to high FGF23 are associated with poor clinical outcomes [8]. In the present study, we found no change in FEP after follow-up. These results suggested the importance of considering not only FEP but also other mineral metabolic parameters in the early stages of CKD. The ratio of FEP to FGF23 may thus be regarded as a parameter of renal sensitivity to FGF23. From (2),

$$Up \times V = nephron\ index \times FGF23 \qquad (4)$$

and substitute $nephron\ index \times FGF23$ for $Up \times V$ in (3):

$$FEP = \frac{nephron\ index \times FGF23}{Ccr \times Pp} \qquad (5)$$

$$\therefore \frac{FEP}{FGF23} = nephron\ index \times \frac{1}{Ccr \times Pp} \qquad (6)$$

Equation (6) indicates that the renal sensitivity to FGF23 (the ratio of FEP to FGF23) correlates with the nephron number when the renal function (Ccr) and serum phosphate levels (Pp) are constant. In other words, CKD patients with reduced renal sensitivity to FGF23—probably because their residual nephron number is low—are associated with poor clinical outcomes. However, one report of moderately

progressed CKD patients during 5-year follow-up found that FEP did not modify the relation between FGF23 and renal and vascular outcome [9]. In another study, a low FEP/FGF23 ratio was associated with the severity of aortic calcification in CKD stages 3–4 patients [10]. Contrastingly, Haruhara et al. revealed that the glomerular density (the number of glomeruli per total renal cortical area) evaluated by renal biopsy specimens was decreased in patients with hypertensive nephrosclerosis with a preserved eGFR compared with that in kidney transplant donors [11]. This result suggested that even if eGFR was preserved, low glomerular density is an important characteristic in hypertensive patients. Particularly, diabetic kidneys presented both glomerular changes and tubular injury before microalbuminuria or macroalbuminuria [12, 13]. We consider that diabetes decreases the number of nephrons, even when eGFR is preserved and impairs renal sensitivity to FGF23. FGF23 elevation in early CKD is an adaptive response to maintain phosphate metabolism by its phosphaturic action. Simultaneously the expression of α-klotho, a coreceptor for FGF23, is reduced in the kidney, leading to FGF23 hyporesponsiveness, namely, FGF23 resistance in kidney [4, 5]. Nephron index could be a novel early CKD marker and useful index for estimating FGF23 resistance in kidney.

There were some limitations of the present study. The first limitation of our study is its small number and retrospective observational nature. Large-size, prospective studies are necessary to verify whether the nephron index is a useful predictor of the decline of CKD. Second, we could not examine the pathological analysis by using human kidney specimen. Pathological examination is necessary to validate whether nephron index reflects exact nephron numbers. Finally, we enrolled only uncontrolled type 2 diabetic patients who had undergone a second admission for diabetes control. In that sense, the participants of this study were highly selected, and the follow-up period was limited. Moreover, it will be necessary to compare the present results of nephron index with those in other renal diseases, such as glomerular diseases.

In summary, the nephron index—defined as the ratio of urinary phosphate excretion to serum FGF23—holds promise as an indicator for clinical outcomes among CKD patients with similar renal function and as a noninvasive estimation of the residual nephron number. We might estimate residual nephron number by using nephron index and nephron index could be an early intervention target for CKD patients with type 2 diabetes. Further prospective and interventional studies using the nephron index are essential to establish its usefulness in the management of CKD patients.

Acknowledgments

The authors thank Taeko Otani for the assistance with the ELISA technique. Makoto Kuro-o was supported by research grants from AMED-CREST, JST, MEXT-Supported Program for the Strategic Research Foundation at Private Universities, and Vehicle Racing Commemorative Foundation. This research was supported by a grant from the Kidney Foundation, Japan (JKFB17-18), to Hodaka Yamada. The authors would like to acknowledge Enago (www.enago.jp) for the English language review.

References

[1] T. Isakova, P. Wahl, G. S. Vargas et al., "Fibroblast growth factor 23 is elevated before parathyroid hormone and phosphate in chronic kidney disease," *Kidney International*, vol. 79, no. 12, pp. 1370–1378, 2011.

[2] L. Salanova Villanueva, C. Sánchez González, J. A. Sánchez Tomero, A. Aguilera, and E. Ortega Junco, "Bone mineral disorder in chronic kidney disease: Klotho and FGF23; cardiovascular implications," *Nefrología*, vol. 36, no. 4, pp. 368–375, 2016.

[3] K. Yoda, Y. Imanishi, M. Yoda et al., "Impaired response of FGF-23 to oral phosphate in patients with type 2 diabetes: A possible mechanism of atherosclerosis," *The Journal of Clinical Endocrinology & Metabolism*, vol. 97, no. 11, pp. E2036–E2043, 2012.

[4] M. Kuro-O, "A phosphate-centric paradigm for pathophysiology and therapy of chronic kidney disease," *Kidney International Supplements*, vol. 3, no. 5, pp. 420–426, 2013.

[5] M. Kuro-o, "Klotho, phosphate and FGF-23 in ageing and disturbed mineral metabolism," *Nature Reviews Nephrology*, vol. 9, no. 11, pp. 650–660, 2013.

[6] H. Yamada, M. Kuro-o, K. Hara et al., "The urinary phosphate to serum fibroblast growth factor 23 ratio is a useful marker of atherosclerosis in early-stage chronic kidney disease," *PLoS ONE*, vol. 11, no. 8, Article ID e0160782, 2016.

[7] Y. Kanda, "Investigation of the freely available easy-to-use software "EZR" for medical statistics," *Bone Marrow Transplantation*, vol. 48, no. 3, pp. 452–458, 2013.

[8] J. R. Dominguez, M. G. Shlipak, M. A. Whooley, and J. H. Ix, "Fractional excretion of phosphorus modifies the association between fibroblast growth factor-23 and outcomes," *Journal of the American Society of Nephrology*, vol. 24, no. 4, pp. 647–654, 2013.

[9] A. P. Bech, A. Bouma-de Krijger, A. D. van Zuilen et al., "Impact of fractional phosphate excretion on the relation of FGF23 with outcome in CKD patients," *Journal of Nephrology*, vol. 28, no. 4, pp. 477–484, 2015.

[10] L. Craver, A. Dusso, M. Martinez-Alonso, F. Sarro, J. M. Valdivielso, and E. Fernández, "A low fractional excretion of Phosphate/Fgf23 ratio is associated with severe abdominal Aortic calcification in stage 3 and 4 kidney disease patients," *BMC Nephrology*, vol. 14, 221 pages, 2013.

[11] K. Haruhara, N. Tsuboi, G. Kanzaki et al., "Glomerular Density in Biopsy-Proven Hypertensive Nephrosclerosis," *American Journal of Hypertension*, vol. 28, no. 9, pp. 1164–1171, 2015.

[12] E. I. Ekinci, G. Jerums, A. Skene et al., "Renal structure in normoalbuminuric and albuminuric patients with type 2 diabetes and impaired renal function," *Diabetes Care*, vol. 36, no. 11, pp. 3620–3626, 2013.

[13] V. S. Vaidya, M. A. Niewczas, L. H. Ficociello et al., "Regression of microalbuminuria in type 1 diabetes is associated with lower levels of urinary tubular injury biomarkers, kidney injury molecule-1, and N-acetyl-β-D-glucosaminidase," *Kidney International*, vol. 79, no. 4, pp. 464–470, 2011.

32

Acute Kidney Injury and Atypical Features during Pediatric Poststreptococcal Glomerulonephritis

Rose M. Ayoob and Andrew L. Schwaderer

Division of Nephrology, Department of Pediatrics, Nationwide Children's Hospital, Columbus, OH, USA

Correspondence should be addressed to Andrew L. Schwaderer; andrew.schwaderer@nationwidechildrens.org

Academic Editor: Frank Park

The most common acute glomerulonephritis in children is poststreptococcal glomerulonephritis (PSGN) usually occurring between 3 and 12 years old. Hypertension and gross hematuria are common presenting symptoms. Most PSGN patients do not experience complications, but rapidly progressive glomerulonephritis and hypertensive encephalopathy have been reported. This paper reports 17 patients seen in 1 year for PSGN including 4 with atypical PSGN, at a pediatric tertiary care center. Seventeen children (11 males), mean age of 8 years, were analyzed. Ninety-four percent had elevated serum BUN levels and decreased GFR. Four of the hospitalized patients had complex presentations that included AKI along with positive ANA or ANCAs. Three patients required renal replacement therapy and two were thrombocytopenic. PSGN usually does not occur as a severe nephritis. Over the 12-month study period, 17 cases associated with low serum albumin in 53%, acute kidney injury in 94%, and thrombocytopenia in 18% were treated. The presentation of PSGN may be severe and in a small subset have associations similar to SLE nephritis findings including AKI, positive ANA, and hematological anomalies.

1. Introduction

The most common form of acute glomerulonephritis in children is poststreptococcal glomerulonephritis (PSGN) which usually occurs between 3 and 12 years old. PSGN occurs following infection with a nephritogenic strain of group A *Streptococcus* (GAS) in around 15% of cases [1]. PSGN is now recognized to be a immunologically mediated, nonsupporative complication of GAS [2]. Gross hematuria is present in 30–70% of patients while microscopic hematuria is present in all patients and hypertension occurs in 70% of patients requiring hospitalization [1]. Severe PSGN complications, hypertensive encephalopathy, and rapidly progressing glomerulonephritis occur in <10% and 1% of children hospitalized for PSGN, respectively [1]. The diagnosis is likely when hypocomplementemia is present during an acute glomerulonephritis and improves spontaneously within a few months [2]. Here we report a case series of severe PSGN cases seen at a pediatric tertiary care center over one year.

2. Methods

2.1. Study Type. One-year case series of children referred to a children's tertiary care hospital for PSGN.

2.2. Patients. After obtaining IRB approval (IRB09-00444), children seen with PSGN at Nationwide Children's Hospital (NCH) in Columbus, Ohio, between July 1, 2010, and June 30, 2011, were identified. Children between the ages of 3–18 years diagnosed with acute PSGN (ICD-9 code 580.0) seen in both inpatient and outpatient settings were identified. All patients included had hematuria based on urine dipstick, low serum complement (C3) that subsequently returned to normal within 3 months, and laboratory documentation of a streptococcal infection or household contact with a streptococcal infection. Patients with clinical or histological evidence of other underlying renal diseases were excluded.

2.3. Data Collection. Data obtained from medical records included age, sex, height, and weight as well as clinical course and complications. Labs recorded included complete blood counts, serum chemistries, and any additional serology or immunology collected at diagnosis or the following 4 months. For all patients, estimated glomerular filtration rate (eGFR) was calculated with the 2009 Schwartz formula [9].

2.4. Culture Isolates. Culture isolates were collected and transported to the Center for Disease Control and Prevention (CDC) Streptococcal Research Laboratory. The sample from *Patient 12* was collected from a throat culture and *Patient B* from fluid drained from a peritonsillar abscess. At the CDC, specimens were *emm* typed by sequencing polymerase chain reaction products [10]. Subtypes were assigned according to the CDC *emm* sequence database [11].

2.5. Renal Pathology. Percutaneous renal biopsies under ultrasound guidance were performed in 4 of the patients with unusual presentations or more severe disease. Specimens were fixed and embedded in paraffin using standard procedures and sections 1-2 μm in thickness were stained with haematoxylin-eosin (HE), periodic acid-Schiff (PAS), Jones methenamine silver, and Masson's trichrome for pathologist examination under light microscopy. Immunofluorescence studies were performed for IgG, IgA, IgM, C1q, C3, and C4 antibodies and electron microscopy was performed on Epon embedded tissue stained with uranyl acetate and lead citrate.

2.6. Statistical Analysis. Descriptive statistics were reported as mean ± standard deviation for normally distributed data. Binomial variables were compared with a Fischer exact test if expected cell frequencies were less than 5; otherwise the Chi-square test was used. Continuous variables were evaluated by Student's *t*-test and considered significant for $P < 0.05$.

3. Results

3.1. Patient Demographics. After review of inpatient and outpatient records, 17 patients met inclusion criteria (Table 1). The mean age of included patients was 8 years and 65% (11/17) were male. Seventy-one percent (12/17) of the children presented between November and April and 88% (15/17) were Caucasian. All of the children examined had a current or preceding pharyngitis but none had a documented skin infection.

3.2. BP and Urine Lab Findings. Presentation and follow-up of BP and urine findings are presented in Table 2. A systolic and/or diastolic blood pressure (BP) ≥95th% tile for age, height, and sex at the time of presentation was noted in 88% (15/17) of patients and persisted into follow-up in 3 patients. All patients had hematuria.

3.3. Serum Lab Findings. Serum lab findings are presented in Table 3. All patients had C3 <80 mg/dL that normalized on follow-up. The mean nadir eGFR was 44.5 ± 22.9 mL/min/1.73 m^2 that improved to 105 ± 19.4 on follow-up, although 18% (3/17) had eGFR that remained <80 on follow-up. Fifty-three percent (9/17) had serum albumin levels ≤3 g/dL.

TABLE 1: Patient demographics.

Patient	Sex	Age (yr)	f/u time (yr)
1	M	6	<1
2	M	7	<1
3	M	8	1
4	F	15	1
5	F	6	<1
6	M	6	<1
7	M	7	0
8	F	8	2
9	M	6	<1
10	M	8	5
11	F	6	1
12	M	12	1
13	M	11	<1
14	F	11	<1
15	F	5	<1
16	M	7	<1
17	M	10	<1

TABLE 2: BP and urine findings during acute PSGN and at follow-up.

Patient	BP (mmHg)		BP%$^\wedge$		Urine heme/RBCs per HPF	
	Initial	f/u	Initial	f/u	Initial	f/u
1	116/76		95	NA	409	79
2	90/60	111/67	50	90	44	Large
3	119/86	107/69	95	95	1011	Trace
4	173/123	126/68	99	90	LRG	Large
5	119/72	107/65	99	90	LRG	28
6	109/74	109/74	90	90	401	Large
7	81/59	89/60	50	25	236	Trace
8	123/66	100/60	99	50	266	Neg
9	138/80	113/62	99	90	776	Large
10	118/73	118/65	95	75	307	Neg
11	114/76	95/60	95	75	1481	Neg
12	141/73	113/63	99	80	573	Neg
13	137/83	128/69	99	96	99	Large
14	131/92	104/67	99	50	247	15
15	149/106	104/70	99	85	LRG	Mod
16	127/53	113/59	99	89	117	Mod
17	136/74	116/65	99	95	23	Small

NA: not available; $^\wedge$BP% by age, height, and gender.

Additionally sixty-five percent (11/17) of the patients had hemoglobin levels <11 g/dL and 18% (3/17) presented with thrombocytopenia.

TABLE 3: Serum lab results during acute PSGN and at follow-up.

Patient	Creatine (mg/dL)		eGFR (mL/min/1.73 m^2)		BUN		Albumin		C3 (mg/dL)	
	Peak	f/u	Nadir	f/u	Peak	f/u	Peak	f/u	Initial	f/u
1	0.91	0.55	56	93	28	16	3.3	4.6	11	90
2	0.64	0.55	83	96	20	NA	3.8	3.8	42	97
3	7.03	0.56	8	104	120	21	2.6	4.4	29	110
4	1.39	0.87	48	75	36	15	3.2	3.7	17	127
5	0.8	NA	56	NA	18	NA	3.2	NA	15	123
6	0.7	0.45	74	115	22	NA	3.9	NA	20	137
7	0.67	0.48	73	102	26	8	2.6	NA	27	91
8	2.45	0.49	22	115	52	12	2.4	4.2	9	123
9	0.99	0.46	52	110	29	12	3.1	4.7	40	168
10	10.4	0.97	6	69	208	22	2.2	4.1	30	119
11	3.51	0.39	14	136	93	13	3.1	4.1	25	120
12	3.62	0.45	16	130	91	NA	2.5	4	7	123
13	1.64	0.58	40	114	82	13	2.8	4.4	6	139
14	1.8	0.78	36	75	92	14	3.1	NA	15	93
15	0.73	0.45	64	101	26	13	3.1	NA	12	125
16	3.43	0.45	16	119	105	12	NA	NA	11	93
17	1.29	0.48	48	128	46	21	4	4	21	114

NA: not available.

TABLE 4: Patients with atypical PSGN.

Pt	eGFR	BUN initial : peak	K$^+$ initial : peak	% fluid overload	BP initial : peak	RRT indication	% crescents	Serology	Atypical findings
3	10	113 : 120	5.6 : 5.6	10.8	119/86 : 145/106	AKI, fluid overload, anuria	66%	ANA +1 : 160	Thrombocytopenia
10	6	208 : 208	6.1 : 6.1	1.9	118/73 : 131/85	AKI, hyperK$^+$	85%	ANA +1 : 80	Seizures
11	18	36 : 93	4.7 : 6.6	7.5	114/76 : 131/70	No RRT, hyperK$^+$, HTN responded to medical management	30%	cANCA +1 : 20	Mental status changes, neck mass
12	24	64 : 91	4.0 : 5.8	12	141/73 : 159/106	AKI, HTN urgency	None	ANA +1 : 160	Thrombocytopenia

4. Atypical PSGN

Of the 13 patients hospitalized, 4 patients underwent renal biopsy due to concern for rapidly progressive glomerulonephritis. Additional serologic abnormalities were also found in these patients. Patients 3, 10, and 12 had positive antinuclear antibody (ANA) tests but negative *Crithidia* and each required renal replacement therapy (RRT) during their hospitalization (Table 4). Renal replacement therapy was performed on 3 patients and consisted of acute hemodialysis for the indications of fluid overload and/or uremia. The thrombocytopenia, when present, was not severe, with nadirs of 95 and 51 K/mm^3 for patients 3 and 12, respectively. Patient 11 did not require RRT but did test positive for cytoplasmic anti-neutrophil cytoplasmic antibody (c-ANCA). All

ANCA testing mentioned in this case series was performed by indirect immunofluorescence at the Ohio State Wexner Medical Center Laboratories. Patient 10 had new onset seizures of undetermined etiology. The glomeruli in all the biopsies showed diffuse proliferative glomerulonephritis with prominent infiltration of neutrophils and cellular crescents were found in 3 of the biopsies (Table 4). The throat culture collected from *Patient D* had GAS strain that was T nontypeable, M protein gene subtype 44.0 (*emm* 44.0). *Patient B*'s GAS strain from the fluid drained from a peritonsillar abscess was T type 2, *emm* 2.0.

4.1. Comparison to Past Studies. Comparison to past studies are presented in Table 5. In general our cohort appears to

TABLE 5: Comparison of study patients with historical studies in poststreptococcal glomerulonephritis.

Parameter	Study patients	Historical studies	P value
BUN > 20 mg/dL	16/17 (94%)	18/45 (40%) [3]	*<0.001
		48/138 (35%) [4]	*<0.001
		21/35 (60%) [5]	*0.01
		36/46 (78%) [6]	0.26
eGFR < 80 mL/min/1.73 m^2	16/17 (94%)	14/32 (44%) [7]	*0.002
		14/29 (48%) [8]	*0.004
Hypertensive complications	7/17 (41%)	13/50 (26%) [7]	0.38
		10/35 (28%) [5]	0.55

* refers to statistical significance.

be more likely to have elevated BUN and lower GFR while hypertensive complications were similar.

5. Discussion

Our study was comparable to historical references with respect to presenting symptoms and mean age of presentation [2]. With respect to acute changes in renal function, our cohort noted higher BUN values and lower eGFR values. In the current study, 76% (13/17) of children had BUN >20 mg/dL and 94% (16/17) had eGFR <80 mL/min/1.73 m^2 with the mean eGFR 45 mL/min/1.73 m^2. Our patients also had more hypertensive complications.

A previous pediatric study of 153 children with PSGN reported that more than 50% of patients had hemoglobin ≤11 g/dL [12]. In our study, 52% (11/16) had levels at or below 11 g/dL. Significantly lower mean platelet levels were found compared to patients treated as outpatients in our study. Thrombocytopenia has only been associated with PSGN in a few case reports. The triad of hemolytic anemia, thrombocytopenia, and acute kidney injury occurred in a 13-year-old African American boy with a high ASO and low C3 [13]. A four-year-old Japanese boy was reported to have a low C3, "mild glomerulonephritis," a negative throat culture and thrombocytopenia with platelet antigen-specific Fab fragment autoantibodies [14]. None of the patients in our series had elevated LDH or haptoglobin levels to suggest a hemolytic process. The anemia and/or thrombocytopenia created a diagnostic dilemma particularly when combined with a positive ANA titer or ANCA antibodies as the possibility of an underlying autoimmune or vasculitic process. Recent studies have indicated a higher rate of severe glomerulonephritis [15, 16]. Because the thrombocytopenia resolved around the same time as the nephritis, the patients with low platelets in our case series were not tested for thrombotic microangiopathies so we cannot rule out that underlying complement disorders may have been present. In the aforementioned publications from New Zealand, AKI was present in 67% of patients. Interestingly patients of Pacific Island and Maori descent were disproportionately affected and those of European descent were spared.

Streptococcus pyogenes, a beta-hemolytic bacterium of the Lancefield serogroup A, is also referred to as group A streptococci. Group A streptococci are usually typed based

on their surface M proteins which function as virulence factors [17]. The common pharyngitis associated nephritogenic strains include M types 1, 4, and 25 and some M12 strains [2]. Over the last 40 years in the United States, an apparent decline in the incidence of PSGN is assumed to be due to the near eradication of streptococcal pyoderma due to improved hygiene and/or decreased prevalence of skin infection associated nephritogenic M serotypes [18]. Virtually no epidemiologic data, however, has been published on the M serotypes since the near disappearance of pyoderma associated PSGN in developed countries. We were unable to find prior reports of the *emm* 44 subtype found in *Patient D*.

Certain factors have been associated with susceptibility to and severity of PSGN. For instance, low birth weights and high BMIs were reported to be associated with increased albuminuria in the Australian aboriginal population which experiences high rates of PSGN [19]. Early life risk factors were not included in our analysis which may be important considerations to identify PSGN patients at risk for complications. A recent case series reported a high rate of AKI in children of Maori or Pacific Islander ancestry with children of European ancestry relatively spared; however GFR was not calculated or BUN presented so direct comparison to our study is not possible [15]. According to the United States 2010 Census, the race/ethnicity demographics of the Columbus, Ohio metropolitan area, is approximately 61.5% non-Hispanic Caucasian, 28% African American, 4% Asian, 5.6% Hispanic, and 0.4% Native American or Pacific Islander. Because the mean GFR ± SD in our series was 45 ± 23 mL/min/1.73 m^2, our results highlight that children in the United States population may also frequently experience AKI during PSGN. The role of race or ethnicity in PSGN susceptibility remains an area for future investigation.

The PSGN patients in our series who had positive ANA or ANCA titers had particularly severe courses which often included the need for acute hemodialysis. On review of the literature a cluster of severe postinfectious glomerulonephritis cases was reported in Brazil following outbreak caused by group C *Streptococcus zooepidemicus* [20]. The frequency of severe PSGN over time from group A organisms has not been studied to our knowledge; however other populations did report the association between severe PSGN and increased ANCA levels [21].

The study is limited by potential selection bias. We cannot exclude that mild cases of PSGN were cared for by community primary care providers or outside hospitals. This study was also limited by the absence of 24-hour urines to quantify proteinuria in the setting of AKI and our inability to obtain race, ethnicity, gestational age at birth, and birth weights in our medical records.

In the current era, no epidemiologic studies have been published on M types in PSGN. Different strains and virulence factors may be the cause of more severe disease seen in the past. It is not known whether the increased rate of severe PSGN will be isolated to the reported year. We submit that the relevance of the described cohort to PSGN patients includes that PSGN should be considered in cases of severe nephritis even when the presentation is consistent with other types of nephritis. Additionally thrombocytopenia may be associated with PSGN; however it is not clear if the PSGN alone is causative. Testing for thrombotic microangiopathies may be a consideration for future patients with both PSGN and low platelets. Additionally determination of M serotype of organisms resulting in severe PSGN may be helpful in determining if a severe clinical course is based on the infecting organism or underlying patient characteristics.

Acknowledgments

The authors are grateful to Bernard Beall, Centers for Disease Control and Prevention, Atlanta, GA, for expert technical assistance in providing *emm* typing data. The authors also would like to thank Mario J. Marcon, Director of the Clinical/Molecular Microbiology, Virology, Immunoserology Department at Nationwide Children's Hospital, Columbus, OH, for his work on the culture isolates.

References

[1] V. Tasic, "Postinfectious glomerulonephritis," in *Comprehensive Pediatric Nephrology*, F. Geary DaS, Ed., pp. 309–319, Mosby Elsevier, Philadelphia, Pa, USA, 2008.

[2] T. M. Eison, B. H. Ault, D. P. Jones, R. W. Chesney, and R. J. Wyatt, "Post-streptococcal acute glomerulonephritis in children: clinical features and pathogenesis," *Pediatric Nephrology*, vol. 26, no. 2, pp. 165–180, 2011.

[3] M. Ilyas and A. Tolaymat, "Changing epidemiology of acute post-streptococcal glomerulonephritis in Northeast Florida: a comparative study," *Pediatric Nephrology*, vol. 23, no. 7, pp. 1101–1106, 2008.

[4] T. Kasahara, H. Hayakawa, S. Okubo et al., "Prognosis of acute poststreptococcal glomerulonephritis (APSGN) is excellent in children, when adequately diagnosed," *Pediatrics International*, vol. 43, no. 4, pp. 364–367, 2001.

[5] S. Roy III, J. A. pitcock, and J. N. Etteldorf, "Prognosis of acute poststreptococcal glomerulonephritis in childhood: prospective study and review of the literature," *Advances in Pediatrics*, vol. 23, pp. 35–69, 1976.

[6] J. E. Lewy, L. Salinas-Madrigal, P. B Herdson, C. L. Pirani, and J. Metcoff, "Clinico-pathologic correlations in acute poststreptococcal glomerulonephritis. A correlation between renal functions, morphologic damage and clinical course of 46 children with acute poststreptococcal glomerulonephritis," *Medicine*, vol. 50, no. 6, pp. 453–501, 1971.

[7] O. Becquet, J. Pasche, H. Gatti et al., "Acute post-streptococcal glomerulonephritis in children of French Polynesia: a 3-year retrospective study," *Pediatric Nephrology*, vol. 25, no. 2, pp. 275–280, 2010.

[8] M. Herthelius and U. Berg, "Renal function during and after childhood acute poststreptococcal glomerulonephritis," *Pediatric Nephrology*, vol. 13, no. 9, pp. 907–911, 1999.

[9] G. J. Schwartz, A. Muñoz, M. F. Schneider et al., "New equations to estimate GFR in children with CKD," *Journal of the American Society of Nephrology*, vol. 20, no. 3, pp. 629–637, 2009.

[10] S. T. Shulman, R. R. Tanz, W. Kabat et al., "Group A streptococcal pharyngitis serotype surveillance in North America, 2000–2002," *Clinical Infectious Diseases*, vol. 39, pp. 325–332, 2004.

[11] B. Beall, R. Facklam, and T. Thompson, "Sequencing emm-specific PCR products for routine and accurate typing of group A streptococci," *Journal of Clinical Microbiology*, vol. 34, no. 4, pp. 953–958, 1996.

[12] S. Sanjad, A. Tolaymat, J. Whitworth, and S. Levin, "Acute glomerulonephritis in children: a review of 153 cases," *Southern Medical Journal*, vol. 70, no. 10, pp. 1202–1206, 1977.

[13] C. R. Medani, P. L. Pearl, and M. Hall-Craggs, "Acute renal failure, hemolytic anemia, and thrombocytopenia in poststreptococcal glomerulonephritis," *Southern Medical Journal*, vol. 80, no. 3, pp. 370–373, 1987.

[14] T. Muguruma, T. Koyama, T. Kanadani, M. Furujo, H. Shiraga, and Y. Ichiba, "Acute thrombocytopenia associated with poststreptococcal acute glomerulonephritis," *Journal of Paediatrics and Child Health*, vol. 36, no. 4, pp. 401–402, 2000.

[15] W. Wong, M. C. Morris, and J. Zwi, "Outcome of severe acute post-streptococcal glomerulonephritis in New Zealand children," *Pediatric Nephrology*, vol. 24, no. 5, pp. 1021–1026, 2009.

[16] W. Wong, D. R. Lennon, S. Crone, J. M. Neutze, and P. W. Reed, "Prospective population-based study on the burden of disease from post-streptococcal glomerulonephritis of hospitalised children in New Zealand: epidemiology, clinical features and complications," *Journal of Paediatrics and Child Health*, vol. 49, no. 10, pp. 850–855, 2013.

[17] M. W. Cunningham, "Pathogenesis of group A streptococcal infections," *Clinical Microbiology Reviews*, vol. 13, no. 3, pp. 470–511, 2000.

[18] B. Schwartz, R. R. Facklam, and R. F. Breiman, "Changing epidemiology of group A streptococcal infection in the USA," *The Lancet*, vol. 336, no. 8724, pp. 1167–1171, 1990.

[19] W. E. Hoy, A. V. White, B. Tipiloura et al., "The multideterminant model of renal disease in a remote Australian Aboriginal population in the context of early life risk factors: lower birth weight, childhood post-streptococcal glomerulonephritis, and current body mass index influence levels of albumi," *Clinical Nephrology*, vol. 83, pp. 75–81, 2015.

[20] S. W. L. Pinto, G. Mastroianni-Kirsztajn, and R. Sesso, "Ten-year follow-up of patients with epidemic post infectious glomerulonephritis," *PLoS ONE*, vol. 10, no. 5, Article ID e0125313, 2015.

[21] H. Kanai, E. Sawanobori, K. Koizumi, R. Ohashi, and K. Higashida, "Pediatric case of crescentic post-streptococcal glomerulonephritis with myeloperoxidase anti-neutrophil cytoplasmic antibody," *Clinical Nephrology*, vol. 83, no. 4, pp. 243–248, 2015.

33

Transforming Growth Factor-β Protects against Inflammation-Related Atherosclerosis in South African CKD Patients

Muzamil Olamide Hassan ⓘ,[1] Raquel Duarte ⓘ,[2] Therese Dix-Peek ⓘ,[2] Caroline Dickens ⓘ,[2] Sagren Naidoo,[1] Ahmed Vachiat,[3] Sacha Grinter,[3] Pravin Manga,[3] and Saraladevi Naicker[4]

[1]Division of Nephrology, Department of Internal Medicine, Faculty of Health Sciences, University of the Witwatersrand, South Africa
[2]Internal Medicine Research Laboratory, Department of Internal Medicine, Faculty of Health Sciences, University of the Witwatersrand, South Africa
[3]Division of Cardiology, Department of Internal Medicine, Faculty of Health Sciences, University of the Witwatersrand, South Africa
[4]Department of Internal Medicine, Faculty of Health Sciences, University of the Witwatersrand, South Africa

Correspondence should be addressed to Muzamil Olamide Hassan; muzlamide@yahoo.com

Academic Editor: Jochen Reiser

Background. Transforming growth factor-β (TGF-β) may inhibit the development of atherosclerosis. We evaluated serum levels of TGF-β isoforms concurrently with serum levels of endotoxin and various inflammatory markers. In addition, we determined if any association exists between polymorphisms in the *TGF-β1* gene and atherosclerosis in South African CKD patients. *Methods.* We studied 120 CKD patients and 40 healthy controls. Serum TGF-β1, TGF-β2, TGF-β3, endotoxin, and inflammatory markers were measured. Functional polymorphisms in the *TGF-β1* genes were genotyped using a polymerase chain reaction-sequence specific primer method and carotid intima media thickness (CIMT) was assessed by B-mode ultrasonography. *Results.* TGF-β isoforms levels were significantly lower in the patients with atherosclerosis compared to patients without atherosclerosis (p<0.001). Overall, TGF-β isoforms had inverse relationships with CIMT. TGF-β1 and TGF-β2 levels were significantly lower in patients with carotid plaque compared to those without carotid plaque [TGF-β1: 31.9 (17.2 – 42.2) versus 45.9 (35.4 – 58.1) ng/ml, p=0.016; and TGF-β2: 1.46 (1.30 – 1.57) versus 1.70 (1.50 – 1.87) ng/ml, p=0.013]. In multiple logistic regression, age, TGF-β2, and TGF-β3 were the only independent predictors of subclinical atherosclerosis in CKD patients [age: odds ratio (OR), 1.054; 95% confidence interval (CI): 1.003 – 1.109, p=0.039; TGF-β2: OR, 0.996; 95% CI: 0.994–0.999, p=0.018; TGF-β3: OR, 0.992; 95% CI: 0.985–0.999, p=0.029). *TGF-β1* genotypes did not influence serum levels of TGF-β1 and no association was found between the *TGF-β1* gene polymorphisms and atherosclerosis risk. *Conclusion.* TGF-β isoforms seem to offer protection against the development of atherosclerosis among South African CKD patients.

1. Introduction

Chronic kidney disease (CKD) patients are more likely to develop cardiovascular disease (CVD) than age-matched counterparts in the general population. As a consequence, the risk of death in CKD patients due to cardiovascular disease is much higher than the risk of requiring dialysis [1, 2].

Chronic inflammation is directly related to several complications of CKD, including accelerated atherosclerosis and left ventricular hypertrophy [2, 3]. Chronic low-grade inflammation is common in patients with coexisting CKD and CVD and plays a pivotal role in the development of atherosclerotic plaques by driving oxidative stress and stimulating production of inflammatory cytokines leading to activation of chemokines and adhesion molecules [3–5].

Endotoxin (lipopolysaccharide), a glycolipid that comprises most of the outer wall of gram-negative bacteria, is a potential source of inflammation in CKD patients [6, 7]. It is reported that circulating endotoxaemia constitutes a strong risk factor for atherosclerotic CVD [8–10]. This finding suggests that chronic exposure to endotoxins may be related to subclinical atherosclerosis and represents a reversible CVD risk factor in CKD patients.

Atherosclerosis is a complex disease process in which inflammation plays a central role in various pathogenetic mechanisms that contribute to the progressive structural changes that are characteristic of atherogenesis [11, 12]. Besides promoting atherosclerosis, inflammation also plays a significant role in the process of plaque rupture and arterial thrombosis, leading to vascular occlusion and infarction [13]. Thus, inflammation has been found to be a significant predictor of cardiovascular mortality in CKD patients [14].

Transforming growth factor-β (TGF-β), a multifunctional inflammatory cytokine, is produced by many inflammatory cells including leucocytes, macrophages, smooth muscle cells, and platelets [15–18]. There are three isoforms of TGF-β: TGF-β1, TGF-β2, and TGF-β3. Transforming growth factor-β1, the most extensively studied of these three isoforms, exhibits anti-inflammatory and antiproliferative properties by inhibiting the synthesis of tumour necrosis factor-α (TNF-α) or by downregulating the proinflammatory effects of IL-1β and interferon-γ [19, 20]. In turn, this leads to reduction of inflammatory cytokine-induced vascular cell adhesion molecule-1 (VCAM-1), chemotaxis, leucocyte adhesion to vascular endothelial lining, and decreased macrophage activity [19, 21]. Previous studies have suggested that low serum levels of TGF-β1 are a risk factor for atherosclerosis in non-CKD [22, 23] and CKD patients [10]. However, there is a paucity of data on whether TGF-β2 and TGF-β3 contribute to the susceptibility and the severity of atherosclerosis in CKD patients.

The TGF-β1 gene, located on the long arm of chromosome 19, contains six common single nucleotide polymorphisms (SNPs), namely, C-988A, G-800A, C-509T, T-869C, G-915C, and C-11929T [24, 25]. Previous studies have shown that TGF-β1 gene polymorphisms predicted serum levels of TGF-β1 [26–28]. However, the role of TGF-β1 gene polymorphisms in atherosclerotic cardiovascular disease in CKD patients remains controversial. While some studies have linked polymorphisms in the genes encoding TGF-β1 to increased risk of atherosclerosis [29–31], studies in other populations were negative [32–34]. It is against this background that we performed measurements of serum levels of TGF-β isoforms concurrently with serum levels of endotoxin and some inflammatory markers (lipoprotein binding protein, serum CD14, and monocyte chemoattractant protein-1) and examined anti-inflammatory and atheroprotective effects of TGF-β isoforms in South African CKD patients. In addition, we determined if any association exists between polymorphisms in the TGF-β1 gene and atherosclerosis in South African CKD patients.

2. Materials and Methods

2.1. Study Population.
The study was approved by the University of the Witwatersrand, Human Research Ethics Committee. A total of 160 participants, comprising 40 stage 3 CKD patients, 40 peritoneal dialysis (PD) patients, 40 haemodialysis (HD) patients, and 40 controls, were included in this study. Exclusion criteria included clinical signs of active or chronic infection, diabetes mellitus, seropositive status for hepatitis B, C and HIV, autoimmune disease, liver dysfunction, malignancy, heart failure, and use of anti-inflammatory or immunosuppressive therapy at least three months prior to enrolment. Using a structured interview form, information on age, race, gender, and tobacco use was documented. Patients were classified as smokers if they were current smokers, former smokers if they stopped smoking for at least six months prior to the study, and nonsmokers if they had never smoked.

2.2. Blood Pressure Measurement.
Blood pressure for HD patients was recorded noninvasively in the arm without the A-V fistula with an Accoson mercury sphygmomanometer in the sitting position before a dialysis session commenced. Blood pressure was estimated by averaging all pre-dialysis and post-dialysis blood pressure recordings taken during the month before the study (3 measurements per week for a total of 12 measurements, that is, 3/week). Among PD and CKD patients, blood pressure was recorded at the time of the clinic visit. The blood pressure average of four clinic visits was taken as the patient's actual BP. In control patients, blood pressure was measured in the sitting position after resting for 5 minutes and an average of three readings recorded 5 minutes apart was used. Pulse pressure was calculated as systolic blood pressure (SBP) minus diastolic blood pressure (DBP). Mean arterial blood pressure (MABP) was calculated as diastolic blood pressure plus one-third pulse pressure.

2.3. Blood Sample Collection.
Following an overnight fast, 10mls of blood was collected into anticoagulant-free tubes and kept on ice until the serum was separated within 30 minutes of collection and centrifuged at 3000 rpm for 10 minutes at room temperature. Serum was subsequently separated and stored in appropriate endotoxin-free Eppendorf tubes at -70°C until analysis. Serum creatinine, albumin, total cholesterol, high density lipoprotein (HDL), low density lipoprotein (LDL) and triglyceride (TG) levels were measured using ADVIA^R auto-analyzers (Siemens Healthcare Diagnostics Inc, USA).

2.4. Transforming Growth Factor-β1, β2, and β3 Concentrations.
Serum TGF-β1, 2, and 3 levels were determined using BioPlex Pro$^{(TM)}$ TGF-β Assay kits (Bio-RAD Laboratories, Inc., Hercules, CA, USA). Assays were carried out in accordance with the manufacturer's instructions. The sample dilution was 1:16. Fluorescence was measured on the Bio-Plex$^{(TM)}$ 200 system (Bio-Rad) and concentrations were generated automatically with Bio-Plex manager software, version 5.0 (Bio-Rad Laboratories Inc).

2.5. Endotoxin Levels.
Circulating endotoxin was measured using the Limulus amebocyte lysate QCL-1000 assay (Lonza, Walkersville, USA) according to manufacturer's instructions, using a previously described method [34]. Absorbance was

measured using an ELx800 microplate reader (BioTek Instruments, Inc, VT, USA).

2.6. Lipopolysaccharide Binding Protein (LBP) Concentrations. Lipopolysaccharide binding protein levels were assayed using a commercial human LBP ELISA kit, Hycult HK315 (Hycult Biotechnology, Uden, Netherlands), in accordance with the manufacturer's instructions.

2.7. Inflammatory Marker Assays. Serum high sensitivity C-reactive protein (hs-CRP), serum CD14 (sCD14), and monocyte chemoattractant protein 1 (MCP-1) were analyzed using Luminex® Performance Assay multiplex kits (R&D Systems, Inc., Minneapolis, USA). Assays were carried out in accordance with the manufacturer's instructions. For hs-CRP measurements, the sample dilution was 1:1000 while samples for sCD14 measurements were diluted 1:50. Samples for MCP-1 were not diluted. Fluorescence was measured on the Bio-Plex™ 200 system (Bio-Rad) and concentrations were generated automatically with Bio-Plex manager software, version 5.0 (Bio-Rad Laboratories Inc).

2.8. Carotid Intima Media Thickness Measurement. Carotid intima media thickness was assessed using high resolution B-mode ultrasonography with the aid of L3-11 MHz linear array transducer (Philips Corporation USA) according to American Society of Echocardiography guidelines [35, 36]. Carotid intima media thickness was measured in plaque-free areas. Carotid plaque was defined as the echogenic structure protruding into the lumen with the distance between the media adventitia interface and the internal side of the lesion ≥ 1.2 mm. All measurements were performed by the same sonographer who was blinded to the clinical details and laboratory data of the participants.

2.9. DNA Extraction and TGF-β1 Genotyping. All procedures were carried out at room temperature (15-25°C). Genomic DNA was extracted from whole blood using a modified salting out method as previously described [37]. Genotyping was performed on the study groups and the controls using a cytokine genotyping tray kit (One Lambda Inc., Los Angeles, USA). The preoptimized primers were presented lyophilised in different wells of a 96-well 0.2ml thin-walled tube tray for polymerase chain reaction (PCR), to which DNA samples (100 ng), recombinant Taq polymerase (5U/μL HotStarTaq DNA Polymerase, Qiagen, Hilden, Germany), and specially formulated dNTP-buffer mix (D-mix) were added as per the manufacturer's protocol. The PCR products were amplified on a thermocycler (MJ Mini Thermal cycler, Bio-Rad) using the One Lambda PCR program (1 cycle: 96°C for 120s; 10 cycles: 96°C for 10s, 63°C for 60s; 20 cycles: 96°C for 10s, 59°C for 50s, 72°C for 30s; hold at 4°C) according to manufacturer's instructions. All the PCR products were visualized on a 2% agarose gel stained with ethidium bromide, with the aid of an image analyzer (Gel Doc™ EZ Imager, Bio-Rad). *TGF-β1* SNPs were assessed based on the sizes of the amplified products with negative amplifications scored only if the internal control product was present.

2.10. Data Analysis. Data analyses were performed using the statistical package for social sciences (SPSS) 16 (SPSS, Inc., Chicago IL). Variables were presented as mean ± SD and median (interquartile range, IQR) for normally and nonnormally distributed continuous data, respectively, and percentages and frequencies for categorical data. Results were analyzed using a t-test with the Tukey post hoc test for normally distributed data and the chi-square test and Kruskal Wallis test for nonparametric data. Correlation between variables was assessed by the Spearman correlation coefficients. Genotype frequencies were determined by gene counting method and expressed as percentages. The frequencies were compared using Fisher's exact test. Further analysis was performed to assess the influence of various genotypes of *TGF-β1* on the serum levels of TGF-β1 and CIMT. A P-value <0.05 (two-tailed) was considered significant.

3. Results

3.1. Demographic and Clinical Data. Patients' demographics and clinical and laboratory data are shown in Table 1. This study consisted of 120 patients comprising PD, HD, and stage 3 CKD patients, with mean ages of 40.6±9.9, 40.6±10.1, and 42.1±10.6 years, respectively. In each group, male patients comprised 55% of the studied population. Of the patients, 106 (88.3%) were Black, 8 (6.7%) were White, 3 (2.5%) were Indian, and 3 (2.5%) were of mixed race. The controls were matched for age and gender. There were 22 (55%) male and 18 (45%) female controls. The mean age for the controls was 42.2±10.1 years. The aetiology of CKD was hypertension-attributed in 59/120 (49.2%), chronic glomerulonephritis in 36/120 (30%), polycystic kidney disease in 8/120 (6.7%), reflux nephropathy in 4/120 (3.3%), congenital abnormalities of the kidneys in 4/120 (3.3%) patients, obstructive uropathy in 3/120 (2.5%), and unknown in 7 (5%) patients. Hypertension as the primary cause of CKD was present in 52/59 (88.1%) of black patients and only in 7/52 (11.9%) in other race groups.

One hundred and two patients (85%) received various combinations of antihypertensive agents. Calcium channel blockers were taken by 81/120 (67.5%) patients, beta blockers by 40/120 (33.3%), angiotensin-II receptor blockers or angiotensin-converting enzyme inhibitors (ARB/ACEI) by 27/120 (22.5%), diuretics by 22/120 (18.3%), and alpha blockers by 16/120 13.3%) of the patients. Regarding patients that were treated with antihypertensive medications, 43/102 (42.2%) were on monotherapy, 39/102 (38.2%) on double, 15/102 (14.7%) on triple, and 3/102 (2.9%) on quadruple agents while 2/102 (1.96%) patients received 5 agents in various combination. In addition, patients received other medications for ESRD management including phosphate binders in 104/120 (86.7%), statins in 28/120 (23.3%), and aspirin in 9/120 (7.5%) of cases.

3.2. Transforming Growth Factor-Beta Isoform Levels in CKD Patients. The median concentrations of the three TGF-β isoforms are presented in Table 1. Of the three TGF-β isoforms, TGF-β1 had the highest levels. The lowest TGF-β isoform concentrations were present in HD patients compared to the PD, CKD patients, and controls. Female

TABLE 1: Demographics and clinical and laboratory data of the study population.

Parameter	All patients (N=120)	PD (N=40)	HD (N=40)	CKD stage 3 (N=40)	Control (N=40)	*P value
Age (years; mean ± SD)	41.1 ± 10.2	40.6 ± 9.9	40.6 ± 10.1	42.1 ± 10.6	42.2 ± 10.1	0.494[a]
Sex (Male/Female)	60/40	22/18	22/18	22/18	22/18	0.784[b]
Race (Black/Non-Black)	106/14	37/3	37/3	35/5	31/9	0.091[b]
Smoking (Yes/No)	17/103	9/31	5/35	3/37	2/38	0.121[b]
MABP (mmHg)	134.8 (118.8-150.0)	143.3 (130.0-163.8)	144.7 (135.2-157.3)	136.2 (119.5-148.6)	117.0 (107.8-130.6)	<0.001[c]
Serum creatinine (mmol/L)	262.5 (92.3-766.0)	1175.5 (877.0-1363.0)	513.0 (401.5-727.0)	124.0 (105.5-166.8)	71.5 (60.5-86.0)	<0.001[c]
eGFR (ml/min/1.73m^2)	-	NA	NA	47.5 (44.0-50.0)	96.5 (83-119)	-
Serum albumin (g/L)	40.0 (36.0-43.0)	35.5 (33.0-40.0)	38.5 (35.0-41.0)	41.5 (38.3-44.0)	43.0 (40.3-44)	<0.001[c]
Total cholesterol (mmol/L)	4.20 (3.43 – 5.18)	5.20 (4.20 – 5.90)	3.40 (3.00 – 3.70)	4.40 (4.00 – 5.10)	4.00 (3.33 – 4.88)	0.519[c]
HDL (mmol/L)	1.20 (0.90 – 1.40)	1.2 (0.90 – 1.40)	1.00 (0.90 – 1.20)	1.30 (1.10 – 1.40)	1.25 (1.03 – 1.40)	0.421[c]
LDL (mmol/L)	2.30 (1.80 – 3.00)	3.00 (2.40 – 4.10)	1.80 (1.40 – 2.20)	2.50 (1.90 – 3.00)	2.20 (1.60 – 2.98)	0.456[c]
TG (mmol/L)	1.20 (0.80 – 1.70)	1.30 (1.00 – 2.00)	0.80 (0.60 – 1.20)	1.30 (1.00 – 1.90)	0.95 (0.63 – 1.60)	0.172[c]
TGF-β1 (ng/ml)	45.0 (33.5-56.9)	45.1 (33.8-52.3)	36.0 (25.2-44.4)	59.0 (46.1-66.9)	66.3 (57.7-75.4)	<0.001[c]
TGF-β2 (ng/ml)	1.7 (1.5-1.9)	1.6 (1.4-1.9)	1.6 (1.5-1.8)	1.7 (1.5-1.9)	1.8 (1.6-1.9)	0.062[c]
TGF-β3 (ng/ml)	0.45 (0.39-0.50)	0.44 (0.38-0.50)	0.40 (0.36-0.45)	0.48 (0.44-0.60)	0.52 (0.48-0.65)	<0.001[c]
MCP-1 (pg/ml)	9.0 (4.8-17.0)	12.3 (7.2-19.3)	7.2 (4.5-10.9)	6.8 (4.6-12.2)	3.6 (2.2-7.3)	<0.001[c]
sCD14 (µg/m³)	1.8 (1.3-2.2)	2.0 (1.5-2.6)	1.8 (1.4-2.1)	1.5 (1.0-1.9)	1.2 (1.0-1.4)	<0.001[c]
Hs-CRP (mg/dL)	0.7 (0.2-1.4)	1.1 (0.5-1.9)	1.0 (0.4-1.6)	0.7 (0.2-1.4)	0.2 (0.1-0.7)	<0.001[c]
Endotoxin (EU/ml)	0.46 (0.30-0.67)	0.56 (0.44-0.75)	0.51 (0.28-0.78)	0.52 (0.31-0.70)	0.33 (0.26-0.41)	<0.001[c]
LBP (ng/ml)	1.2 (0.9-1.6)×10^5	1.4 (1.2-1.7)×10^5	1.4 (1.1-1.7)×10^5	1.2 (0.9-1.4)×10^5	0.9 (0.8-1.1)×10^5	<0.001[c]
CIMT (mm)	0.6 (0.47-0.61)	0.6 (0.54-0.71)	0.5 (0.49-0.61)	0.5 (0.47-0.61)	0.4 (0.42-0.52)	<0.001[c]
Plaques (Present; %)	8 (6.7%)	2 (5%)	5 (12.5%)	1 (2.5%)	0 (0%)	<0.001[b]

PD, peritoneal dialysis; HD, haemodialysis; CKD, chronic kidney disease; MABP, mean arterial blood pressure; HDL, high density lipoprotein; LDL, low density lipoprotein; TG, triglycerides; MCP-1, monocyte chemoattractant protein-1; sCD14, serum CD14; TGF, transforming growth factor; Hs-CRP, high sensitivity C-reactive protein; LBP, lipopolysaccharide binding protein; CIMT, carotid intima media thickness. Continuous data were expressed as mean ± SD or median (IQR) and categorical data as percentages. * P-values compare all CKD patients (n=120) to controls (n=40).

[a] p-value calculated using Student's *t*-test.

[b] p-values calculated using Chi-square test.

[c] p-values calculated using Mann–Whitney test.

TABLE 2: Correlation between transforming growth factor β isoforms, renal function, lipoprotein particles, inflammation, and markers of atherosclerosis.

Variables	TGF-β1		TGF-β2		TGF-β3	
	r value	p value	r value	p value	r value	p value
MABP	− 0.248	0.006	− 0.028	0.763	− 0.136	0.137
Serum creatinine	− 0.348	< 0.001	− 0.237	0.009	− 0.316	< 0.001
Serum albumin	0.247	0.007	0.192	0.036	0.257	0.005
Total cholesterol	0.322	< 0.001	0.226	0.013	0.356	< 0.001
HDL	0.258	0.004	0.262	0.004	0.229	0.012
LDL	0.248	0.006	0.155	0.091	0.263	0.004
TG	0.221	0.016	0.142	0.121	0.269	0.003
Hs-CRP	− 0.183	0.046	− 0.153	0.096	− 0.320	0.001
MCP-1	− 0.212	0.020	− 0.069	0.457	− 0.184	0.045
sCD14	− 0.347	< 0.001	− 0.313	0.001	− 0.318	< 0.001
Endotoxins	− 0.196	0.032	− 0.207	0.023	− 0.139	0.130
LBP	− 0.281	0.002	− 0.402	< 0.001	− 0.403	< 0.001
CIMT	− 0.614	< 0.001	− 0.547	< 0.001	− 0.430	< 0.001

MABP; mean arterial blood pressure; HDL, high density lipoprotein; LDL, low density lipoprotein, TG, triglycerides; Hs-CRP, high sensitivity C-reactive protein; MCP-1, monocyte chemoattractant protein-1; sCD14, serum CD14, LBP, lipopolysaccharide binding protein; CIMT, carotid intima media thickness; TGF, transforming growth factor. Correlation was assessed by Spearman's correlation coefficient.

TABLE 3: Multiple linear regression analysis of determinants of serum TGF-β1 levels.

Variables	Unstandardized coefficients (β)	Standardized coefficients (Beta)	95% Confidence interval	P value
CIMT	− 81439.078	− 0.593	− 107604.8 – −55273.3	< 0.001
Creatinine	− 3.111	− 0.095	− 8.484 – 2.262	0.254
sCD14	0.000	− 0.006	− 0.005 – 0.005	0.965
LBP	− 0.026	− 0.096	− 0.082 – 0.031	0.374
MABP	− 122.815	− 0.174	− 226.892 – − 18.739	0.021
Albumin	304.912	0.095	− 227.427 – − 837.251	0.259
MCP-1	258.890	0.181	− 13.286 – 531.066	0.062
Hs-CRP	− 230.671	− 0.011	− 3758.684 – 3297.342	0.897

CIMT, carotid intima media thickness; MABP; mean arterial blood pressure; sCD14, serum CD14; LBP, lipopolysaccharide binding protein; MCP-1, monocyte chemoattractant protein-1; Hs-CRP, high sensitivity C-reactive protein.

CKD patients had significantly higher levels of TGF-β1 as compared to male patients (TGF-β1: 49.6 (41.2-60.2) ng/ml versus 39.4 (31.1-49.3) ng/ml, p=0.001). No relationship was found between any of the TGF-β isoforms and age. Both TGF-β1 and TGF-β3 isoforms levels were significantly lower in HD patients compared to other study groups including the controls (p<0.05), while, in the subanalysis of TGF-β2 concentrations, there was no difference between HD and PD patients (p>0.05). In CKD patients (HD, PD, and stage 3 CKD), TGF-β isoforms levels were not associated with the aetiology of the CKD. Even though angiotensin-converting enzyme inhibitor was previously shown to lower serum TGF-β1 levels in patients with diabetic nephropathy [38, 39], this current study, however, did not show any significant differences in TGF-β isoforms levels between CKD patients who were treated with ARB/ACEI and those not treated with ARB/ACEI [TGF-β1: 46.7 (36.7 – 53.6) versus 44.1 (33.7 – 65.1) ng/ml, p=0.259; TGF-β2: 1.63 (1.44 – 1.85) versus 1.68 (1.50 – 1.86) ng/ml, p=0.453; and TGF-β3: 0.47 (0.43 – 0.57) versus 0.44 (0.38 – 0.50), p=0.120 ng/ml]. As shown in Table 1, CKD patients had significantly lower concentrations

of TGF-β1 and TGF-β3 compared to the controls (p<0.001), while there was no difference in the concentration of TGF-β2 between CKD patients and controls (p=0.062).

3.3. Relationship Between TGF-β, Inflammatory Cytokines, Lipoprotein Particles, and Blood Pressure. Table 2 shows the relationship between TGF-β isoforms, renal function, inflammation, and CIMT. When TGF-β1 was correlated with mediators of the endotoxin signalling pathway, a modest relationship was demonstrated between TGF-β3 and LBP (r=−0.403, p<0.001), and serum CD14 (r=−0.318, p<0.001). Transforming growth factor-β1 showed a weak relationship with MCP-1 (r=−0.212, p=0.020). Transforming growth factor-β3 demonstrated a weak negative correlation with hs-CRP (r=−0.320, p<0.001) while TGF-β1 showed an inverse relationship with MABP (r=−0.248, p=0.006). TGF-β3 showed a weak positive correlation with albumin (r=0.256, p=0.005). Furthermore, TGF-β3 had a positive correlation with total cholesterol, LDL, HDL, and TG. Multiple linear regression analysis showed that CIMT and MABP were independent predictors of TGF-β1 levels (r^2=0.41, p<0.001) (Table 3) and CIMT and MCP-1

(a)

(b)

(c)

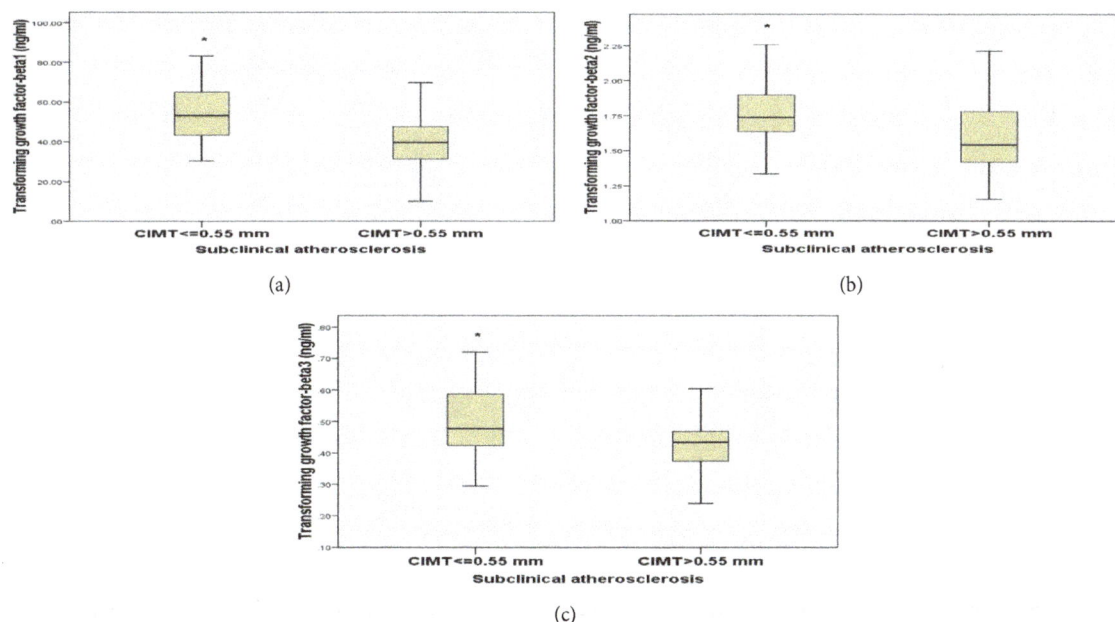

FIGURE 1: **Comparison of serum transforming growth factor-β1 (a), β2 (b), and β3 (c) between patients with subclinical atherosclerosis and those without atherosclerosis.** The boxes indicate median, 25th, and 75th percentile; whiskers represent data range; whisker caps indicate 5th and 95th percentile. Transforming growth factor-β1, β2, and β3 levels were analyzed with Bio-Plex Pro™ TGF-β Assays kit. Carotid intima media thickness was measured using B-mode ultrasound. Serum transforming growth factor-β1, β2, and β3 levels were compared between CKD patients and controls, ∗ P < 0.001 compared to controls.

were independent determinants of serum TGF-β2 (r^2=0.39; p<0.001) while CIMT was the only predictor of serum TGF-β3 levels (r^2=0.33; p<0.001).

3.4. Atherosclerosis and Transforming Growth Factor-β Isoforms. Sixty-seven CKD patients (55.8%) had subclinical atherosclerosis (CIMT of > 0.55 mm). Carotid plaques were present in 5% of PD, 12.5% of HD, and 2.5% of nondialytic CKD patients, but not in any of the controls (Table 1). Transforming growth factor-β isoforms concentrations were significantly lower in the patients with subclinical atherosclerosis compared to patients without atherosclerosis [TGF-β1: 39.1 (30.6 – 47.5) versus 53.9 (44.1 – 65.1) ng/ml, p<0.001; TGF-β2: 1.51 (1.42 – 1.73) versus 1.83 (1.64 – 1.96) ng/ml, p<0.001; and TGF-β3: 0.43 (0.37 – 0.46) versus 0.50 (0.42 – 0.62), p<0.001 ng/ml] (Figure 1). Furthermore, TGF-β1 and TGF-β2 levels were significantly lower in patients with carotid plaque compared to those without carotid plaque [TGF-β1: 31.9 (17.2 – 42.2) versus 45.9 (35.4 – 58.1) ng/ml, p=0.016; and TGF-β2: 1.46 (1.30 – 1.57) versus 1.70 (1.50 – 1.87) ng/ml, p=0.013] (Figure 2). However, there was no difference in the levels of TGF-β3 between patients with carotid plaque and those without plaque [0.41 (0.34 – 0.50) versus 0.44 (0.39 – 0.52) ng/ml, p=0.330] (Figure 2). Overall, TGF-β isoforms had inverse relationships with CIMT (Table 2). Age, smoking, MABP, HDL, LDL, TG, hs-CRP, serum creatinine (marker of kidney function), TGF-β1, TGF-β2, and TGF-β3 levels were entered into the multiple logistic regression analysis as covariates to determine their contribution to the risk of atherosclerosis. Age, TGF-β2, and TGF-β3 were the only

independent predictors of subclinical atherosclerosis in CKD patients in the regression model [age: Odds ratio (OR), 1.054; 95% confidence interval (CI): 1.003 – 1.109, p=0.039; TGF-β2: OR, 0.996; 95% CI: 0.994–0.999, p=0.018; TGF-β3: OR, 0.992; 95% CI: 0.985–0.999, p=0.029) (Table 4).

3.5. Circulating Endotoxaemia and CIMT in CKD Patients. Carotid intima media thickness was significantly greater in CKD patients (median, 0.60 mm; IQR, 0.47-0.61 mm) compared to controls (median, 0.40 mm; IQR, 0.42-0.52 mm), p<0.001. Patients with elevated circulating endotoxaemia (> 0.5 EU/ml) had significantly higher CIMT compared to patients with lower endotoxin levels (≤ 0.5 EU/ml) (p<0.001). Carotid intima media thickness correlated with endotoxin (r=0.313, p=0.001) and LBP (r=0.311, p=0.001). On univariate analysis, atherosclerosis was associated with endotoxin levels (OR, 4.16; 95% CI: 1.04 – 16.6), p=0.044), with excess risk confined to the group with high endotoxin levels.

3.6. TGF-β1 Polymorphisms, TGF-β1 Levels, and Atherosclerosis. The distribution of the *TGF-β1* SNPs [T-869C (rs1800470) and G-915C (rs1800471)] and their genotyping frequencies in the CKD patients and the controls are shown in Table 5. The *TGF-β1* genotypes did not differ between controls and the CKD patients (p>0.05). Further analysis was done to determine whether the presence of *TGF-β1* genotypes influence the levels of TGF-β1 in the sera of the study participants. Although serum levels TGF-β1 were higher among the high producers compared to the intermediate producers and the low producers, they were

(a)

(b)

(c)

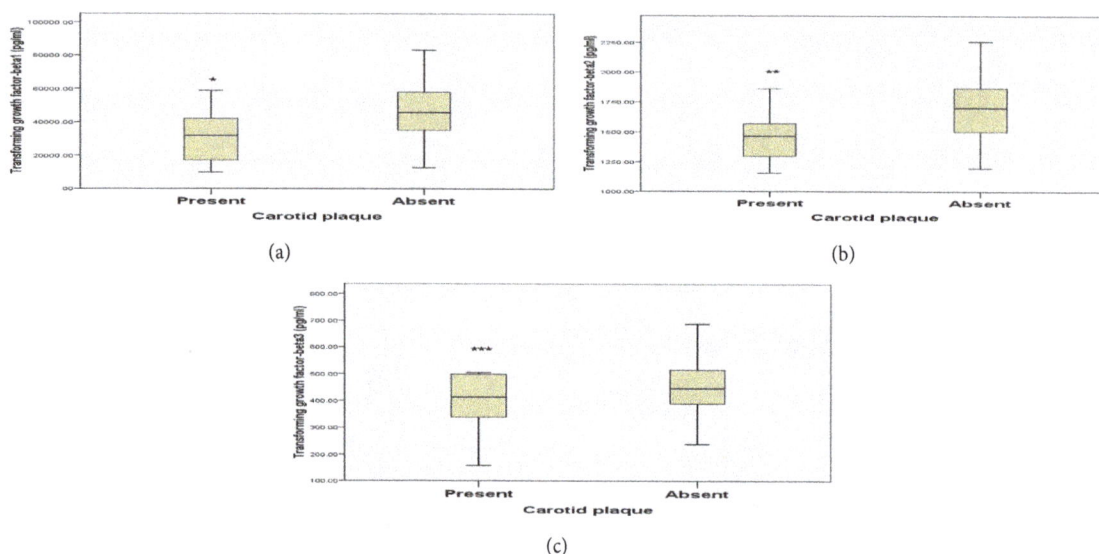

FIGURE 2: **Comparison of serum transforming growth factor-β1 (a), β2 (b), and β3 (c) between patients with carotid plaque and those without plaques.** The boxes indicate median, 25th, and 75th percentile; whiskers represent data range; whisker caps indicate 5th and 95th percentile. Transforming growth factor-β1, β2, and β3 levels were analyzed with Bio-Plex Pro™ TGF-β Assays kit. Carotid plaque was defined as the echogenic structure protruding into the lumen with the distance between the media adventitia interface and the internal side of the lesion $\geq$ 1.2 mm. Serum transforming growth factor-β1, β2, and β3 levels were compared between patients with carotid plaques and those without plaque, $*$P = 0.016, $**$ P = 0.013, and $***$P = 0.330 compared to those patients without plaque.

TABLE 4: Multiple logistic regression analysis of risk factors for atherosclerosis in CKD patients.

Variables	B	Standard error of β	Odds ratio	95% Confidence interval	P value
Age	0.053	0.026	1.054	1.003 – 1.109	0.039
Smoking	0.961	0.775	2.615	0.573 – 11.939	0.215
MABP	− 0.005	0.011	0.995	0.974 – 1.017	0.678
HDL	− 0.436	0.564	0.647	0.214 –1.953	0.440
LDL	0.392	0.269	1.480	0.874 – 2.507	0.144
TG	0.579	0.371	1.784	0.862 – 3.690	0.119
Hs-CRP	− 0.505	0.356	0.604	0.300 – 1.213	0.156
Serum Creatinine	0.000	0.001	1.000	0.998 – 1.001	0.468
TGF-β1	0.000	0.000	1.000	1.000 – 1.000	0.046
TGF-β2	− 0.004	0.001	0.996	0.994 – 0.999	0.018
TGF-β3	− 0.008	0.004	0.992	0.985 – 0.999	0.029

HDL, high density lipoprotein; LDL, low density lipoprotein, TG, triglycerides; Hs-CRP, high sensitivity C-reactive protein; TGF, transforming growth factor.

TABLE 5: *TGF-β1* T-869C and G-915C SNPs distribution and frequency in study participants.

SNPs /Producer	CKD patients (n=79)	Controls (n=32)	P-value
T/T G/G (high)	16 (20.3%)	7 (21.9%)	1.00
T/C G/G (high)	41 (51.9%)	17 (53.1%)	1.00
T/C G/C (intermediate)	6 (7.6%)	5 (15.6%)	0.29
C/C G/G (intermediate)	9 (11.4%)	1 (3.1%)	0.28
T/T G/C (intermediate)	1 (1.3%)	0 (0%)	1.00
C/C G/C (low)	5 (6.3%)	2 (6.3%)	1.00
T/C C/C (low)	1 (1.3%)	0 (0%)	1.00

TGF-β1, transforming growth factor β1; T-869C, rs1800470; G-915C, rs1800471. P-values were calculated using Chi-square and Fisher's exact test where applicable. From the analysis of the SNPs, there was no difference between CKD patients and the controls (p>0.05).

TABLE 6: Producer status and transforming growth factor-β1 in genotyped study participants (n=111).

Producer status	High	Intermediate	Low	*P-value
Frequency	81 (73.0%)	22 (19.8%)	8 (7.2%)	0.649
TGF-β1 levels (ng/ml)(Median; IQR)	52.9 (41.8 – 64.6)	45.8 (35.8 – 68.0)	46.8 (42.8 – 82.5)	

TGF-β1: transforming growth factor β1. *P-value was calculated using Kruskal-Wallis test and compared TGF-β1 levels across the three comparison groups. Post hoc analysis did not showed any significant difference among the three comparison groups (p>0.05).

TABLE 7: Relationship between *TGF-β1* gene polymorphisms (T-869C and G-915C) and atherogenesis in CKD patients.

TGF-β1 SNPs /Producer	Odds Ratio	95% Confidence Interval	P-value	Risk of Atherogenesis
T/T G/G (high)	1.26	0.53-3.01	0.406	No association
T/C G/G (high)	0.98	0.64-1.51	0.560	No association
T/C G/C (intermediate)	6.29	0.77-51.4	0.057	No association
C/C G/G (intermediate)	0.36	0.08-1.62	0.144	No association
T/T G/C (intermediate)	1.02	0.98-1.07	0.562	No association
C/C G/C (low)	0.31	0.04-2.69	0.259	No association
T/C C/C (low)	0.97	0.91-1.03	0.440	No association

TGFβ1: transforming growth factor β1. Odds ratios, 95% confidence interval, and p-value were derived from analyses of the strength of association between *TGF-β1* gene polymorphisms and subclinical atherosclerosis in CKD patients with atherosclerosis compared to those without atherosclerosis (reference group).

not statistically significant (Table 6). In the CKD group, no association was found between the *TGF-β1* genotypes and subclinical atherosclerosis (Table 7).

4. Discussion

This study has demonstrated that serum levels of TGF-β1, TGF-β2, and TGF-β3 are significantly reduced in CKD patients compared to the control group, especially in patients with subclinical atherosclerosis and carotid plaque. This is in agreement with previous studies in non-CKD patients, stage 3 CKD patients, and dialysis patients [10, 28, 40]. It has also been demonstrated that there is reduced expression of TGF-β1 by peripheral leucocytes in patients who had acute myocardial infarction [41]. Furthermore, our finding is also in support of a previous study that showed that TGF-β1 expression inversely correlated with ankle-brachial index (another surrogate marker of atherosclerosis) in patients with peripheral arterial disease [16]. In agreement with our observations, Janda and colleagues identified age and TGF-β1 as independent predictors of common carotid artery intima media thickness (CCA-IMT) among end-stage renal disease patients treated with peritoneal dialysis; however, they observed a positive correlation between TGF-β1 and CCA-IMT [42].

The inverse relationship between TGF-β isoforms and accelerated atherosclerosis in the CKD patients may be related to the antiproliferative and cardioprotective properties of these immunomodulatory cytokines. Transforming growth factor-β1, the most extensively studied of the three closely related isoforms of TGF-β, counteracts vascular inflammation by inhibiting the synthesis of tumour necrosis factor-α [14]. Furthermore, by downregulating the proinflammatory effects of IL-1β and interferon-γ, it leads to reduction of inflammatory cytokine-induced VCAM-1, chemotaxis, leucocyte adhesion to vascular endothelial lining, and decreased macrophage activity [19, 21]. Thus, TGF-β1 is important in the maintenance of normal vascular integrity.

Transforming growth factor-β1 has been shown previously by Arciniegas and colleagues to induce the differentiation of aortic endothelial cells into contractile, synthetic, and luminal smooth muscle cells in TGF-β1-treated cultures [43]. The authors further demonstrated that TGF-β1 inhibited cell proliferation and induced morphological changes, resulting in decreased expression of factor VIII-related antigen and increased expression of α-smooth muscle actin (contractile protein) in smooth muscle cells which, in turn, play a vital role in the maintenance of healthy blood vessels [43]. Taken together, these *in vitro* functions of TGF-β1 are consistent with the hypothesis that TGF-β1 may play a role in the process of atherogenesis.

There is no consensus about the role of TGF-β1 in the process of atherosclerosis and restenosis. Some studies have reported an association between elevated TGF-β1 levels and vascular restenosis lesions [30, 44]. In contrast, other authors have showed that decreased expression of TGF-β1 contributes to progression of atherosclerosis [10, 22, 23]. Nevertheless, the absence of the antiproliferative effects of TGF-β1 in the blood vessels leads to increased chemotaxis, deposition of extracellular matrix, proliferation of vascular smooth muscle cells, and decreased apoptosis, thereby facilitating progression of atherosclerosis [45, 46]. Moreover, the negative associations between TGF-β isoforms and inflammatory mediators (LBP, sCD14, MCP-1) observed in the current study further highlight the anti-inflammatory effect of TGF-β1.

In this study, serum levels of TGF isoforms predicted reduced risk for subclinical atherosclerosis in patients with CKD. These findings are compatible with the hypothesis that TGF-β, an anti-inflammatory cytokine, is implicated in the pathogenesis of atherosclerosis [40, 47]. However, our study rules out the possibility that biologic variations in

TGF-β1 gene affect serum levels of TGF-β1 and the development of atherosclerosis. This result suggests that, given the complexity and the variety of the TGF-β superfamily of ligands, receptors, and binding proteins, *TGF-β1* gene polymorphisms alone may not sufficiently explain the reduced susceptibility and severity of atherosclerosis observed among studied CKD patients. Therefore, future studies targeted at exploring potential defects in the activation and signalling pathway of TGF-β might well hold the key to understanding the mechanisms leading to low serum TGF-β isoform levels in CKD patients with atherosclerotic CVD.

Hypertension, an established risk factor for myocardial infarction, showed weak but significant association with TGF-β1 levels. This observation was supported by the report of an inverse relationship between *TGF-β1* polymorphisms/hypomorphs and hypertension in previous human and animal studies [48, 49]. Likewise, gender to some extent affected TGF-β1 concentrations in this study. This finding is in support of a previous study in non-CKD patients that reported an association between TGF-β1 levels and gender [50]. The authors postulated that serum TGF-β1 levels in women may be under the control of antioestrogen hormones, ultimately resulting in the secretion of TGF-β1 by fetal human fibroblasts.

The finding that TGF-β1 levels demonstrated a modest significant correlation with hs-CRP and albumin (a marker of malnutrition) was consistent with the report of Stefoni et al. [40]. Furthermore, previous studies had suggested a link between malnutrition, inflammation, and cardiovascular disease morbidity and mortality in end-stage renal disease patients [51–54]. Therefore, the association between serum TGF-β1 levels and hs-CRP may suggest the degree of vascular inflammation, while correlation with low serum albumin may suggest a state of malnutrition which is very common in CKD patients [35].

The low levels of TGF-β in haemodialysis patients observed in this study may be due to subclinical endothelial damage or a result of heparin-mediated activation of TGF-β signalling pathways leading to exhaustion of TGF-β from the repeated binding of TGF-β to various TGF-β receptors [51]. However, heparin-mediated activation of TGF-β pathways does not explain the low levels of TGF-β in peritoneal dialysis and stage 3 CKD patients, since these groups of patients are not exposed to heparin. Moreover, multiple linear regression analysis showed that subclinical atherosclerosis is an independent determinant of TGF-β levels in all CKD patients. It is therefore plausible that subclinical endothelial damage leading to progression of atherosclerosis may provide an explanation for the lower levels of TGF-β isoforms in the CKD patients compared to the controls. Nonetheless, additional studies are needed to explore the complex biology of TGF-β signalling pathways in CKD patients.

There are some important limitations of our study. Firstly, the sample size is relatively small. This may have limited the statistical power of the study to detect any association between TGF-β1 polymorphisms and serum TGF-β1 levels as well as subclinical atherosclerosis. A larger study in a more diverse CKD population in sub-Saharan Africa is needed to determine if our findings are generalizable. A second important limitation is that the study design was essentially a cross-sectional one and the measurements were only carried out at one point. Therefore, our results can only be regarded as preliminary. A prospective epidemiological study is needed to determine the potential protective role of TGF-β on the risk of incident atherosclerosis in the African populations.

In conclusion, we demonstrated that serum levels of TGF-β isoforms were significantly lower in patients with subclinical atherosclerosis and predicted reduced risk for subclinical atherosclerosis in South African patients with CKD. Given the cross-sectional design of this study, the cause and effect relationship between serum TGF-β isoform levels and atherosclerosis remains to be established. In this context, low serum TGF-β isoforms levels can only be considered an important, but not a sufficient risk factor for inflammation-related atherosclerosis in CKD patients. Future prospective longitudinal controlled studies will be needed to evaluate the role of TGF-β1 on the risk of incident atherosclerotic CVD among indigenous African CKD populations.

Disclosure

Raquel Duarte and Saraladevi Naicker are joint senior authors. This work was presented in abstract form at the South African Renal Society (SARS) 2016 Congress, September 9-11, 2016, Cape Town, South Africa.

Acknowledgments

This work was carried out by Dr. Hassan during his ISN Fellowship at the University of the Witwatersrand, South Africa. This work was supported by funding from the National Research Foundation, AstraZeneca Research Trust, and the Division of Nephrology.

References

[1] C. Daly, "Is early chronic kidney disease an important risk factor for cardiovascular disease? A background paper prepared for the UK Consensus Conference on early chronic kidney disease," *Nephrology Dialysis Transplantation*, vol. 22, supplement 9, pp. ix19–ix25, 2007.

[2] United States Renal Data System, *2015 USRDS Annual Data Report: Epidemiology of Kidney Disease in the United States*. Bethesda MNIoH, National Institute of Diabetes and Digestive and Kidney Diseases, 2015.

[3] M. O. Hassan, R. Duarte, T. Dix-Peek et al., "Correlation between volume overload, chronic inflammation, and left ventricular dysfunction in chronic kidney disease patients," *Clinical Nephrology*, vol. 86, no. S1, pp. 131–135, 2016.

[4] C. W. McIntyre, L. E. A. Harrison, M. T. Eldehni, H. J. Jefferies, and C. Szeto, "Circulating endotoxaemia: a novel factor in systemic inflammation and cardiovascular disease in chronic kidney disease," *Clin J Am Soc Nephrol*, vol. 6, pp. 133–141, 2011.

[5] O. M. Akchurin and F. Kaskel, "Update on inflammation in chronic kidney disease," *Blood Purification*, vol. 39, no. 1–3, pp. 84–92, 2015.

[6] A. Ramezani and D. S. Raj, "The gut microbiome, kidney disease, and targeted interventions," *Journal of the American Society of Nephrology*, vol. 25, no. 4, pp. 657–670, 2014.

[7] A. S. Andreasen, K. S. Krabbe, R. Krogh-Madsen, S. Taudorf, B. K. Pedersen, and K. Møller, "Human endotoxemia as a model of systemic inflammation," *Current Medicinal Chemistry*, vol. 15, no. 17, pp. 1697–1705, 2008.

[8] C.-C. Szeto, B. C.-H. Kwan, K.-M. Chow et al., "Circulating bacterial-derived DNA fragment level is a strong predictor of cardiovascular disease in peritoneal dialysis patients," *PLoS ONE*, vol. 10, no. 5, Article ID e0125162, 2015.

[9] S. Kiechl, G. Egger, M. Mayr et al., "Chronic infections and the risk of carotid atherosclerosis: prospective results from a large population study," *Circulation*, vol. 103, no. 8, pp. 1064–1070, 2001.

[10] M. O. Hassan, R. Duarte, T. Dix-Peek, S. Naidoo, and A. Vachiat, "Transforming Growth Factor-β Isoforms Protect against Endotoxaemia Related Atherosclerosis in Chronic Kidney Disease Patients (P18)," in *African Journal of Nephrology*, vol. 19, pp. 17–75, South African Renal Society 2016 Congress Proceedings, Cape Town, South Africa, 2016.

[11] M. Varma, L. A. Mundkur, and V. V. Kakkar, "Autoimmune diseases and atherosclerosis: The inflammatory connection," *Current Immunology Reviews*, vol. 8, no. 4, pp. 297–306, 2012.

[12] C. Weber and H. Noels, "Atherosclerosis: current pathogenesis and therapeutic options," *Nature Medicine*, vol. 17, no. 11, pp. 1410–1422, 2011.

[13] I. Tabas, G. García-Cardeña, and G. K. Owens, "Recent insights into the cellular biology of atherosclerosis," *The Journal of Cell Biology*, vol. 209, no. 1, pp. 13–22, 2015.

[14] Q. Cai, V. K. Mukku, and M. Ahmad, "Coronary artery disease in patients with chronic kidney disease: A clinical update," *Current Cardiology Reviews*, vol. 9, no. 4, pp. 331–339, 2013.

[15] N. G. Frangogiannis, "The role of transforming growth factor (TGF)-β in the infarcted myocardium," *Journal of Thoracic Disease*, vol. 9, pp. S52–S63, 2017.

[16] D. M. Ha, L. C. Carpenter, P. Koutakis et al., "Transforming growth factor-beta 1 produced by vascular smooth muscle cells predicts fibrosis in the gastrocnemius of patients with peripheral artery disease," *Journal of Translational Medicine*, vol. 14, no. 1, article no. 39, 2016.

[17] A. Ostriker, H. N. Horita, J. Poczobutt, M. C. Weiser-Evans, and R. A. Nemenoff, "Vascular Smooth Muscle Cell-Derived Transforming Growth Factor- Promotes Maturation of Activated, Neointima Lesion-Like Macrophages," *Arteriosclerosis, Thrombosis, and Vascular Biology*, vol. 34, no. 4, pp. 877–886, 2014.

[18] D. Nurgazieva, A. Mickley, K. Moganti, W. Ming, I. Ovsyi, A. Popova et al., "Platelet expression of transforming growth factor beta 1 is enhanced and associated with cardiovascular prognosis in patients with acute coronary syndrome," *Atherosclerosis*, vol. 237, no. 2, pp. 754–759, 2014.

[19] S. Park, W. S. Yang, S. K. Lee et al., "TGF-β1 down-regulates inflammatory cytokine-induced VCAM-1 expression in cultured human glomerular endothelial cells," *Nephrology Dialysis Transplantation* , vol. 15, no. 5, pp. 596–604, 2000.

[20] G. Arango Duque and A. Descoteaux, "Macrophage cytokines: involvement in immunity and infectious diseases," *Frontiers in Immunology*, vol. 5, article 491, 2014.

[21] I. Toma and T. A. McCaffrey, "Transforming growth factor-β and atherosclerosis: Interwoven atherogenic and atheroprotective aspects," *Cell and Tissue Research*, vol. 347, no. 1, pp. 155–175, 2012.

[22] S. Redondo, J. Navarro-Dorado, M. Ramajo et al., "Age-dependent defective TGF-beta1 signaling in patients undergoing coronary artery bypass grafting," *Journal of Cardiothoracic Surgery*, vol. 9, no. 1, article no. 24, 2014.

[23] H. A. Bolayır, "The Effect of Serum IL-12 and TGF-β1 Levels on the Prevalence of Atherosclerosis," *Cumhuriyet Medical Journal*, vol. 38, no. 3, p. 195, 2016.

[24] J.-H. Park, L. Li, and K.-H. Baek, "Study of the association of the T869C polymorphism of the transforming growth factor-β1 gene with polycystic ovary syndrome," *Molecular Medicine Reports*, vol. 12, no. 3, pp. 4560–4565, 2015.

[25] Z. Peng, L. Zhan, S. Chen, and E. Xu, "Association of transforming growth factor-β1 gene C-509T and T869C polymorphisms with atherosclerotic cerebral infarction in the Chinese: a case-control study," *Lipids in Health and Disease*, vol. 10, no. 1, p. 100, 2011.

[26] J. Ma, Y. C. Liu, Y. Fang, Y. Cao, and Z. L. Liu, "TGF-ß1 polymorphism 509 C>T is associated with an increased risk for hepatocellular carcinoma in HCV-infected patients," *Genet Mol Res*, vol. 14, no. 2, pp. 4461–4481, 2015.

[27] R. A. Najar, S. M. Ghaderian, and A. S. Panah, "Association of Transforming Growth Factor-β1 Gene Polymorphisms With Genetic Susceptibility to Acute Myocardial Infarction," *The American Journal of the Medical Sciences*, vol. 342, no. 5, pp. 365–370, 2011.

[28] D. J. Grainger, K. Heathcote, M. Chiano et al., "Genetic control of the circulating concentration of transforming growth factor type β1," *Human Molecular Genetics*, vol. 8, no. 1, pp. 93–97, 1999.

[29] D. R. Morris, J. V. Moxon, E. Biros, S. M. Krishna, and J. Golledge, "Meta-analysis of the association between transforming growth Factor-Beta polymorphisms and complications of coronary heart disease," *PLoS ONE*, vol. 7, no. 5, Article ID e37878, 2012.

[30] S. Uluçay, F. S. Çam, M. B. Batır, R. Sütçü, Ö. Bayturan, and K. Demircan, "A novel association between TGFβ1 and ADAMTS4 in coronary artery disease: A new potential mechanism in the progression of atherosclerosis and diabetes," *Anadolu Kardiyoloji Dergisi*, vol. 15, no. 10, pp. 823–829, 2015.

[31] Y. Li, Y. Zhou, G. Gong, H. Geng, and X. Yang, "TGF-β1 Gene -509C/T Polymorphism and Coronary Artery Disease: An Updated Meta-Analysis Involving 11,701 Subjects," *Frontiers in Physiology*, vol. 8, 2017.

[32] T. Osadnik, A. Lekston, K. Bujak, J. K. Strzelczyk, L. Poloński, and M. Gąsior, "The Relationship between VEGFA and TGFB1 Polymorphisms and Target Lesion Revascularization after Elective Percutaneous Coronary Intervention," *Disease Markers*, vol. 2017, 2017.

[33] T. Osadnik, J. K. Strzelczyk, A. Lekston et al., "The association of functional polymorphisms in genes encoding growth factors for endothelial cells and smooth muscle cells with the severity of coronary artery disease," *BMC Cardiovascular Disorders*, vol. 16, no. 1, article no. 218, 2016.

[34] M. P. S. Sie, A. G. Uitterlinden, M. J. Bos et al., "TGF-β1 polymorphisms and risk of myocardial infarction and stroke: The Rotterdam study," *Stroke*, vol. 37, no. 11, pp. 2667–2671, 2006.

[35] M. O. Hassan, R. Duarte, T. Dix-Peek et al., "Volume overload and its risk factors in South African chronic kidney disease

patients: An appraisal of bioimpedance spectroscopy and inferior vena cava measurements," *Clinical Nephrology*, vol. 86, no. 1, pp. 27–34, 2016.

[36] J. H. Stein, C. E. Korcarz, R. T. Hurst et al., "Use of Carotid Ultrasound to Identify Subclinical Vascular Disease and Evaluate Cardiovascular Disease Risk: a Consensus Statement from the American Society of Echocardiography Carotid Intima-Media Thickness Task Force Endorsed by the Society for Vascular Medicine," *Journal of the American Society of Echocardiography*, vol. 21, no. 2, pp. 93–111, 2008.

[37] H. Nasiri, M. Forouzandeh, M. J. Rasaee, and F. Rahbarizadeh, "Modified salting-out method: High-yield, high-quality genomic DNA extraction from whole blood using laundry detergent," *Journal of Clinical Laboratory Analysis*, vol. 19, no. 6, pp. 229–232, 2005.

[38] D. Pohlers, J. Brenmoehl, I. Löffler et al., "TGF-β and fibrosis in different organs—molecular pathway imprints," *Biochimica et Biophysica Acta*, vol. 1792, no. 8, pp. 746–756, 2009.

[39] K. Sharma, B. O. Eltayeb, T. A. McGowan et al., "Captopril-induced reduction of serum levels of transforming growth factor-β1 correlates with long-term renoprotection in insulin-dependent diabetic patients," *American Journal of Kidney Diseases*, vol. 34, no. 5, pp. 818–823, 1999.

[40] S. Stefoni, G. Cianciolo, G. Donati et al., "Low TGF-β1 serum levels are a risk factor for atherosclerosis disease in ESRD patients," *Kidney International*, vol. 61, no. 1, pp. 324–335, 2002.

[41] K. Kempf, G. Haltern, R. Füth et al., "Increased TNF-α and Decreased TGF-β Expression in Peripheral Blood Leukocytes after Acute Myocardial Infarction," *Hormone and Metabolic Research*, vol. 38, no. 5, pp. 346–351, 2006.

[42] K. Janda, M. Krzanowski, P. Dumnicka, B. Kuśnierz-Cabala, A. Kraśniak, and W. Sułowicz, "Transforming growth factor beta 1 as a risk factor for cardiovascular diseases in end-stage renal disease patients treated with peritoneal dialysis," *Clinical Laboratory*, vol. 60, no. 7, pp. 1163–1168, 2014.

[43] E. Arciniegas, A. B. Sutton, T. D. Allen, and A. M. Schor, "Transforming growth factor beta 1 promotes the differentiation of endothelial cells into smooth muscle-like cells in vitro," *Journal of Cell Science*, vol. 103, part 2, pp. 521–529, 1992.

[44] M. Wildgruber, W. Weiss, H. Berger, O. Wolf, H.-H. Eckstein, and P. Heider, "Association of Circulating Transforming Growth Factor beta, Tumor Necrosis Factor alpha and Basic Fibroblast Growth Factor with Restenosis after Transluminal Angioplasty," *European Journal of Vascular and Endovascular Surgery*, vol. 34, no. 1, pp. 35–43, 2007.

[45] E. Pardali and P. ten Dijke, "TGFβ signaling and cardiovascular diseases," *International Journal of Biological Sciences*, vol. 8, no. 2, pp. 195–213, 2012.

[46] K. Aihara, Y. Ikeda, S. Yagi, M. Akaike, and T. Matsumoto, " Transforming Growth Factor- ," *Cardiology Research and Practice*, vol. 2011, pp. 1–9, 2011.

[47] M. Goumans and P. ten Dijke, "TGF-β Signaling in Control of Cardiovascular Function," *Cold Spring Harbor Perspectives in Biology*, vol. 10, no. 2, p. a022210, 2018.

[48] F. Cambien, S. Ricard, A. Troesch et al., "Polymorphisms of the transforming growth factor-β1 gene in relation to myocardial infarction and blood pressure: the etude cas-temoin de l'infarctus du myocarde (ECTIM) study," *Hypertension*, vol. 28, no. 5, pp. 881–887, 1996.

[49] M. Kakoki, O. M. Pochynyuk, C. M. Hathaway et al., "Primary aldosteronism and impaired natriuresis in mice underexpressing TGF 1," *Proceedings of the National Acadamy of Sciences of*

the United States of America, vol. 110, no. 14, pp. 5600–5605, 2013.

[50] D. J. Grainger, P. R. Kemp, J. C. Metcalfe et al., "The serum concentration of active transforming growth factor-β is severely depressed in advanced atherosclerosis," *Nature Medicine*, vol. 1, no. 1, pp. 74–79, 1995.

[51] P. Stenvinkel, "Malnutrition and chronic inflammation as risk factors for cardiovascular disease in chronic renal failure," *Blood Purification*, vol. 19, no. 2, pp. 143–151, 2001.

[52] B. B. Kirushnan, B. Subba Rao, R. Annigeri et al., "Impact of malnutrition, inflammation, and atherosclerosis on the outcome in hemodialysis patients," *Indian Journal of Nephrology*, vol. 27, no. 4, pp. 277–283, 2017.

[53] A. A. Allawi, "Malnutrition, inflamation and atherosclerosis (MIA syndrome) in patients with end stage renal disease on maintenance hemodialysis (a single centre experience)," *Diabetes & Metabolic Syndrome: Clinical Research & Reviews*, vol. 12, no. 2, pp. 91–97, 2018.

[54] M. Maraj, B. Kuśnierz-Cabala, P. Dumnicka et al., "Malnutrition, Inflammation, Atherosclerosis Syndrome (MIA) and Diet Recommendations among End-Stage Renal Disease Patients Treated with Maintenance Hemodialysis," *Nutrients*, vol. 10, no. 1, p. 69, 2018.

Permissions

List of Contributors

Chie Saito and Kunihiro Yamagata
Department of Nephrology, Faculty of Medicine, University of Tsukuba, 1-1-1 Tennodai, Tsukuba, Ibaraki 305-8575, Japan

Kei Nagai
Department of Nephrology, Faculty of Medicine, University of Tsukuba, 1-1-1 Tennodai, Tsukuba, Ibaraki 305-8575, Japan
Comprehensive Human Sciences, Faculty of Medicine, University of Tsukuba, 1-1-1 Tennodai, Tsukuba, Ibaraki 305-8575, Japan

Asako Zempo-Miyaki
Comprehensive Human Sciences, Faculty of Medicine, University of Tsukuba, 1-1-1 Tennodai, Tsukuba, Ibaraki 305-8575, Japan

Atsushi Ueda
Tsukuba University Hospital Hitachi Medical Education and Research Center, Jonan-cho 2-1-1, Hitachi, Ibaraki 317-0077, Japan

B. L. Goh and K. L. Ang
1 Clinical Research Centre, Serdang Hospital, Kajang 43000, Malaysia

A. Soraya and A. Goh
Azmi Burhani Consulting, Petaling Jaya 47820, Malaysia

Claudio Bazzi
D'Amico Foundation for Renal Disease Research, 20145 Milan, Italy

Elena Tagliabue and Sara Raimondi
Division of Epidemiology and Biostatistics, European Institute of Oncology, 20141 Milan, Italy

Virginia Rizza
Biochemical Laboratory, San Carlo Borromeo Hospital, 20153 Milan, Italy

Daniela Casellato
Nephrology and Dialysis Unit, San Carlo Borromeo Hospital, 20153 Milan, Italy

Masaomi Nangaku
Division of Nephrology and Endocrinology, University of Tokyo School of Medicine, Tokyo 113-8655, Japan

Jennifer E. Flythe
Department of Medicine, Renal Division, Brighamand Women's Hospital, Boston, MA, USA
Department of Medicine, Division of Nephrology and Hypertension, University of North Carolina Kidney Center, UNC School of Medicine, 7024 Burnett-Womack CB No. 7155, Chapel Hill, NC 27599-7155, USA

Steven M. Brunelli
Department of Medicine, Renal Division, Brighamand Women's Hospital, Boston, MA, USA
DaVita Clinical Research, Minneapolis, MN, USA

Nien-Chen Li, Shu-Fang Lin, Jeffrey Hymes and Eduardo Lacson Jr.
Fresenius Medical Care North America, Waltham, MA, USA

Andreia Freire de Menezes, Douglas Rafanelle Moura de Santana Motta and Fernanda Oliveira de Carvalho
Postgraduate Program in Health Sciences, Federal University of Sergipe, São Cristóvão, SE, Brazil

Kleyton de Andrade Bastos
Postgraduate Program in Health Sciences, Federal University of Sergipe, São Cristóvão, SE, Brazil
Clinese Clínica de Nefrologia de Sergipe Ltda., Aracaju, SE, Brazil
Department of Medicine, Federal University of Sergipe, São Cristóvão, SE, Brazil

Eduesley Santana-Santos
Nursing Department, Federal University of Sergipe, São Cristóvão, SE, Brazil

Manoel Pacheco de Andrade Júnior
Clinese Clínica de Nefrologia de Sergipe Ltda., Aracaju, SE, Brazil

Mirela Farias Figueirôa and Maria Isabel Teles Farias
Department of Medicine, Federal University of Sergipe, São Cristóvão, SE, Brazil

Nilgül Akalin, Özlem Harmankaya and Sibel Koçak Yücel
Department of Nephrology, Bakırk¨oy Dr. Sadi Konuk Training and Research Hospital, Istanbul 34147, Turkey

Yıldız Okuturlar and Selçuk Sezıklı
Department of Internal Medicine, Bakırk˙oy Dr. Sadi Konuk Training and Research Hospital, Istanbul 34147, Turkey

Asuman Gedıkbaşi
Department of Biochemistry, Bakırköy Dr. Sadi Konuk Training and Research Hospital, Istanbul 34147, Turkey

Christian M. Beilstein, John R. Prowle and Christopher J. Kirwan
Adult Critical Care Unit, The Royal London Hospital, Barts Health NHS Trust, Whitechapel Road, London E1 1BB, UK

Ahmed Hassaan Qavi and Rida Kamal
Shifa College of Medicine, Shifa Tameer-e-Millat University, Pitras Bukhari Road, Sector H-8/4, Islamabad 44000, Pakistan

Robert W. Schrier
Division of Renal Diseases and Hypertension, University of Colorado School of Medicine, 12700 East 19th Avenue C281, Research Building 2, Room 7001, Aurora, CO 80045, USA

Aibek E. Mirrakhimov and Adam Gray
Department ofMedicine, University of Kentucky College of Medicine, Lexington, KY, USA

Aram Barbaryan
Department of Internal Medicine, University of Kansas Medical Center, Kansas City, KS, USA

Taha Ayach
Division of Nephrology, Bone and Mineral Metabolism, University of Kentucky College of Medicine, Lexington, KY, USA

Bancha Satirapoj, Pamila Tasanavipas and Ouppatham Supasyndh
Division of Nephrology, Department of Medicine, Phramongkutklao Hospital and College of Medicine, Bangkok 10400, Thailand

Sana R. Akbar, Umair S. Ahmed, Hafiz I. Iqbal and Cheryl Dalton
Division of Nephrology, Department of Medicine, West Virginia University School of Medicine, Morgantown, WV, USA

Dustin M. Long
Division of Biostatistics, West Virginia University School of Medicine, Morgantown, WV, USA

Kashif Hussain, Ahmad Alhajhusain and Ailia W. Ali
Division of Pulmonary and Critical Care Medicine, Department of Medicine, West Virginia University School of Medicine, Morgantown, WV, USA

Rachel Leonard
Department of Medicine, West Virginia University School of Medicine, Morgantown, WV, USA

Maisarah Jalalonmuhali, Maw Pin Tan, Soo Kun Lim and Kok Peng Ng
Department of Medicine, University of Malaya Medical Centre, 59100 Kuala Lumpur, Malaysia

Salma Mohamed Abouzriba Elagel
Management and Science University, 40100 Shah Alam, Selangor, Malaysia

Robert Nee, Ian Rivera, Dustin J. Little, Christina M. Yuan and Kevin C. Abbott
Department of Nephrology, Walter Reed National Military Medical Center, 8901Wisconsin Avenue, Bethesda, MD 20889-5600, USA

Mohamed S. Al Riyami, Badria Al Ghaithi, Nadia Al Hashmi and Naifain Al Kalbani
Pediatric Nephrology Unit, Department of Child Health, Royal Hospital, 111 Muscat, Oman

Maija Suvanto, Timo Jahnukainen and Hannu Jalanko
Children's Hospital, University of Helsinki and Helsinki University Hospital, 00290 Helsinki, Finland

Marjo Kestilä
Department of Chronic Disease Prevention, National Institute for Health andWelfare, 00271 Helsinki, Finland

Biruh Workeneh and William E. Mitch
Division of Nephrology, Baylor College of Medicine, Houston, TX 77030, USA

Danielle Guffey and Charles G. Minard
Dan L. Duncan Institute for Clinical and Translational Research, Baylor College of Medicine, Houston, TX 77030, USA

Bianca Ballarin Albino, Mariele Gobo-Oliveira and André Luís Balbi
Botucatu School of Medicine, University of São Paulo State (UNESP), Brazil

Daniela Ponce
Botucatu School of Medicine, University of São Paulo State (UNESP), Brazil
Course of Medicine, University of São Paulo (USP), Bauru, Brazil

Aibek E. Mirrakhimov, Taha Ayach, Goutham Talari, Romil Chadha and Adam Gray
Department of Medicine, University of Kentucky College of Medicine, Lexington, KY, USA

Aram Barbaryan
University of Kansas Medical Center, Kansas City, KS, USA

Sandawana William Majoni
Royal Darwin Hospital, Department of Nephrology, Division of Medicine, Tiwi, Darwin, NT, Australia
Northern Territory Medical Programme, Flinders University School of Medicine, Tiwi, Darwin, NT, Australia
Wellbeing and Preventable Chronic Disease Division, Menzies School of Health Research, Charles Darwin University, Casuarina, NT, Australia

Jaquelyne T. Hughes
Royal Darwin Hospital, Department of Nephrology, Division of Medicine, Tiwi, Darwin, NT, Australia
Wellbeing and Preventable Chronic Disease Division, Menzies School of Health Research, Charles Darwin University, Casuarina, NT, Australia

Paul D. Lawton, Federica Barzi and Alan Cass
Wellbeing and Preventable Chronic Disease Division, Menzies School of Health Research, Charles Darwin University, Casuarina, NT, Australia

Sanjeevan Sriskandarajah
Department of Clinical Medicine, University of Bergen, Bergen, Norway

Leif Bostad
Department of Clinical Medicine, University of Bergen, Bergen, Norway
Department of Pathology, Haukeland University Hospital, Bergen, Norway

Rune Bjørneklett
Department of Clinical Medicine, University of Bergen, Bergen, Norway
Emergency Care Clinic, Haukeland University Hospital, Bergen, Norway

Tor Åge Myklebust and Bjørn Møller
Department of Clinical and Registry-Based Research, Cancer Registry of Norway, Institute of Population-Based Cancer Research, Oslo, Norway

Steinar Skrede
Department of Clinical Science, University of Bergen, Bergen, Norway
Department of Medicine, Haukeland University Hospital, Bergen, Norway

Jun Odaka, Takahiro Kanai, Takane Ito, Takashi Saito, Jun Aoyagi, Hiroyuki Betsui and Takanori Yamagata
Department of Pediatrics, Jichi Medical University, 3311-1 Yakushiji, Shimotsuke, Tochigi 329-0498, Japan

Silvi Shah
Department of Nephrology and Hypertension, University of Cincinnati, Cincinnati, OH, USA

Prasoon Verma
Division of Neonatal/Perinatal Medicine, Brown University, Providence, RI, USA

John T. Sanders
Sanford Children's Hospital, Sioux Falls, SD 57117, USA

Zoran Bursac
University of Tennessee Health Sciences Center, Memphis, TN 38013, USA

M. Colleen Hastings and Robert J. Wyatt
University of Tennessee Health Sciences Center, Memphis, TN 38013, USA
Children's Foundation Research Institute, Memphis, TN 38013, USA

Zina Moldoveanu, Jan Novak and Bruce A. Julian
University of Alabama at Birmingham, Birmingham, AL 35294, USA

Kazunori Washio
Saiyu Kawaguchi Clinic, Kawaguchi, Japan

Hiroya Takami
Saiyu Kawaguchi Clinic, Kawaguchi, Japan
Saitama Honoka Clinic, Saitama, Japan

Hiromichi Gotoh
3Saiyu Souka Clinic, Souka, Japan

Manish Suneja and PhilipM. Polgreen
Department of Internal Medicine, University of Iowa Hospitals and Clinics, Iowa City, IA 52242, USA

Fan Tang and Joseph E. Cavanaugh
Department of Biostatistics, University of Iowa, Iowa City, IA 52242, USA

Linnea A. Polgreen
Department of Pharmacy Practice and Science, University of Iowa, Iowa City, IA 52242, USA

Murat Tuğcu
Department of Nephrology, Marmara University Pendik Training and Research Hospital, Istanbul, Turkey

Umut Kasapoğlu
Department of Nephrology, Ağrı Public Hospital, Ağrı, Turkey

Gülizar Fahin
Department of Nephrology, Sultan Abdulhamid Han Training and Research Hospital, Istanbul, Turkey

Süheyla Apaydın
Department of Nephrology, Bakirkoy Sadi Konuk Training and Research Hospital, Istanbul, Turkey

Kerstin Benz, Christoph Daniel and Kerstin Amann
Department of Nephropathology, Friedrich-Alexander University (FAU) Erlangen-Nürnberg, Germany

Karl-Friedrich Hilgers
Department of Nephrology and Hypertension, Friedrich-Alexander University (FAU) Erlangen-Nürnberg, Germany

M. S. Sayapina, S. G. Averinova, T. V. Zacharova, A. V. Kashkadaeva and S. V. Shiryaev
N.N. Blokhin Russian Cancer Research Center, Ministry of Health of Russia, 23 Kashirskoe Shosse, Moscow 115478, Russia

M. V. Poluectova and O. A. Vorobéva
A. Tsyb Medical Radiological Research Centre, Branch of the National Medical Research Radiological Centre of The Ministry of Health ofThe Russian Federation, 10 Zhukov St., Obninsk, Kaluga 249036, Russia

Mohd Rizal Abdul Manaf and Naren Kumar Surendra
Department of Community Health, Faculty of Medicine, Pusat Perubatan Universiti Kebangsaan Malaysia, Jalan Yaacob Latif, Bandar Tun Razak, 56000 Cheras, Kuala Lumpur, Malaysia

Abdul Halim Abdul Gafor
Nephrology Unit, Faculty of Medicine, Pusat Perubatan Universiti Kebangsaan Malaysia, Jalan Yaacob Latif, Bandar Tun Razak, 56000 Cheras, Kuala Lumpur, Malaysia

Lai Seong Hooi
Hospital Sultanah Aminah, Jalan Persiaran Abu Bakar Sultan, 80100 Johor Bahru, Johor, Malaysia

Sunita Bavanandan
Hospital Kuala Lumpur, Jalan Pahang, 50586 Kuala Lumpur, Malaysia

Amnuay Sirisopha, Bunyong Phakdeekitcharoen, Amornpan Lertrit and Chagriya Kitiyakara
Department of Medicine, Faculty of Medicine Ramathibodi Hospital, Mahidol University, Bangkok 10400, Thailand

Somlak Vanavanan and Anchalee Chittamma
Department of Pathology, Faculty of Medicine Ramathibodi Hospital, Mahidol University, Bangkok 10400, Thailand

Ammarin Thakkinstian
Section for Clinical Epidemiology and Biostatistics, Faculty of Medicine Ramathibodi Hospital, Mahidol University, Bangkok 10400, Thailand

Nuankanya Sathirapongsasuti
Graduate Program in Translational Medicine, Research Center, Faculty of Medicine Ramathibodi Hospital, Mahidol University, Bangkok 10400, Thailand

Hodaka Yamada, Shunsuke Funazaki, Masafumi Kakei and Kazuo Hara
Department of Medicine, Division of Endocrinology and Metabolism, Jichi Medical University Saitama Medical Center, 1-847 Amanuma-cho, Omiya-ku, Saitama 330-8503, Japan

Makoto Kuro-o
Center for MolecularMedicine, Jichi Medical University, 3311-1 Yakushiji Shimotsuke, Tochigi 329-0498, Japan

San-e Ishikawa
Division of Endocrinology and Metabolism, International University of Health andWelfare Hospital, 537-3 Iguchi, Nasushiobara, Tochigi 329-2763, Japan

Rose M. Ayoob and Andrew L. Schwaderer
Division of Nephrology, Department of Pediatrics, Nationwide Children's Hospital, Columbus, OH, USA

Muzamil Olamide Hassan and Sagren Naidoo
Division of Nephrology, Department of Internal Medicine, Faculty of Health Sciences, University of the Witwatersrand, South Africa

Raquel Duarte, Therese Dix-Peek and Caroline Dickens
Internal Medicine Research Laboratory, Department of Internal Medicine, Faculty of Health Sciences, University of the Witwatersrand, South Africa

Ahmed Vachiat, Sacha Grinter and Pravin Manga
Division of Cardiology, Department of Internal Medicine, Faculty of Health Sciences, University of the Witwatersrand, South Africa

Saraladevi Naicker
Department of Internal Medicine, Faculty of Health Sciences, University of theWitwatersrand, South Africa

Index